Chemical and Molecular Approach to Tumor Metastases

Special Issue Editors

Gianni Sava
Alberta Bergamo

MDPI • Basel • Beijing • Wuhan • Barcelona • Belgrade

MDPI

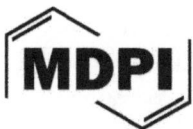

Special Issue Editors
Gianni Sava
University of Trieste
Italy

Alberta Bergamo
Callerio Foundation Onlus
Italy

Editorial Office
MDPI
St. Alban-Anlage 66
Basel, Switzerland

This edition is a reprint of the Special Issue published online in the open access journal *International Journal of Molecular Sciences* (ISSN 1422-0067) from 2017–2018 (available at: http://www.mdpi.com/journal/ijms/special_issues/Tumor_Metastases).

For citation purposes, cite each article independently as indicated on the article page online and as indicated below:

Lastname, F.M.; Lastname, F.M. Article title. *Journal Name* **Year**, *Article number*, page range.

First Editon 2018

Cover photo courtesy of Paul Dyson.

ISBN 978-3-03842-895-4 (Pbk)
ISBN 978-3-03842-896-1 (PDF)

Table of Contents

About the Special Issue Editors   v

Preface to "Chemical and Molecular Approach to Tumor Metastases" vii

Alberta Bergamo and Gianni Sava
Chemical and Molecular Approach to Tumor Metastases
doi: 10.3390/ijms19030843   1

Huijun Xie, Guihui Tong, Yupei Zhang, Shu Liang, Kairui Tang and Qinhe Yang
PGK1 Drives Hepatocellular Carcinoma Metastasis by Enhancing Metabolic Process
doi: 10.3390/ijms18081630   3

Kangyun Lan, Yuni Zhao, Yue Fan, Binbin Ma, Shanshan Yang, Qin Liu, Hua Linghu and
Hui Wang
Sulfiredoxin May Promote Cervical Cancer Metastasis via Wnt/β-Catenin Signaling Pathway
doi: 10.3390/ijms18050917 14

Kosuke Toda, Gen Nishikawa, Masayoshi Iwamoto, Yoshiro Itatani, Ryo Takahashi,
Yoshiharu Sakai and Kenji Kawada
Clinical Role of ASCT2 (SLC1A5) in KRAS-Mutated Colorectal Cancer
doi: 10.3390/ijms18081632 27

Alysha K. Croker, Mauricio Rodriguez-Torres, Ying Xia, Siddika Pardhan, Hon Sing Leong,
John D. Lewis and Alison L. Allan
Differential Functional Roles of ALDH1A1 and ALDH1A3 in Mediating Metastatic Behavior
and Therapy Resistance of Human Breast Cancer Cells
doi: 10.3390/ijms18102039 40

Hsiang-Cheng Chi, Chung-Ying Tsai, Ming-Ming Tsai, Chau-Ting Yeh and Kwang-Huei Lin
Roles of Long Noncoding RNAs in Recurrence and Metastasis of Radiotherapy-Resistant
Cancer Stem Cells
doi: 10.3390/ijms18091903 58

Laura Mercatali, Federico La Manna, Giacomo Miserocchi, Chiara Liverani, Alessandro De Vita,
Chiara Spadazzi, Alberto Bongiovanni, Federica Recine, Dino Amadori, Martina Ghetti
and Toni Ibrahim
Tumor-Stroma Crosstalk in Bone Tissue: The Osteoclastogenic Potential of a Breast Cancer
Cell Line in a Co-Culture System and the Role of EGFR Inhibition
doi: 10.3390/ijms18081655 87

Ana Cavaco, Maryam Rezaei, Stephan Niland and Johannes A. Eble
Collateral Damage Intended—Cancer-Associated Fibroblasts and Vasculature Are Potential
Targets in Cancer Therapy
doi: 10.3390/ijms18112355 102

Sung-Ying Huang, Shu-Fang Chang, Kuan-Fu Liao and Sheng-Chun Chiu
Tanshinone IIA Inhibits Epithelial-Mesenchymal Transition in Bladder Cancer Cells via
Modulation of STAT3-CCL2 Signaling
doi: 10.3390/ijms18081616 145

Keyan Cheng and Min Hao
Metformin Inhibits TGF-β1-Induced Epithelial-to-Mesenchymal Transition via PKM2
Relative-mTOR/p70s6k Signaling Pathway in Cervical Carcinoma Cells
doi: 10.3390/ijms17122000 . . . . **159**

**Bo-Gyoung Kim, Jin-Wook Kim, Soo-Min Kim, Ryeo-Eun Go, Kyung-A Hwang and
Kyung-Chul Choi**
3,3′-Diindolylmethane Suppressed Cyprodinil-Induced Epithelial-Mesenchymal Transition
and Metastatic-Related Behaviors of Human Endometrial Ishikawa Cells via an Estrogen
Receptor-Dependent Pathway
doi: 10.3390/ijms19010189 . . . . **173**

**Coralie Genevois, Arnaud Hocquelet, Claire Mazzocco, Emilie Rustique, Franck Couillaud
and Nicolas Grenier**
In Vivo Imaging of Prostate Cancer Tumors and Metastasis Using Non-Specific Fluorescent
Nanoparticles in Mice
doi: 10.3390/ijms18122584 . . . . **186**

**Yan Lu, Liping Wang, Hairi Li, Yanru Li, Yang Ruan, Dongjing Lin, Minlan Yang,
Xiangshu Jin, Yantong Guo, Xiaoli Zhang and Chengshi Quan**
SMAD2 Inactivation Inhibits CLDN6 Methylation to Suppress Migration and Invasion of
Breast Cancer Cells
doi: 10.3390/ijms18091863 . . . . **196**

Thaiz F. Borin, Kartik Angara, Mohammad H. Rashid, Bhagelu R. Achyut and Ali S. Arbab
Arachidonic Acid Metabolite as a Novel Therapeutic Target in Breast Cancer Metastasis
doi: 10.3390/ijms18122661 . . . . **211**

**Ronald F. S. Lee, Stéphane Escrig, Catherine Maclachlan, Graham W. Knott, Anders Meibom,
Gianni Sava and Paul J. Dyson**
The Differential Distribution of RAPTA-T in Non-Invasive and Invasive Breast Cancer Cells
Correlates with Its Anti-Invasive and Anti-Metastatic Effects
doi: 10.3390/ijms18091869 . . . . **234**

**Stefano Guadagni, Giammaria Fiorentini, Marco Clementi, Giancarlo Palumbo, Paola Palumbo,
Alessandro Chiominto, Stefano Baldoni, Francesco Masedu, Marco Valenti, Ambra Di Tommaso,
Bianca Fabi, Camillo Aliberti, Donatella Sarti, Veronica Guadagni and Cristina Pellegrini**
Does Locoregional Chemotherapy Still Matter in the Treatment of Advanced Pelvic Melanoma?
doi: 10.3390/ijms18112382 . . . . **242**

About the Special Issue Editors

Gianni Sava, full Professor of Pharmacology. Born on September 9, 1952 at Gemona del Friuli, Udine, Italy. Since 1992, Prof. Sava is the scientific director of the Callerio Foundation Onlus, a non-profit, private research organisation active in the bio-pharmacological research in the Life Sciences. Prof. Sava has long standing experience in the pharmacology of compounds active on metastases of solid tumours. His research activity at the University of Trieste and at the Callerio Foundation also comprises the study of oral formulations of critical drugs, the pharmacological effects of lysozyme in cancer and diabetes, and the set-up of a totally in vitro device to mimic the spontaneous metastasis formation of solid tumours. 278 full-length papers (HI 66, total citations 12904, Google Scholar, updated March 2018).

Alberta Bergamo is researcher at the Callerio Foundation Onlus, a private, non-profit research institute. She holds a degree in Chemical and Technological Pharmacy and a II level Masters in "Regulatory Disciplines and Drug Policy". Her main areas of interest are: pharmacology, cancer chemotherapy, pharmacogenomics, and nutraceutics. She has considerable experience in the field of Medicinal Inorganic Chemistry, having focused her research on the study of metallodrugs against solid tumour metastases and tumour microenvironments. In this context, she dealt also with the development of in vitro systems as alternatives of in vivo animal models. More recently, she has undertaken research on the production and biological/pharmacological characterization of devices that are destined to oral administration for the microencapsulation of active ingredients such as lysozyme and are beneficial for the prevention of infections in breeding fish, of diabetic nephropathy complications, and of age-related afflictions.

Preface to "Chemical and Molecular Approach to Tumor Metastases"

The study of cancer metastasis is gaining particular attention, given the impact that this disseminated disease has on the success of tumour therapy. This special issue draws attention to the biochemical and molecular aspects of metastatic diseases, but also to potential targets and some specific emerging treatment opportunities.

The work of Huijnun Xie et al. presents the role of phosphoglycerate kinase 1, an important enzyme involved in glycolysis, in the progression of the hepatocellular carcinoma. An interesting warning is presented by Kangyun Lan et al. regarding the excess of antioxidants, such as sulphoredoxin, which can promote cancer growth and metastases. Kosuke Toda el al. demonstrate that KRAS mutated colorectal cancer is maintained by the overexpression of the ASCT2 (SLC1A5) aminoacid transporter, suggesting its potential role as a specific target for the pharmacological control of this tumour. Alysha K. Croker et al. point out that aldehyde deydrogenase activity and CD44 expression are responsible for the metastatic progression of therapy-resistant human breast cancer, and Hsiang-Cheng Chi et al. review the literature on the roles of noncoding RNAs in relation to the resistance to radiotherapy of cancer stem cells in metastatic foci. Laura Mercatali et al. stress the role of the relationships between tumour cells and the extracellular matrix, showing how EGFR is crucial to the osteoclastogenic effect in breast cancer. The work of Ana Cavaco et al. focuses on a similar aspect, indicating that stroma-producing fibroblasts and the tumour vasculature can be promising targets for cancer therapy. In this context, Sung-Ying Huang et al. and Bo-Gyoung Kim et al. report on the Epithelial to Mesenchymal Transition and demonstrate the role of inhibition of this process with an extract of a traditionally used herbal Chinese medicine and with 3,3'-diindolylmethane. Metformine also plays an important role in this process, report Keyang Cheng and Min Hao, throughout the TGF-beta1 influence on the mTOR signalling activity. From another point of view, Coralie Genevois presents an imaging model based on the use of non-specific nanoparticles to visualize prostate cancer tumours and their metastases in vivo.

Yan Lu et al. point out on the importance of inactivating SMAD2, with inhibition of CLDN6 methylation, leading to the control of the processes of migration and invasion of breast cancer, and Thaiz F. Borin et al. suggest the targeting of 20-hydroxyeicosanotetraenoic acid as a novel therapy approach to breast cancer metastases. Ronald F.S. Lee et al. present data on the cell distribution of an innovative inorganic compound for the treatment of metastatic tumours. Stefano Guadagni et al. conclude the series of presentations of this special issue, discussing whether the locoregional chemotherapy for the treatment of advanced melanomas is still a valid therapeutic option.

Gianni Sava and **Alberta Bergamo**

Special Issue Editors

International Journal of
Molecular Sciences

MDPI

Editorial

Chemical and Molecular Approach to Tumor Metastases

Alberta Bergamo [1] and Gianni Sava [2],*

[1]   Callerio Foundation Onlus, 34127 Trieste, Italy; a.bergamo@callerio.org
[2]   Department of Life Sciences, University of Trieste, 34127 Trieste, Italy
*   Correspondence: gsava@units.it; Tel.: +39-040-558-8633

Received: 1 March 2018; Accepted: 12 March 2018; Published: 14 March 2018

Tumours are not merely masses of abnormally proliferating cancer cells. Today, we have a clearer view of cancer complexity in which the participation of cancer and host cells leads to a tremendous heterogeneity of neoplastic diseases concerning the genetics, epigenetics, proteomics and biochemistry of the tumour [1]. Such intra-tumour heterogeneity provides the basis for inter-metastatic heterogeneity among different metastatic lesions of the same patient, each originating from a founder cell, or small group of cells, with a very different mutation kit, and likely originating from different and distinct primary tumour areas [1]. This situation has important implications regarding chemotherapeutic sensitivity and responses. In addition, the offspring of the founder cell(s) can generate heterogeneity among the cells of an individual metastasis, affecting the response to systemic therapies and providing the seeds for drug resistance.

Correspondingly, drug treatment is progressively shifting from the use of chemicals producing toxics effects in general processes of cell division, with the goal of killing the tumour cell, to compounds targeting specific cell behaviours with the goal of disarming the malignancy of the tumour cell (Figure 1) [2,3]. This new strategy implies the use of novel systems of drug design, particularly those concerning biological drugs leading to compounds capable of targeting specific molecules expressed only by selected tumour cells [4–6]. The main aim of this novel era of drug development is the response to the need of overcoming the heavy toxicity of the "conventional" chemotherapy that poorly distinguishes between cancer and healthy cells, therefore, causing severe side effects that often hamper the compliance of the patient.

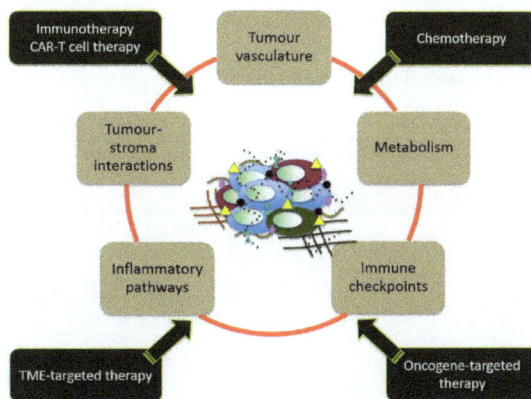

Figure 1. Graphical representation of the tumour/metastasis heterogeneity and of the main targets and therapeutic approaches (CAR-T = Chimeric Antigen Receptor T cell; TME = Tumour Micro Environment).

Int. J. Mol. Sci. **2018**, *19*, 843

Metastasis is the primary target for cancer chemotherapy, independently of the kind of drug being used. The main reason is that the primary tumour can often, if not always, be aggressed by surgery and/or radiotherapy whereas metastases, spread in several tissues and organs, are believed to be better reached with drugs that follow the pharmacological rules of distribution in the body.

The generation of these novel drugs, whether selective and specific monoclonal antibodies or small organic molecules, requires a deep knowledge of the nature of the tumour cell and particularly of tumour metastasis. Similarly, to the primary lesions, tumour metastases are characterised by the interactions with healthy cells and extracellular matrix leading to a complex microenvironment in dynamic evolution but extremely important for the metastatic growth [7,8].

The twin research that joins the biochemistry and molecular biology of cancer metastasis with the study of novel targets and novel approaches to combat their growth is even more mandatory in a scientific era in which the improvements of human health are transforming cancers into chronic diseases and therefore significantly prolonging the life-time expectancy.

Conflicts of Interest: The authors declare no conflict of interest.

References

1. Yachida, S.; Jones, S.; Bozic, I.; Antal, T.; Leary, R.; Fu, B.; Kamiyama, M.; Hruban, R.H.; Eshleman, J.R.; Nowak, M.A.; et al. Distant metastasis occurs late during the genetic evolution of pancreatic cancer. *Nature* **2010**, *467*, 1114–1117. [CrossRef] [PubMed]
2. Hanahan, D.; Weinberg, R.A. The hallmarks of cancer. *Cell* **2000**, *100*, 57–70. [CrossRef]
3. Palumbo, M.O.; Kavan, P.; Miller, W.H., Jr.; Panasci, L.; Assouline, S.; Johnson, N.; Cohen, V.; Patenaude, F.; Pollak, M.; Jagoe, R.T.; et al. Systemic cancer therapy: Achievements and challenges that lie ahead. *Front. Pharmacol.* **2013**, *4*, 57. [CrossRef] [PubMed]
4. He, Q.; Guo, S.; Qian, Z.; Chen, X. Development of Individualized Anti-Metastasis Strategies by Engineering Nanomedicines. *Chem. Soc. Rev.* **2015**, *44*, 6258–6286. [CrossRef] [PubMed]
5. Park, G.-T.; Choi, K.-C. Advanced new strategies for metastatic cancer treatment by therapeutic stem cells and oncolytic virotherapy. *Oncotarget* **2016**, *7*, 58684–58695. [CrossRef] [PubMed]
6. Sun, Y.; Ma, L. The emerging molecular machinery and therapeutic targets of metastasis. *Trends Pharmacol. Sci.* **2015**, *36*, 349–359. [CrossRef] [PubMed]
7. Hanahan, D.; Weinberg, R.A. Hallmarks of cancer: The next generation. *Cell* **2011**, *144*, 646–674. [CrossRef] [PubMed]
8. Kitamura, T.; Qian, B.-Z.; Pollard, J.W. Immune cell promotion of metastasis. *Nat. Rev. Immunol.* **2015**, *15*, 73–86. [CrossRef] [PubMed]

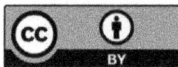

International Journal of
Molecular Sciences

MDPI

Article

PGK1 Drives Hepatocellular Carcinoma Metastasis by Enhancing Metabolic Process

Huijun Xie [1,†], Guihui Tong [2,†], Yupei Zhang [1], Shu Liang [1], Kairui Tang [1] and Qinhe Yang [1,*]

1   College of Traditional Chinese medicine, Jinan University, Guangzhou 510632, China;
    huijunxie@jnu.edu.cn (H.X.); zyp6115@jnu.edu.cn (Y.Z.); liangshu2830145@gmail.com (S.L.);
    tangkarry1991@gmail.com (K.T.)
2   Department of Pathology, Guangdong Provincial Key Laboratory of Molecular Tumor Pathology
    and School of Basic Medical Sciences, Southern Medical University, Guangzhou 510515, China;
    tongguihui123@gmail.com
*   Correspondence: tyangqh@jnu.edu.cn; Tel.: +86-20-8522-6197
†   These authors contributed equally to this work.

Received: 16 May 2017; Accepted: 22 July 2017; Published: 27 July 2017

Abstract: During the proliferation and metastasis, the tumor cells prefer glycolysis (Warburg effect), but its exact mechanism remains largely unknown. In this study, we demonstrated that phosphoglycerate kinase 1 (PGK1) is an important enzyme in the pathway of metabolic glycolysis. We observed a significant overexpression of PGK1 in hepatocellular carcinoma tissues, and a correlation between PGK1 expression and poor survival of hepatocellular carcinoma patients. Also, the depletion of PGK1 dramatically reduced cancer cell proliferation and metastasis, indicating an oncogenic role of PGK1 in liver cancer progression. Further experiments showed that PGK1 played an important role in *MYC*-induced metabolic reprogramming, which led to an enhanced Warburg effect. Our results revealed a new effect of PGK1, which can provide a new treatment strategy for hepatocellular carcinoma, as PGK1 is used to indicate the prognosis of hepatocellular carcinoma (HCC).

Keywords: PGK1; *MYC*; hepatocellular carcinoma; metastasis; Warburg effect

1. Introduction

Tumor cells mainly obtain energy in a special metabolic condition, which is called the Warburg effect. This is effective in reducing incidence and mortality [1]. The key enzymes in this process can regulate the metabolism, and metabolites produced by tumor cells significantly affect tumor migration and invasion [2]. In solid tumors, possible metabolic exchange is an important dimension of metabolic heterogeneity [3]. However, the metabolic biology of hepatocellular carcinoma (HCC) is yet to be well characterized.

Phosphoglycerate k inase 1 (PGK1) is an important ATP-generating enzyme in the glycolytic pathway [4]. It catalyzes the reversible transfer of a phosphate group from 1,3-bisphosphoglycerate (1,3-BPG) to ADP that produced 3-phosphoglycerate (3-PG) and ATP [4]. PGK1 is very important in tumorigenesis and progression. PGK1 regulates autophagy to promote tumorigenesis [5]. PGK1 is a predictor of poor survival and a novel prognostic biomarker of chemoresistance to paclitaxel treatment in breast cancer [6]. PGK1 appeared to be a predictor of CXCR4 expression, bone marrow metastases, and survival in neuroblastoma [7]. PGK1 is a promoter of metastasis in colon cancer [8], which might be a potential protein biomarker of intracellular oxidative status in human colon carcinoma cells [9]. PGK1 secreted by prostate cancer regulates bone formation at the metastatic site [10]. PGK1 is a potential marker [11] and a promoting enzyme for peritoneal dissemination in gastric cancer [12].

Involved in the glycolytic pathway, PGK1 promotes invasion and metastasis in HCC [13]. Several proteins associates with PGK1 signaling have already been identified, including ornithine transaminase (OTA) [14] and hypoxia inducible factor 1 (HIF-1) [15]. A recent article shows that acetylation at the K323 site of PGK1, as an important regulatory mechanism, promotes its enzymatic activity and cancer cell metabolism [16]. All of these findings indicate that PGK1 is a potential marker for progression in HCC. However, its role in HCC metastasis remains to be further explored.

On the other side, the structure of human PGK1 (hPGK1) has been well understood. hPGK1, as long as 417 amino acids, is a typical hinge-bending enzyme with two similar sized Rossmann fold domains [17]. When the two substrates are bonded, the hinge flexion moves the enzyme into a closed form to allow the substrate to contact [17]. PGK1 inhibits susceptibility to chemotherapeutic drugs in gastric cancer cells and tumor stem cells [18]. PGK1 might be an advisable target molecule for specific immunotherapy of HLA-A2+ colon cancer patients [19]. All these findings indicate the possibility that PGK1 can be a biomarker in the treatment of hepatocellular carcinoma.

MYC promotes multiple processes, such as uncontrolled cell proliferation, cell growth, and genomic instability for promoting malignant transformation [20]. Importantly, in order to adapt to the tumor microenvironment, *MYC* also joins the metabolic reprogramming, which is essential for cancer cells [20]. *MYC* as a regulator of PGK1 is essential for proliferation of clear cell renal cell carcinoma cells when its pathway is activated [21]. Proto-oncogene *c-MYC* as an upstream regulator links to the tumor-secreted protein PGK1 in the process of breast cancer development [22]. As for hepatocellular carcinoma, there is a hypothesis that *c-MYC* mainly regulates controlling PGK1 expression [16]. Therefore, the role of *MYC* regulates the metabolic function of PGK1 in HCC which needs to be further studied.

Here we utilized a public database and HCC cell lines to assess the expression and to evaluate the significance of PGK1. The results showed that PGK1 not only promoted HCC cell lines proliferation, but also boosted metastasis via *MYC*-dependent PGK1 expression to modulate the HCC cells metabolism. Moreover, PGK1 was overexpressed in HCC, and it was associated with poor prognosis and worse malignancy. These results recommend a new view of PGK1 in HCC development.

2. Results

2.1. Phosphoglycerate Kinase 1 (PGK1) Promotes Proliferation in Hepatocellular Carcinoma (HCC) In Vitro

Concerned with the function of PGK1 protein, Western blotting assays were used to detect endogenous expression of PGK1 in a panel of HCC cell lines and a normal liver cell line, HL7702. The result indicated that SNU449 and HCCLM3 expressed higher levels of PGK1 protein compared to HL7702 cells. While among the HCC cell lines examined, SNU182 and JHH5 expressed the lowest, which was similar to HL7702 (Figure 1A). According to the results of endogenous expression of PGK1 in HCC cell lines, SNU182 and JHH5 were selected for the overexpression of PGK1, SNU182/Vector and JHH5/Vector were used as the normal control; SNU449 and HCCLM3 were selected for knocking down PGK1, then we examined the transfection efficiency by Western blotting with SNU449/NC and HCCLM3/NC as normal controls (Figure 1B).

Cell counting kit-8 (CCK8) assay displayed that the forced PGK1 expression significantly increased the ability of SNU182 and JHH5 cells to proliferate ($p < 0.01$, Figure 1C). As PGK1 was knocked down in SNU449 and HCCLM3 cells, the proliferation rate evidently decreased ($p < 0.01$, Figure 1D). These results were validated by the plate colony formation assay ($p < 0.01$, Figure 1E,F). Thus, PGK1 is adequate to promote the proliferation of HCC cells.

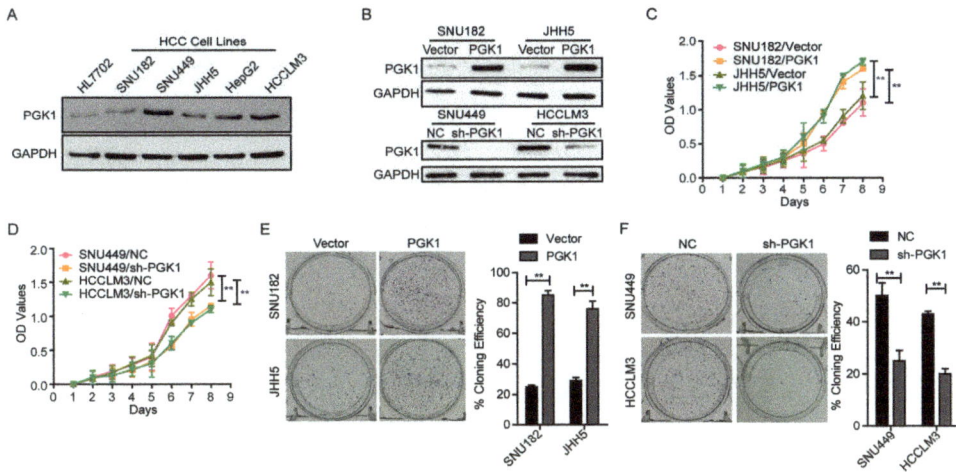

Figure 1. Effect of Phosphoglycerate Kinase 1 (PGK1) on the proliferation of Hepatocellular Carcinoma (HCC) cells. (**A**) Endogenous expression of PGK1 in nomal and five HCC cell lines by Western blotting. Glyceraldehyde 3-phosphate dehydrogenase (GAPDH) was used as internal control. (**B**) Transfection efficiency of PGK1 overexpress and knockdown in HCC. GAPDH was used as internal control. (**C**) Effect of PGK1 on proliferation of SNU182 and JHH5 cells by cell counting kit-8 (CCK8) assay. (**D**) Effect of PGK1 knockdown on proliferation of SNU449 and HCCLM3 cells by CCK8 assay. (**E**) Effect of PGK1 on proliferation of SNU182 and JHH5 cells by plate colony formation assay. (**F**) Effect of PGK1 knockdown on proliferation of SNU449 and HCCLM3 cells by plate colony formation assay. ** $p < 0.01$. NC, negative control; sh-PGK1, short hairpin RNA inhibiting PGK1 gene.

2.2. PGK1 Is Effective in Promoting Tumor Metastasis In Vivo

To investigate the function of PGK1 in tumor growth in vivo, SNU449/sh-PGK1 cells or SNU449/negative control (NC) cells were subcutaneously implanted into nude mice ($n = 6$) and monitored tumor growth. Notably, knocking down PGK1 obviously inhibited tumor growth in vivo ($p < 0.01$, Figure 2A). Additionally, compared to control groups, sh-PGK1 decreased tumor proliferation indices by Ki-67 expression ($p < 0.01$, Figure 2B).

Furthermore, we performed tail vein injecting assay ($n = 6$) in nude mice to evaluate the effect of PGK1 in tumor metastasis in vivo. We injected SNU449/sh-PGK1 cells or SNU449/NC cells into node mice's tail veins. As shown in Figure 2C, the metastatic lung nodules of sh-PGK1 group was larger than the control group ($p < 0.01$). These results declared that PGK1 is sufficient to promote tumor metastasis in vivo.

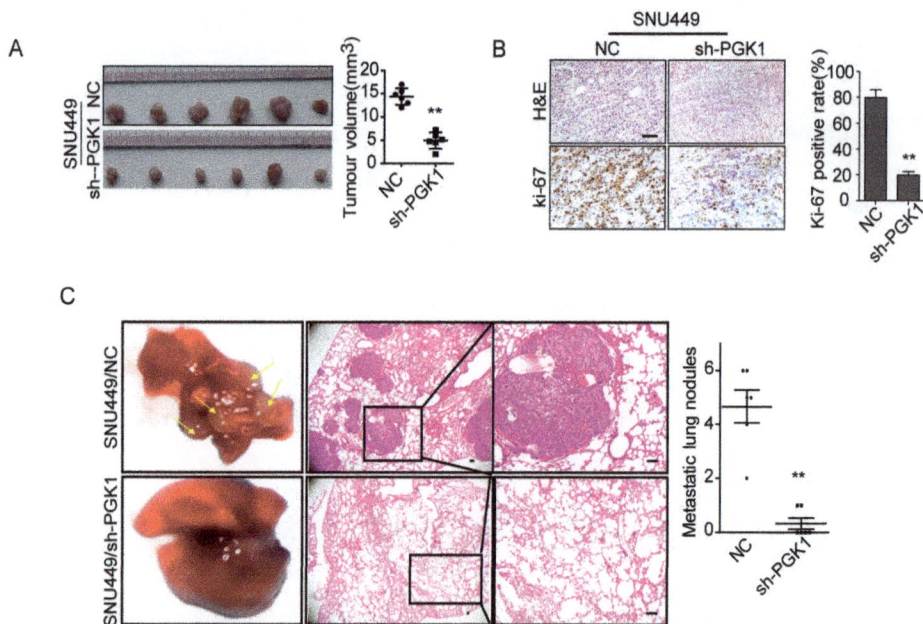

Figure 2. Effect of PGK1 on proliferation and metastasis in vivo. (**A**) Effect of PGK1 knockdown in HCC cell proliferation in vivo. PGK1 knockdowning SNU449 cells and control cells were implanted subcutaneously into nude mice to perform xenograft assay (*n* = 6). Tumor volumes were measured on the indicated days. Data points are presented as the mean tumor volume ± SD. (**B**) Histopathological analysis of xenograft tumors. The tumor sections were stained with H&E or subjected to IHC staining using an antibody against Ki-67. (**C**) Effect of PGK1 knockdown on CRC metastasis in vivo. 1×10^6 cells knockdowning PGK1 or control vector were injected into each nude mouse through tail vein. The number of lung metastasis nodules was counted under the microscope. Error bars represent mean ± SD. The tumor sections were stained with H&E. ** *p* < 0.01.

2.3. MYC-Dependent PGK1 Modulates Metabolic Reprogramming of HCC Cells

PGK1 is a major metabolic enzyme in the glycolysis pathway, and *c-MYC* is the main regulator in controlling PGK1 expression [16]. Therefore, we explored the rescue experiment to detect the metabolic process in HCC. Western blotting analysis was performed to assess the expression of solute carrier family 2 facilitated glucose transporter member 4, SLC2A4 gene (GLUT4), hexokinase 2 (HK2), and lactate dehydrogenase A (LDHA) in the rescue experiment. Results revealed that PGK1 significantly increased the expression of GLUT4, HK2, and LDHA in SNU182 cells, while si-*MYC* could not rescue this effect (Figure 3A). Knockdown of PGK1 decreased the expression of GLUT4, HK2 and LDHA in SNU449 cells, while *MYC* could not rescue this effect (Figure 3A). However, knockdown of *MYC* decreased the expression of GLUT4, HK2, and LDHA in SNU182 cells; while PGK1 could rescue this effect (Figure 3A). These results support that the knockdown of *MYC* decreases the expression of GLUT4, HK2, and LDHA by PGK1 inhibition.

Extracellular acidification measurement was used to determine the metabolic condition of HCC. Knockdown of PGK1 decreased cellular glucose uptake in SNU449 cells, while *MYC* could not rescue this effect (*p* < 0.01, Figure 3B). PGK1 significantly increased glucose uptake in SNU182 cells, while si-*MYC* could not rescue this effect (*p* < 0.01, Figure 3B). However, *MYC* significantly increased glucose uptake in SNU449 cells, while sh-PGK1 could rescue this effect (*p* < 0.01, Figure 3B). The knockdown of *MYC* decreased cellular glucose uptake in SNU182 cells, while PGK1 could rescue this effect ($p < 0.01$, Figure 3B). Analogous results were observed in lactate production and ATP levels (Figure 3C,D). *MYC* induces PGK1 to improve metabolic efficiency in HCC. We hypothesize that this improved metabolic efficiency is one of the mechanisms by which PGK1 promotes the proliferation and metastasis of HCC.

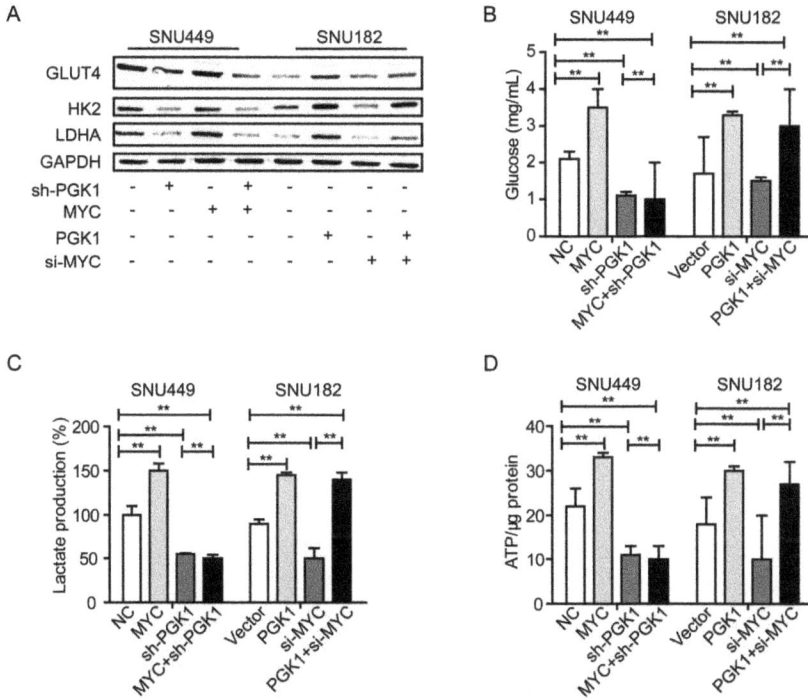

Figure 3. PGK1 modulated Warburg effects of HCC cells. (**A**) Western blot analysis of the expression of GLUT4, hexokinase 2 (HK2), and lactate dehydrogenase A (LDHA of PGK1, sh-PGK1, si-*MYC*, or *MYC* cells. GAPDH was used as internal control. (**B**) Glucose uptake levels of SNU449 and SNU182 cells with PGK1 overpression, sh-PGK1, si-*MYC*, or *MYC* overpression. (**C**) Lactate production of SNU449 and SNU182 cells with PGK1 overpression, sh-PGK1, si-*MYC*, or *MYC* overpression. (**D**) ATP levels of SNU449 and SNU182 cells with PGK1 overpression, sh-PGK1, si-*MYC*, or *MYC* overpression. ** $p < 0.01$.

2.4. PGK1 Is Overexpressed in Human Hepatocellular Carcinoma Specimens

The clinical relevance of PGK1 expression was determined by three online databases. First, we analyzed the PGK1 protein expression in clinical specimens from the human protein atlas (www.proteinatlas.org). We found that PGK1 had the positive strong expression in HCC, and negative weak expression in normal liver (Figure 4A). Secondly, in the Roesser liver database (Compendia Biosciences, www.oncomine.org), PGK1 mRNA level was superior in HCC tissues to normal liver tissues ($p < 0.001$, $n = 22$, Figure 4B). At last, we exploited the TCGA Research Network: http://cancergenome.nih.gov/ to evaluate the results of survival data. The results showed that patients with high PGK1 expression may have a significantly shorter 10-year survival time ($p = 0.0401$, Figure 4C). These results suggest that PGK1 upregulation in HCC tissue is closely related to the prognosis of HCC patients.

A B C

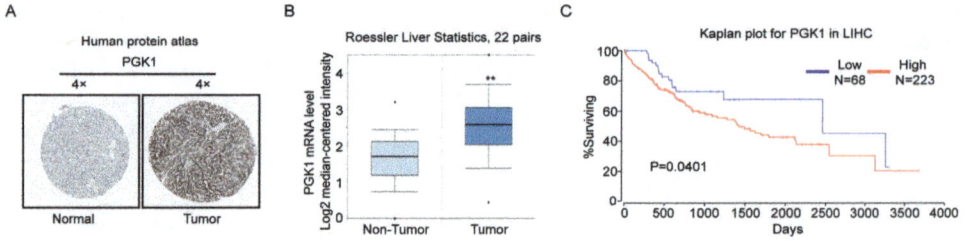

Figure 4. PGK1 is upregulated in human hepatocellular carcinoma specimens. (**A**) PGK1 expression in normal liver tissue and hepatocellular carcinoma specimens. Images were taken from the Human Protein Atlas online database. (**B**) Oncomine data showing PGK1 expression in normal vs. tumor of liver (*n* = 22). (**C**) Kaplan Meier survival analysis of HCC patients with high and lowPGK1 expression based upon data generated by the TCGA Research Network (*p* = 0.0401). ** *p* < 0.01. LIHC, Liver hepatocellular carcinoma.

3. Discussion

Metabolic reprogramming was thought to be a sign of cancer [23], and had been a popular research field for the past decade. The Warburg effect was not only beneficial to the growth of cancer cells, but also conducive to tumor migration and invasion.

The carcinogenic signaling pathway directly promoted the acquisition of nutrients and promoted the decomposition of carbon into macromolecules (lipids, proteins, and nucleic acids) when nutrient-enriched for the proliferation of cancer cells. These net effects of conducts were expected to strengthen growth and cell proliferation [3]. In the hierarchical structure of the tumor alteration pathway, the mutations of *MYC*, TP53, Ras-related oncogene, LKB1-AMP kinase (AMPK) and PI3K kinase (PI3K) signaling pathway were always invoved in glucose and glutamine metabolism [3]. The increase in *MYC* caused a number of metabolic effects by reprogramming gene expression, including promoted glycolysis, partial activation by LDHA transcription [24], improved mitochondrial biogenesis [25], and increased glutamine catabolism [26,27], eventually achieving biomass assimilation. The intersection of glucose and glutamine in many aspects reflected their richness and they both could enter the central metabolic multiple nodes. Glutamine was necessary for growth, as it provided two nitrogen atoms to synthesize hexosamine, nucleotides, and amino acids [28].

However, for resisting the physical environment of solid tumors, cancer cells must optimize nutritional use due to the scarce resources. Some works highlighted the importance of culturing cells and metabolic flexibility in vivo. For instance, in colon cancer cells, the deprivation of glucose or subcutaneous space in mice grown in a harsh environment caused selective stress on KRAS mutations [29].

Here, KRAS mutation allowed the cells to tolerate low glucose conditions. Cancer cells usually employ a nutrient to pack another nutrient normally provided into the metabolite pool, which can recombine their metabolism to remunerate the loss of glucose or glutamine in the culture [30–32]. As a means of sustaining growth, high-throughput screening showed that long-term exposure to low glucose cells required oxidative phosphorylation [33]. Similarly, a subset of lymphomas was preferentially used and it perfered to depend on oxidative metabolism in a classic glycolytic phenotype [34]. Thus, hypoxia-inducible factor (HIF1) activation, lactate released and redox production, these metabolic transitions caused by cancer cells, changed by associating with the development of invasive cancers [2]. A mathematical model provided an acid-mediated hypothesis of invasion of tumor [35]. Through this model, due to the additional glucose production and glucose metabolism changes, the H+ flow concentration gradient generated adjacent to the normal organization. The release of cathepsin B and other proteolytic enzymes to normal cells caused cellular death and extracellular matrix degradation, resulting in chronic exposure to the acidic microenvironment of the surrounding normal tissue. All of these allow cancer cells to invade adjacent normal tissues [2]. In addition, glycolytic enzymes are very important to the migration of tumor cells. GLUT4 is a member of the solute carrier family 2 (promotes glucose transporter) family and transmits glucose through the cell membrane. HK2 is the key enzyme for the first step in most glucose metabolic pathways. As a key metabolic enzyme, lactate dehydrogenase (LDH) catalyzes pyruvate conversely to lactate. LDHA is a subunit of LDH. LDHA was essential for maintaining glycolysis and improving the cancer cells' invasive activity [2].

Here we showed that PGK1 was overexpressed in human HCC tissues, and *MYC* induced PGK1 to improve the metabolic efficiency in HCC. We demonstrated that, in HCC cells, more and more glucoses were transported into cells by improved GLUT4, which induced by *MYC*-dependent PGK1. Then with the over expressed of HK2 and LDHA (they are both the key enzymes in glycolysis) induced by *MYC*-dependent PGK1, the rate of glycolysis was accelerated. After that, more and more ATP and lactate were produced. Finally, a large amount of ATP provided energy required for HCC proliferation, and lactate promoted metastasis and had a interrelation with poor hepatic carcinoma overall survival and patient prognosis (Figure 5). Our results demonstrated that oncogenic PGK1 enhanced expression of GLUT4 to stimulate glucose uptaken; on the other hand, PGK1 utilizated the glucose by anabolic pathways. *MYC* upregulated PGK1, resulting in more metabolic product and ultimately cell survival and growth. Moreover, the structure of Human PGK1 was well understood. Our findings strongly suggest that targeting PGK1 is a therapeutic strategy for HCC.

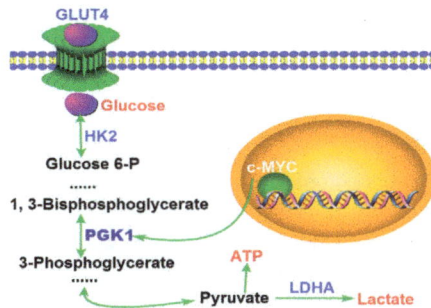

Figure 5. A model for the role of PGK1 in human hepatocellular carcinoma. PGK1 had an important role in metabolic reprogramming induced by *MYC*, leading to an enhanced Warburg effect.

4. Materials and Methods

4.1. Cell Culture

Human HCC cell lines (SNU182, SNU449, JHH5, HepG2, and HCCLM3) and normal liver cell line HL7702 were acquired from Cell Bank of Type Culture Collection (Shanghai City, China). The cells were cultured in DMEM (Hyclone, Los Angeles, CA, USA) with 10% FBS under 5% CO_2 at 37 °C.

4.2. Cell Transfection with siRNAs and Plasmids

All the primers for PGK1 and *MYC* detection assays were purchased from Ribobio. Transfection of *MYC* siRNA and negative control (NC) were conducted via siRNA kit (RIBOBIO, Guangzhou, China) according to the manufacturer's protocol.

The steps of PGK1 and *MYC* overexpression are as follows: the CDS full length of human PGK1 and *MYC* genes was synthesized and cloned into Pez-Lv105 vector by GeneCopoeia (Guangzhou, China). The vectors were transfected into lentiviral packaged 293T cell lines. Then 1 mL of viral supernatant (containing 4 Attograms (Ag) of polybrene) was added into HCC cell lines for 14 days.

To eliminate PGK1, a lentivirus with shRNA vector targeting PGK1 was transfected into HEK293T cells, and 1 mL of virus supernatant (containing 4 Ag of polybrene) was added to the HCC cell line. Western blotting detected PGK1 expression after 72 h.

4.3. Western Blotting

First, cells were lyzed on ice in a radioimmunoprecipitation (RIPA) buffer with a protease inhibitor then quantified by quinolinic acid (BCA) assay. Second, SDS-PAGE isolated a total of 50 μg of protein lysate, which was then transferred to a PVDF membrane (Millipore Corp, Billerica, MA, USA). Third, the membrane was blocked with 5% fat-free milk, then incubated with PGK1 (ABclonal Biotech Co., Woburn, MA, USA, 1:100), *MYC* (ABclonal Biotech Co., Woburn, MA, USA, 1:100), LDHA (ABclonal Biotech Co., Woburn, MA, USA, 1:100), HK2 (ABclonal Biotech Co., Woburn, MA, USA, 1:100), GLUT4 (ABclonal Biotech Co., Woburn, MA, USA, 1:100), or glyceraldehyde 3-phosphate dehydrogenase (GAPDH) (ABclonal Biotech Co., Woburn, MA, USA, 1:1000) at 4 °C overnight. After that, the membranes were incubated with secondary antibodies. Then, ECL test reagent (Fudebio, China) was used to show the bands.

4.4. Cell Proliferation Assay

8×10^2 cells were suspended in 100 μL medium, then seeded in 96-well plates and incubated for seven days. 10 μL of CCK8 (Dojindo Molecular Technologies, Inc., Kumamoto, Japan) added in the new 100 μL medium was added to every well and the cells were incubated with 5% CO_2 at 37 °C for 2 h. Then the absorbance values were measured with a microplate reader set at 570 nm. Each experiment was conducted for three times.

4.5. Plate Colony Formation Assay

2×10^2 cells were suspended in 2 mL medium, then seeded in 6-well plates and incubated at 37 °C with 5% CO_2 for 14 days, then stained with hematoxylin. After that, counting colonies containing more than 50 cells. Last, a calculated with the formula—plate clone formation efficiency = (number of colonies/number of cells inoculated) × 100% was applied.

4.6. Proliferation and Metastasis in Mouse Model

For assessing tumor growth in vivo, 2×10^6 cells were subcutaneously injected into the left abdomen or right abdomen of the six-week-old non-obese diabetic (NOD)/severe combined immunodeficiency (SCID) mice, each group had six mice. After 28 days, the tumor was measured with a caliper to assess the tumor volume.

For assessing tumor transfer in vivo, 2×10^6 cells were injected into the tail vein of six-week-old NOD/SCID mice, each group had six mice. After eight weeks, the animals were euthanized; the thoracic, peritoneum, and peritoneal cavity of the various organs removed, washed, fixed, and then underwent pathological examination. The number of metastatic lung nodules was determined.

4.7. Glucose Uptake, Lactate Production, ATP Level Detection

In glucose uptake assay, first, cells were cultured in 6-well plates. Then according to the manufacturer's protocol, glucose uptake was determined using a glucose assay kit (Biovision Inc., Milpitas, CA, USA).

In lactate production measurement, according to the manufacturer's protocol, first cells were seeded into 96-well plates with phenol red-free medium, then determined using a lactate assay kit (Biovision Inc., Milpitas, CA, USA).

In ATP levels assay, an ATP assay kit (Biovision Inc., Milpitas, CA, USA) was used according to the manufacturer's protocol.

4.8. Analysis of PGK1 Expression in Human HCC

In HCC tissues and normal tissues, PGK1 protein expression was determined from the human protein atlas (www.proteinatlas.org). HCC PGK1 gene expression was determined through analysis of Roessler and TCGA databases, which are available through Oncomine (Compendia Biosciences, www.oncomine.org) and UCSC (http://xena.ucsc.edu/getting-started/). Survival analysis for the gene expression data were performed using OncoLnc [36].

4.9. Statistical Analysis

Statistical analysis was carried out by SPSS 13.0 software. Utilizated Student's *t*-test to compare the groups in the cell experiments. The data were expressed as the mean $\pm$ SEM of the three independent experiments. $p < 0.05$ was considered statistically significant.

Acknowledgments: This work was financially supported by the National Natural Science Foundation of China (81602152).

Author Contributions: Huijun Xie conceived and designed the experiments, and wrote the manuscript; Guihui Tong, Shu Liang, and Kairui Tang performed the experiments; Yupei Zhang analysised the data; Qinhe Yang conceived and designed the study, and reviewed the manuscript.

Conflicts of Interest: The authors declare no conflict of interest.

References

1. Ryerson, A.B.; Eheman, C.R.; Altekruse, S.F.; Ward, J.W.; Jemal, A.; Sherman, R.L.; Henley, S.J.; Holtzman, D.; Lake, A.; Noone, A.M.; et al. Annual report to the Nation on the Status of Cancer, 1975–2012, featuring the increasing incidence of liver cancer. *Cancer* **2016**, *122*, 1312–1337. [CrossRef] [PubMed]
2. Han, T.; Kang, D.; Ji, D.; Wang, X.; Zhan, W.; Fu, M.; Xin, H.B.; Wang, J.B. How does cancer cell metabolism affect tumor migration and invasion? *Cell Adhes. Migr.* **2013**, *7*, 395–403. [CrossRef] [PubMed]
3. Boroughs, L.K.; DeBerardinis, R.J. Metabolic pathways promoting cancer cell survival and growth. *Nat. Cell Biol.* **2015**, *17*, 351–359. [CrossRef] [PubMed]
4. Li, X.; Zheng, Y.; Lu, Z. PGK1 is a new member of the protein kinome. *Cell Cycle* **2016**, *15*, 1803–1804. [CrossRef] [PubMed]
5. Qian, X.; Li, X.; Lu, Z. Protein kinase activity of the glycolytic enzyme PGK1 regulates autophagy to promote tumorigenesis. *Autophagy* **2017**, 1–2. [CrossRef] [PubMed]
6. Sun, S.; Liang, X.; Zhang, X.; Liu, T.; Shi, Q.; Song, Y.; Jiang, Y.; Wu, H.; Jiang, Y.; Lu, X.; et al. Phosphoglycerate kinase-1 is a predictor of poor survival and a novel prognostic biomarker of chemoresistance to paclitaxel treatment in breast cancer. *Br. J. Cancer* **2015**, *112*, 1332–1339. [CrossRef] [PubMed]
7. Ameis, H.M.; Drenckhan, A.; von Loga, K.; Escherich, G.; Wenke, K.; Izbicki, J.R.; Reinshagen, K.; Gros, S.J. PGK1 as predictor of CXCR4 expression, bone marrow metastases and survival in neuroblastoma. *PLoS ONE* **2013**, *8*, e83701. [CrossRef] [PubMed]
8. Ahmad, S.S.; Glatzle, J.; Bajaeifer, K.; Bühler, S.; Lehmann, T.; Königsrainer, I.; Vollmer, J.P.; Sipos, B.; Ahmad, S.S.; Northoff, H.; et al. Phosphoglycerate kinase 1 as a promoter of metastasis in colon cancer. *Int. J. Oncol.* **2013**, *43*, 586–590. [CrossRef] [PubMed]
9. Jang, C.H.; Lee, I.A.; Ha, Y.R.; Lim, J.; Sung, M.K.; Lee, S.J.; Kim, J.S. PGK1 induction by a hydrogen peroxide treatment is suppressed by antioxidants in human colon carcinoma cells. *Biosci. Biotechnol. Biochem.* **2008**, *72*, 1799–1808. [CrossRef] [PubMed]
10. Younghun, J.; Yusuke, S.; Jianhua, W.; Jingcheng, W.; Zhuo, W.; Pedersen, E.A.; Lee, C.H.; Hall, C.L.; Hogg, P.J.; Krebsbach, P.H.; et al. Taichman expression of PGK1 by prostate cancer cells induces bone formation. *Mol. Cancer Res.* **2009**, *7*, 1595–1604. [CrossRef]
11. Zieker, D.; Königsrainer, I.; Traub, F.; Nieselt, K.; Knapp, B.; Schillinger, C.; Stirnkorb, C.; Fend, F.; Northoff, H.; Kupka, S.; et al. PGK1 a potential marker for peritoneal dissemination in gastric cancer. *Cell. Physiol. Biochem.* **2008**, *21*, 429–436. [CrossRef] [PubMed]

12. Zieker, D.; Königsrainer, I.; Tritschler, I.; Löffler, M.; Beckert, S.; Traub, F.; Nieselt, K.; Bühler, S.; Weller, M.; Gaedcke, J.; et al. Phosphoglycerate kinase 1 a promoting enzyme for peritoneal dissemination in gastric cancer. *Int. J. Cancer* **2010**, *126*, 1513–1520. [CrossRef] [PubMed]
13. Ai, J.; Huang, H.; Lv, X.; Tang, Z.; Chen, M.; Chen, T.; Duan, W.; Sun, H.; Li, Q.; Tan, R.; et al. FLNA and PGK1 are two potential markers for progression in hepatocellular carcinoma. *Cell. Physiol. Biochem.* **2011**, *27*, 207–216. [CrossRef] [PubMed]
14. Hundhausen, C.; Boesch-Saadatmandi, C.; Matzner, N.; Lang, F.; Blank, R.; Wolffram, S.; Blaschek, W.; Rimbach, G. Ochratoxin a lowers mRNA levels of genes encoding for key proteins of liver cell metabolism. *Cancer Genom. Proteom.* **2008**, *5*, 319–332.
15. Okino, S.T.; Chichester, C.H.; Whitlock, J.P., Jr. Hypoxia-inducible mammalian gene expression analyzed in vivo at a TATA-driven promoter and at an initiator-driven promoter. *J. Biol. Chem.* **1998**, *273*, 23837–23843. [CrossRef] [PubMed]
16. Hu, H.; Zhu, W.; Qin, J.; Chen, M.; Gong, L.; Li, L.; Liu, X.; Tao, Y.; Yin, H.; Zhou, H.; et al. Acetylation of PGK1 promotes liver cancer cell proliferation and tumorigenesis. *Hepatology* **2017**, *65*, 515–528. [CrossRef] [PubMed]
17. Valentini, G.; Maggi, M.; Pey, A.L. Protein stability, folding and misfolding in human PGK1 deficiency. *Biomolecules* **2013**, *3*, 1030–1052. [CrossRef] [PubMed]
18. Schneider, C.C.; Archid, R.; Fischer, N.; Bühler, S.; Venturelli, S.; Berger, A.; Burkard, M.; Kirschniak, A.; Bachmann, R.; Königsrainer, A.; et al. Metabolic alteration—Overcoming therapy resistance in gastric cancer via PGK-1 inhibition in a combined therapy with standard chemotherapeutics. *Int. J. Surg.* **2015**, *22*, 92–98. [CrossRef] [PubMed]
19. Shichijo, S.; Azuma, K.; Komatsu, N.; Ito, M.; Maeda, Y.; Ishihara, Y.; Itoh, K. Two proliferation-related proteins, TYMS and PGK1, could be new cytotoxic T lymphocyte-directed tumor-associated antigens of HLA-A2+ colon cancer. *Clin. Cancer Res.* **2004**, *10*, 5828–5836. [CrossRef] [PubMed]
20. Wahlstrom, T.; Henriksson, M.A. Impact of MYC in regulation of tumor cell metabolism. *Biochim. Biophys. Acta* **2015**, *1849*, 563–569. [CrossRef] [PubMed]
21. Tang, S.W.; Chang, W.H.; Su, Y.C.; Chen, Y.C.; Lai, Y.H.; Wu, P.T.; Hsu, C.I.; Lin, W.C.; Lai, M.K.; Lin, J.Y. MYC pathway is activated in clear cell renal cell carcinoma and essential for proliferation of clear cell renal cell carcinoma cells. *Cancer Lett.* **2009**, *273*, 35–43. [CrossRef] [PubMed]
22. Xu, D.; Aka, J.A.; Wang, R.; Lin, S.X. 17beta-hydroxysteroid dehydrogenase type 5 is negatively correlated to apoptosis inhibitor GRP78 and tumor-secreted protein PGK1, and modulates breast cancer cell viability and proliferation. *J. Steroid Biochem. Mol. Biol.* **2017**, *171*, 270–280. [CrossRef] [PubMed]
23. Hanahan, D.; Weinberg, R.A. Hallmarks of cancer: The next generation. *Cell* **2011**, *144*, 646–674. [CrossRef] [PubMed]
24. Shim, H.; Dolde, C.; Lewis, B.C.; Wu, C.S.; Dang, G.; Jungmann, R.A.; Dalla-Favera, R.; Dang, C.V. c-MYC transactivation of LDH-A: Implications for tumor metabolism and growth. *Proc. Natl. Acad. Sci. USA* **1997**, *94*, 6658–6663. [CrossRef] [PubMed]
25. Li, F.; Wang, Y.; Zeller, K.I.; Potter, J.J.; Wonsey, D.R.; O'Donnell, K.A.; Kim, J.W.; Yustein, J.T.; Lee, L.A.; Dang, C.V. MYC stimulates nuclearly encoded mitochondrial genes and mitochondrial biogenesis. *Mol. Cell. Biol.* **2005**, *25*, 6225–6234. [CrossRef] [PubMed]
26. Wise, D.R.; DeBerardinis, R.J.; Mancuso, A.; Sayed, N.; Zhang, X.Y.; Pfeiffer, H.K.; Nissim, I.; Daikhin, E.; Yudkoff, M.; McMahon, S.B.; et al. MYC regulates a transcriptional program that stimulates mitochondrial glutaminolysis and leads to glutamine addiction. *Proc. Natl. Acad. Sci. USA* **2008**, *105*, 18782–18787. [CrossRef] [PubMed]
27. Gao, P.; Tchernyshyov, I.; Chang, T.C.; Lee, Y.S.; Kita, K.; Ochi, T.; Zeller, K.I.; de Marzo, A.M.; van Eyk, J.E.; Mendell, J.T.; et al. c-MYC suppression of miR-23a/b enhances mitochondrial glutaminase expression and glutamine metabolism. *Nature* **2009**, *458*, 762–765. [CrossRef] [PubMed]
28. DeBerardinis, R.J.; Cheng, T. Q's next: The diverse functions of glutamine in metabolism, cell biology and cancer. *Oncogene* **2010**, *29*, 313–324. [CrossRef] [PubMed]
29. Yun, J.; Rago, C.; Cheong, I.; Pagliarini, R.; Angenendt, P.; Rajagopalan, H.; Schmidt, K.; Willson, J.K.; Markowitz, S.; Zhou, S.; et al. Glucose deprivation contributes to the development of KRAS pathway mutations in tumor cells. *Science* **2009**, *325*, 1555–1559. [CrossRef] [PubMed]

30. Le, A.; Lane, A.N.; Hamaker, M.; Bose, S.; Gouw, A.; Barbi, J.; Tsukamoto, T.; Rojas, C.J.; Slusher, B.S.; Zhang, H.; et al. Glucose-independent glutamine metabolism via TCA cycling for proliferation and survival in B cells. *Cell Metab.* **2012**, *15*, 110–121. [CrossRef] [PubMed]

31. Yang, C.; Sudderth, J.; Dang, T.; Bachoo, R.M.; McDonald, J.G.; DeBerardinis, R.J. Glioblastoma cells require glutamate dehydrogenase to survive impairments of glucose metabolism or Akt signaling. *Cancer Res.* **2009**, *69*, 7986–7993. [CrossRef] [PubMed]

32. Cheng, T.; Sudderth, J.; Yang, C.; Mullen, A.R.; Jin, E.S.; Matés, J.M.; DeBerardinis, R.J. Pyruvate carboxylase is required for glutamine-independent growth of tumor cells. *Proc. Natl. Acad. Sci. USA* **2011**, *108*, 8674–8679. [CrossRef] [PubMed]

33. Birsoy, K.; Possemato, R.; Lorbeer, F.K.; Bayraktar, E.C.; Thiru, P.; Yucel, B.; Wang, T.; Chen, W.W.; Clish, C.B.; Sabatini, D.M. Metabolic determinants of cancer cell sensitivity to glucose limitation and biguanides. *Nature* **2014**, *508*, 108–112. [CrossRef] [PubMed]

34. Caro, P.; Kishan, A.U.; Norberg, E.; Stanley, I.A.; Chapuy, B.; Ficarro, S.B.; Polak, K.; Tondera, D.; Gounarides, J.; Yin, H.; et al. Metabolic signatures uncover distinct targets in molecular subsets of diffuse large B cell lymphoma. *Cancer Cell* **2012**, *22*, 547–560. [CrossRef] [PubMed]

35. Gatenby, R.A.; Gawlinski, E.T.; Gmitro, A.F.; Kaylor, B.; Gillies, R.J. Acid-mediated tumor invasion: A multidisciplinary study. *Cancer Res.* **2006**, *66*, 5216–5223. [CrossRef] [PubMed]

36. Anaya, J. OncoLnc: Linking TCGA survival data to mRNAs, miRNAs, and lncRNAs. *PeerJ* **2016**, *32*, 1–8. [CrossRef]

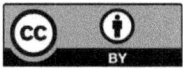

International Journal of
Molecular Sciences

MDPI

Article

Sulfiredoxin May Promote Cervical Cancer Metastasis via Wnt/β-Catenin Signaling Pathway

Kangyun Lan, Yuni Zhao, Yue Fan, Binbin Ma, Shanshan Yang, Qin Liu, Hua Linghu and Hui Wang *

Department of Obstetrics and Gynecology, The First Affiliated Hospital of Chongqing Medical University, Chongqing 400016, China; kangyun_lan@126.com (K.L.); tutoo250@sina.com (Y.Z.); lemon.1993@163.com (Y.F.); 13220309803@163.com (B.M.); yss133yss133@126.com (S.Y.); liudier771@126.com (Q.L.); linghu_hua@126.com (H.L.)
* Correspondence: cqhrong@tom.com; Tel./Fax: +86-23-8901-1082

Academic Editors: Gianni Sava and Alberta Bergamo
Received: 19 March 2017; Accepted: 22 April 2017; Published: 27 April 2017

Abstract: The abnormal elevation of sulfiredoxin (Srx/SRXN1)—an antioxidant enzyme whose main function is to protect against oxidative stress—has been shown to be closely correlated with the progression of several types of cancer, including human cervical cancer. However, the molecular mechanism by which Srx promotes tumor progression, especially cancer metastasis in cervical cancer, has not been elucidated. Here, we show that Srx expression gradually increases during the progression of human cervical cancer and its expression level is closely correlated with lymph node metastasis. Our study also reveals a significant positive correlation between the expression of Srx and β-catenin in cervical cancer tissues. Loss-of-function studies demonstrate that Srx knockdown using a lentiviral vector-mediated specific shRNA decreases the migration and invasion capacity in HeLa (human papilloma virus 18 type cervical cancer cell line) and SiHa SiHa (cervical squamous cancer cell line). Notably, the exact opposite effects were observed in gain-of-function experiments in C-33A cells. Mechanistically, downregulation or upregulation of Srx leads to an altered expression of proteins associated with the Wnt/β-catenin signaling pathway. Furthermore, blockage of the Wnt/β-catenin signaling pathway contributed to attenuated Srx expression and resulted in significant inhibition of cell migration and invasion in cervical cancer cell lines. Combined, Srx might be an oncoprotein in cervical cancer, playing critical roles in activating the Wnt/β-catenin signaling pathway; it may therefore be a therapeutic target for cervical cancer.

Keywords: sulfiredoxin; cervical cancer; metastasis; Wnt/β-catenin signaling

1. Introduction

Cervical cancer is the second leading cause of death among young women aged 19–39 years [1], and the fourth leading cause of mortality in females worldwide [2]. Many patients with cervical carcinoma metastasis previously treated with surgery or chemotherapy will develop recurrent disease which seriously affects the quality of life of patients [3]. Thus, it is critical to elucidate the molecular and biologic mechanisms in the development of cervical tumor and develop better therapeutic strategies in cervical cancer.

Sulfiredoxin (Srx) is a novel discovered antioxidant enzyme [4,5], which was initially identified in yeast. The main role of Srx is to reduce its downstream target gene hyperoxidized peroxiredoxin (Prx; a member of antioxidant protein) back to active peroxidases in the presence of ATP [6–8], and then counteract the excessive reactive oxygen species (ROS) to protect the host organism from oxidative damages [9]. However, this property of Srx becomes a damaging effect to host cells when it starts protecting the survival of cancer cells [10,11]. As per published literature and the data from the microarray database, Srx is altered in multiple types of cancer and plays critical roles in carcinogenesis by modulating cell signal transduction involved in cell proliferation, migration and metastasis [10]. It has been reported that Srx was upregulated in several human cancers, including colorectal cancer [12], skin malignancies [13], lung cancer [14] and human cervical cancer [15], suggesting the potential role of Srx in tumor. As we mentioned above, Srx is associated with cancer metastasis. For example, Srx can modulate cancer cell motility via redox sensitive interaction with non-muscle myosin IIA (NMIIA) and S100A4 [16], and promotes colorectal cancer cell adhesion and migration through a mechanism of enhancing EGFR (epidermal growth factor receptor) signaling [12]. These studies indicate that Srx plays a critical role in cancer progression and metastasis. However, the complicated function and molecular mechanism of Srx in cervical cancer metastasis has remained largely undiscovered.

Wnt/β-catenin signaling, which activates β-catenin to initiate the transcription of its downstream target genes, has been reported to be associated with carcinogenesis and progression in cervical cancer [17–19]. A study showed that Prx, a target gene of Srx [20], has been implicated in the regulation of the Wnt/β-catenin signaling pathway. For example, knockdown of Prx inhibits the growth of colorectal cells by downregulating the Wnt/β-catenin signaling [21]. Our previously study revealed a significant positive correlation between the expression of Srx and E-catenin (an upstream molecule of the Wnt/β-catenin signaling pathway) in cervical cancer tissues [15].

In light of these observation, we hypothesize that Srx may be an important molecule in human cervical cancer development and progression. We assessed Srx expression in human cervical tissue specimens, including normal cervical squamous cell epithelium tissues (NC), cervical intraepithelial neoplasia tissues (CIN) and human cervical cancer tissues; investigated the biological function of Srx in cervical cancer; and examined whether these effects are mediated by the Wnt/β-catenin signaling pathway.

2. Results

Srx and β-catenin are overexpressed and correlated with metastasis in cervical cancer, and the expression of the two proteins is positively correlated.

We evaluated the expression of Srx and β-catenin in 20 normal cervical samples (NC), 30 cervical intraepithelial neoplasia (CIN) and 90 human cervical cancer tissues by immunohistochemistry. The results showed that Srx was predominantly localized in the cytoplasm of cervical cancer tissues (Figure 1(Ac)), and was rarely found in NC tissues (Figure 1(Aa)). Based on the expression scores, the percentage of Srx positive expression samples increased gradually from 15% in NC, to 46.7% in CIN to 73.3% in cervical cancer (Table 1). β-catenin was located in the membrane of the cell in NC (Figure 1(Ad)). However, its location transfers to the cytoplasm and nucleus in cervical cancer (Figure 1(Af)). The positive rate of β-catenin in cervical cancer (78.9%) and CIN (53.3%) was higher than in NC (20%) (Table 1). The differences in the positive expression rate of Srx or β-catenin in NC, CIN, and cervical cancer groups were statistically significant ($p < 0.05$). Then, we evaluated the expression of Srx and β-catenin in five NC, five CIN and five cervical cancer tissues by Western blotting, and the results showed that the two proteins significantly upregulated in both NC and CIN tissues, compared to the NC group ($p < 0.05$; Figure 1B). These findings indicated that Srx and β-catenin are highly expressed in human cervical cancer tissues (Figure 1 and Table 1). Next, we assessed the correlation between the expression of the two proteins and the clinicopathological features of cervical cancer, respectively. In these 90 patients with cervical cancer, there were significant associations between Srx expression and lymph node metastasis ($p < 0.05$) or infiltration of the haemal tube ($p < 0.05$), but we did not find a correlation between Srx expression and age, tumor size, degree of histologic differentiation, clinical stage or depth of cancer invasion ($p > 0.05$) (Table 2). The data also revealed that expression of β-catenin was closely associated with lymph node metastasis ($p < 0.05$) (Table 2). Furthermore, Spearman's rank correlation analysis showed a significant positive correlation between Srx expression and β-catenin expression in human cervical cancer tissues ($r = 0.365$, $p = 0.000$) (Table 3).

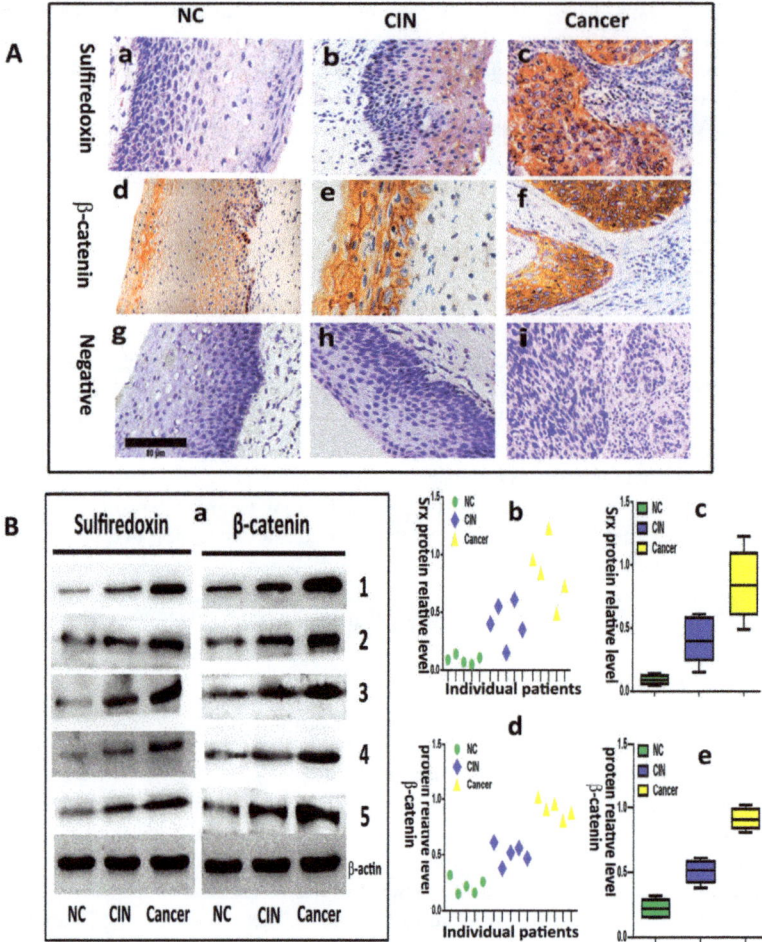

Figure 1. Sulfiredoxin (Srx) and β-catenin are highly expressed in human cervical cancer tissues. (**A**) Immunohistochemical staining to detect Srx and β-catenin. (**a**) Normal cervical (NC) tissues without Srx expression; (**b**) Cervical intraepithelial neoplasia (CIN) with mild expression of Srx; (**c**) Strong positive staining for Srx was observed in cervical cancer tissues; (**d**) Cytomembrane expression of β-catenin in NC tissues; (**e**) Partial defect of β-catenin in cytomembrane from CIN; (**f**) Cytoplasmic and nuclear strong positive staining of β-catenin in cervical cancer tissues; (**g–i**) No measurable staining of PBS (phosphate belanced solution)was used as a negative control; (**a–i**) Original magnification 200×. All the images in the Figure 2B have the same scale bar; (**B**) The protein expression of Srx and β-catenin in NC, CIN and cervical cancer tissues was assayed by Western blotting. (**a**) Western blotting showing the expression of Srx in NC, CIN and cervical cancer tissues; (**b**) Dot plot of individual patients and their corresponding Srx protein relative level; (**c**) Box plot shows median, lower and upper quartiles, and minimum and maximum values of Srx protein relative level for NC cases, CIN cases and cervical cancer cases; (**d**) Dot plot of individual patients and their corresponding β-catenin protein relative level; (**e**) Box plot shows median, lower and upper quartiles, and minimum and maximum of β-catenin protein relative level for NC cases, CIN cases and cervical cancer cases. Srx and β-catenin expression was significantly increased in cervical cancer tissues. ($p < 0.05$, NC vs. CIN; $p < 0.01$, NC vs. Cancer). The expression of β-actin was used as a loading control.

Table 1. Expression of Srx and β-catenin in different cervical tissues.

Sample	Case	Expression of Srx				Expression of β-Catenin			
		+ (%)	− (%)	χ^2	*p*	+ (%)	− (%)	χ^2	*p*
NC	20	3(15.0)	17(85.0)			4(20)	16(80.0)		
CIN	30	14(46.7)	16(53.3)			16(53.3)	14(46.7)		
CINI	5	1(20.0)	4(80.0)			1(20.0)	3(80.0)		
CINII	12	5(41.7)	7(58.3)			6(50.0)	6(50.0)		
CINIII	13	8(61.5)	5(38.5)			9(69.2)	4(30.8)		
CSCC	90	66(73.3)	22(26.7)			71(78.9)	19(21.1)		
NC vs. CIN				3.980	0.021			4.253	0.018
CINvs. Cancer				7.200	0.013			7.370	0.010
NC vs. Cancer				21.386	0.000			23.514	0.000
NC vs. CIN vs. Cancer				26.476	0.000			27.037	0.000

CINI (Cervical intra-epithelial-neoplasia1); CINII (Cervical intra-epithelial-neoplasia2); CINIII (Cervical intra-epithelial-neoplasia3). CIN = CINI + CINII + CINIII.

Table 2. Correlation between the expression of the two proteins and clinical pathological features of cervical cancer.

Variable	N	Expression of Srx			Expression of β-Catenin		
		+ (%)	− (%)	*p*	+ (%)	− (%)	*p*
Age (year)							
≥45	42	33(78.6)	9(21.4)	0.209	36(85.7)	6(14.3)	0.110
<45	48	33(68.7)	15(31.3)		35(72.9)	13(27.1)	
FIGO stage							
I	70	49(70.0)	21(30.0)	0.146	52(74.3)	18(25.7)	0.037
II	20	17(85.0)	3(15.0)		19(95.0)	1(5.0)	
Tumor size (cm)							
≥4	10	6(60.0)	4(40.0)	0.255	6(60.0)	4(40.0)	0.129
<4	80	60(75.0)	20(25.0)		65(81.2)	15(18.8)	
Histologic differentiation							
Well and moderate	63	44(69.8)	19(30.2)	0.190	46(73.0)	17(27.0)	0.030
Poor	27	22(81.5)	5(18.5)		25(92.6)	2(7.4)	
Lymph node metastasis							
+	27	24(88.9)	3(11.1)	**0.023**	25(92.6)	2(7.4)	**0.030**
−	63	42(66.7)	21(33.3)		46(73.0)	17(27.0)	
Infiltration of haemal tube							
+	21	19(90.5)	2(9.5)	**0.034**	15(71.4)	6(28.6)	0.252
−	69	47(68.1)	22(31.9)		56(81.2)	13(18.8)	
Depth of cancer invasion							
Light layer	54	36(66.7)	18(33.3)	0.064	41(75.9)	13(24.1)	0.284
Deep layer	36	30(83.3)	6(6.7)		30(83.3)	16(16.7)	

FIGO (International Federation of Gynecology and Obstetrics); "+" means positive expression; "−" means negative expression. Bold values are statistically significant.

Table 3. Correlation of Srx and β-catenin expression in cervical cancer tissues.

Expression of β-Catenin	Expression of Srx	
	Positive (*n* = 66)	Negative (*n* = 24)
Positive (*n* = 71)	58	13
Negative (*n* = 19)	8	11

2.1. Srx Promotes the Migration and Invasion of Cervical Cancer Cells

The correlation between Srx and human cervical cancer metastasis suggested that Srx may play a role in the process of cervical cancer migration and invasion. To test this hypothesis, we subsequently established an effective cell model and performed the transwell assay to measure it. First, we examined the expression of Srx in HeLa, SiHa and C33A cervical cancer cells by Western blotting and qRT-PCR, and results showed that Srx was highly expressed in the HeLa and SiHa cells (Figure 2A). Then, we knocked down Srx in HeLa and SiHa cells by transfecting lentiviruses containing Srx shRNA (Srx-shRNA) (Figure 2B–D), and explored loss-of-function of Srx in human cervical cancer cell lines. The transwell assay showed that cell migration (Figure 3A) ($p < 0.05$) and invasion (Figure 3B) ($p < 0.05$) were significantly reduced with Srx knockdown in HeLa cell lines. The role of Srx knockdown in SiHa cells was similar to that in HeLa cells. Knockdown of Srx inhibited migration (Figure 3A) ($p < 0.05$) and invasion (Figure 3B) ($p < 0.05$) in SiHa cells. Gain-of-function of Srx in C33A cell lines by transfecting lentiviruses containing Srx (Srx-LV) (Figure 2B–D) revealed that overexpression of Srx promoted C33A cell migration (Figure 3A) ($p < 0.05$) and invasion (Figure 3B) ($p < 0.05$).

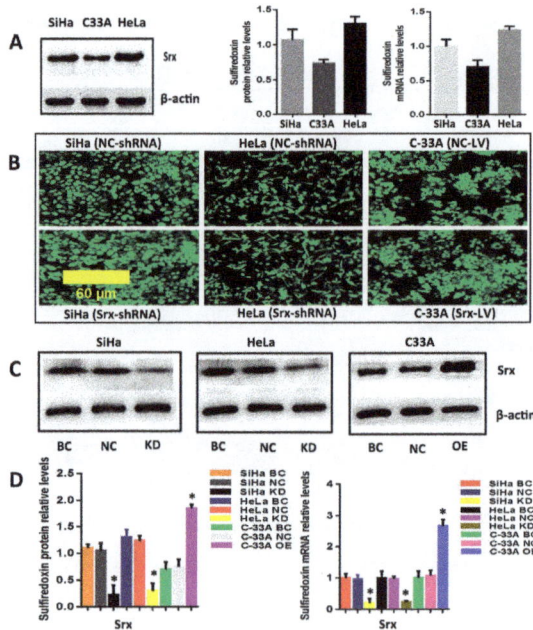

Figure 2. Srx was knocked down by Srx-shRNA and overexpressed by Srx-LV efficiently in cervical cancer cell lines. (**A**) Western blotting (left panel) and qRT-PCR (right panel) were used to detect the expression of Srx in HeLa (human papilloma virus 18 type cervical cancer cell line), SiHa (cervical squamous cancer cell line).and C33A cervical cancer cell lines; (**B**) HeLa and SiHa cells were transduced with lentivirus containing Srx-shRNA, and C33A cells were transduced with lentivirus containing Srx-LV for 72 h, respectively. GFP signals were measured by fluorescence microscopy (100×) and showed that lentiviruses were successfully transduced into cervical cancer cell lines. All the images in the Figure 2B have the same scale bar; (**C,D**) Overexpressed and knockdown efficiency of Srx were confirmed by Western blotting (**C** and the left panel of **D**) and qRT-PCR (the right panel of **D**). The NC-LV-transduced cells (NC-LV) and NC-shRNA-transduced cells (NC-shRNA) were used as negative control (NC). Non-transduced cells were used as blank control (BC). The results are expressed as mean ± S.D. * $p < 0.05$.

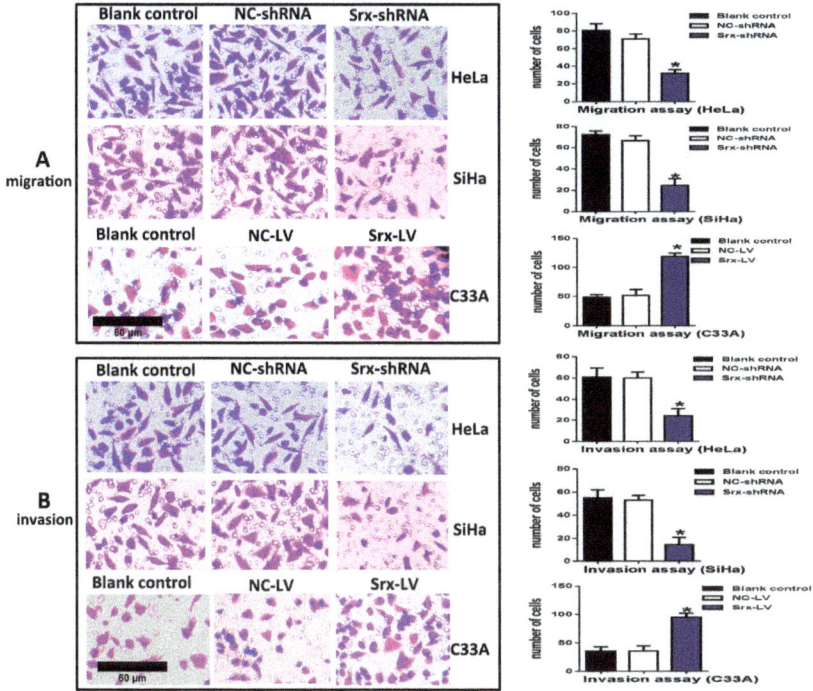

Figure 3. Srx promoted the migration and invasion of cervical cancer cells by the transwell assay. (**A**) The migration of HeLa (upper panels) and SiHa cells (middle panels) was significantly inhibited with Srx knockdown in comparison to the blank control (BC) and NC-shRNA-transduced negative control (NC) group cells. C33A cell (lower panels) migration was markedly increased with Srx overexpression in comparison to the BC and NC-LV-transduced negative control (NC) group cells, as determined by the transwell assay without Matrigel; (**B**) The invasion of HeLa (upper panels) and SiHa cells (middle panels) was significantly inhibited with Srx knockdown in comparison to BC and NC group cells. C33A cell (lower panels) invasion was markedly increased with Srx overexpression in comparison to the BC and NC group cells, as determined by the transwell assay coated with Matrigel. The cells on transwell chambers were fixed, dyed and photographed after culture for 24 h (invasion) or 22 h (migration). All the images in the Figure 2A,B have the same scale bar. The values are expressed as the mean ± SD. (* $p < 0.05$ vs. control).

2.2. Silencing or Overexpression of Srx Resulted in Alteration of Proteins Levels Associated with Wnt/β-Catenin Signaling Pathway

To explore whether Srx promotes the migration and invasion of cervical cancer cells via Wnt/β-catenin signaling, Srx was silenced in HeLa and SiHa cell lines by lentiviruses containing Srx shRNA, and overexpressed in C33A cell lines by lentiviruses containing Srx-LV. In the present study, with the alteration of Srx expression, we focused on the changing of β-catenin and GSK-3β activity, and the transcriptional activity of target genes. Following over-expression of Srx, total expression of intracellular β-catenin was significantly increased in C33A cells ($p < 0.05$; Figure 4A). In addition, the phosphorylated β-catenin (P-β-catenin), which was generated to break down the Wnt signal, was appreciably decreased with Srx over-expression ($p < 0.05$; Figure 4A). Furthermore, GSK/3β, a critical factor of the Wnt signal, was decreased when Srx was overexpressed in C33A cells, whereas the level of phosphorylated GSK/3b (p-GSK/3b) was notably increased with Srx upregulated in C33A cells ($p < 0.05$; Figure 4A). CD44, a target gene of the Wnt signal, was remarkably increased with Srx over-expression in C33A cells ($p < 0.05$; Figure 4A). Notably, the exact opposite effects were observed in loss-of-function experiments in HeLa and SiHa cells. β-Catenin, p-GSK/3b and CD44 were significantly reduced by knocking down the expression of Srx in HeLa and SiHa cells. We also found that treatment of HeLa and SiHa cells with Srx shRNA significantly increased the expression of GSK-3β and P-β-catenin ($p < 0.05$; Figure 4). These findings indicated that Srx may be involved in the regulation of the Wnt/β-catenin signal pathway in human cervical cancer cells.

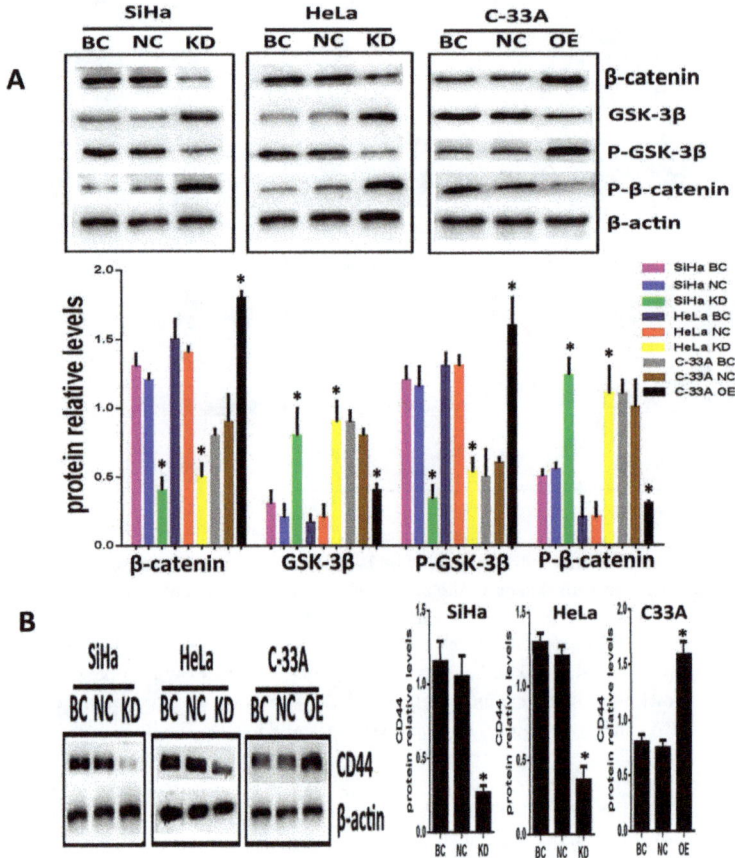

Figure 4. Knockdown of Srx expression inhibits the activation of Wnt/β-catenin signal pathways and upregulation of Srx level promotes the activation of Wnt/β-catenin signal pathways. (**A**) The expression of β-catenin, P-β-catenin, GSK-3β and p-GSK-3β in Srx-depleted HeLa and SiHa cells and Srx-upregulated C33A cells were determined by Western blotting; (**B**) The expression of CD44 (Wnt/β-catenin pathway target genes) in Srx-depleted HeLa and SiHa cells and Srx-upregulated C33A cells were measured by Western blotting. β-Actin was used as the loading controls (* $p < 0.05$ vs. controls).

2.3. The Suppression of Wnt/β-Catenin Signaling Pathway by XAV-939 Inhibits Migration, Invasion and Srx Expression in Cervical Cancer Cell Lines

To further confirm that the canonical Wnt signaling is the pathway where Srx promotes the migration and invasion of human cervical cancer, XAV-939 (an inhibitor of the canonical Wnt signaling pathway) was used to block Wnt/β-catenin signaling in HeLa, SiHa and Srx-over-expressing C33A

(LV-C33A) cell lines. When HeLa, SiHa and LV-C33A cell lines were treated with XAV-939, β-catenin was obviously reduced compared to those in the two cell lines treated with DMSO by Western blotting ($p < 0.05$, Figure 5C). In addition, the inhibition of this pathway caused remarkable suppression of Srx expression ($p < 0.05$, Figure 5C) and highly degreased the migration ($p < 0.05$, Figure 5A) and invasion ($p < 0.05$, Figure 5B) in HeLa, SiHa and LV-C33A cell lines. Taken together, these results suggest that Srx promotes the migration and invasion of cervical cancer cells and may be involved in the activation of the Wnt/β-catenin signaling pathway.

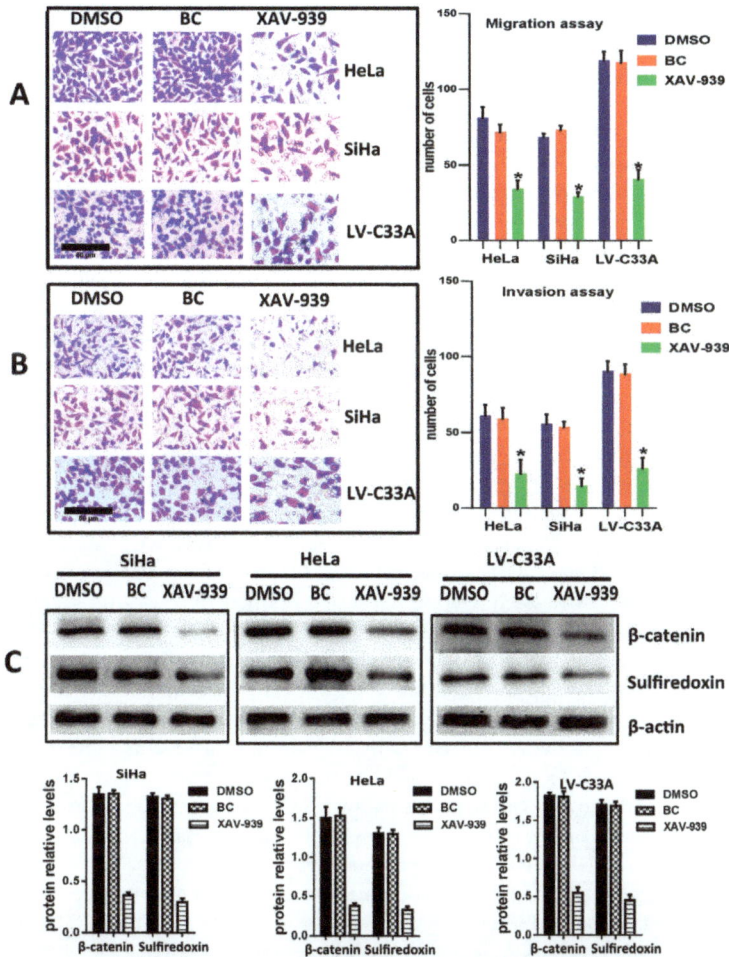

Figure 5. Inhibition of the Wnt/β-catenin signal decreases migration, invasion and Srx expression in cervical cancer cell lines. (**A**) The migration of HeLa, SiHa and LV-C33A cells was markedly inhibited after treatment with XAV-939, an inhibitor of β-catenin, in comparison to the DMSO negative control and blank control (BC), as determined by the transwell assay (* $p < 0.05$ vs. control); (**B**) The effects of XAV-939 on the invasion of HeLa, SiHa and LV-C33A cells were evaluated by the transwell assay, in comparison to the DMSO and BC control (* $p < 0.05$ vs. control); (**C**) Western blotting showed that treatment with XAV-939 in HeLa, SiHa and LV-C33A cells resulted in significant inhibition of β-catenin and Srx expression, in comparison to DMSO and BC control (* $p < 0.05$ vs. control).

3. Discussion

The abnormally elevated expression of Srx was shown to be associated with carcinogenesis in colorectal cancer [22], skin malignancies [23], lung cancer [24], etc. Subsequently, the overexpression of Srx has already been demonstrated to promote cancer metastasis in multiple cancers [10], including those cancers we just mentioned. It is well documented that cancer cells are known to bring about numerous ROS. Thus, it is not difficult to understand that the elevated expression of antioxidant protein such as Srx could be of benefit to cancer cell survival. Furthermore, it is not difficult to understand that cancer treatment may via controlling Srx expression in cancer cells. Based on these observations, our purposes were to elucidate the molecular mechanism by which Srx regulates the metastasis of cervical cancer and establishes the associated signaling mechanisms.

In our present study, the expression of Srx was found to be gradually enhanced from NC tissues to CIN tissues and then to cervical cancer tissues, in agreement with the results of previous studies of cervical cancer [15]. Then, to further explore the function of Srx in cervical carcinogenesis, the correlation between the expression of Srx and clinical pathological features in cervical cancer tissues was analyzed. Furthermore, the results showed that there were significant associations between Srx expression and lymph node metastasis and the infiltration of the haemal tube in cervical cancer tissues. Srx is highly expressed in colorectal cancer cells and is required for colorectal cancer adhesion and migration [12,16], which provides us with evidence that Srx is associated with cancer metastasis. Subsequently, we knocked down Srx in HeLa and SiHa cells by transfecting lentiviruses containing Srx shRNA and upregulated Srx in C33A cell lines by transfecting lentiviruses containing Srx to further confirm that Srx expression might be associated with metastasis in cervical cancer. The results showed that Srx significantly promoted the migration and invasion of cervical cancer cells.

The Wnt/β-catenin signaling pathway, which activates β-catenin to initiate the transcription of its specific downstream target genes [25], has been reported to be associated with numerous cancers [26–29]. Aberrant activation of the canonical Wnt pathway plays a significant role in human cervical cancer. However, limited data show the correlation between the cancer clinical pathological characteristics and the key molecules such as β-catenin. In our study, we confirmed that β-catenin, indeed, is highly expressed in cervical carcinoma tissues and its expression level was closely associated with lymph node metastasis, which was similar to the findings of other investigators [30]. Based on the published literature, in order to take part in the regulation of serious cancer development, the Wnt/β-catenin signaling pathway does not always stay in the same situation, and is regulated by lots of factors. Here, we suppose that Srx is involved in the regulation of the Wnt/β-catenin signaling pathway. Srx is an antioxidant enzyme that exclusively reduces over-oxidized typical 2-Cys Prx [31], and the reduction of hyperoxidized Prx by Srx can be considered as a rate limiting step in the reduction of hyperoxidized Prx [32]. Individual components of the Srx–Prx axis play critical roles in carcinogenesis by modulating the cell signaling pathway involved in cell migration and metastasis [10]. For example, knockdown of Prx inhibits the growth of colorectal cancer cells via downregulating Wnt/β-catenin signaling [21]. In our study, Spearman's rank correlation analysis showed a significant positive correlation between Srx expression and β-catenin expression in human cervical cancer tissues. Then, we confirmed that the Wnt/β-catenin pathway was stimulated by Srx in HeLa, SiHa and C33A cells, with activation of CD44—its target genes—resulting in the promotion of invasion and migration in cervical cancer cell lines. All of these studies and evidence offer proof that Srx really is involved in the regulation of the Wnt/β-catenin signaling pathway in human cancer.

4. Methods and Materials

4.1. Clinical Patient Specimens

A total of 140 cervical specimens, including 20 normal cervical epithelia (NC), 30 cervical intraepithelial neoplasia (CIN) and 90 human cervical cancer tissues, were obtained from the First Affiliated Hospital of Chongqing Medical University (Chongqing, China) from 2010 to 2016.

The histological classifications and clinical stages were based on the International Federation of Gynecology and Obstetrics (FIGO) criteria. None of the patients had received chemotherapy, radiotherapy or immunotherapy before specimen collection. All patients voluntarily signed the informed consent before operation. This study protocol was approved by the ethics committee of Chongqing Medical University in 2 March 2015. No. 2015-0302. This study protocol was approved by the ethics committee of Chongqing Medical University.

4.2. Cell Lines and Reagents

Human cervical cancer cell lines (HeLa (human papilloma virus 18 type cervical cancer cell line) C33A) were purchased from the Shanghai Cell Bank, Chinese Academy of Sciences (Shanghai, China). Human cervical cancer cell line (SiHa (cervical squamous cancer cell line)) was obtained from Proteintech Group (Wuhan, China). These cell lines were cultured in Dulbecco's Modified Eagle's Medium (DMEM; Gibco, Grand Island, NY, USA), respectively supplemented with 10% fetal bovine serum (FBS; Hyclone, Shanghai, China). All cell lines were maintained at 37 °C with 5% CO_2. XAV-939 was purchased from Sigma-Aldrich (St. Louis, MO, USA), and was added to the cells for 12 h treatment at a final concentration of 5 μM. Culture media were changed after 12 h.

4.3. Immunohistochemistry (IHC)

IHC staining was performed using the Immunohistochemical SABC kit (Boster, Wuhan, China) according to the manufacturer's instructions. The paraffin sections of tissues were deparaffinized as routine. Endogenous peroxidase was removed by 3% H_2O_2 for 10 min at 37 °C and antigen was retrieved by citrate buffer (pH 6.0) at 95 °C for 15 min. To prevent non-specific binding, tissues were blocked with 5% bovine serum albumin (BSA) for 20 min at room temperature. Next, tissues were incubated with anti-Srx (1:100; Proteintech; Cat No: 14273-1-AP) and anti-β-catenin (1:100; Proteintech; Cat No: 51067-2-AP) primary rabbit monoclonal antibodies overnight at 4 °C, then goat anti-rabbit secondary antibody for 1 h at 37 °C. Then, the tissues were stained with DAB (diaminobenzidine) dehydrated, fixed and photographed.

Srx and β-catenin expression levels were evaluated based on the staining intensity (0, no staining; 1, light yellow; 2, brown; and 3 dark brown) and the percentage of positive cells (0, <10%; 1, 10–25%; 2, 25–50%; 3, 50–75%; and 4, >75%). Protein staining positivity was calculated by using the following formula: immunoreactivity score (IRS) = intensity score × quantity score. The final score was defined as follows: negative, final score ≤3; weak positive, final score >3; strong positive, final score <6.

4.4. Lentiviral Transduction and Establishment of Stable Cell Lines

All lentiviruses, including those containing Srx (Srx-LV) and Srx shRNA (Srx-shRNA) for overexpressing and knocking down Srx, respectively, and control (ctrl-LV) were purchased from GenePharma Co., Ltd. (Shanghai, China). The targeting sequences are Srx-LV (5′-atggggctgcgtgcag gaggaacgctgggcagggccggcgcgggtcggggggcgcccgaggggcccgggccgagcggcggcgcgcagggcggcagcatccactcgg gccgcatcgccgcggtgcacaacgtgccgctgagcgtgctcatccggccgctgccgtccgtgttggaccccgccaaggtgcagagcctcgtggac acgatccgggaggacccagacagcgtgccccccatcgatgtcctctggatcaaaggggcccagggaggtgactacttctactcctttgggggctgcc accgctacgcggcctaccagcaactgcagcgagagaccatccccgccaagcttgtccagtccactctctcagacctaagggtgtacctgggagcatc cacaccagacttgcagtag-3′) and Srx-shRNA (5′-TCGATGTCCTCTGGATCAA-3′). All the transfection experiments were performed according to the manufacturer's instructions. Srx-LV was transduced into C33A cells at a multiplicity of infection (MOI) of 60 and Srx-shRNA was transduced into HeLa and SiHa cells at a MOI of 30. Polybrene (GenePharma, Shanghai, China) was added in each well at a final concentration of 5 μg/mL to enhance infection solution. The effects of gene interference on Srx overexpression or silencing were validated using real-time quantitative polymerase chain reaction (RT-qPCR) and Western blotting.

4.5. RT-qPCR

Total RNA was extracted using the TRIzol reagent (TaKaRa, Dalian, China) and then reversely transcribed into cDNA using the Prime Script RT Reagent Kit (TakaRa), according to the manufacturer's instructions. RT-qPCR was performed with the CFX96™ Real-Time System (Bio-Rad, Hercules, California, USA) using SYBR Green (SYBR Premix Ex Taq™ II; TaKaRa) for fluorescent quantification. The following cycling conditions were used for RT-qPCR: pre-denaturation (95 °C, 30 s), denaturation (95 °C, 5 s, 35 cycles), annealing (55–60 °C, 30 s), extension (72 °C, 1 min) and final extension (72 °C, 10 min). The relative mRNA expression was calculated using the $2^{-\Delta\Delta Ct}$ method. The primers were used as follows: Srx (Forward 5′-AAGGTGCAGAGCCTCGTGG-3′ and Reverse 5′-GCTACTGCAAGTCTGGTGTGGA-3′); and β-actin (Forward 5′-CCACGAAACTACCTTCA ACTCC-3′ and Reverse 5′-GTGATCTCCTTCTGCATCCTGT-3′).

4.6. Western Blot Analysis (WB)

Total Proteins were extracted from tissues and cells by the Protein Extraction Kit (Beyotime, Haimen, China) and the protein concentrations were determined with a BCA (Bicinchoninic acid) protein assay kit (Pierce Biotechnology, Shanghai, China), according to the manufacturer's instructions. Equal amounts of protein (50 µg) were separated by 10% sodium dodecyl sulfatepolyacrylamide gel electrophoresis (SDS-PAGE) and transferred onto poplvinylidene fluoride (PVDF) membrane. Next, the PVDF membrane was blocked with 5% *w/v* non-fat milk for 2 h at room temperature, then incubated with primary antibodies to Srx (1:300; Proteintech), β-catenin (1:500; Cell Signaling Technology, Shanghai, China), GSK/3β (1:500; Cell Signaling Technology), P-β-catenin (1:1000; Cell Signaling Technology), p-GSK/3β (1:1000; Cell Signaling Technology), CD44 (1:1000; Proteintech) and β-actin (1:1000; Abcam, Shanghai, China) at 4 °C with gentle shaking, overnight. After washing with PBS (phosphate belanced solution; PBS) containing 0.05% Tween 20, membranes were incubated with HRP-labeled secondary antibodies (1:2000) for 1.5 h at 37 °C. To calculate protein expression levels, chemiluminescent signals were captured by a chemiluminescence detection system (ChemiDoc™ XRS imager, (Bio-Rad, Hercules, California, USA) and the signal intensity of each PVDF membrane was detected by Fusion software (Vilber Lourmat, Marne-laVallée CEDEX, Shanghai, China).

4.7. Cell Migration and Invasion Assay

For cell migration assay, HeLa, SiHa and C33A cells were re-suspended in serum-free DMEM medium and then seeded into the upper chamber of transwell chambers (Corning Costar, Corning, NY, USA). DMEM medium with 10% FBS was added into the lower chamber as a chemoattractant. After 20 h, the chamber was washed three times with PBS and non-invading cells were removed using a soft cotton swab. Migrated cells on the lower membrane surface were fixed in 4% paraformaldehyde, stained with crystal violet, and photographed at 100× selected in a random manner from five different fields of each sample. Cell invasion assay is basically similar to cell migration assay. The difference is that the transwell chambers used in the cell invasion assay are coated with Matrigel (BD Biosciences, Hercules, CA, USA) and the time of incubation is 24 h. The values for cell migration and invasion were obtained through the mean counting of cells in five fields per membrane. The results are presented as the average of three independent experiments.

4.8. Statistical Analyses

All data from these experiments were assessed with statistical software SPSS 20.0 (SPSS, Chicago, IL, USA). The results, not including correlation analysis, from immunohistochemistry were analysis by Pearson's Chi-Square or Fisher's exact tests. The correlation between Srx and β-catenin expression was examined by Spearman's rank correlation. The analysis of variance (ANOVA) was applied to evaluate the significant differences. The data are presented as the mean $\pm$ standard deviation. $p < 0.05$ was considered statistically significant. Each experiment was repeated in triplicate.

5. Conclusions

In conclusion, our findings indicated that Srx promotes cell invasion and migration in cervical cancer via activating the Wnt/β-catenin signaling pathway. More in-depth mechanistic studies in the future will help to unravel inter weaved behavior of Srx and lead to the development of better therapeutic strategies for cancer prevention and treatment.

Acknowledgments: The authors gratefully thank Tumor Central Laboratory of Chongqing Medical University for providing equipment support. The current work was partly supported by a research grant from Chongqing science and technology commission (cstc2015shmszx10007).

Author Contributions: Hui Wang designed the study; KangYun Lan and Hui Wang analyzed the data; Kangyun Lan wrote the main manuscript text; Hui Wang revised the manuscript; All authors reviewed and approved the manuscript; Kangyun Lan, Qin Liu, Binbin Ma, Shanshan Yang, Yuni Zhao, Hua Linghu and Yue Fan collected and checked the information of eligible articles.

Conflicts of Interest: The authors declare no conflict of interest.

References

1. Fei, L.; Wang, T.; Tang, S. SOX14 promotes proliferation and invasion of cervical cancer cells through Wnt/β-catenin pathway. *Int. J. Clin. Exp. Pathol.* **2015**, *8*, 1698–1704.
2. Qian, C.; Zheng, P.S.; Yang, W.T. EZH2-mediated repression of GSK-3β and TP53 promotes Wnt/β-catenin signaling-dependent cell expansion in cervical carcinoma. *Oncotarget* **2016**, *7*, 36115–36129.
3. Cheng, Y.; Guo, Y.; Zhang, Y.; You, K.; Li, Z.; Geng, L. MicroRNA-106b is involved in transforming growth factor β1-induced cell migration by targeting disabled homolog 2 in cervical carcinoma. *J. Exp. Clin. Cancer Res.* **2016**, *35*, 36116–36129. [CrossRef] [PubMed]
4. Baek, J.Y.; Han, S.H.; Sung, S.H.; Lee, H.E.; Kim, Y.M.; Noh, Y.H.; Bae, S.H.; Rhee, S.G.; Chang, T.S. Sulfiredoxin protein is critical for redox balance and survival of cells exposed to low steady-state levels of H_2O_2. *J. Biol. Chem.* **2012**, *287*, 81–89. [CrossRef] [PubMed]
5. Findlay, V.J.; Tapiero, H.; Townsend, D.M. Sulfiredoxin: A potential therapeutic agent? *Biomed. Pharmacother.* **2005**, *59*, 374–379. [CrossRef] [PubMed]
6. Jeong, W.; Bae, S.H.; Toledano, M.B.; Rhee, S.G. Role of sulfiredoxin as a regulator of peroxiredoxin function and regulation of its expression. *Free Radic. Biol. Med.* **2012**, *53*, 447–456. [CrossRef] [PubMed]
7. Jeong, W.; Park, S.J.; Chang, T.S.; Lee, D.Y.; Rhee, S.G. Molecular mechanism of the reduction of cysteine sulfinic acid of peroxiredoxin to cysteine by mammalian sulfiredoxin. *J. Biol. Chem.* **2006**, *281*, 14400–14407. [CrossRef] [PubMed]
8. Biteau, B.; Labarre, J.; Toledano, M.B. ATP-dependent reduction of cysteine-sulphinic acid by *S. cerevisiae* sulphiredoxin. *Nature* **2003**, *425*, 980–984. [CrossRef] [PubMed]
9. Li, Q.; Yu, S.; Wu, J.; Zou, Y.Y.; Zhao, Y. Sulfiredoxin-1 protects PC12 cells against oxidative stress induced by hydrogen peroxide. *J. Neurosci. Res.* **2013**, *91*, 861–870. [CrossRef] [PubMed]
10. Mishra, M.; Jiang, H.; Wua, L.; Chawsheena, H.A.; Wei, Q. The sulfiredoxin–peroxiredoxin (Srx–Prx) axis in cell signal transduction and cancer development. *Cancer Lett.* **2015**, *366*, 150–159. [CrossRef] [PubMed]
11. Kim, H.; Lee, G.R.; Kim, J.; Baek, J.Y.; Jo, Y.J.; Hong, S.E.; Kim, S.H.; Lee, J.; Lee, H.I.; Park, S.K.; et al. Sulfiredoxin inhibitor induces preferential death of cancer cells through reactive oxygen species-mediated mitochondrial damage. *Free Radic. Biol. Med.* **2016**, *91*, 264–274. [CrossRef] [PubMed]
12. Jiang, H.; Wu, L.; Chen, J.; Mishra, M.; Chwsheen, H.A.; Zhu, H.; Wei, Q. Sulfiredoxin promotes colorectal cancer cell invasion and metastasis through a novel mechanism of enhancing EGFR signaling. *Mol. Cancer Res.* **2015**, *13*, 1554–1566. [CrossRef] [PubMed]
13. Wu, L.; Jiang, H.; Chwsheen, H.A.; Mishra, M.; Young, M.R.; Gerard, M.; Toledano, M.B.; Colburn, N.H.; Wei, Q. Tumor promoter-induced sulfiredoxin is required for mouse skin tumorigenesis. *Carcinogenesis* **2014**, *35*, 1177–1184. [CrossRef] [PubMed]
14. Kim, Y.S.; Lee, H.L.; Lee, K.B.; Park, J.H.; Chung, W.Y.; Lee, K.S.; Sheen, S.S.; Park, K.J.; Hwang, S.C. Nuclear factor E2-related factor 2 dependent overexpression of sulfiredoxin and peroxiredoxin III in human lung cancer. *Korean J. Intern. Med.* **2011**, *26*, 304–313. [CrossRef] [PubMed]

15. Yan, C.X.; Qin, L.; Lan, K.Y.; Wang, S.; Wang, H. The expression and clinical significance of Srx- and E-cadherin in cervical squamous cell carcinoma tissue. *Immunol. J.* **2015**, *31*, 1067–1071.

16. Bowers, R.R.; Manevich, Y.; Townsend, D.M.; Tew, K.D. Sulfiredoxin redox-sensitive interaction with S100A4 and non-muscle myosin IIA regulates cancer cell motility. *Biochemistry* **2012**, *51*, 7740–7754. [CrossRef] [PubMed]

17. Rath, G.; Jawanjal, P.; Salhan, S.; Nalliah, M.; Dhawan, I. Clinical significance of inactivated glycogen synthase kinase 3β in HPV-associated cervical cancer: Relationship with Wnt/β-catenin pathway activation. *Am. J. Reprod. Immunol.* **2015**, *73*, 460–478. [CrossRef] [PubMed]

18. Wei, H.; Wang, N.; Zhang, Y.; Wang, S.; Pang, X.; Zhang, S. Wnt-11 overexpression promoting the invasion of cervical cancer cells. *Tumour Biol.* **2016**, *37*, 11789–11798. [CrossRef] [PubMed]

19. Zhou, Y.; Huang, Y.; Cao, X.; Xu, J.; Zhang, L.; Wang, J.; Huang, L.; Huang, S.; Yuan, L.; Jia, W.; et al. Wnt2 promotes cervical carcinoma metastasis and induction of epithelial-mesenchymal transition. *PLoS ONE* **2016**, *11*, e0160414. [CrossRef] [PubMed]

20. Puerto-Galan, L.; Perez-Ruiz, J.M.; Guinea, M.; Cejudo, F.J. The contribution of NADPH thioredoxin reductase C (NTRC) and sulfiredoxin to 2-Cys peroxiredoxin overoxidation in arabidopsis thaliana chloroplasts. *J. Exp. Bot.* **2015**, *66*, 2957–2966. [CrossRef] [PubMed]

21. Lu, W.; Fu, Z.; Wang, H.; Feng, J.; Wei, J.; Guo, J. Peroxiredoxin 2 knockdown by RNA interference inhibits the growth of colorectal cancer cells by downregulating Wnt/β-catenin signaling. *Cancer Lett.* **2014**, *343*, 190–199. [CrossRef] [PubMed]

22. Wei, Q.; Jiang, H.; Baker, A.; Dodge, L.K.; Gerard, M.; Young, M.R.; Toledano, M.B.; Colburn, N.H. Loss of sulfiredoxin renders mice resistant to azoxymethane/dextran sulfate sodium-induced colon carcinogenesis. *Carcinogenesis* **2013**, *34*, 1403–1410. [CrossRef] [PubMed]

23. Wei, Q.; Jiang, H.; Matthews, C.P.; Colburn, N.H. Sulfiredoxin is an AP-1 target gene that is required for transformation and shows elevated expression in human skin malignancies. *Proc. Natl. Acad. Sci. USA* **2008**, *105*, 19738–19743. [CrossRef] [PubMed]

24. Wei, Q.; Jiang, H.; Xiao, Z.; Baker, A.; Young, M.R.; Veenstra, T.D.; Colburn, N.H. Sulfiredoxin–peroxiredoxin IV axis promotes human lung cancer progression through modulation of specific phosphokinase signaling. *Proc. Natl. Acad. Sci. USA* **2011**, *108*, 7004–7009. [CrossRef] [PubMed]

25. Maryam, K.; Mohammed, C.S.; Wang, J.; Wei, Q.; Wang, X.; Collier, Z.; Tang, S.; Liu, H.; Zhang, F.; Huang, J.; et al. Wnt/β-catenin signaling plays an ever-expanding role in stem cell self-renewal, tumorigenesis and cancer chemoresistance. *Genes Dis.* **2016**, *3*, 11–40.

26. Aminuddin, A.; Ng, P.Y. Promising druggable target in head and neck squamous cell carcinoma: Wnt signaling. *Front. Pharmacol.* **2016**, *7*, 244–257. [CrossRef] [PubMed]

27. Liang, S.; Zhang, S.; Wang, P.; Yang, C.; Shang, C.; Yang, J.; Wang, J. LncRNA, TUG1 regulates the oral squamous cell carcinoma progression possibly via interacting with Wnt/β-catenin signaling. *Gene* **2017**, *608*, 49–57. [CrossRef] [PubMed]

28. Clevers, H.; Nusse, R. Wnt/β-catenin signaling and disease. *Cell* **2012**, *149*, 1192–1205. [CrossRef] [PubMed]

29. Liang, J.; Liang, L.; Ouyang, K.; Li, Z.; Yi, X. MALAT1 induces tongue cancer cells' EMT and inhibits apoptosis through Wnt/β-catenin signaling pathway. *J. Oral Pathol. Med.* **2017**, *46*, 98–105. [CrossRef] [PubMed]

30. Gang, W.H.; Fu, Y.S.; Zhou, K.M.; Guo, Y.; Yuan, M.; Dong, H.J. The expression of β-catenin and galectin-3 in cervical carcinoma and its clinical pathological significances. *West. China Med. J.* **2015**, *30*, 1452–1456.

31. Moon, J.C.; Kim, G.M.; Kim, E.K.; Lee, H.N.; Ha, B.; Lee, S.Y.; Jiang, H.H. Reversal of 2-Cys peroxiredoxin oligomerization by sulfiredoxin. *Biochem. Biophys. Res. Commun.* **2013**, *432*, 291–295. [CrossRef] [PubMed]

32. Noh, Y.H.; Baek, J.Y.; Jeong, W.; Rhee, S.G.; Chang, T.S. Sulfiredoxin translocation into mitochondria plays a crucial role in reducing hyperoxidized peroxiredoxin III. *J. Biol. Chem.* **2009**, *284*, 8470–8477. [CrossRef] [PubMed]

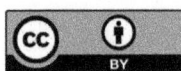

International Journal of
Molecular Sciences

MDPI

Article

Clinical Role of ASCT2 (SLC1A5) in KRAS-Mutated Colorectal Cancer

Kosuke Toda [†], Gen Nishikawa [†], Masayoshi Iwamoto, Yoshiro Itatani, Ryo Takahashi, Yoshiharu Sakai and Kenji Kawada *

Department of Surgery, Graduate School of Medicine, Kyoto University, Kyoto 606-8507, Japan;
kotoda@kuhp.kyoto-u.ac.jp (K.T.); gnishika@kuhp.kyoto-u.ac.jp (G.N.); iwamoto@kuhp.kyoto-u.ac.jp (M.I.);
itatani@kuhp.kyoto-u.ac.jp (Y.I.); ryotak@kuhp.kyoto-u.ac.jp (R.T.); ysakai@kuhp.kyoto-u.ac.jp (Y.S.)
* Correspondence: kkawada@kuhp.kyoto-u.ac.jp; Tel.: +81-75-366-7595; Fax: +81-75-366-7642
† These authors contributed equally to this work.

Received: 29 June 2017; Accepted: 24 July 2017; Published: 27 July 2017

Abstract: Mutation in the *KRAS* gene induces prominent metabolic changes. We have recently reported that *KRAS* mutations in colorectal cancer (CRC) cause alterations in amino acid metabolism. However, it remains to be investigated which amino acid transporter can be regulated by mutated *KRAS* in CRC. Here, we performed a screening of amino acid transporters using quantitative reverse-transcription polymerase chain reaction (RT-PCR) and then identified that ASCT2 (*SLC1A5*) was up-regulated through KRAS signaling. Next, immunohistochemical analysis of 93 primary CRC specimens revealed that there was a significant correlation between *KRAS* mutational status and ASCT2 expression. In addition, the expression level of ASCT2 was significantly associated with tumor depth and vascular invasion in *KRAS*-mutant CRC. Notably, significant growth suppression and elevated apoptosis were observed in *KRAS*-mutant CRC cells upon *SLC1A5*-knockdown. ASCT2 is generally known to be a glutamine transporter. Interestingly, *SLC1A5*-knockdown exhibited a more suppressive effect on cell growth than glutamine depletion. Furthermore, *SLC1A5*-knockdown also resulted in the suppression of cell migration. These results indicated that ASCT2 (*SLC1A5*) could be a novel therapeutic target against *KRAS*-mutant CRC.

Keywords: colorectal cancer; KRAS; ASCT2; SLC1A5

---

1. Introduction

Colorectal cancer (CRC) is one of the most common cancers worldwide; therefore, development of novel diagnostic measures and treatment is very important [1]. *KRAS* mutations are found in approximately 40% of CRC cases [2–4]. A number of clinical trials have shown that *KRAS* mutations in CRC can predict a lack of responses towards anti-epidermal growth factor receptor (EGFR)-based therapy [2–4]. Therefore, development of new therapy for CRC with mutated *KRAS* has been desired clinically. Some studies have investigated the correlation between *KRAS* mutations and metabolic alterations in pancreatic and lung cancers [5–9] as well as in CRC [10–15]. We have recently reported that, using metabolome analysis, concentration of amino acids is elevated in CRC cells with mutated *KRAS* compared to CRC cells with wild-type *KRAS* [12]. The increase in glucose transporter 1 (GLUT1) expression and glucose uptake was critically dependent on mutated *KRAS* [16–18]. However, it remains to be investigated which amino acid transporter is specifically regulated by mutated *KRAS* in CRC. In the present study, we performed a screening of amino acid transporters in *KRAS*-mutant CRC cells transfected by si*KRAS* and found that ASCT2 (*SLC1A5*) was particularly up-regulated through KRAS signaling.

The *SLC1A5* gene encodes alanine-serine-cysteine amino acid transporter (ASCT2), which is an essential glutamine transporter. ASCT2 over-expression has been reported in several cancers [19–31].

However, the role of ASCT2 in CRC has not yet been reported. In addition to glucose, glutamine is an essential source of cellular building blocks to fuel cell proliferation. Recent studies have established a better understanding about the importance of glutamine as a critical nutrient in fast growing cancer cells [32–34]. In the present study, we investigated the significance of ASCT2 expression in CRC using in vitro cultures and clinical samples.

2. Results

2.1. SLC1A5 (ASCT2) Is Regulated through KRAS Signaling in KRAS-Mutant CRC Cells

We have recently reported that mutated *KRAS* induces metabolic alterations in many amino acids [12]. Therefore, we hypothesized that the expression of amino acid transporters might be regulated by mutated *KRAS*. Several amino acid transporters (*SLC1A5*, *SLC7A5*, *SLC7A11*, *SLC3A2*, and *SLC43A1*) have been reported to be up-regulated in different cancers [32]. To determine the specific transporter that could be regulated by mutated *KRAS*, we introduced two different small interfering RNAs (siRNAs) targeting *KRAS* in *KRAS*-mutant CRC cell lines (HCT116 and DLD-1). We confirmed that si*KRAS* significantly reduced the mRNA levels of *KRAS* in both cell lines (Figure S1a). Interestingly, *KRAS*-knockdown significantly reduced *SLC1A5* expression in both *KRAS*-mutant cell lines (Figure 1a). *SLC1A5* (ASCT2) is a known glutamine transporter. Next, we investigated whether glutamine transporters other than *SLC1A5* (i.e., *SLC1A4*, *SLC38A1*, *SLC38A2*, *SLC38A3*, and *SLC38A5*) could be regulated by KRAS signaling [33]. Expression levels of *SLC1A4* and *SLC38A1* were decreased after *KRAS*-knockdown in HCT116; however, their expression was not decreased in DLD-1 (Figure 1b). We also found that *KRAS*-knockdown significantly reduced protein expression of ASCT2 in both *KRAS*-mutant cell lines (Figure 1c). The mutated *KRAS* continuously activates both Raf/MEK/ERK and PI3K/Akt/mTOR pathways. To investigate which pathway regulates ASCT2 expression, we used specific inhibitors of each pathway. Western blot analysis revealed that ASCT2 expression was dramatically reduced in *KRAS*-mutant CRC cell lines by addition of LY 294002 (PI3K inhibitor) or rapamycin (mTOR inhibitor), which suggested that KRAS signaling may regulate ASCT2 expression in CRC mainly via the PI3–Akt–mTOR pathway (Figure 1d).

2.2. Relationship between ASCT2 Expression and KRAS Mutational Status in CRC Clinical Samples

We next performed immunohistochemistry (IHC) to evaluate the relationship between ASCT2 expression and *KRAS* mutational status in clinical specimens of human primary CRC. Regarding the expression levels of ASCT2, we classified the clinical specimens into four groups; score 0 (0–10%), score 1+ (10–40%), score 2+ (40–70%), and score 3+ ($\geq$70%). Score 0 was found in 12 patients (12.9%), score 1+ in 22 patients (23.6%), score 2+ in 29 patients (31.2%), and score 3+ in 30 patients (32.3%) (Figure 2a). We defined score 3+ as the high expression group, while score 0, 1+, and 2+ were categorized as the low expression group. Regarding *KRAS* mutational status, mutated *KRAS* and wild-type *KRAS* were found in 39 and 54 patients, respectively. ASCT2 expression was high in 43.6% (17 of 39) of CRC patients with mutated *KRAS*, whereas in 24.1% (13 of 54) of CRC patients with wild-type *KRAS*, which indicated that there was a significant correlation between high ASCT2 expression and *KRAS* mutation (risk ratio: 1.62, 95%; confidence interval (CI): 1.02–2.57, $p = 0.047$, Figure 2b).

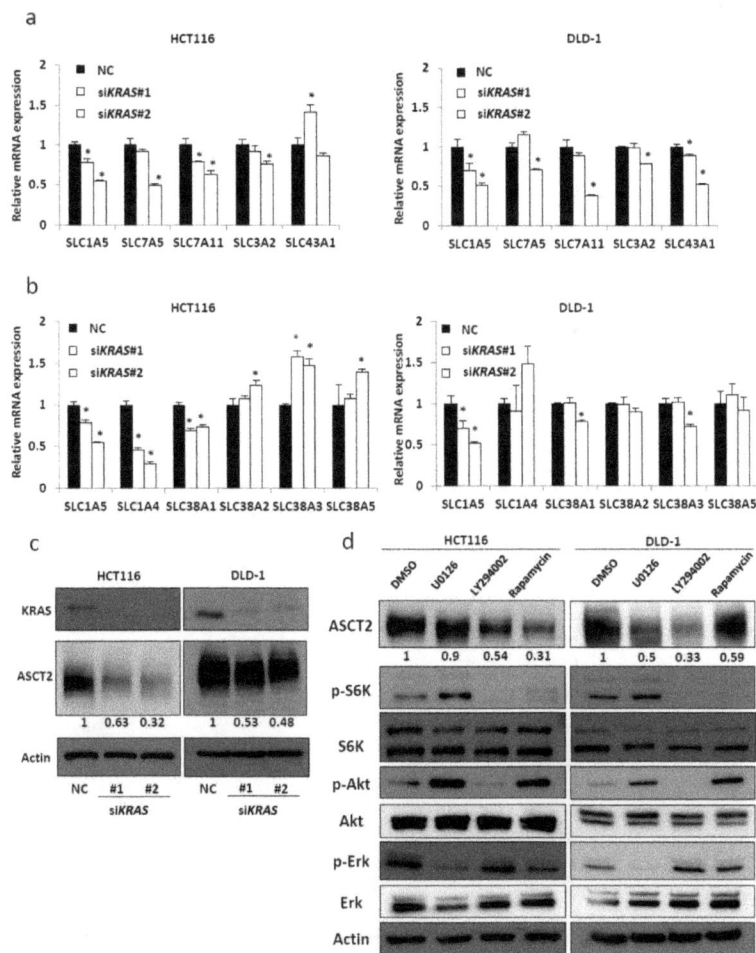

Figure 1. Identification of the amino acid transporter regulated by mutated *KRAS*. (**a**) Relative mRNA levels of amino acid transporters that are reported to be associated with cancer; (**b**) relative mRNA levels of amino acid transporters that are involved in glutamine transport. HCT116 cells (left) and DLD-1 cells (right) were treated separately with two independent siRNA constructs (#1 and #2) targeting *KRAS* and negative control (NC) siRNA. Mean; bars, ± SD, $n = 3$ (Student's t-test; * $p < 0.05$); (**c**) Western blotting for KRAS, ASCT2, and β-actin (Actin). The relative ASCT2 expression levels for three independent experiments are shown by quantitative analysis normalized to β-actin (Actin); (**d**) CRC cells (HCT116 and DLD-1) were treated with 0.1% dimethyl sulfoxide (DMSO), 20 μM U0126 (MEK inhibitor), and 50 μM LY294002 (PI3K inhibitor) or 20 nM rapamycin (mTOR inhibitor) for 48 h. Protein levels of ASCT2 were normalized to β-actin (Actin). Densitometry values were expressed as fold change compared with DMSO-treated cells.

a

b

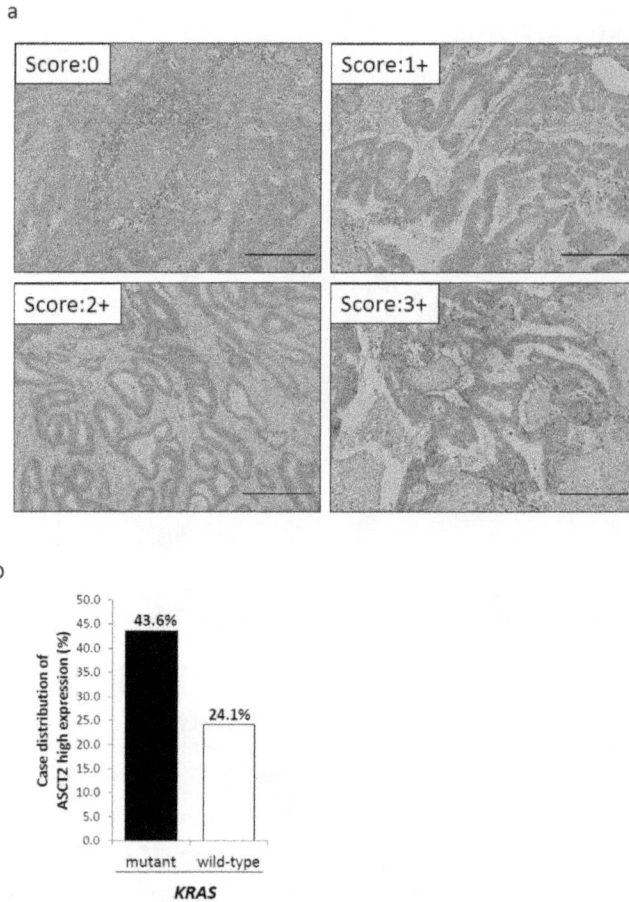

Figure 2. Immunohistochemical staining for ASCT2 of primary colorectal cancer (CRC) specimens. (a) Representative picture. Scale bar, 200 μm (200× magnification); (b) Relationship between *KRAS* mutational status and ASCT2 expression.

2.3. Knockdown of SLC1A5 (ASCT2) Results in Suppression of Cell Growth

To investigate the role of *SLC1A5* (ASCT2) in CRC cell lines with mutated *KRAS*, we introduced non-silencing siRNA and two different siRNAs targeting *SLC1A5* (referred as si*SLC1A5*#1 and si*SLC1A5*#2) into CRC cell lines (Figure S2). Knockdown of *SLC1A5* (ASCT2) significantly suppressed the cell growth in all the 3 cell lines with mutated *KRAS* (HCT116, DLD-1, and SW480), whereas in 1 out of 3 cell lines with wild-type *KRAS* (RKO) (Figure 3a). Furthermore, we investigated the knockdown effect of *SLC1A5* on cell apoptosis. Knockdown of *SLC1A5* induced a significant increase in caspase 3/7 activities in all the 3 cell lines with mutated *KRAS* (HCT116, DLD-1, and SW480), whereas in 2 out of 3 cell lines with wild-type *KRAS* (HT29 and RKO) (Figure 3b). Oncogenic *PIK3CA* mutations were reported to reprogram glutamine metabolism in CRC [35]. *PIK3CA* mutations are observed in HCT116 (a H1047R mutation), DLD-1 (E545K; D549N mutations), HT29 (a P449T mutation), WiDR (a P449T mutation), and RKO (a H1047R mutation), whereas the *PIK3CA* status is wild-type in SW480. The *PIK3CA* status might be related to the differences in the knockdown effect of *SLC1A5* between cell lines.

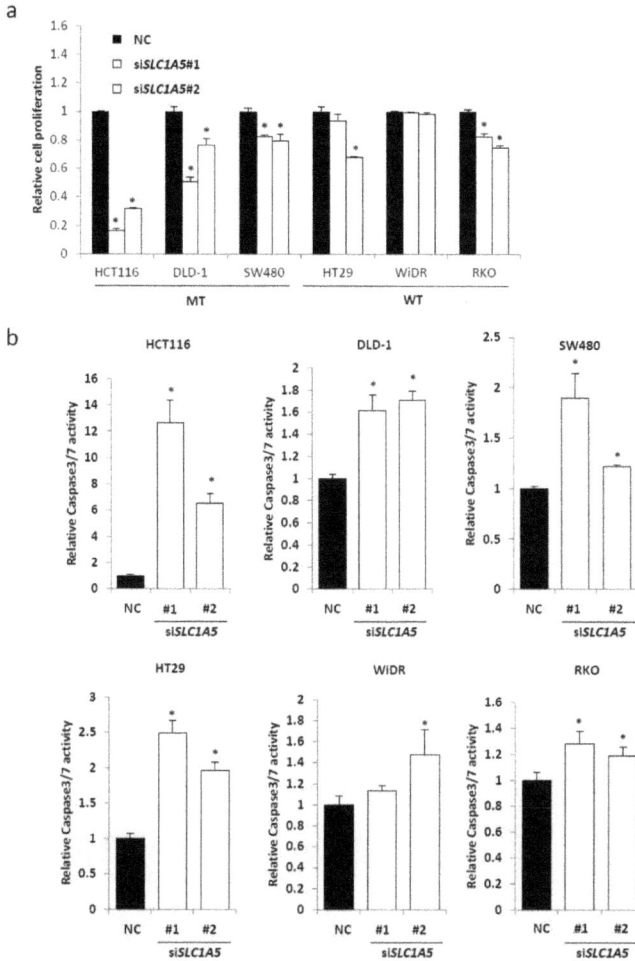

Figure 3. *SLC1A5* knockdown inhibits cell proliferation and induces cell apoptosis of CRC cells. (**a**) Cell proliferation measured by CCK-8 assay. CRC cells were transfected with negative control (NC) or two independent si*SLC1A5* and cultured for 72 h. Viability in each si*SLC1A5* was normalized to that in NC. Student's *t*-test; * $p < 0.05$; (**b**) caspase 3/7 activities measured by Caspase-Glo assay. CRC cells transfected with negative control (NC) or two independent si*SLC1A5* were cultured for 72 h. Caspase 3/7 activity was normalized to the cell viability measured by CCK-8 assay under the same density and conditions. Mean; bars, ± SD, $n = 3$ (Student's *t*-test; * $p < 0.05$).

2.4. Role of SLC1A5 (ASCT2) in KRAS-Mutant CRC Cells

SLC1A5 (ASCT2) is generally regarded as a glutamine transporter. In a *KRAS*-mutant CRC cell line (HCT116), glutamine depletion resulted in decreased cell proliferation and enhanced caspase 3/7 activities. Importantly, even in the presence of glutamine, si*SLC1A5* dramatically suppressed cell proliferation and up-regulated caspase 3/7 activities (Figure 4a,b), which indicated that the effect of *SLC1A5*-knockdown was more prominent on cell growth and apoptosis than glutamine depletion. To further investigate the functional role of *SLC1A5*, we established stable HCT116 transfectant cell lines in which *SLC1A5* was knocked down by shRNA constructs targeting *SLC1A5* (referred as sh*SLC1A5*#1 and sh*SLC1A5*#2) (Figure S3). In the clonogenic assay, *SLC1A5*-knockdown significantly suppressed colony number as compared to the control (Figure 4c). Moreover, in the wound healing assay, *SLC1A5*-knockdown significantly inhibited wound closure as compared to the control (Figure 4d). Taken together, these results indicate that the inhibition of *SLC1A5* (ASCT2) could be a therapeutic target in *KRAS*-mutant CRC.

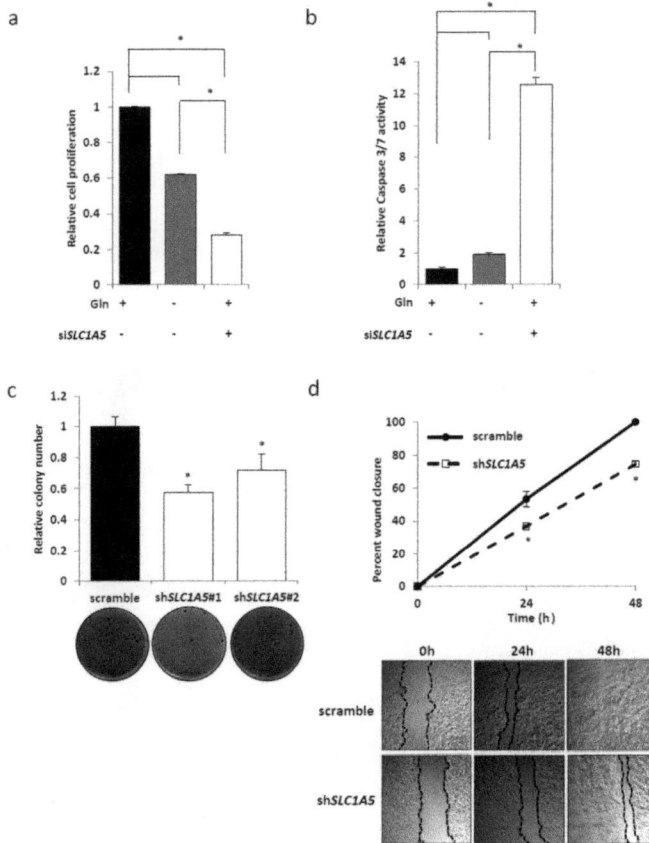

Figure 4. The role of *SLC1A5* (ASCT2) in *KRAS*-mutant CRC cells. *SLC1A5* knockdown exhibited more effective on suppressing cell growth (**a**) and inducing apoptosis (**b**) than under glutamine deprivation. Mean; bars, ± SD, $n = 3$ (Student's *t*-test; * $p < 0.05$); (**c**) clonogenic assay with HCT116 transfected with control or two independent sh*SLC1A5* vectors. Cells were maintained under 4 mM glutamine condition containing 10% fetal bovine serum (FBS) for 10 days. Mean; bars, ± SD, $n = 3$ (Student's *t*-test; * $p < 0.05$); (**d**) wound healing assay with HCT116 transfected with control or sh*SLC1A5* vector. Cells were photographed at 50× magnification at 0, 24, and 48 h. Wound closure (%) was evaluated. Mean; bars, ± SD, $n = 3$ (Student's *t*-test; * $p < 0.05$).

2.5. Tumor Characteristics and ASCT2 Expression in CRC Clinical Samples

Table 1 shows the relationship between ASCT2 expression and clinicopathologic variables. ASCT2 expression was significantly correlated with tumor location, but not with age, sex, tumor size, stage, T-/N-/M-category, lymphatic invasion, or vascular invasion. We further investigated the clinical significance of ASCT2, based on the *KRAS* mutational status. Interestingly, we found that high ASCT2 expression was significantly associated with tumor depth and vascular invasion in *KRAS*-mutant CRC, which was not observed in wild-type *KRAS* CRC.

Table 1. Correlation between ASCT2 expression and clinicopathological variables (* p < 0.05).

Variables	Total			KRAS Wild-Type			KRAS Mutant		
	ASCT2			ASCT2			ASCT2		
	High (n = 30)	Low (n = 63)	p-value	High (n = 13)	Low (n = 41)	p-value	High (n = 17)	Low (n = 22)	p-value
Age, mean ± SD (y)	71.2 ± 9.4	68.0 ± 10.7	0.16	69.8 ± 10.5	67.2 ± 10.6	0.42	72.2 ± 9.8	69.4 ± 11.1	0.41
Sex									
Male	16	39	0.43	8	28	0.65	8	11	0.86
Female	14	24		5	13		9	11	
Location									
Left	18	50	0.049 *	9	33	0.45	9	17	0.11
Right	12	13		4	8		8	5	
Tumor size (mm)									
≥50	12	25	0.98	5	15	0.9	12	25	0.98
<50	18	38		8	26		18	38	
UICC-TMN stage									
I/II	14	33	0.61	7	23	0.89	7	10	0.79
III/IV	16	30		6	18		10	12	
T-category									
1/2	5	25	0.16	4	10	0.72	1	9	0.024 *
3/4	25	44		9	31		16	13	
M-category									
Negative	25	53	0.92	10	35	0.67	15	18	0.75
Positive	5	10		3	6		2	4	
N-category									
Negative	16	35	0.84	8	23	0.73	8	12	0.64
Positive	14	28		5	18		9	10	
Lymphatic invasion									
Negative	18	39	0.86	6	25	0.35	12	14	0.65
Positive	12	24		7	16		5	8	
Vascular invasion									
Negative	6	19	0.3	3	8	1	3	11	0.049 *
Positive	24	44		10	33		14	11	

2.6. Patients' Prognosis

To evaluate the relationship between ASCT2 expression and patients' prognosis, we performed the log-rank test analysis with CRC patients who underwent curative resection of primary CRC ($n = 90$). Kaplan–Meier survival curves indicated that ASCT2 expression was not significantly correlated with recurrence-free survival (RFS) in all cases (Figure 5a). However, in *KRAS*-mutant CRC cases ($n = 38$), the estimated RFS rate at 5-year tended to be lower in the high ASCT2 group than in the low ASCT2 group (52.9% vs. 70.2%; $p = 0.251$) (Figure 5b, right). On the other hand, in wild-type *KRAS* CRC cases ($n = 52$), the estimated RFS rate at 5-year was almost similar between the high and low ASCT2 groups (84.6% vs. 75.8%; $p = 0.513$) (Figure 5b, left). Taken together, high ASCT2 expression can be one of the crucial prognostic factors in *KRAS*-mutant CRC.

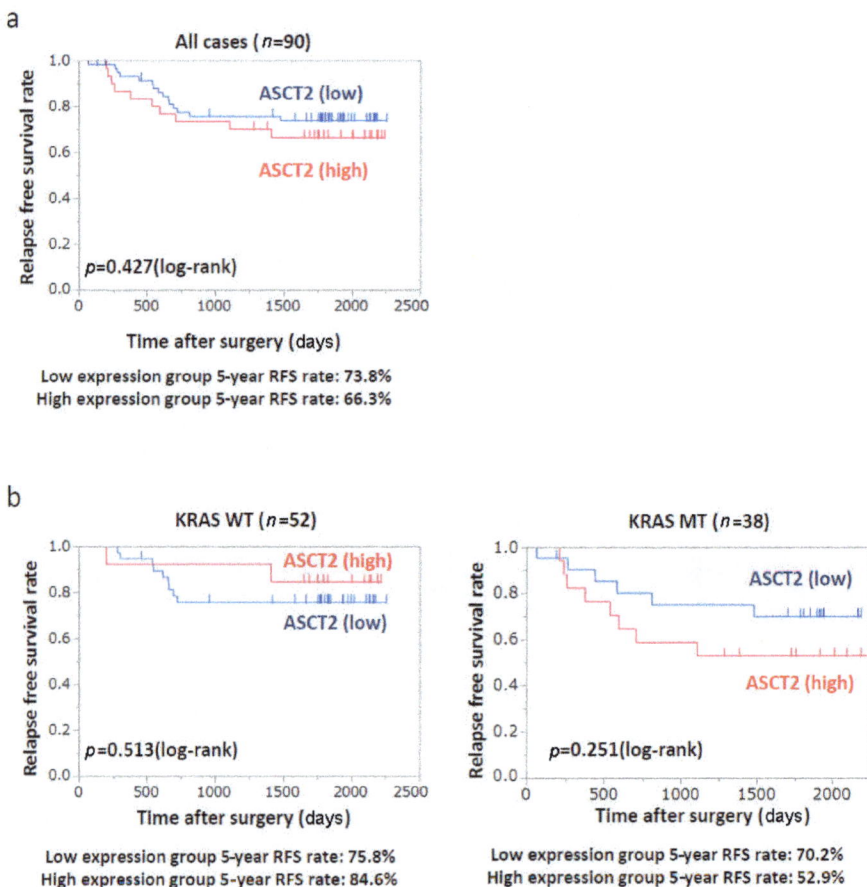

Figure 5. Kaplan–Meier analysis of relapse-free survival (RFS) according to ASCT2 expression and *KRAS* status. (**a**) RFS according to ASCT2 expression in total patients; (**b**) RFS according to ASCT2 expression in *KRAS*-mutant cases (right) and wild-type *KRAS* cases (left).

3. Discussion

KRAS mutations are found in a variety of human cancers, including pancreatic cancer, non-small cell lung cancer, and CRC. Recent studies have shown that mutated *KRAS* promotes metabolic reprogramming through nutrients uptake, glycolysis, glutaminolysis, and synthesis of nucleotides and fatty acids. The mechanism by which mutated *KRAS* coordinates the metabolic reprogramming to promote tumor growth remains to be investigated. The International CRC Subtyping Consortium has suggested that CRC can be divided into four subtypes with distinguished features: CMS1, CMS2, CMS3, and CMS4 [15]. Notably, CMS3 is characterized by metabolic dysregulation and is strongly associated with *KRAS* mutations. Using a comprehensive metabolomics analysis with isogenic CRC cell lines harboring mutated or wild-type *KRAS*, we have recently reported that mutated *KRAS* induces some metabolic alterations in glycolysis, the pentose phosphate pathway (PPP), the tricarboxylic acid (TCA) cycle, and most significantly in the amino acid pathway [12]. We identified that mutated *KRAS* regulated asparagine synthetase (ASNS), an enzyme that is involved in de novo synthesis of asparagine from aspartate, and that *KRAS*-mutant CRC cells could become adaptive to glutamine depletion through ASNS-dependent asparagine biosynthesis. There is also some evidence from other groups that *KRAS* mutations in CRC are associated with glutamine metabolism. Wong et al. reported that *SLC25A22* (a mitochondrial glutamine transporter) was a synthetic lethal metabolic gene in *KRAS*-mutant CRC cells and that expression of *SLC25A22* was correlated with poor prognosis in patients harboring *KRAS* mutations [11]. Miyo et al. reported that glutamine dehydrogenase 1 (GLUD1) and *SLC25A13* (a mitochondrial aspartate-glutamate carrier) played an essential role in cell survival of CRC cells under glucose-deprived conditions, and that combined expression of GLUD1 and *SLC25A13* was significantly associated with tumor aggressiveness and poorer prognosis in CRC patients [13]. These results indicate that the amino acid metabolism including glutaminolysis is more essential for cell survival in *KRAS*-mutant CRC than in wild-type *KRAS* CRC.

In this study, we focused on the amino acid transporter which was exclusively regulated by mutated *KRAS*, although several amino acid transporters have been reported to be up-regulated in cancer [32]. Herein, we identified *SLC1A5* as a novel target gene regulated by mutated *KRAS* in CRC. Expressions of *SLC25A22* and *SLC25A13* were not affected by *KRAS*-knockdown in our experiments (Figure S1b). Up-regulation of *SLC1A5* (ASCT2) and its clinical significance has been reported in a variety of human cancers [19–31]. In the present study, we demonstrated that *SLC1A5* (ASCT2) expression was regulated through KRAS signaling, and that *SLC1A5*-knockdown resulted in reduced cell growth and increased cell apoptosis in *KRAS*-mutant CRC cells (Figures 1 and 3). Importantly, the effect of *SLC1A5*-knockdown was more prominent on cell growth and apoptosis than that of glutamine depletion (Figure 4a,b), which indicates that *SLC1A5* (ASCT2) plays a critical role in the malignant progression of *KRAS*-mutant CRC. Furthermore, *SLC1A5*-knockdown resulted in the suppression of cell migration (Figure 4d). In primary CRC clinical specimens, we found that ASCT2 expression was significantly associated with tumor depth and vascular invasion in *KRAS*-mutant CRC, but not in wild-type *KRAS* CRC (Table 1). In conclusion, our data indicates that *SLC1A5* (ASCT2) could be a novel biomarker as well as a potential therapeutic target in *KRAS*-mutant CRC.

4. Materials and Methods

4.1. Cell Lines and Reagents

HCT116, DLD-1, SW480, SW620, HT29, RKO, and WiDR cells were obtained from American Type Culture Collection. All cell lines were cultured in Dulbecco's Modified Eagle Medium (DMEM) (glucose 25 mM, glutamine 4 mM) (043-30085, Wako, Tokyo, Japan) supplemented with 10% FBS and penicillin–streptomycin. Media without glutamine were prepared by using glutamine-free DMEM (glucose 25 mM, glutamine 0 mM) (045-32245, Wako) supplemented with 10% FBS. The identity of each cell line was confirmed by STR analysis (Takara Bio, Shiga, Japan). U0126 was purchased from Calbiochem, LY294002 and rapamycin were from Wako.

4.2. Quantitative Reverse Transcription Polymerase Chain Reaction (RT-PCR) Analysis

Total RNAs were extracted from cells with High Pure RNA Isolation Kit (Roche, Mannheim, Germany) according to the manufacturer's instructions. RNA was reverse transcribed to cDNA with

Transcriptor First Strand cDNA Synthesis Kit (Roche) according to the manufacturer's instructions. The relative levels of respective genes were quantified using StepOnePlusTM Real-Time PCR System (Applied Biosystems, Foster City, CA, USA). The respective mRNA levels were normalized to that for ACTB. Primer sequences were found in Table S1.

4.3. Western Blot Analysis

Cells were washed with ice-cold phosphate-buffered saline and lysed in sodium dodecyl sulfate lysis buffer supplemented with inhibitor cocktails of protease and phosphatase. Primary antibodies can be found in Table S2.

4.4. Small Interfering RNA and Short Hairpin RNA

FlexiTube GeneSolutions for si*SLC1A5* (#1: SI05141017, #2: SI00079730) and non-silencing control siRNA (AllStars negative control siRNA, SI03650318) were purchased from Qiagen (Hilden, Germany). The siRNA (10 nM) was transfected with Lipofectamine RNAiMAX (Invitrogen, Carlsbad, CA, USA) according to the manufacturer's reverse-transfection protocol. *SLC1A5* shRNA vectors were made from the same sequence of si*SLC1A5* (#1, #2), and cloned into pLKO.1 vectors. pLKO.1-scramble vector (Addgene) was used as control.

4.5. Cell Proliferation Assay

A cell proliferation assay was measured by Cell Counting Kit-8 (Dojindo, Kumamoto, Japan) according to the manufacturer's instruction. Cells transfected with siRNA were cultured in 96-well plates at a density of 5000 cells/well for 72 h.

4.6. Clonogenic Assay

Cells were seeded in 6-well plates at a density of 100 cells per well in complete media. At the end point, colonies were fixed in 1% glutaraldehyde and stained with 0.2% crystal violet for 30 min, and number of colonies was counted. A colony was defined as a cluster of at least 50 cells.

4.7. Apoptosis Assay

The activity of Caspase-3 and -7 was measured by using Caspase-Glo 3/7 assay (Promega, Madison, WI, USA) according to the manufacturer's protocol. Caspase activity was normalized to the cell number counted by CCK-8 cell proliferation assay under the same density and conditions.

4.8. Wound Healing Assay

Cell lines were seeded into 12-well plates and grew until 80–90% confluence. Confluent cultures were scratched with sterile tips, washed with PBS, and cultured in DMEM containing 5% FBS. Cells were photographed by a 50× magnification at 0, 24, and 48 h. Wound closure (%) was evaluated using the ImageJ software.

4.9. Immunohistochemistry

Formalin-fixed, paraffin-embedded sections were stained with anti-rabbit ASCT2 (Sigma-Aldrich, St. Louis, MO, USA) antibody. Antigen retrieval was achieved with microwave in citrate buffer (pH: 6.0). For primary CRC tissue, ASCT2 immunoreactivity score was determined by the proportion, as previously described [30]. The proportion was scored based on the positively rate as "0" (0–10%), "1" (10–40%), "2" (40–70%), "3" (>70%). Scores of 0, 1, and 2 were defined as low expression, whereas 3 was high expression.

Two researchers (Kosuke Toda and Gen Nishikawa) independently evaluated all immunohistochemistry samples without prior knowledge of other data. The slides with different evaluations among them were reinterpreted at a conference to reach the consensus.

Int. J. Mol. Sci. **2017**, *18*, 1632

4.10. Patients, Clinicopathological Data

93 patients were collected from patients who underwent primary colorectal cancer resection at Kyoto University Hospital between April 2009 and September 2013.

No patients received chemotherapy and/or radiation therapy. *KRAS* mutational status in all patients was analyzed by using an ABI 3130 Genetic Analyzer (Applied Biosystems, foster City, CA, USA), as described previously. Pathologic staging was categorized in accordance with the 7th edition of Union for International Cancer Control (UICC) classification of malignant tumors.

4.11. Statistical Analysis

All values were expressed as mean ± standard deviation (SD). Statistical analyses were conducted with the JMP Pro 12 (SAS Institute, Inc., Cary, NC, USA). Student's *t*-test was used for comparing means between two groups. In clinical data, the statistical significance of differences between variables of two groups was determined by student's *t*-test, chi-squared test, or Fisher's exact test. Relapse-free survival (RFS) rates were evaluated by the Kaplan–Meier survival curve and log-rank test. All analyses were two-sided, and differences with a p value of less than 0.05 were considered statistically significant in all analyses.

Supplementary Materials: Supplementary materials can be found at www.mdpi.com/1422-0067/18/8/1632/s1.

Acknowledgments: This work was supported by grants from the Ministry of Education, Culture, Sports, Science and Technology of Japan, and from KOTOSUGI CO. Ltd.

Author Contributions: Kenji Kawada and Kosuke Toda contributed to the planning of study design and interpretation of the data; Kosuke Toda and Gen Nishikawa performed the experiments; Kenji Kawada, Kosuke Toda and Gen Nishikawa performed the data analysis; Kenji Kawada, Kosuke Toda, and Gen Nishikawa wrote the manuscript; Masayoshi Iwamoto, Yoshiro Itatani, Ryo Takahashi and Yoshiharu Sakai reviewed the manuscript for important intellectual content.

Conflicts of Interest: The authors declare no conflict of interest.

Abbreviations

ASCT2	Alanine-serine-cysteine amino acid transporter
ASNS	Asparagine synthetase
CRC	Colorectal cancer
EGFR	Epidermal growth factor receptor
GLUD1	Glutamine dehydrogenase 1
GLUT1	Glucose transporter 1
PPP	Pentose phosphate pathway
RFS	Recurrence-free survival (RFS)
RT-PCR	Reverse-transcription polymerase chain reaction
siRNA	Small interfering RNA
TCA cycle	Tricarboxylic acid cycle

References

1. Siegel, R.L.; Miller, K.D.; Jemal, A. Cancer statistics, 2017. *CA Cancer J. Clin.* **2017**, *67*, 7–30. [CrossRef] [PubMed]
2. Misale, S.; Yaeger, R.; Hobor, S.; Scala, E.; Janakiraman, M.; Liska, D.; Valtorta, E.; Schiavo, R.; Buscarino, M.; Siravegna, G.; et al. Emergence of KRAS mutations and acquired resistance to anti-EGFR therapy in colorectal cancer. *Nature* **2012**, *486*, 532–536. [CrossRef] [PubMed]
3. Bokemeyer, C.; Bondarenko, I.; Makhson, A.; Hartmann, J.T.; Aparicio, J.; de Braud, F.; Donea, S.; Ludwig, H.; Schuch, G.; Stroh, C.; et al. Fluorouracil, leucovorin, and oxaliplatin with and without cetuximab in the first-line treatment of metastatic colorectal cancer. *J. Clin. Oncol.* **2009**, *27*, 663–671. [CrossRef] [PubMed]

4. Karapetis, C.S.; Khambata-Ford, S.; Jonker, D.J.; O'Callaghan, C.J.; Tu, D.; Tebbutt, N.C.; Simes, R.J.; Chalchal, H.; Shapiro, J.D.; Robitaille, S.; et al. K-Ras mutations and benefit from cetuximab in advanced colorectal cancer. *N. Engl. J. Med.* **2008**, *359*, 1757–1765. [CrossRef] [PubMed]

5. Bryant, K.L.; Mancias, J.D.; Kimmelman, A.C.; Der, C.J. KRAS: Feeding pancreatic cancer proliferation. *Trends Biochem. Sci.* **2014**, *39*, 91–100. [CrossRef] [PubMed]

6. Son, J.; Lyssiotis, C.A.; Ying, H.; Wang, X.; Hua, S.; Ligorio, M.; Perera, R.M.; Ferrone, C.R.; Mullarky, E.; Shyh-Chang, N.; et al. Glutamine supports pancreatic cancer growth through a KRAS-regulated metabolic pathway. *Nature* **2013**, *496*, 101–105. [CrossRef] [PubMed]

7. Ying, H.; Kimmelman, A.C.; Lyssiotis, C.A.; Hua, S.; Chu, G.C.; Fletcher-Sananikone, E.; Locasale, J.W.; Son, J.; Zhang, H.; Coloff, J.L.; et al. Oncogenic Kras maintains pancreatic tumors through regulation of anabolic glucose metabolism. *Cell* **2012**, *149*, 656–670. [CrossRef] [PubMed]

8. Davidson, S.M.; Papagiannakopoulos, T.; Olenchock, B.A.; Heyman, J.E.; Keibler, M.A.; Luengo, A.; Bauer, M.R.; Jha, A.K.; O'Brien, J.P.; Pierce, K.A.; et al. Environment impacts the metabolic dependencies of Ras-driven non-small cell lung cancer. *Cell Metab.* **2016**, *23*, 517–528. [CrossRef] [PubMed]

9. Kimmelman, A.C. Metabolic dependencies in RAS-driven cancers. *Clin. Cancer Res.* **2015**, *21*, 1828–1834. [CrossRef] [PubMed]

10. Yun, J.; Rago, C.; Cheong, I.; Pagliarini, R.; Angenendt, P.; Rajagopalan, H.; Schmidt, K.; Willson, J.K.; Markowitz, S.; Zhou, S.; et al. Glucose deprivation contributes to the development of KRAS pathway mutations in tumor cells. *Science* **2009**, *325*, 1555–1559. [CrossRef] [PubMed]

11. Wong, C.C.; Qian, Y.; Li, X.; Xu, J.; Kang, W.; Tong, J.H.; To, K.F.; Jin, Y.; Li, W.; Chen, H.; et al. SLC25A22 Promotes proliferation and survival of colorectal cancer cells with KRAS mutations and xenograft tumor progression in mice via intracellular synthesis of aspartate. *Gastroenterology* **2016**, *151*, 945–960. [CrossRef] [PubMed]

12. Toda, K.; Kawada, K.; Iwamoto, M.; Inamoto, S.; Sasazuki, T.; Shirasawa, S.; Hasegawa, S.; Sakai, Y. Metabolic alterations caused by KRAS mutations in colorectal cancer contribute to cell adaptation to glutamine depletion by upregulation of asparagine synthetase. *Neoplasia* **2016**, *18*, 654–665. [CrossRef] [PubMed]

13. Miyo, M.; Konno, M.; Nishida, N.; Sueda, T.; Noguchi, K.; Matsui, H.; Colvin, H.; Kawamoto, K.; Koseki, J.; Haraguchi, N.; et al. Metabolic adaptation to nutritional stress in human colorectal cancer. *Sci. Rep.* **2016**, *6*, 38415. [CrossRef] [PubMed]

14. Yun, J.; Mullarky, E.; Lu, C.; Bosch, K.N.; Kavalier, A.; Rivera, K.; Roper, J.; Chio, I.I.; Giannopoulou, E.G.; Rago, C.; et al. Vitamin C selectively kills KRAS and BRAF mutant colorectal cancer cells by targeting GAPDH. *Science* **2015**, *350*, 1391–1396. [CrossRef] [PubMed]

15. Guinney, J.; Dienstmann, R.; Wang, X.; de Reynies, A.; Schlicker, A.; Soneson, C.; Marisa, L.; Roepman, P.; Nyamundanda, G.; Angelino, P.; et al. The consensus molecular subtypes of colorectal cancer. *Nat. Med.* **2015**, *21*, 1350–1356. [CrossRef] [PubMed]

16. Kawada, K.; Toda, K.; Nakamoto, Y.; Iwamoto, M.; Hatano, E.; Chen, F.; Hasegawa, S.; Togashi, K.; Date, H.; Uemoto, S.; et al. Relationship between 18F-FDG PET/CT scans and KRAS mutations in metastatic colorectal cancer. *J. Nucl. Med.* **2015**, *56*, 1322–1327. [CrossRef] [PubMed]

17. Iwamoto, M.; Kawada, K.; Nakamoto, Y.; Itatani, Y.; Inamoto, S.; Toda, K.; Kimura, H.; Sasazuki, T.; Shirasawa, S.; Okuyama, H.; et al. Regulation of 18F-FDG accumulation in colorectal cancer cells with mutated KRAS. *J. Nucl. Med.* **2014**, *55*, 2038–2044. [CrossRef] [PubMed]

18. Kawada, K.; Nakamoto, Y.; Kawada, M.; Hida, K.; Matsumoto, T.; Murakami, T.; Hasegawa, S.; Togashi, K.; Sakai, Y. Relationship between 18F-fluorodeoxyglucose accumulation and KRAS/BRAF mutations in colorectal cancer. *Clin. Cancer Res.* **2012**, *18*, 1696–1703. [CrossRef] [PubMed]

19. Van Geldermalsen, M.; Wang, Q.; Nagarajah, R.; Marshall, A.D.; Thoeng, A.; Gao, D.; Ritchie, W.; Feng, Y.; Bailey, C.G.; Deng, N.; et al. ASCT2/SLC1A5 controls glutamine uptake and tumour growth in triple-negative basal-like breast cancer. *Oncogene* **2016**, *35*, 3201–3208. [CrossRef] [PubMed]

20. Sun, H.W.; Yu, X.J.; Wu, W.C.; Chen, J.; Shi, M.; Zheng, L.; Xu, J. GLUT1 and ASCT2 as predictors for prognosis of hepatocellular carcinoma. *PLoS ONE* **2016**, *11*, e0168907. [CrossRef] [PubMed]

21. Honjo, H.; Kaira, K.; Miyazaki, T.; Yokobori, T.; Kanai, Y.; Nagamori, S.; Oyama, T.; Asao, T.; Kuwano, H. Clinicopathological significance of LAT1 and ASCT2 in patients with surgically resected esophageal squamous cell carcinoma. *J. Surg. Oncol.* **2016**, *113*, 381–389. [CrossRef] [PubMed]

22. Yazawa, T.; Shimizu, K.; Kaira, K.; Nagashima, T.; Ohtaki, Y.; Atsumi, J.; Obayashi, K.; Nagamori, S.; Kanai, Y.; Oyama, T.; et al. Clinical significance of coexpression of L-type amino acid transporter 1 (LAT1) and ASC amino acid transporter 2 (ASCT2) in lung adenocarcinoma. *Am. J. Transl. Res.* **2015**, *7*, 1126–1139. [PubMed]

23. Ren, P.; Yue, M.; Xiao, D.; Xiu, R.; Gan, L.; Liu, H.; Qing, G. ATF4 and *N*-Myc coordinate glutamine metabolism in MYCN-amplified neuroblastoma cells through ASCT2 activation. *J. Pathol.* **2015**, *235*, 90–100. [CrossRef] [PubMed]

24. Nikkuni, O.; Kaira, K.; Toyoda, M.; Shino, M.; Sakakura, K.; Takahashi, K.; Tominaga, H.; Oriuchi, N.; Suzuki, M.; Iijima, M.; et al. Expression of amino acid transporters (LAT1 and ASCT2) in patients with stage III/IV laryngeal squamous cell carcinoma. *Pathol. Oncol. Res.* **2015**, *21*, 1175–1181. [CrossRef] [PubMed]

25. Liu, Y.; Yang, L.; An, H.; Chang, Y.; Zhang, W.; Zhu, Y.; Xu, L.; Xu, J. High expression of solute carrier family 1, member 5 (SLC1A5) is associated with poor prognosis in clear-cell renal cell carcinoma. *Sci. Rep.* **2015**, *5*, 16954. [CrossRef] [PubMed]

26. Hassanein, M.; Qian, J.; Hoeksema, M.D.; Wang, J.; Jacobovitz, M.; Ji, X.; Harris, F.T.; Harris, B.K.; Boyd, K.L.; Chen, H.; Clark, J.E.; et al. Targeting SLC1a5-mediated glutamine dependence in non-small cell lung cancer. *Int. J. Cancer* **2015**, *137*, 1587–1597. [CrossRef] [PubMed]

27. Toyoda, M.; Kaira, K.; Ohshima, Y.; Ishioka, N.S.; Shino, M.; Sakakura, K.; Takayasu, Y.; Takahashi, K.; Tominaga, H.; Oriuchi, N.; et al. Prognostic significance of amino-acid transporter expression (LAT1, ASCT2, and xCT) in surgically resected tongue cancer. *Br. J. Cancer* **2014**, *110*, 2506–2513. [CrossRef] [PubMed]

28. Shimizu, K.; Kaira, K.; Tomizawa, Y.; Sunaga, N.; Kawashima, O.; Oriuchi, N.; Tominaga, H.; Nagamori, S.; Kanai, Y.; Yamada, M.; et al. ASC amino-acid transporter 2 (ASCT2) as a novel prognostic marker in non-small cell lung cancer. *Br. J. Cancer* **2014**, *110*, 2030–2039. [CrossRef] [PubMed]

29. Scalise, M.; Pochini, L.; Panni, S.; Pingitore, P.; Hedfalk, K.; Indiveri, C. Transport mechanism and regulatory properties of the human amino acid transporter ASCT2 (SLC1A5). *Amino Acids* **2014**, *46*, 2463–2475. [CrossRef] [PubMed]

30. Huang, F.; Zhao, Y.; Zhao, J.; Wu, S.; Jiang, Y.; Ma, H.; Zhang, T. Upregulated SLC1A5 promotes cell growth and survival in colorectal cancer. *Int. J. Clin. Exp. Pathol.* **2014**, *7*, 6006–6014. [PubMed]

31. Wang, Q.; Hardie, R.A.; Hoy, A.J.; van Geldermalsen, M.; Gao, D.; Fazli, L.; Sadowski, M.C.; Balaban, S.; Schreuder, M.; Nagarajah, R.; et al. Targeting ASCT2-mediated glutamine uptake blocks prostate cancer growth and tumour development. *J. Pathol.* **2015**, *236*, 278–289. [CrossRef] [PubMed]

32. Bhutia, Y.D.; Babu, E.; Ramachandran, S.; Ganapathy, V. Amino acid transporters in cancer and their relevance to "glutamine addiction": Novel targets for the design of a new class of anticancer drugs. *Cancer Res.* **2015**, *75*, 1782–1788. [CrossRef] [PubMed]

33. Wise, D.R.; Thompson, C.B. Glutamine addiction: A new therapeutic target in cancer. *Trends Biochem. Sci.* **2010**, *35*, 427–433. [CrossRef] [PubMed]

34. DeBerardinis, R.J.; Cheng, T. Q's next: The diverse functions of glutamine in metabolism, cell biology and cancer. *Oncogene* **2010**, *29*, 313–324. [CrossRef] [PubMed]

35. Hao, Y.; Samuels, Y.; Li, Q.; Krokowski, D.; Guan, B.J.; Wang, C.; Jin, Z.; Dong, B.; Cao, B.; Feng, X.; et al. Oncogenic PIK3CA mutations reprogram glutamine metabolism in colorectal cancer. *Nat. Commun.* **2016**, *7*, 11971. [CrossRef] [PubMed]

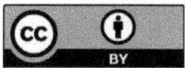

International Journal of
Molecular Sciences

MDPI

Article

Differential Functional Roles of ALDH1A1 and ALDH1A3 in Mediating Metastatic Behavior and Therapy Resistance of Human Breast Cancer Cells

Alysha K. Croker [1,2], Mauricio Rodriguez-Torres [1,2], Ying Xia [1], Siddika Pardhan [3], Hon Sing Leong [3], John D. Lewis [4] and Alison L. Allan [1,5,6,*]

[1]   London Regional Cancer Program, London Health Sciences Centre, 790 Commissioners Road East,
      London, ON N6A 4L6, Canada; alysha.croker@gmail.com (A.K.C.); rodrimauricio@gmail.com (M.R.-T.);
      ying.xia@lhsc.on.ca (Y.X.)
[2]   Department of Anatomy & Cell Biology, Schulich School of Medicine & Dentistry, Western University,
      London, ON N6A 5C1, Canada
[3]   Department of Surgery, Schulich School of Medicine & Dentistry, Western University,
      London, ON N6A 5C1, Canada; siddika15@gmail.com (S.P.); honsing.leong@gmail.com (H.S.L.)
[4]   Department of Oncology, University of Alberta, 5-142C Katz Group Building, 114th St. and 87th Ave. S.,
      Edmonton, AB T6G 2E1, Canada; jdlewis@ualberta.ca
[5]   Department of Oncology and Anatomy & Cell Biology, Schulich School of Medicine & Dentistry,
      Western University, London, ON N6A 5C1, Canada
[6]   Cancer Research Laboratory Program, Lawson Health Research Institute, 750 Base Line Road, Suite 300,
      London, ON N6C 2R5, Canada
*   Correspondence: alison.allan@lhsc.on.ca; Tel.: +1-519-685-8600 (ext. x55134)

Received: 5 September 2017; Accepted: 18 September 2017; Published: 22 September 2017

Abstract: Previous studies indicate that breast cancer cells with high aldehyde dehydrogenase (ALDH) activity and CD44 expression (ALDH^{hi}CD44$^+$) contribute to metastasis and therapy resistance, and that ALDH1 correlates with poor outcome in breast cancer patients. The current study hypothesized that ALDH1 functionally contributes to breast cancer metastatic behavior and therapy resistance. Expression of ALDH1A1 or ALDH1A3 was knocked down in MDA-MB-468 and SUM159 human breast cancer cells using siRNA. Resulting impacts on ALDH activity (Aldefluor® assay); metastatic behavior and therapy response in vitro (proliferation/adhesion/migration/colony formation/chemotherapy and radiation) and extravasation/metastasis in vivo (chick chorioallantoic membrane assay) was assessed. Knockdown of ALDH1A3 but not ALDH1A1 in breast cancer cells decreased ALDH activity, and knockdown of ALDH1A1 reduced breast cancer cell metastatic behavior and therapy resistance relative to control ($p < 0.05$). In contrast, knockdown of ALDH1A3 did not alter proliferation, extravasation, or therapy resistance, but increased adhesion/migration and decreased colony formation/metastasis relative to control ($p < 0.05$). This is the first study to systematically examine the function of ALDH1 isozymes in individual breast cancer cell behaviors that contribute to metastasis. Our novel results indicate that ALDH1 mediates breast cancer metastatic behavior and therapy resistance, and that different enzyme isoforms within the ALDH1 family differentially impact these cell behaviors.

Keywords: breast cancer; metastasis; therapy resistance; ALDH1A1; ALDH1A3

---

1. Introduction

Breast cancer is a leading cause of death in women, due primarily to ineffective treatment of metastatic disease. In order to reduce mortality from breast cancer, it is therefore essential to learn more about the metastatic process, and in particular, mechanisms that may contribute to therapy resistance and disease progression [1,2].

Metastasis is a complex process that involves tumor dissemination from the primary tumor to distant sites throughout the body, arrest and extravasation at secondary organ sites, and initiation and maintenance of growth of metastatic lesions [1,3,4]. Given the multi-step nature of this process, it is not surprising that metastasis is highly inefficient, with the main rate-limiting steps being initiation of growth at the secondary site from single tumor cells to micrometastases, and maintenance of that growth into clinically detectable macrometastases [1,3–5]. Given the heterogeneous nature of breast cancer, this metastatic inefficiency suggests that only a small subpopulation of tumor cells can successfully navigate the entire metastatic process to successfully form metastases. We have previously identified such a subset of breast cancer cells with high aldehyde dehydrogenase (ALDH) activity and expression of CD44, and demonstrated that these $ALDH^{hi}CD44^+$ cells have enhanced tumor-initiating and metastatic abilities both in vitro and in vivo [6]. Subsequent studies by Charafe-Jauffret et al. (2009, 2010) supported our findings, indicating that $ALDH^{hi}CD44^+$ cells may have a role as metastasis-initiating cells [7,8]. We have also demonstrated that these $ALDH^{hi}CD44^+$ cells are significantly more resistant to chemotherapy and radiation therapy, and that the observed therapy resistance may occur, at least in part, via ALDH-dependent mechanisms [9].

The ALDH superfamily of enzymes is involved in detoxification and/or bioactivation of various intracellular aldehydes in a $NAD(P)^+$-dependent manner [10,11]. Of particular biological importance, the ALDH1 family of enzymes (namely ALDH1A1 and ALDH1A3) plays an important role in oxidizing vitamin A (retinal) to retinoic acid (RA) through an alcohol intermediary. RA functions as a ligand for nuclear retinoid receptors and leads to transactivation and transrepression of target genes, and is finally degraded by CYP26 enzymes [12]. ALDH activity has been shown to be involved in self-protection of normal stem cells and in resistance to the chemotherapeutic drug cyclophosphamide [13]. In the treatment of acute promyelocytic leukemia (APL), the differentiation agent all-*trans* retinoic acid (ATRA) is used clinically in combination with chemotherapy [14,15]. Increased levels of RA signaling from ATRA treatment have been shown to indirectly suppress *ALDH1* promoter activity in liver cells [16], as well as driving the differentiation of promyelocytes into neutrophils, causing enhanced cell-cycle arrest and apoptosis [17]. Additionally, ATRA has been shown to modulate cell growth, apoptosis, and differentiation of breast cancer cells [18]. In terms of therapy resistance, Tanei et al. (2009) conducted a clinical study looking at 108 breast cancer patients who received neoadjuvant paclitaxel and epirubicin-based chemotherapy [19]. When $ALDH1A1^+$ and $CD24^-CD44^+$ expression was compared between core needle biopsies (pre-treatment) and subsequent excision (post-treatment), there was a significant increase in ALDH1A1 positive cells, but no change in $CD24^-CD44^+$ cells, indicating that $ALDH1A1^+$ cells may play a significant role in resistance to chemotherapy.

High ALDH1 expression has been shown to correlate with poor prognosis in breast cancer patients [20], and has been associated with early relapse, metastasis development, therapy resistance and poor clinical outcome [7,8,21–23]. The ALDH1A1 isozyme has been shown to have increased expression in breast cancer patients who present with positive lymph nodes and in patients who succumb to their disease [24]. In a meta-analysis that looked at almost 900 breast cancer cases compared to over 1800 control samples, Zhou et al. (2010) found that ALDH1A1 expression was significantly associated with a high histological grade, ER/PR negativity, HER2 positivity, and worse overall survival [25]. Furthermore, when $ALDH^{bright}$ cells in various tumors, including breast, are treated with ALDH1A1-specific $CD8^+$ T cells which target and eliminate ALDH1A1-positive cells, inhibition of tumorigenic and metastatic growth is observed [26]. In contrast, Marcato et al. (2011) demonstrated that ALDH1A3 (but not ALDH1A1) expression in patient breast tumors correlates significantly with tumor grade, metastasis, and cancer stage, indicating that even within the ALDH1 family, alternate isozymes may function differently [27]. Thus, in addition to the classical role of ALDH as a detoxification enzyme, growing evidence suggests that it may also be playing an additional role in disease progression.

The goal of the current study was to test the hypothesis that ALDH1 is not simply a marker of highly aggressive breast cancer cells and poor patient prognosis, but that it also contributes functionally to metastatic behavior and therapy resistance. Importantly, we wanted to begin to elucidate the differential roles of ALDH1 isozymes, namely ALDH1A1 and ALDH1A3. The novel findings presented here indicate that ALDH1 is functionally involved in breast cancer metastasis and therapy resistance, and that different isozymes within the ALDH1 family differentially impact these cell behaviors.

2. Results

2.1. Treatment with DEAB (Diethylaminobenzaldehyde) Reduces Breast Cancer Cell Proliferation, Adhesion, Migration, and Colony Formation In Vitro

We first investigated whether treating cells with previously established chemical inhibitors of ALDH would have a functional effect on malignant breast cancer cell behavior in vitro, including proliferation, adhesion, migration, and colony formation. This included treatment with a direct competitive substrate of ALDH (diethylaminobenzaldehyde (DEAB)) [28]), as well as the differentiation agent ATRA which has been shown to reduce ALDH promoter activity [9,16]. We observed that cells treated with either ATRA or DEAB demonstrated decreased growth in normal culture relative to respective vehicle control (EtOH) treated cells ($p < 0.05$) (Figure 1A). MDA-MB-468 cells treated with DEAB were significantly less adherent (Figure 1A) and migratory (Figure 1C) than vehicle control cells, and DEAB-treated SUM159 cells also demonstrated a significant decrease in migration ($p < 0.05$) (Figure 1C). In contrast, MDA-MB-468 and SUM159 cells treated with ATRA were observed to be significantly more adherent ($p < 0.01$) (Figure 1B) and migratory (Figure 1C) than respective control cells ($p < 0.05$). Finally, in keeping with the proliferation results, cells treated with either ATRA or DEAB demonstrated decreased colony formation in soft agar relative to vehicle control cells ($p < 0.05$) (Figure 1D).

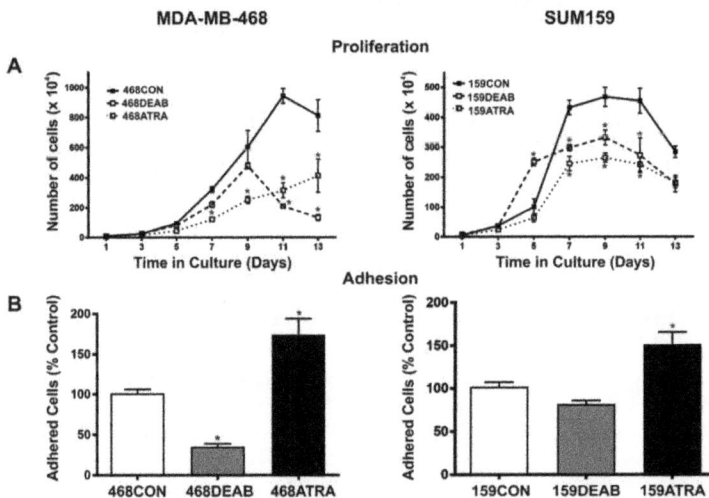

Figure 1. *Cont.*

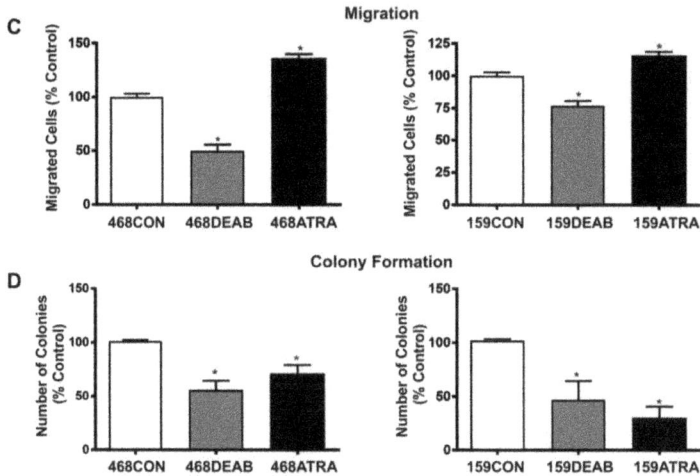

Figure 1. Treatment with diethylaminobenzaldehyde (DEAB) reduces breast cancer cell (**A**) proliferation, (**B**) adhesion, (**C**) migration, and (**D**) colony formation in vitro. MDA-MB-468 (left panels) and SUM159 (right panels) human breast cancer cells were treated with 5 µM all-*trans* retinoic acid (ATRA), 100 µM DEAB or ethanol (EtOH) as a vehicle control (CON). In all cases, data represents the mean ± standard error of the mean (SEM) normalized to vehicle control. * = significantly different than respective vehicle control treatment ($p < 0.05$).

2.2. Decreased Expression of ALDH1A3 but Not ALDH1A1 Reduces ALDH Activity as Measured by the ALDEFLUOR® Assay

Rather than being direct inhibitors of ALDH isozyme expression, DEAB is a competitive substrate of ALDH [28] and ATRA inhibits ALDH promoter activity indirectly through the retinoic acid pathway. In support of this, we did not observe any significant effect of these inhibitors on directly reducing ALDH1A1 or ALDH1A3 protein expression (Figure S1). However, given that previous studies have demonstrated that expression of ALDH1A1 versus ALDH1A3 isozymes have differential correlation with tumor grade, metastasis, and cancer stage in breast cancer patients [27], we wanted to test the hypothesis that directly inhibiting ALDH using the alternative approach of targeted knockdown of ALDH1A1 or ALDH1A3 would also reduce proliferation, adhesion, migration, and colony formation of breast cancer cells.

siRNA was used to knockdown expression of two ALDH1 isozymes (ALDH1A1 and ALDH1A3) in MDA-MB-468 and SUM159 breast cancer cells and generate the following cell populations: 468CON, 468ALDH1A1^{low}, 468ALDH1A3^{low}, 159CON, 159ALDH1A1^{low}, and 159ALDH1A3^{low}. Knockdown of RNA and protein expression was confirmed by quantitative real-time polymerase chain reaction (RT-PCR) and immunoblotting respectively (Figure 2A–C).

There has been some debate over which ALDH1 isozyme is responsible for the ALDH enzymatic activity measured in the ALDEFLUOR® assay. (StemCell Technologies, Vancouver, BC, Canada), with some groups suggesting that ALDH1A1 is responsible, while others believe that it is ALDH1A3 [27,29]. Compared to respective siRNA scrambled controls, we observed that 468ALDH1A3^{low} and 159ALDH1A3^{low} cell populations did demonstrate a significant decrease in ALDH activity ($p < 0.001$), while 468ALDH1A1^{low} and 159ALDH1A1^{low} cell populations did not exhibit a change in ALDH activity ($p > 0.05$) (Figure 2D). This data is further supported by the observation that *ALDH1A3* mRNA expression is higher than *ALDH1A1* mRNA expression in sorted ALDH^{hi} versus unsorted cell populations (Figure S2). Our data also supports previous observations by Marcato et al. (2011), and

43

indicates that the ALDH1A3 isozyme is the major contributor to ALDH activity in breast cancer cells as measured by the ALDEFLUOR® assay [27].

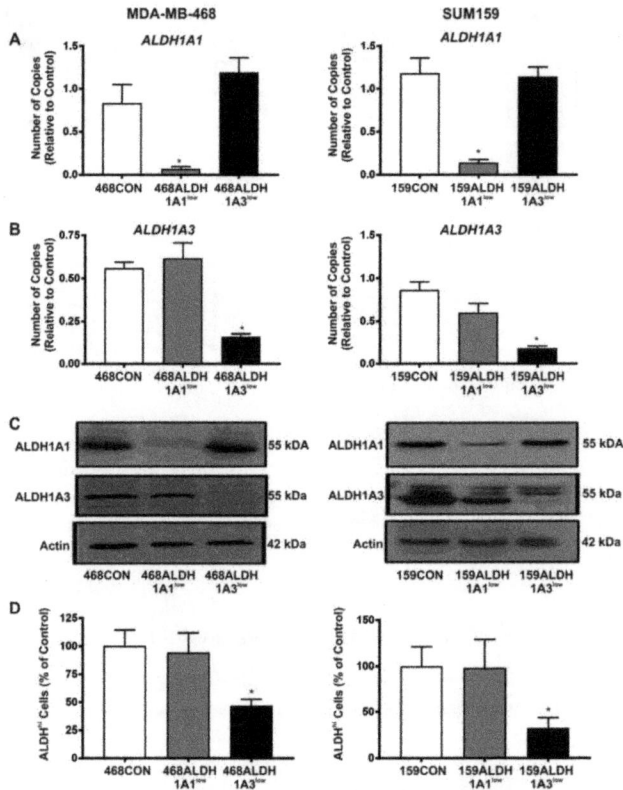

Figure 2. Decreased expression of ALDH1A3 but not ALDH1A1 reduces ALDH activity as measured by the Aldefluor® assay. MDA-MB-468 (left panels) or SUM159 (right panels) human breast cancer cells were transfected with 100 pmol siRNA pool targeted towards ALDH1A1, ALDH1A3, or a scrambled control using Lipofectamine to generate the following cell lines: 468CON, 468ALDH1A1[low], 468ALDH1A3[low], 159CON, 159ALDH1A1[low], and 159ALDH1A3[low]. After 4 days, RNA, cell lysates, or cells were collected and (**A,B**) qRT-PCR, (**C**) immunoblotting, or (**D**) Aldefluor® assays were performed to assess *ALDH1* gene expression, ALDH1 protein expression, and ALDH enzyme activity (respectively). Data represents the mean ± SEM. * = significantly different than respective siCON, 468CON, or 159CON scrambled control cells ($p < 0.05$).

2.3. Decreased Expression of ALDH1A1 Reduces Breast Cancer Cell Proliferation, but Adhesion and Migration of Human Breast Cancer Cells Is Differentially Influenced by ALDH1A1 versus ALDH1A3 In Vitro

Malignant breast cancer cell behavior in vitro was assessed in response to direct knockdown of ALDH1A1 or ALDH1A3 by siRNA (Figure 3). 468ALDH1A1[low] and 159ALDH1A1[low] cells demonstrated significantly decreased growth in normal culture relative to respective control cells ($p < 0.05$), whereas 468ALDH1A3[low] and 159ALDH1A3[low] cells showed no difference in proliferation compared to control cells. Lag times (time to reach exponential growth phase) were also observed to be longer for 468ALDH1A1[low] and 159ALDH1A1[low] cells versus respective control cells (9 days vs. 5 days for MDA-MB-468 cells; 5 days vs. 3 days for SUM159 cells) (Figure 3A). We next assessed the influence of ALDH1A1 and ALDH1A3 knockdown on breast cancer cell adhesion and migration in vitro

(Figure 3B,C). 468ALDH1A1^{low} and 159ALDH1A1^{low} cells were observed to be significantly less adherent (Figure 3B), and less migratory (Figure 3C) than respective control cells ($p < 0.05$). In contrast, 468ALDH1A3^{low} and 159ALDH1A3^{low} cells were observed to be significantly more adherent and more migratory (Figure 3B,C) than respective control cells ($p < 0.05$), suggesting that adhesion and migration of human breast cancer cells is differentially influenced by ALDH1A1 versus ALDH1A3. Knockdown of either ALDH1A1 or ALDH1A3 resulted in reduced colony formation in soft agar relative to control cells ($p < 0.05$) (Figure 3D). It should be noted that the adhesion and migration assays (Figure 3B,C) are performed over time periods of 24 h or less when siRNA knockdown is strong. However, in the proliferation and colony-forming assays (Figure 3A,D), the studies extend well past when the knockdown would be expected to persist. This suggests that the influence of ALDH1 on proliferation and colony formation is an early but important effect that then has a "feed-forward" or downstream effect on the ability of breast cancer cells to proliferate or form established/persistent colonies.

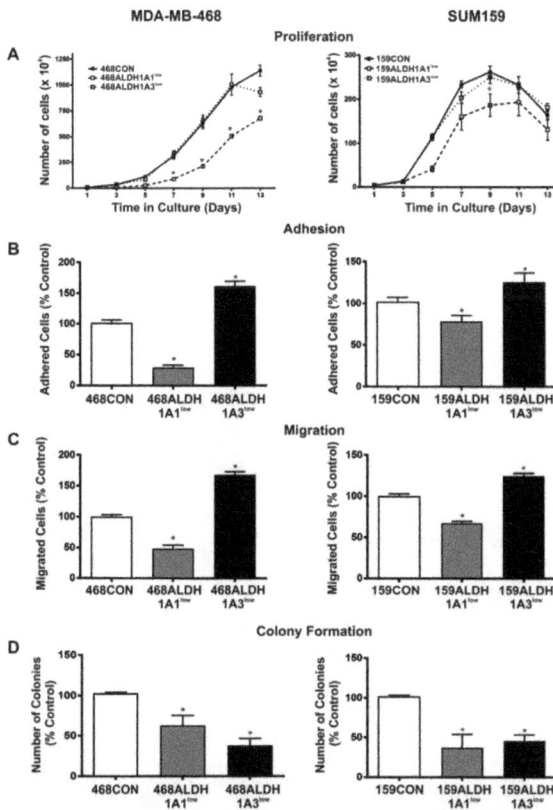

Figure 3. Decreased expression of ALDH1A1 reduces breast cancer cell proliferation, but adhesion and migration of human breast cancer cells is differentially influenced by ALDH1A1 versus ALDH1A3 in vitro. MDA-MB-468 (left panels) and SUM159 (right panels) human breast cancer cells were treated with control siRNA (siCON) or ALDH-specific siRNA (siALDH1A1 or siALDH1A3) for 96 h to generate the following cell lines: 468CON, 468ALDH1A1^{low}, 468ALDH1A3^{low}, 159CON, 159ALDH1A1^{low}, 159ALDH1A3^{low}. (**A**) Proliferation; (**B**) adhesion assays; (**C**) migration; and (**D**) colony formation. In all cases, data represents the mean ± SEM normalized to respective scrambled control. * = significantly different than respective scrambled control ($p < 0.05$).

2.4. Decreased Expression of ALDH1A1 and ALDH1A3 Reduces In Vivo Metastatic Ability of Breast Cancer Cells in the Chick Chorioallantoic Membrane (CAM) Assay

In order to assess the metastatic ability of ALDH-deficient cell populations in vivo, GFP-labeled MDA-MB-468 cell populations (468CON, 468ALDH1A1^{low}, 468ALDH1A3^{low} cells) or CMFDA-labeled SUM159 cell populations (159CON, 159ALDH1A1^{low}, 159ALDH1A3^{low} cells) were inoculated on the CAM of 9- or 12-day-old chicken embryos, and the percentage of breast cancer cell extravasation into the CAM and formation of micrometastases in the chicken embryo were analyzed (Figure 4). 468ALDH1A1^{low} and 159ALDH1A1^{low} cells demonstrated a significant decrease in extravasation compared to respective control cells ($p < 0.05$), whereas there was no significant difference observed in the extravasation of 468ALDH1A3^{low} or 159ALDH1A3^{low} cells compared to control (Figure 4A). In contrast, Both ALDH1A1^{low} and ALDH1A3^{low} cell populations from both MDA-MB-468 and SUM159 cell lines demonstrated a significant decrease in the number of micrometastatic tumors that were able to form compared to control ($p < 0.05$) (Figure 4B).

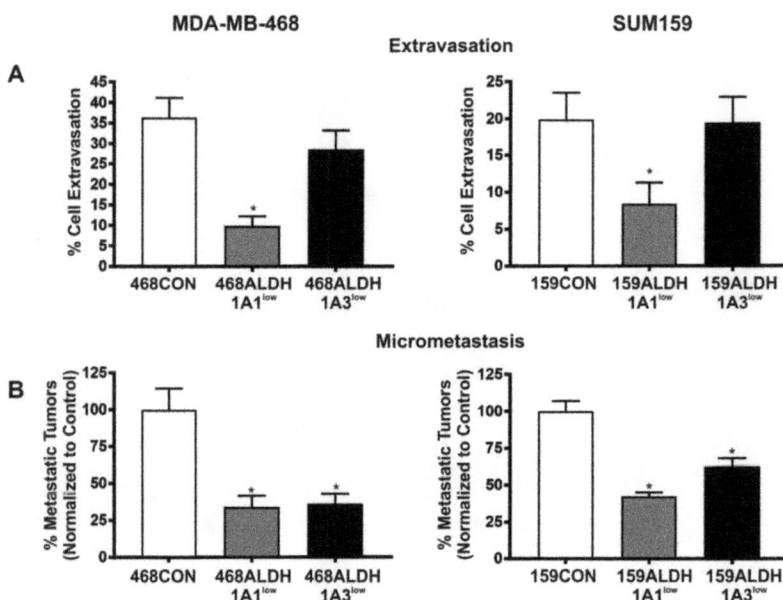

Figure 4. Decreased expression of ALDH1A1 and ALDH1A3 reduces in vivo metastatic ability of breast cancer cells in the chick CAM assay. GFP-labeled MDA-MB-468 or CMFDA-labeled SUM159 cell populations were transfected with 100 pmol (MDA-MB-468) or 400 pmol (SUM159) siRNA targeted towards ALDH1A1, ALDH1A3, or scrambled control using Lipofectamine to generate the following cell lines: 468CON, 468ALDH1A1^{low}, 468ALDH1A3^{low}, 159CON, 159ALDH1A1^{low}, 159ALDH1A3^{low}. After 4 days, 1×10^5 (extravasation assay) or 2×10^5 (micrometastasis assay) cells were injected into chicken embryos and (**A**) cell extravasation was observed after 24 h, or (**B**) micrometastatic formation was observed after 7days. Data represents the mean ± SEM normalized to control cells. * = significantly different than respective 468CON and 159CON cells ($p < 0.05$).

2.5. Decreased Expression of ALDH1A1 but Not ALDH1A3 Sensitizes Breast Cancer Cells to Chemotherapy and Radiation In Vitro

Finally, we have previously observed that breast cancer cells with high ALDH activity and CD44 expression (ALDH^{hi}CD44$^+$ phenotype) are significantly more resistant to chemotherapy and radiation therapy, and that this therapy resistance may occur, at least in part, via ALDH1-dependent mechanisms [9]. Taken together with the known role of ALDH activity in cellular self-protection and detoxification [30], we hypothesized that a siRNA-mediated reduction in ALDH1 expression would sensitize MDA-MB-468 and SUM159 cells to chemotherapy and radiation. We observed that knockdown of ALDH1A1 caused a significant sensitization of both MDA-MB-468 and SUM159 cells to paclitaxel (Figure 5A), doxorubicin (Figure 5B), and radiation therapy (Figure 5C) ($p < 0.05$). In contrast, ALDH1A3 knockdown did not reduce therapy resistance compared to control cells (Figure 5A–C).

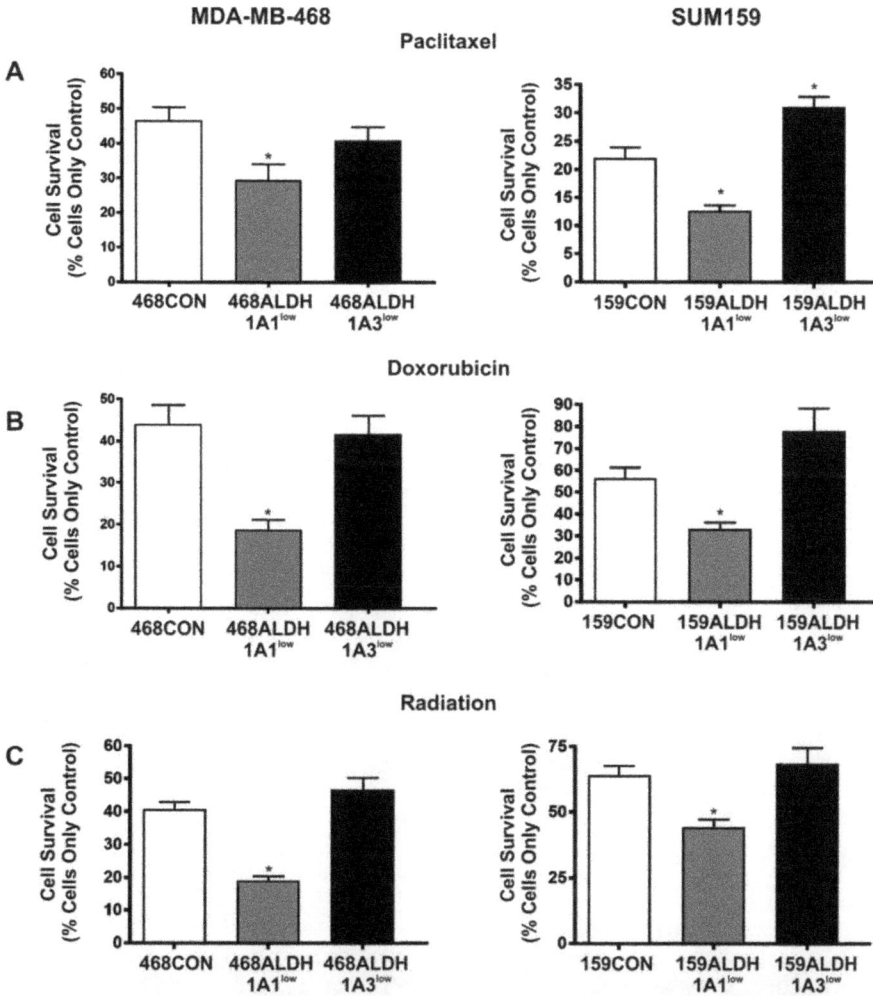

Figure 5. Decreased expression of ALDH1A1 but not ALDH1A3 sensitizes breast cancer cells to chemotherapy and radiation. MDA-MB-468 cells (left panels) and SUM159 cells (right panels) were treated with control siRNA (siCON) or ALDH-specific siRNA (ALDH1A1 or ALDH1A3) for 96 h to generate the following cell lines: 468CON, 468ALDH1A1low, 468ALDH1A3low, 159CON, 159ALDH1A1low, 159ALDH1A3low. Cell populations were treated with (**A**) paclitaxel (0.2 μg/mL), (**B**) doxorubicin (0.2 μg/mL), or (**C**) radiation (2 × 5Gy; MDA-MB-468 or 2 × 15Gy; SUM159). Data represents the mean ± SEM normalized to respective control cells. * = significantly different than respective 468CON or 159CON cells treated with paclitaxel, doxorubicin, or radiation ($p < 0.01$).

3. Discussion

Breast cancer is a leading cause of death in women, primarily due to ineffective treatment of metastatic disease [1,2]. Our group has previously demonstrated that stem-like ALDH^{hi}CD44$^+$ cells play a key role in breast cancer metastasis [6] and are highly resistant to chemotherapy and radiation compared to their ALDH^{low}CD44$^-$ counterparts, potentially as a result of ALDH-dependent mechanisms [9]. Additionally, it has been shown that ALDH1 expression is correlated with early recurrence, worse prognosis, and a higher incidence of metastasis in breast cancer patients [7,20,21,27]. While this suggests that ALDH is an important player in breast cancer metastasis; the actual functional contribution of ALDH1 (in particular its isozymes ALDH1A1 and ALDH1A3) in breast cancer metastasis requires further elucidation, and this was the goal of the current study.

Although the Aldefluor$^®$ assay is often used to isolate ALDH^{hi} cancer cells [6–9,20,31,32], the specific ALDH isozymes that contribute to this activity remain a subject of debate. In this assay, cells are incubated in a buffer containing a fluorescent aldehyde substrate (bodipy-aminoacetylaldehyde). The aminoacetylaldehyde is taken up into the cells via passive diffusion. Once inside the cell, intracellular ALDH oxidizes the aminoacetylaldehyde into aminoacetate, which is negatively charged, and therefore retained inside the cell, causing the cells to fluoresce [32]. When ALDH1A1 was knocked down in both MDA-MB-468 and SUM159 cell lines, there was no observable change in ALDH activity as measured by the Aldefluor$^®$ assay; however, when ALDH1A3 was knocked down, there was an approximate 50% reduction in ALDH activity measured by the Aldefluor$^®$ assay. This is consistent with breast cancer studies done by Marcato et al. (2011), who observed that ALDH1A3 knockdown was better correlated with a decrease in Aldefluor$^®$ activity compared to ALDH1A1 and ALDH2 [27]. Additional studies have reported that ALDH1A1, ALDH7A1, ALDH2 and/or ALDH1A2 are responsible for driving Aldefluor$^®$ activity in other tumor types [32–34], indicating that the ALDH isoform(s) responsible for Aldefluor$^®$ activity may be tumor-specific. Furthermore, in the present study, even after ALDH1A3 knockdown, there was still approximately 50% normal ALDH activity, indicating that other ALDH isozymes might be involved in the context of breast cancer. Taken together, these results suggest that many ALDH isozymes may contribute to the ALDH activity measured by the Aldefluor$^®$ assay, and potentially that different isozymes may contribute to ALDH activity in different tumor types.

We previously reported that ALDH^{hi}CD44$^+$ cells demonstrated enhanced proliferation, adhesion, and migration [6]. Additional work in lung and liver cancer cells has suggested that a decrease in ALDH expression can result in a decrease in proliferation [35–37]. In the current study, we treated breast cancer cells with DEAB (a direct competitive substrate of ALDH [28]) and observed a decrease in cell proliferation, as well as in adhesion and migration in vitro compared to control cells, suggesting that ALDH may potentially contribute to these processes. In order to determine whether ALDH1 isozymes were also involved in these processes, we used siRNA to specifically knockdown ALDH1A1 or ALDH1A3 and observed that ALDH1A1^{low} cells demonstrated decreased proliferation, adhesion, and migration in vitro. In contrast, cells in which ALDH1A3 had been knocked down showed no change in proliferation and in fact demonstrated increased levels of adhesion and migration in vitro.

ALDH1 expression has been clinically correlated with an increased incidence of metastasis [7,20,27]. We used the chick CAM assay to elucidate whether ALDH1A1 and/or ALDH1A3 functionally contributed to metastasis. Cells with decreased ALDH1A1 expression demonstrated decreased abilities to invade/extravasate; whereas cells with decreased ALDH1A3 expression demonstrated no change in invasive capabilities compared to control cells in vivo. However, in terms of the actual formation of metastases in vivo; both ALDH1A1^{low} and ALDH1A3^{low} cells demonstrated a decrease in metastatic potential, with an approximate 50% reduction in the number of micrometastases that were able to form in the chick CAM compared to control cells.

Finally, we have previously observed that that ALDH^{hi}CD44$^+$ cells demonstrate high levels of therapy resistance, and that pre-treatment targeting of ALDH activity using DEAB or ATRA can sensitize these resistant cells to both anthracycline and taxane chemotherapy, as well as radiation [9].

Int. J. Mol. Sci. **2017**, *18*, 2039

In the current study, we directly targeted specific ALDH1 isozymes using siRNA and tested the effect on therapy response. Notably, when ALDH1A1 expression was decreased, there was a significant sensitization of the cancer cells to both chemotherapy and radiation. Cells with decreased ALDH1A3 expression, however, showed no change in therapy resistance to either chemotherapy or radiation. These results suggest that the ALDH1A1 isozyme is an important contributor to therapy resistance in breast cancer cells, not only to cyclophosphamide chemotherapy (as previously reported [13,38]), but also to other classes of chemotherapy and radiotherapy.

Our study is the first in the literature to systematically examine the functional roles of ALDH1 isozymes on individual breast cancer cell behaviors that collectively contribute to the metastatic process. The combined in vitro and in vivo data presented in this study suggests that ALDH1A1 and ALDH1A3 both contribute functionally to various steps in the breast cancer metastatic cascade; however, they may do so in different ways (summarized in Table 1). For example, it appears that ALDH1A1 may mediate the adhesion, migration, extravasation, and initial colonization steps; whereas ALDH1A3 may only participate in colonization and sustainment of metastatic growth. This data both supports and contradicts previous work by Marcato et al. (2011), who reported that ALDH1A3 and not ALDH1A1 correlated with metastatic disease in breast cancer patients [27]. More recent work by this group led to the observation that overexpression of ALDH1A3 in MDA-MB-231 human breast cancer cells increases in vitro invasion and in vivo primary tumor growth and lung metastasis in mice, likely due to changes in RA signaling [39]. Although they observed that knockdown of either ALDH1A1 or ALDH1A3 in MDA-MB-231 cells did not have an effect on malignant behavior, this was not surprising given that this cell line has very low levels of these isozymes to begin with [27]. In contrast, it was somewhat surprising that their knockdown of ALDH1A1 in MDA-MB-468 cells (one of the cell lines used in the present study) actually increased primary tumor growth in mice, which is somewhat in contrast with our observed reduction in proliferation, colony-formation, and in vivo metastasis data presented in the current study. Overall, Marcato et al. [39] observed cell line-specific differences with regards to ALDH1A3 function in malignancy and metastasis. In contrast, our data shows that knockdown of ALDH1A1 consistently reduces most steps in the metastatic cascade except for basic proliferation in two different human breast cancer cell lines with different genetic backgrounds and differing metastatic ability. These experimental findings are supported by clinical data, which demonstrates that ALDH1A1 expression is often associated with worse prognosis in breast and other cancers [7,20,24,40–43].

Overall, the results of this study support the concept that ALDH1 plays a functional role in both breast cancer metastasis and therapy resistance; although the ALDH1A1 and ALDH1A3 isozymes seemed to contribute to these behaviors in different ways. In order to determine the underlying reasons for the differential influence of ALDH1 on different malignant behaviors, in-depth mechanistic studies will need to be carried out in the future. In addition, the observation that ALDH1A3 knockdown only caused a 50% reduction in ALDH activity suggests that other ALDH isozymes must be involved in Aldefluor® activity in breast cancer cells. It would therefore be interesting in the future to determine the functional role of other ALDH isozymes in breast cancer metastasis (i.e., ALDH7A1, ALDH1A2, and/or ALDH2) [33], as well as to assess corresponding changes in genes, transcription factors, and epigenetic modifiers that may ultimately be driving the process of metastasis. Elucidation of the mechanisms by which ALDH1A1, ALDH1A3 and other ALDH isozymes contribute to disease progression could have potentially important implications for the management and treatment of breast cancer in the future. Furthermore, additional investigation of ALDH1A1-specific therapy resistance mechanisms is required, and translating this knowledge into the clinic through development of either a direct, specific ALDH1A1 inhibitor or an ALDH1A1-related inhibitor that is safe for human use could have important implications for the management of both primary and metastatic breast cancer. Finally, it is well known that treating breast cancer before metastasis is observed (i.e., in the adjuvant setting) is significantly correlated with better patient survival [6,9,44]. Given that ALDH1 has been both correlated with metastatic disease and shown to functionally contribute to metastasis, it may be beneficial to use assessment of ALDH1 expression in the primary tumor as a clinical tool for identifying breast cancer patients with a high risk of metastasis and stratifying them for aggressive therapy to prevent disease recurrence or progression.

Table 1. Summary of functional consequences of ALDH1A1 and ALDH1A3 knockdown in MDA-MB-468 and SUM159 human breast cancer cells.

Functional Behavior/Activity	ALDH1A1 Knockdown	ALDH1A3 Knockdown
ALDH Activity (Aldeflour)	No effect	↓
Proliferation	↓	No effect
Adhesion	↓	↑
Migration	↓	↑
Colony Formation	↓	↓
Extravasation	↓	No effect
Metastasis	↓	↓
Therapy Resistance	↓	No effect

↑ = increase in respective functional behavior/activity; ↓ = decrease in respective functional behavior/activity.

4. Materials and Methods

4.1. Cell Culture, Reagents, and Therapy Conditions

MDA-MB-468 cells were a kind gift from Dr. Janet Price, M.D. Anderson Cancer Center, (Houston, TX, USA) [45], and were maintained in αMEM +10% fetal bovine serum (FBS). The 468 subline expressing green fluorescent protein (GFP) was generated previously as described [46]. SUM159 cells [47] were obtained from Asterand (Detriot, MI, USA) and maintained in Hams: F12 + 5% FBS. CellTracker™ 5-chloromethylfluorescein diacetate (CMFDA; Invitrogen, Carlsbad, CA, USA) was used to label SUM159 cells for the CAM assay. All cell lines were authenticated via third party testing of 9 short tandem repeat (STR) loci on 11 April 2103. (CellCheck, RADIL, Columbia, MO, USA). All media was obtained from Invitrogen. FBS was obtained from Sigma (St. Louis, MO, USA). Tissue culture plastic was obtained from NUNC (Roskilde, Denmark).

All-*trans* retinoic acid (ATRA) and diethylamino-benzaldehyde DEAB (Sigma) were constituted in 100% ethanol and diluted in either Hams:F12 (SUM159 cells) or α-MEM (MDA-MB-468 cells) at 5 µM (ATRA) or 100 µM (DEAB). Doxorubicin (Novopharm Limited, Toronto, ON, Canada) and paclitaxel (Biolyse Pharma Corporation, St. Catherines, ON, Canada) were diluted in either Hams: F12 or α-MEM to the concentrations noted below. Radiation was administered at the doses noted below using a Cobalt-60 irradiator (Theratron 60, Atomic Energy of Canada Limited, Chalk River, ON, Canada). All treatment doses were selected based on LC_{50} values determined in previous experiments [9].

4.2. Cell Proliferation Assays

Breast cancer cells were counted and plated at a density of 5.0×10^4 cells/60 mm plate ($n = 3$ per time point) and maintained in regular growth media. Every 48 h for 14 days, cultures ($n = 3$) were trypsinized and counted using a hemocytometer. Doubling time of each cell population was estimated during the exponential growth phase according to $T_d = 0.693t/\ln (N_t/N_0)$, where t is time (in hours), N_t is the cell number at time t, and N_0 is the cell number at initial time.

4.3. Cell Adhesion Assays

Breast cancer cells were plated onto sterile 96-well non-tissue culture plates (Titertek, Flow Laboratories Inc.; McLean, VA, USA) that had been treated with one of: 20 µg/mL of human laminin (Sigma; SUM159 cells), 5 µg/mL of human vitronectin (Sigma; MDA-MB-468 cells), or PBS (negative control), using 1×10^4 cells/well ($n = 3$) for each cell population. Laminin and vitronectin were chosen based on previous experiments in our laboratory that have demonstrated that SUM159 and MDA-MB-468 cells differentially express integrin receptors for vitronectin and laminin respectively [48,49]. Cells were allowed to adhere for 5 h, after which non-adhered cells were rinsed away. Adhered cells were fixed with 2% gluteraldehyde and stained using Harris' hematoxylin. Five high powered fields (HPF) (200×) were counted for each well, and mean numbers of adhered cells/field were calculated and normalized to control cell populations.

4.4. Cell Migration Assays

Transwell plates (8 µm pore size, 6.5 mm; Becton Dickinson; Franklin Lakes, NJ, USA) were coated with 6 µg/well of gelatin (Sigma) [50,51]. Chemoattractant (5% FBS) or control (0.01% BSA) media was placed in the bottom portion of each well. For each cell population, 5×10^4 cells were plated on top of the transwells. After 24 h, the upper transwell was removed, inverted, fixed with 1% gluteraldehyde, and stained with Harris' hematoxylin. A cotton swab was used to carefully remove non-migrated cells on the inner surface of the transwell. For each well, five HPF were counted and mean numbers of migrated cells/field were calculated and normalized to control cell populations.

4.5. Colony Forming Assays

Dishes (60 mm) were coated with 1% agarose (Bioshop; Burlington, ON, Canada) in normal growth media and allowed to solidify for 1 hr. Breast cancer cell suspensions (1.0×10^4 cells/60 mm plate) were prepared using 0.6% agarose in normal growth media and plated on top of the base agarose base layer ($n = 4$ for each time point). Normal growth media was added on top of the cell layer and changed every 3–4 days for 4 weeks, after which the media was removed and plates were fixed in 10% neutral-buffered formalin (EM Sciences, Gladstone, NJ, USA). For each dish, 5 HPF were counted and mean number of colonies per field were calculated and normalized to control cell populations.

4.6. siRNA Knockdown of ALDH1A1 and ALDH1A3

ON-TARGET plus SMART pool small interfering RNAs (siRNA) (Dharmacon Thermo Scientific, Lafayette, CO, USA) were used to transiently transfect human ALDH1A1 and ALDH1A3 into MDA-MB-468 and SUM149 cells. All siRNAs were suspended in sterile RNAse-free water at a concentration of 25 µM. Scrambled control (20–50 µL/mL), ALDH1A1 (20 µL/mL), ALDH1A3 (50 µL/mL) siRNAs and Lipofectamine RNAiMax reagent (20 µL/mL; Invitrogen) were diluted into serum-free Opti-MEM (Invitrogen). Lipofectamine and siRNA concentrations were determined based on preliminary experiments which indicated the greatest knockdown of the proteins of interest [49]. The transfections yielded the following cell populations used in further experiments: 468CON, 468ALDH1A1^{low}, 468ALDH1A3^{low}, 159CON, 159ALDH1A1^{low}, and 159ALDH1A3^{low}.

4.7. RNA Isolation and Quantitative RT-PCR

Total RNA was extracted using TRIzol (Invitrogen) according to the manufacturer's protocol. Total RNA was reverse transcribed using Superscript III (Invitrogen) and the Eppendorf Mastercycler Gradient (Eppendorf, Hamburg, Germany). Primers and cycling conditions used for *ALDH1A1*, *ALDH1A3*, and *GAPDH* are provided in Table 2. Relative quantification of *ALDH1A1* and *ALDH1A3* gene expression in MDA-MB-468 and SUM159 breast cancer cells was determined by quantitative PCR using Brilliant® II SYBR® Green qPCR Low ROX Master Mix (Agilent Technologies, Eugene, OR, USA) and the delta Ct method. *GAPDH* was used for normalization.

Table 2. Primers and qPCR conditions.

Gene	Primer Sequence	qPCR Cycling Conditions	Number of Cycles	Product Size (bp)
ALDH1A1	Fwd: 5′-CGT TGG TTA TGC TCA TTT GGA A-3′ Rev: 5′-TGA TCA ACT TGC CAA CCT CTG T-3′	60 s 55 °C 60 s 72 °C 60 s 95 °C	45	22 bp
ALDH1A3	Fwd: 5′-ATG TGG GAA AAC CCC CTG TG-3′ Rev: 5′-GAA TGG TCC CAC CTT CAC CT-3′	60 s 57 °C 60 s 72 °C 60 s 95 °C	45	20 bp
GAPDH	Fwd: 5′-CAT GTT CGT CAT GGG TGT GAA CCA-3′ Rev: 5′-ATG GCA TGG ACT GTG GTC ATG AGT -3′	45 s 60 °C 45 s 72 °C 60 s 95 °C	40	24 bp

4.8. Immunoblotting

Cell lysates were extracted and protein (10 µg) was subjected to sodium dodecyl sulfate polyacrylamide gel electrophoresis (SDS-PAGE, 12%) and transferred onto polyvinylidene difluoride membranes (PVDF; Immobilon™, Millipore; Bedford, MA, USA). Blocking and antibody dilution was done using 5% skim milk in Tris-buffered saline with 0.1% Tween-20 (TBST). Anti-human primary antibodies included mouse monoclonal ALDH1A1 (clone IG6; 1:1000) and rabbit polyclonal ALDH1A3 (1:500) (Abcam, Cambridge, MA, USA). Secondary antibodies included goat anti-mouse and mouse anti-rabbit antibodies conjugated to horseradish peroxidase (Calbiochem, Gibbstown, NJ, USA) (1:2000). Protein expression was visualized using Amersham ECL Plus (GE Healthcare, Baie d'Urfe, QC, Canada) using β-actin (Sigma, 1:5000) as a loading control.

4.9. ALDEFLUOR® Assay

The ALDEFLUOR® assay (StemCell Technologies, Vancouver, BC, Canada) was used to assess ALDH activity as described previously [52–54]. Briefly, cells were harvested, placed in ALDEFLUOR® assay buffer (2×10^6/mL), and incubated with ALDEFLUOR® substrate for 45 min at 37 °C to allow substrate conversion. As a negative control for all experiments, an aliquot of ALDEFLUOR®-stained cells was immediately quenched with 1.5-mM diethylaminobenzaldehyde (DEAB), a specific ALDH inhibitor. Cells were analyzed using the green fluorescence channel (FL1) on a Beckman Coulter EPICS XL-MCL flow cytometer.

4.10. Chick Embryo Chorioallantoic Membrane (CAM) Assay

For assessment of in vivo extravasation and metastasis, chick embryo chorioallantoic membrane (CAM) assays were used as described previously [55,56]. Briefly, fertilized chicken eggs (McKinley Hatchery, St. Mary's, ON, Canada) were removed from their shell, placed in covered dishes, and maintained *ex ovo* at 37 °C with 90% humidity. Embryos were used at day 9 (micrometastasis assay) and day 12 (extravasation assay). Green-fluorescent protein (GFP) labeled MDA-MB-468 or CellTracker™ CMFDA-labeled SUM159 cell populations were injected intravenously (i.v.) into the CAM as described previously [55,56] using 1×10^5 (extravasation assay) or 2×10^5 (micrometastasis assay) cells/egg (*n* = 8–17 eggs per treatment group). For the extravasation assay, a portion of the CAM was sectioned off using aluminum foil and the number of cells arrested in the sectioned-off area was manually counted using a fluorescence microscope at 20× magnification. Embryos were then returned to the incubator for 24 h, after which time the number of extravasated cells in the sectioned off area were manually counted using a fluorescence microscope. Percent extravasation was calculated by dividing the number of initial cells by the number of successfully extravasated cells in the CAM. For the micrometastasis assay, embryos were returned to the incubator for 7 days after cell injection to allow the formation of metastases. After 7 days, the number of micrometastatic tumors that developed following the i.v. injection were manually counted using a fluorescence microscope at 4× magnification.

Int. J. Mol. Sci. **2017**, *18*, 2039

4.11. Chemotherapy and Radiation Treatment

Cell populations were plated at a density of 5×10^5 cells in 6-well plates ($n = 3$/treatment group) and maintained in normal growth medium for 24 h. Cells were then treated with either normal media alone (control), chemotherapy (paclitaxel (0.2 µM); doxorubicin (0.4 µM)), or radiation (2×5Gy, MDA-MB-468; or 2×15Gy, SUM159) and cultured for a further 72 h. Cells were then harvested and viable cells were quantified using trypan blue exclusion and manual counting on a hemocytometer using light microscopy.

4.12. Statistical Analysis

All experiments were performed following at least three separate siRNA transfections with at least 3 biological replicates included within each experiment. In all cases, quantitative data was compiled from all experiments. Statistical analysis was performed using GraphPad Prism 4.0 software© (San Diego, CA, USA) using either t-test (for comparison between 2 groups) or analysis of variance (ANOVA) with Tukey post-test (for comparison between more than 2 groups) when groups passed both a normality test and an equal variance test. When this was not the case, the Mann-Whitney Rank-Sum test was used. Unless otherwise noted, data is presented as the mean $\pm$ SEM. In all cases, p values of ≤ 0.05 were regarded as being statistically significant.

Supplementary Materials: Supplementary materials can be found at www.mdpi.com/1422-0067/18/10/2039/s1.

Acknowledgments: This work was supported by grants from the Canadian Breast Cancer Foundation-Ontario Region and the Canada Foundation for Innovation (#13199). The work was also supported by the Breast Cancer Society of Canada (Alysha K. Croker, Mauricio Rodriguez-Torres, and Alison L. Allan) and by donor support from John and Donna Bristol through the London Health Sciences Foundation (Alison L. Allan). Alysha K. Croker was the recipient of a Canadian Institute of Health Research (CIHR) Banting & Best Doctoral Scholarship. Mauricio Rodriguez-Torres was the recipient of a Vanier Canada Graduate Scholarship. Alison L. Allan was supported by a CIHR New Investigator Award and an Early Researcher Award from the Ontario Ministry of Research and Innovation.

Author Contributions: Alysha K. Croker and Alison L. Allan conceived and designed the experiments; Alysha K. Croker, Mauricio Rodriguez-Torres, Ying Xia, Siddika Pardhan, and Hon Sing Leong performed the experiments; Alysha K. Croker, Mauricio Rodriguez-Torres, Ying Xia and Alison L. Allan analyzed the data; John D. Lewis and Alison L. Allan contributed reagents/materials/analysis tools; and Alysha K. Croker and Alison L. Allan wrote the paper.

Conflicts of Interest: The authors declare no conflict of interest. The funding sponsors had no role in the design of the study; in the collection, analyses, or interpretation of data; in the writing of the manuscript, and in the decision to publish the results.

Abbreviations

ALDH	Aldehyde dehydrogenase
ANOVA	Analysis of variance
APL	Acute promyelocytic leukemia
ATRA	All-*trans* retinoic acid
BSA	Bovine serum albumin
CAM	Choroiallantoic membrane assay
CD	Cluster of differentiation
CMFDA	5-chloromethylfluorescein diacetate
CYP	Cytochrome P450
DEAB	Diethylaminobenzaldehyde
ECL	Enhanced chemiluminescence
ER	Estrogen receptor
EtOH	Ethanol
FBS	Fetal bovine serum
GAPDH	Glyceraldehyde 3-phosphate dehydrogenase

GFP	Green fluorescent protein
Gy	Gray
HPF	High-powered field
LC_{50}	Lethal concentration (50%)
NAD(P)	Nicotinamide adenine dinucleotide phosphate
PBS	Phosphate buffered saline
PCR	Polymerase chain reaction
PR	Progesterone receptor
PVDF	Polyvinylidene fluoride
RA	Retinoic acid
RT	Reverse transcriptase
SDS-PAGE	Sodium dodecyl sulfate polyacrylamide gel electrophoresis
SEM	Standard error of the mean
siRNA	Small interfering RNA
STR	Short tandem repeat
TBST	Tris-buffered saline + Tween-20

References

1. Chambers, A.F.; Groom, A.C.; MacDonald, I.C. Dissemination and growth of cancer cells in metastatic sites. *Nat. Rev. Cancer* **2002**, *2*, 563–572. [CrossRef] [PubMed]
2. Siegel, R.L.; Miller, K.D.; Jemal, A. Cancer statistics, 2017. *CA Cancer J. Clin.* **2017**, *67*, 7–30. [CrossRef] [PubMed]
3. Luzzi, K.J.; MacDonald, I.C.; Schmidt, E.E.; Kerkvliet, N.; Morris, V.L.; Chambers, A.F.; Groom, A.C. Multistep nature of metastatic inefficiency: Dormancy of solitary cells after successful extravasation and limited survival of early micrometastases. *Am. J. Pathol.* **1998**, *153*, 865–873. [CrossRef]
4. Weiss, L. Metastatic inefficiency. *Adv. Cancer Res.* **1990**, *54*, 159–211. [PubMed]
5. Goss, P.; Allan, A.L.; Rodenhiser, D.I.; Foster, P.J.; Chambers, A.F. New clinical and experimental approaches for studying tumor dormancy: Does tumor dormancy offer a therapeutic target? *APMIS* **2008**, *116*, 552–568. [CrossRef] [PubMed]
6. Croker, A.K.; Goodale, D.; Chu, J.; Postenka, C.; Hedley, B.D.; Hess, D.A.; Allan, A.L. High aldehyde dehydrogenase and expression of cancer stem cell markers selects for breast cancer cells with enhanced malignant and metastatic ability. *J. Cell. Mol. Med.* **2009**, *13*, 2236–2252. [CrossRef] [PubMed]
7. Charafe-Jauffret, E.; Ginestier, C.; Iovino, F.; Tarpin, C.; Diebel, M.; Esterni, B.; Houvenaeghel, G.; Extra, J.M.; Bertucci, F.; Jacquemier, J.; et al. Aldehyde dehydrogenase 1-positive cancer stem cells mediate metastasis and poor clinical outcome in inflammatory breast cancer. *Clin. Cancer Res.* **2010**, *16*, 45–55. [CrossRef] [PubMed]
8. Charafe-Jauffret, E.; Ginestier, C.; Iovino, F.; Wicinski, J.; Cervera, N.; Finetti, P.; Hur, M.H.; Diebel, M.E.; Monville, F.; Dutcher, J.; et al. Breast cancer cell lines contain functional cancer stem cells with metastatic capacity and a distinct molecular signature. *Cancer Res.* **2009**, *69*, 1302–1313. [CrossRef] [PubMed]
9. Croker, A.K.; Allan, A.L. Inhibition of aldehyde dehydrogenase (ALDH) activity reduces chemotherapy and radiation resistance of stem-like ALDHhiCD44(+) human breast cancer cells. *Breast Cancer Res. Treat.* **2012**, *133*, 75–87. [CrossRef] [PubMed]
10. Rodriguez-Torres, M.; Allan, A.L. Aldehyde dehydrogenase as a marker and functional mediator of metastasis in solid tumors. *Clin. Exp. Metastasis* **2016**, *33*, 97–113. [CrossRef] [PubMed]
11. Pors, K.; Moreb, J.S. Aldehyde dehydrogenases in cancer: An opportunity for biomarker and drug development? *Drug Discov. Today* **2014**, *19*, 1953–1963. [CrossRef] [PubMed]
12. Collins, C.A.; Watt, F.M. Dynamic regulation of retinoic acid-binding proteins in developing, adult and neoplastic skin reveals roles for β-catenin and notch signalling. *Dev. Biol.* **2008**, *324*, 55–67. [CrossRef] [PubMed]
13. Sladek, N.E. Human aldehyde dehydrogenases: Potential pathological, pharmacological, and toxicological impact. *J. Biochem. Mol. Toxicol.* **2003**, *17*, 7–23. [CrossRef] [PubMed]
14. Fenaux, P.; Castaigne, S.; Dombret, H.; Archimbaud, E.; Duarte, M.; Morel, P.; Lamy, T.; Tilly, H.; Guerci, A.; Maloisel, F.; et al. All-transretinoic acid followed by intensive chemotherapy gives a high complete remission rate and may prolong remissions in newly diagnosed acute promyelocytic leukemia: A pilot study on 26 cases. *Blood* **1992**, *80*, 2176–2181. [PubMed]

15. Sanz, M.A.; Lo-Coco, F. Modern approaches to treating acute promyelocytic leukemia. *J. Clin. Oncol.* **2011**, *29*, 495–503. [CrossRef] [PubMed]
16. Elizondo, G.; Corchero, J.; Sterneck, E.; Gonzalez, F.J. Feedback inhibition of the retinaldehyde dehydrogenase gene *ALDH1* by retinoic acid through retinoic acid receptor alpha and ccaat/enhancer-binding protein β. *J. Biol. Chem.* **2000**, *275*, 39747–39753. [CrossRef] [PubMed]
17. Ozeki, M.; Shively, J.E. Differential cell fates induced by all-*trans* retinoic acid-treated HL-60 human leukemia cells. *J. Leukoc. Biol.* **2008**, *84*, 769–779. [CrossRef] [PubMed]
18. Ginestier, C.; Wicinski, J.; Cervera, N.; Monville, F.; Finetti, P.; Bertucci, F.; Wicha, M.S.; Birnbaum, D.; Charafe-Jauffret, E. Retinoid signaling regulates breast cancer stem cell differentiation. *Cell Cycle* **2009**, *8*, 3297–3302. [CrossRef] [PubMed]
19. Tanei, T.; Morimoto, K.; Shimazu, K.; Kim, S.J.; Tanji, Y.; Taguchi, T.; Tamaki, Y.; Noguchi, S. Association of breast cancer stem cells identified by aldehyde dehydrogenase 1 expression with resistance to sequential paclitaxel and epirubicin-based chemotherapy for breast cancers. *Clin. Cancer Res.* **2009**, *15*, 4234–4241. [CrossRef] [PubMed]
20. Ginestier, C.; Hur, M.H.; Charafe-Jauffret, E.; Monville, F.; Dutcher, J.; Brown, M.; Jacquemier, J.; Viens, P.; Kleer, C.G.; Liu, S.; et al. ALDH1 is a marker of normal and malignant human mammary stem cells and a predictor of poor clinical outcome. *Cell Stem Cell* **2007**, *1*, 555–567. [CrossRef] [PubMed]
21. Zhong, Y.; Lin, Y.; Shen, S.; Zhou, Y.; Mao, F.; Guan, J.; Sun, Q. Expression of ALDH1 in breast invasive ductal carcinoma: An independent predictor of early tumor relapse. *Cancer Cell Int.* **2013**, *13*, 60. [CrossRef] [PubMed]
22. Kida, K.; Ishikawa, T.; Yamada, A.; Shimada, K.; Narui, K.; Sugae, S.; Shimizu, D.; Tanabe, M.; Sasaki, T.; Ichikawa, Y.; et al. Effect of aldh1 on prognosis and chemoresistance by breast cancer subtype. *Breast Cancer Res. Treat.* **2016**, *156*, 261–269. [CrossRef] [PubMed]
23. Miyoshi, Y.; Shien, T.; Ogiya, A.; Ishida, N.; Yamazaki, K.; Horii, R.; Horimoto, Y.; Masuda, N.; Yasojima, H.; Inao, T.; et al. Differences in expression of the cancer stem cell marker aldehyde dehydrogenase 1 among estrogen receptor-positive/human epidermal growth factor receptor type 2-negative breast cancer cases with early, late, and no recurrence. *Breast Cancer Res. BCR* **2016**, *18*, 73. [CrossRef] [PubMed]
24. Khoury, T.; Ademuyiwa, F.O.; Chandrasekhar, R.; Jabbour, M.; Deleo, A.; Ferrone, S.; Wang, Y.; Wang, X. Aldehyde dehydrogenase 1A1 expression in breast cancer is associated with stage, triple negativity, and outcome to neoadjuvant chemotherapy. *Mod. Pathol.* **2012**, *25*, 388–397. [CrossRef] [PubMed]
25. Zhou, L.; Jiang, Y.; Yan, T.; Di, G.; Shen, Z.; Shao, Z.; Lu, J. The prognostic role of cancer stem cells in breast cancer: A meta-analysis of published literatures. *Breast Cancer Res. Treat.* **2010**, *122*, 795–801. [CrossRef] [PubMed]
26. Visus, C.; Wang, Y.; Lozano-Leon, A.; Ferris, R.L.; Silver, S.; Szczepanski, M.J.; Brand, R.E.; Ferrone, C.R.; Whiteside, T.L.; Ferrone, S.; et al. Targeting ALDH(bright) human carcinoma-initiating cells with ALDH1A1-specific CD8(+) T cells. *Clin. Cancer Res.* **2011**, *17*, 6174–6184. [CrossRef] [PubMed]
27. Marcato, P.; Dean, C.A.; Pan, D.; Araslanova, R.; Gillis, M.; Joshi, M.; Helyer, L.; Pan, L.; Leidal, A.; Gujar, S.; et al. Aldehyde dehydrogenase activity of breast cancer stem cells is primarily due to isoform ALDH1A3 and its expression is predictive of metastasis. *Stem Cells* **2011**, *29*, 32–45. [CrossRef] [PubMed]
28. Koppaka, V.; Thompson, D.C.; Chen, Y.; Ellermann, M.; Nicolaou, K.C.; Juvonen, R.O.; Petersen, D.; Deitrich, R.A.; Hurley, T.D.; Vasiliou, V. Aldehyde dehydrogenase inhibitors: A comprehensive review of the pharmacology, mechanism of action, substrate specificity, and clinical application. *Pharmacol. Rev.* **2012**, *64*, 520–539. [CrossRef] [PubMed]
29. Chute, J.P.; Muramoto, G.G.; Whitesides, J.; Colvin, M.; Safi, R.; Chao, N.J.; McDonnell, D.P. Inhibition of aldehyde dehydrogenase and retinoid signaling induces the expansion of human hematopoietic stem cells. *Proc. Natl. Acad. Sci. USA* **2006**, *103*, 11707–11712. [CrossRef] [PubMed]
30. Vasiliou, V.; Nebert, D.W. Analysis and update of the human aldehyde dehydrogenase (ALDH) gene family. *Hum. Genom.* **2005**, *2*, 138–143.
31. Moreb, J.S.; Baker, H.V.; Chang, L.J.; Amaya, M.; Lopez, M.C.; Ostmark, B.; Chou, W. Aldh isozymes downregulation affects cell growth, cell motility and gene expression in lung cancer cells. *Mol. Cancer* **2008**, *7*, 87. [CrossRef] [PubMed]

32. Moreb, J.S.; Zucali, J.R.; Ostmark, B.; Benson, N.A. Heterogeneity of aldehyde dehydrogenase expression in lung cancer cell lines is revealed by aldefluor flow cytometry-based assay. *Cytom. Part B Clin. Cytom.* **2007**, *72*, 281–289. [CrossRef] [PubMed]

33. Hoogen, C.; Horst, G.; Cheung, H.; Buijs, J.T.; Pelger, R.C.M.; Pluijm, G. The aldehyde dehydrogenase enzyme 7A1 is functionally involved in prostate cancer bone metastasis. *Clin. Exp. Metastasis* **2011**, *28*, 615–625. [CrossRef] [PubMed]

34. Moreb, J.S.; Ucar, D.; Han, S.; Amory, J.K.; Goldstein, A.S.; Ostmark, B.; Chang, L.J. The enzymatic activity of human aldehyde dehydrogenases 1A2 and 2 (ALDH1A2 and ALDH2) is detected by aldefluor, inhibited by diethylaminobenzaldehyde and has significant effects on cell proliferation and drug resistance. *Chem. Biol. Interact.* **2012**, *195*, 52–60. [CrossRef] [PubMed]

35. Canuto, R.A.; Muzio, G.; Salvo, R.A.; Maggiora, M.; Trombetta, A.; Chantepie, J.; Fournet, G.; Reichert, U.; Quash, G. The effect of a novel irreversible inhibitor of aldehyde dehydrogenases 1 and 3 on tumour cell growth and death. *Chem. Biol. Interact.* **2001**, *130–132*, 209–218. [CrossRef]

36. Muzio, G.; Maggiora, M.; Paiuzzi, E.; Oraldi, M.; Canuto, R.A. Aldehyde dehydrogenases and cell proliferation. *Free Radic. Biol. Med.* **2012**, *52*, 735–746. [CrossRef] [PubMed]

37. Muzio, G.; Trombetta, A.; Martinasso, G.; Canuto, R.A.; Maggiora, M. Antisense oligonucleotides against aldehyde dehydrogenase 3 inhibit hepatoma cell proliferation by affecting map kinases. *Chem. Biol. Interact.* **2003**, *143–144*, 37–43. [CrossRef]

38. Moreb, J.S.; Mohuczy, D.; Ostmark, B.; Zucali, J.R. Rnai-mediated knockdown of aldehyde dehydrogenase class-1A1 and class-3A1 is specific and reveals that each contributes equally to the resistance against 4-hydroperoxycyclophosphamide. *Cancer Chemother. Pharmacol.* **2007**, *59*, 127–136. [CrossRef] [PubMed]

39. Marcato, P.; Dean, C.A.; Liu, R.Z.; Coyle, K.M.; Bydoun, M.; Wallace, M.; Clements, D.; Turner, C.; Mathenge, E.G.; Gujar, S.A.; et al. Aldehyde dehydrogenase 1A3 influences breast cancer progression via differential retinoic acid signaling. *Mol. Oncol.* **2015**, *9*, 17–31. [CrossRef] [PubMed]

40. Li, T.; Su, Y.; Mei, Y.; Leng, Q.; Leng, B.; Liu, Z.; Stass, S.A.; Jiang, F. ALDH1A1 is a marker for malignant prostate stem cells and predictor of prostate cancer patients' outcome. *Lab. Investig.* **2010**, *90*, 234–244. [CrossRef] [PubMed]

41. Li, X.; Wan, L.; Geng, J.; Wu, C.L.; Bai, X. Aldehyde dehydrogenase 1A1 possesses stem-like properties and predicts lung cancer patient outcome. *J. Thorac. Oncol.* **2012**, *7*, 1235–1245. [CrossRef] [PubMed]

42. Morimoto, K.; Kim, S.J.; Tanei, T.; Shimazu, K.; Tanji, Y.; Taguchi, T.; Tamaki, Y.; Terada, N.; Noguchi, S. Stem cell marker aldehyde dehydrogenase 1-positive breast cancers are characterized by negative estrogen receptor, positive human epidermal growth factor receptor type 2, and high ki67 expression. *Cancer Sci.* **2009**, *100*, 1062–1068. [CrossRef] [PubMed]

43. Neumeister, V.; Agarwal, S.; Bordeaux, J.; Camp, R.L.; Rimm, D.L. In situ identification of putative cancer stem cells by multiplexing ALDH1, CD44, and cytokeratin identifies breast cancer patients with poor prognosis. *Am. J. Pathol.* **2010**, *176*, 2131–2138. [CrossRef] [PubMed]

44. Cristofanilli, M. Advancements in the treatment of metastatic breast cancer (MBC): The role of ixabepilone. *J. Oncol.* **2012**, *2012*, 703858. [CrossRef] [PubMed]

45. Price, J.E.; Polyzos, A.; Zhang, R.D.; Daniels, L.M. Tumorigenicity and metastasis of human breast carcinoma cell lines in nude mice. *Cancer Res.* **1990**, *50*, 717–721. [PubMed]

46. Vantyghem, S.A.; Allan, A.L.; Postenka, C.O.; Al-Katib, W.; Keeney, M.; Tuck, A.B.; Chambers, A.F. A new model for lymphatic metastasis: Development of a variant of the MDA-MB-468 human breast cancer cell line that aggressively metastasizes to lymph nodes. *Clin. Exp. Metastasis* **2005**, *22*, 351–361. [CrossRef] [PubMed]

47. Flanagan, L.; Van Weelden, K.; Ammerman, C.; Ethier, S.P.; Welsh, J. SUM-159PT cells: A novel estrogen independent human breast cancer model system. *Breast Cancer Res. Treat.* **1999**, *58*, 193–204. [CrossRef] [PubMed]

48. Allan, A.L.; George, R.; Vantyghem, S.A.; Lee, M.W.; Hodgson, N.C.; Engel, C.J.; Holliday, R.L.; Girvan, D.P.; Scott, L.A.; Postenka, C.O.; et al. Role of the integrin-binding protein osteopontin in lymphatic metastasis of breast cancer. *Am. J. Pathol.* **2006**, *169*, 233–246. [CrossRef] [PubMed]

49. Croker, A.K.; Allan, A.L. London Regional Cancer Program, London, ON, Canada. Unpublished work, 2011.

50. Schulze, E.B.; Hedley, B.D.; Goodale, D.; Postenka, C.O.; Al-Katib, W.; Tuck, A.B.; Chambers, A.F.; Allan, A.L. The thrombin inhibitor argatroban reduces breast cancer malignancy and metastasis via osteopontin-dependent and osteopontin-independent mechanisms. *Breast Cancer Res. Treat.* **2008**, *112*, 243–254. [CrossRef] [PubMed]

51. Furger, K.A.; Allan, A.L.; Wilson, S.M.; Hota, C.; Vantyghem, S.A.; Postenka, C.O.; Al-Katib, W.; Chambers, A.F.; Tuck, A.B. β(3) integrin expression increases breast carcinoma cell responsiveness to the malignancy-enhancing effects of osteopontin. *Mol. Cancer Res.* **2003**, *1*, 810–819. [PubMed]

52. Hess, D.A.; Craft, T.P.; Wirthlin, L.; Hohm, S.; Zhou, P.; Eades, W.C.; Creer, M.H.; Sands, M.S.; Nolta, J.A. Widespread non-hematopoietic tissue distribution by transplanted human progenitor cells with high aldehyde dehydrogenase activity. *Stem Cells* **2008**, *26*, 611–620. [CrossRef] [PubMed]

53. Hess, D.A.; Meyerrose, T.E.; Wirthlin, L.; Craft, T.P.; Herrbrich, P.E.; Creer, M.H.; Nolta, J.A. Functional characterization of highly purified human hematopoietic repopulating cells isolated according to aldehyde dehydrogenase activity. *Blood* **2004**, *104*, 1648–1655. [CrossRef] [PubMed]

54. Hess, D.A.; Wirthlin, L.; Craft, T.P.; Herrbrich, P.E.; Hohm, S.A.; Lahey, R.; Eades, W.C.; Creer, M.H.; Nolta, J.A. Selection based on CD133 and high aldehyde dehydrogenase activity isolates long-term reconstituting human hematopoietic stem cells. *Blood* **2006**, *107*, 2162–2169. [CrossRef] [PubMed]

55. Leong, H.S.; Chambers, A.F.; Lewis, J.D. Assessing cancer cell migration and metastatic growth in vivo in the chick embryo using fluorescence intravital imaging. *Methods Mol. Biol.* **2012**, *872*, 1–14. [PubMed]

56. Seandel, M.; Noack-Kunnmann, K.; Zhu, D.; Aimes, R.T.; Quigley, J.P. Growth factor-induced angiogenesis in vivo requires specific cleavage of fibrillar type I collagen. *Blood* **2001**, *97*, 2323–2332. [CrossRef] [PubMed]

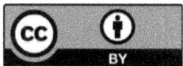

International Journal of
Molecular Sciences

MDPI

Review

Roles of Long Noncoding RNAs in Recurrence and Metastasis of Radiotherapy-Resistant Cancer Stem Cells

Hsiang-Cheng Chi [1], Chung-Ying Tsai [2], Ming-Ming Tsai [3,4], Chau-Ting Yeh [5] and Kwang-Huei Lin [5,6,7,*]

[1] Radiation Biology Research Center, Institute for Radiological Research, Chang Gung University/Chang Gung Memorial Hospital, Linkou, Taoyuan 333, Taiwan; hgchi@mail.cgu.edu.tw

[2] Kidney Research Center and Department of Nephrology, Chang Gung Immunology Consortium, Chang Gung Memorial Hospital, Chang Gung University College of Medicine, Taoyuan 333, Taiwan; monster_0616@yahoo.com.tw

[3] Department of Nursing, Chang-Gung University of Science and Technology, Taoyuan 333, Taiwan; mmtsai@mail.cgust.edu.tw

[4] Department of General Surgery, Chang Gung Memorial Hospital, Chiayi 613, Taiwan

[5] Liver Research Center, Chang Gung Memorial Hospital, Linkou, Taoyuan 333, Taiwan; chautingy@gmail.com

[6] Department of Biochemistry, College of Medicine, Chang-Gung University, Taoyuan 333, Taiwan

[7] Research Center for Chinese Herbal Medicine, College of Human Ecology, Chang Gung University of Science and Technology, Taoyuan 333, Taiwan

*   Correspondence: khlin@mail.cgu.edu.tw; Tel.: +886-3-2118263

Received: 13 July 2017; Accepted: 30 August 2017; Published: 5 September 2017

Abstract: Radiotherapy is a well-established therapeutic regimen applied to treat at least half of all cancer patients worldwide. Radioresistance of cancers or failure to treat certain tumor types with radiation is associated with enhanced local invasion, metastasis and poor prognosis. Elucidation of the biological characteristics underlying radioresistance is therefore critical to ensure the development of effective strategies to resolve this issue, which remains an urgent medical problem. Cancer stem cells (CSCs) comprise a small population of tumor cells that constitute the origin of most cancer cell types. CSCs are virtually resistant to radiotherapy, and consequently contribute to recurrence and disease progression. Metastasis is an increasing problem in resistance to cancer radiotherapy and closely associated with the morbidity and mortality rates of several cancer types. Accumulating evidence has demonstrated that radiation induces epithelial–mesenchymal transition (EMT) accompanied by increased cancer recurrence, metastasis and CSC generation. CSCs are believed to serve as the basis of metastasis. Previous studies indicate that CSCs contribute to the generation of metastasis, either in a direct or indirect manner. Moreover, the heterogeneity of CSCs may be responsible for organ specificity and considerable complexity of metastases. Long noncoding RNAs (lncRNAs) are a class of noncoding molecules over 200 nucleotides in length involved in the initiation and progression of several cancer types. Recently, lncRNAs have attracted considerable attention as novel critical regulators of cancer progression and metastasis. In the current review, we have discussed lncRNA-mediated regulation of CSCs following radiotherapy, their association with tumor metastasis and significance in radioresistance of cancer.

Keywords: radiotherapy; radioresistance; CSCs; EMT; metastasis; LncRNAs

1. Introduction

Radiotherapy has remained one of the mainstay treatments for cancer in the clinic for over 100 years. The principle of the treatment is based on the theory that cancerous regions are more sensitive than normal tissues to radiation because cancer cells have a limited ability to repair damaged DNA and tend to divide more quickly, while the normal tissue parts surrounding tumor lesions can withstand radiotherapy and recover [1]. However, the biological complexity and heterogeneity of cancers lead to certain tumor types being more resistant to radiotherapy. Importantly, resistance to treatment often leads to subsequent recurrence and metastasis of cancer in numerous patients [2,3]. Previous studies have reported that intrinsic cancer stem cells (CSC) representing a small subpopulation of cancer cells existing within heterogeneous tumors are responsible for radioresistance and metastasis in various cancer types [4–6]. In contrast, rather than CSCs, the progeny that differentiates from CSCs accounting for substantial tumor regions is hypothesized to be sensitive to radiotherapy, leading to short-term regression of cancer. Failure to treat and prevent cancer is therefore attributable to the fact that radiotherapy is aimed at the tumor bulk but not CSCs [7]. Findings to date have implied that radiation can paradoxically enhance tumor recurrence and metastasis [3,8,9].

The process of cancer metastasis is thought to consist of several steps. The initial escape from the primary region requires the epithelial tumor cells to become motile and degrade the underlying basement membrane and extracellular matrix (ECM). Activation of epithelial–mesenchymal transition (EMT) is considered necessary to allow epithelial cancer cells local invasion and dissemination at distant organs [10,11]. Moreover, radiation induces EMT in several cancer cell types [12,13]. EMT is closely linked to CSC generation and radioresistance [2,14,15]. As mentioned above, several CSC characteristics are relevant to metastasis, such as motility, invasiveness, and resistance to radiotherapy.

Therefore, regulation of CSCs and therapies that specifically target stem cells are required for prevention of radiation-induced metastasis and developing improved radiotherapeutic strategies. A small fraction of the human genome (~1.5%) codes for proteins [16]. The majority of the remaining noncoding regulatory regions transcribed are defined as noncoding RNAs (ncRNA). ncRNAs have been shown to influence a variety of human diseases, including cancers. Long noncoding RNAs (lncRNAs) are a subclass of ncRNAs implicated in the development and progression of cancers [17]. Several investigations on large clinical cancer samples have demonstrated that specific lncRNAs, such as HOX transcript antisense RNA (*HOTAIR*) and Growth arrest specific 5 (*GAS5*), can influence the outcomes of radiotherapy and act as valuable prognostic biomarkers [18]. Increasing studies have focused on the biological functions and mechanisms of lncRNAs in recurrence or progression following radiotherapy.

While the relationship between lncRNAs and CSCs has gradually become an important topic in cancer research, the specific cellular mechanisms by which these RNAs regulated in the cancer stem cells and subsequently affect recurrence and metastasis of radioresistant cancers remain unclear at present. In the current review, we have summarized recent studies focusing on: (1) the relationship between CSCs and radiotherapy; (2) underlying mechanisms implicated in radiation-induced metastasis, radioresistance and CSC generation; (3) roles of lncRNAs participating in radioresistance and radiotherapy-induced cancer metastasis; and (4) roles of lncRNAs in the progression and metastasis of CSCs. It is speculated that the long noncoding RNAs potentially contribute to radioresistant tumor occurrence and metastasis by affecting the population or behavior of cancer stem cells. Elucidation of the molecular cues underlying the effects of noncoding RNAs on CSCs may thus facilitate the design of effective strategies to improve radiotherapy and prevent cancer metastasis.

2. Cancer Stem Cells and Radiotherapy

Several reports to date have demonstrated that CSCs serve as the crucial contributor to radioresistance and recurrence after radiotherapy in the majority of cancers, including lung cancer, breast cancer and hepatocellular carcinoma (HCC) [4–6,19]. CSCs are defined as a small population of cancer cells within tumors that exhibit self-renewal capacity. These cells can effectively differentiate into the heterogeneous lineages of tumor cells constituting a specific cancer type [20]. At present, it is hypothesized that tumor development is triggered by the capacity of self-renewal and multi-lineage differentiation of CSCs, whereas differentiated offspring of CSCs do not display the ability to self-renew and extensively proliferate, therefore losing tumorigenesis potential [21].

CSCs were initially identified in human acute myeloid leukemia (AML) with the capacity to reconstruct the original disease entirely over several transplantations into immunocompromised mice. In this study, self-renewal and differentiation properties were only detected within the immature CD34$^+$/CD38$^-$ population of cells [22]. CSCs from solid tumors were identified initially in breast tumors [23] and subsequently in a broad spectrum of solid tumors, including colorectal, brain, melanoma, pancreatic, ovarian, lung, prostate and gastric cancers [24]. As CSCs display similar characteristics as normal stem cells with self-renewal and differentiation capacities, they have high clonogenic ability and can generate a serially transplantable phenocopy of the primary tumor in immunocompromised or syngenic animals [20]. At present, however, no reliable markers that allow precise measurement of CSCs in different tumors are available in the clinic. The most widely used strategy for isolation of CSCs is based on specific sets of surface markers [20]. Several specific surface markers of CSCs have been identified in diverse human tumors, including CD133, CD44, CD44$^+$/CD24$^-$ and CD34$^+$/CD38$^-$ [2,24]. Furthermore, specific membrane transporters and activities or expression patterns of enzymes in CSCs are different from those in non-CSCs. For instance, levels of adenosine triphosphate-binding cassette (ABC) transporters on the cell membrane are increased and consequently facilitate efflux of Hoechst dye in CSCs of several cancer types, including ovarian, lung, glioma and nasopharyngeal carcinoma [25–27]. ALDH1 (aldehyde dehydrogenase 1) activity in CSCs is additionally enhanced in several tumor types, such as lung, breast and pancreatic cancers [28–30]. Transcription factors, such as NANOG (Nanog homeobox), OCT4 (POU class 5 homeobox 1, POU5F1), SOX2 (SRY-box 2), c-MYC (MYC proto-oncogene, bHLH transcription factor) and KLF4 (Kruppel like factor 4), and signaling pathways, including WNT (Wingless-type MMTV integration site family), Hh (Hedgehog), Notch, TGF-β (Transforming growth factor beta), PDGF (Platelet derived growth factor) and JAK (Janus kinase 1)/STAT (signal transducer and activator of transcription), play crucial roles in maintaining self-renewal capacity in CSCs and therefore present potential targets in the development of therapeutic strategies [2,31]. In addition to surface markers and functional regulators, CSCs display unique characteristics, including increased levels of anti-apoptotic regulators, enhanced DNA repair efficiency and cellular quiescence [2,31].

The radioresistant ability of CSC markers/regulator-positive cells has been established [2,4,32–34]. Functional markers/regulators, together with the stem cell characteristics, influence the outcomes of radiotherapy [31,35,36]. Moreover, markers of CSCs may serve as predictors of clinical outcomes in patients receiving radiotherapy. In view of the crucial effects of CSCs on radiotherapy, clarification of the underlying mechanisms that mediate radioresistance is an urgent consideration. Generally, radioresistance of CSCs is associated with increased self-renewal capacity, activation of anti-apoptosis genes, enhanced capacity of DNA repair and reduced DNA damage via inhibition of reactive oxygen species (ROS) [36]. Additionally, radiotherapy has been shown to trigger EMT, and, consequently, metastasis and radioresistance of cancer cells [12,13]. The relationship between radiation and EMT is discussed below.

3. Mechanisms Implicated in Radiation-Induced Metastasis, Radioresistance and CSC Generation

3.1. Radiation Promotes Cancer Metastasis and Radioresistance via Induction of EMT

Metastasis is one of the major obstacles to successful cancer therapy [10,37,38] and closely associated with EMT, a biological process critical in embryogenesis, organ fibrosis and wound healing. Moreover, the EMT process confers mesenchymal phenotypes to epithelial cells, characterized by loss of epithelial phenotypes and markers, such as E-Cadherin, ZO-1 (tight junction protein 1, TJP1), and Desmoplakin, and simultaneous gain of mesenchymal markers, including N-cadherin, Vimentin,

Fibronectin, and α-smooth muscle actin (α-SMA). Thus, cancer cells undergoing EMT gain invasive and metastatic abilities [10,11].

Notably, radiation is reported to trigger EMT and promote metastasis of several cancer types. For example, radiation treatment enhances the stability of β-catenin (catenin β 1) via the activation of PI3K (phosphatidylinositol-4,5-bisphosphate 3-kinase)/AKT (AKT Serine/threonine kinase), thereby inducing the expression and secretion of granulocyte colony-stimulating factor (G-CSF). Recent report also indicates that radiation promotes the expressions of Nrf2 and Notch1 to activate EMT process in non-small cell lung cancer (NSCLC) cells. Inhibition of Nrf2-Notch axis reduces EMT but enhanced radiosensitivity of NSCLC, and consequently decreases radiation-induced NSCLC invasion [39]. Another report also suggests that radiation treatment can activate TGF-β1 signaling to induce EMT process in Lewis lung carcinoma [40]. Additionally, irradiation induces EMT of human alveolar type II epithelial carcinoma A549 cells, characterized by elimination of E-cadherin and enhancement of Vimentin expression is mediated via TBK-GSK-3β axis [41].

In esophageal cancer cells, irradiation induces the EMT phenotype accompanied by increased migration, invasion, and radioresistance through the induction of SNAIL (Snail family transcriptional repressor 1), TWIST (Twist family bHLH transcription factor 1), IL-6 (interleukin-6) and STAT3 (signal transducer and activator of transcription 3) signals [42,43]. In glioma cells, sub-lethal doses of radiation have been shown to promote the metastatic ability through inducing the expression of $\alpha_v\beta_3$ integrin, enhancing matrix metalloproteinase (MMP) activity, and altering the ratio of BCL-2 (B cell leukemia/lymphoma 2)/BAX (BCL2 associated X) toward the apoptosis-resistant phenotype [8,44]. Further, radiation treatment induces the expression and activity of MET though ATM (ATM serine/threonine kinase)-NF-κB (nuclear factor kappa-light-chain-enhancer of activated B cells) signaling pathway, and consequently promotes invasion and apoptosis-resistance of breast cancer cells [12]. Similar phenomena have been observed in nasopharyngeal carcinoma, colorectal, lung, and liver cancer subjected to radiation therapy [3,8,13,45,46]. Furthermore, preclinical and clinical evidence suggests that radiation enhances metastatic potential, in both the primary tumor region and normal tissues, under specific circumstances [3,47].

In addition to radiation-induced metastasis, cancer cells that have gained mesenchymal characteristics via EMT are more resistant to radiotherapy, indicating that radiation-induced EMT confers radioresistance, which contributes to relapse [48]. For example, prostate cancer cells have been shown to exhibit EMT phenotypes and become more resistant to radiation after radiotherapy [49]. Similar results have been reported with other cancer types, including nasopharyngeal carcinoma, colorectal cancer (CRC), lung cancer, HCC cells, breast cancer and gastric cancer [45,50–54].

The process of EMT contributes to radioresistance of cancer cells via induction of EMT-related genes/signals, such as PI3K/AKT, PTEN (phosphatase and tensin homolog), mTOR (mechanistic target of rapamycin kinase) and TGF-β, which inhibit cell death signals. Accordingly, silencing the expression of SNAIL and SLUG (Snail family transcriptional repressor 2), crucial EMT inducers, could sensitize cancer cells to genotoxic stress induced by chemo or radiotherapy [55]. In addition, activation of the Notch signaling pathway induces SNAIL and SLUG expression in tumor cells and the phenomenon of EMT, leading to the suppression of p53-mediated apoptosis induced by cancer therapy [14,56]. Therefore, initiation of EMT is accompanied by the activation of crucial gene sets or signals that influence sensitivity to radiotherapy.

As mentioned above, radiotherapy-induced EMT in cancer cells promotes the development of cancer cell radioresistance. Additionally, previous studies have demonstrated that EMT leads to the generation of CSCs generally resistant to therapy with elevated expression of genes involved in free-radical scavenging, DNA repair pathways and drug transporting capacity [57,58]. Interestingly, non-stem cancer cells can spontaneously dedifferentiate into CSCs via EMT. Thus, generation of CSCs after radiation via EMT may be an important factor in the development of resistance of cancer cells to radiotherapy. In conclusion, radiation treatment is prone to damage cancer cells and shrink tumors. However, irradiation triggers a small percentage of cancer cells to adopt the malignant phenotypes including stemness, metastasis and anti-apoptosis through EMT (Figure 1A). The inhibition of the signals associated with EMT represents a potentially efficient strategy for the treatment patients with radioresistant tumors, although further investigation is required.

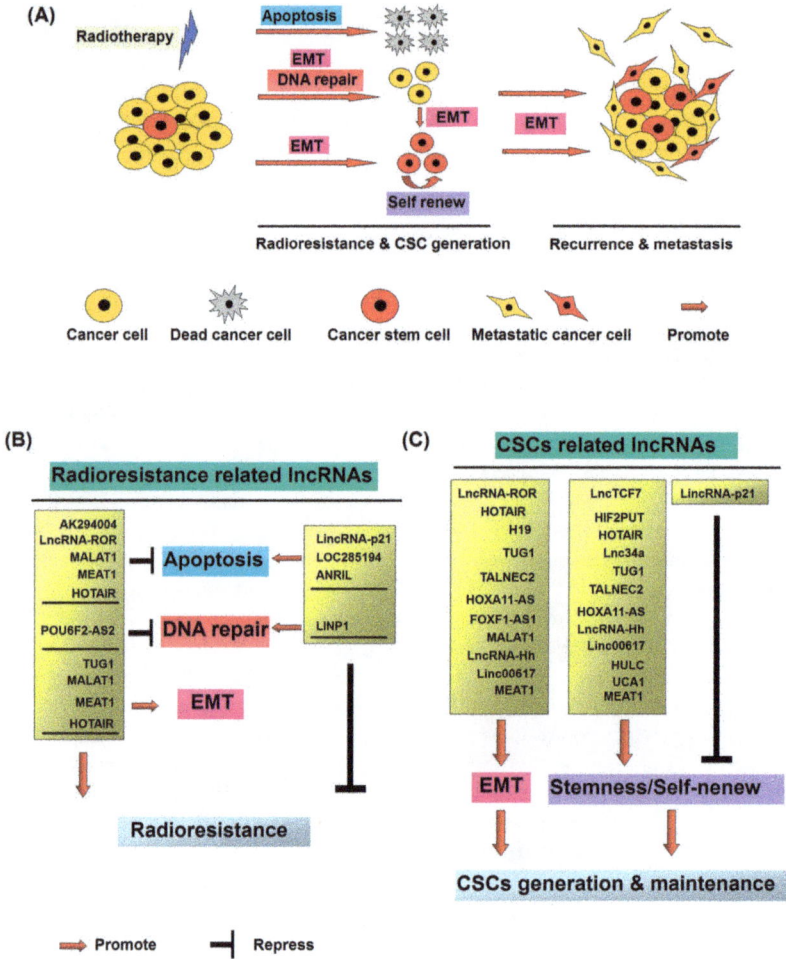

Figure 1. Molecular mechanisms of radiotherapy induced cancer recurrence and metastasis: (**A**) Cancer stem cells (CSCs) representing a small subpopulation of cancer cells existing within heterogeneous tumors are responsible for radioresistance and metastasis. After the radiation treatment, the majority of cancer cells are killed via the induction of apoptosis or mitotic death. However, a small number of non-CSCs exhibit the radioresistant property and dedifferentiate and transform into CSCs through radiation induced epithelial–mesenchymal transition (EMT). The newly generated CSCs from non-CSCs, together with the intrinsic CSCs, consequently contribute to recurrence and metastasis of cancer; (**B**) radioresistant CSC associated long noncoding RNAs (lncRNAs); and (**C**) CSC associated lncRNA.

3.2. Radiation Promotes CSC Generation

Radiation treatment causes enrichment of CSCs both in vitro and in vivo, implying that CSC generation is triggered by radiation. For instance, radiotherapy has been shown to enhance the population of CD44$^+$ cells that display CSC properties in patients with prostate cancer [59]. Another study reported an increase in expression of CSC surface markers in the MDA-MB-231-xenograft model after stimulation with fractionated radiation [60]. Enrichment of breast CSCs via radiation is considered the result of different sensitivities of CSC and non-CSC cancer cells to radiotherapy. Notably, earlier studies have demonstrated that radiation promotes reprogramming of differentiated cancer cells into CSCs. Enrichment of breast CSCs after radiation stimulation is implicated in the induction of stem cell-like characteristics in non-stem cancer cells [61,62]. In these studies, ALDH1$^-$ breast cancer cells in a single cell suspension were isolated from either human breast specimens or established cell lines and subsequently subjected to various doses of radiation. The number of ALDH1$^+$ cells was dramatically increased in a dose-dependent manner after five days of radiation treatment. The results clearly indicate that radiotherapy can induce the CSC phenotype in non-stem breast cancer cells. Moreover, radiation-induced CSCs display better capacity of mammosphere formation and tumorigenicity, and express stem cell-related genes similar to breast CSCs isolated from samples without radiation treatment. In addition to breast cancers, radiotherapy could induce a stem cell-like phenotype in non-stem HCC cells [63]. Non-CSCs isolated from HepG2 and Huh7 cells display better sphere formation ability and express stem cell-related genes after exposure to radiation [63].

Non-stem cancer cells can generate cells with CSC properties via the EMT process [15,64,65]. Additionally, radiation treatment induces cancer cells to undergo EMT, leading to radioresistance [49]. For example, after radiotherapy, resistant cells display a complex phenotype involving a combination of the properties of CSCs and EMT with higher expression of Snail, CD44, CD24, and PDGFR-β (platelet derived growth factor receptor β) in non-small cell lung cancer (NSCLC) cells [6]. Additionally, the subpopulation of CD133$^+$ colorectal or CD24$^+$ ovarian cancer cells exhibits both properties of CSC and EMT, characterized as increased SNAIL, TWIST, and Vimentin along with decreased E-cadherin expression [66,67]. EMT is reported to induce transcriptional regulators or signaling pathways, such as SNAIL, STAT3, NF-κB, Notch and PI3K/AKT and the MAPK (mitogen-activated protein kinase) cascade, indicative of a critical role in radiation-induced CSC properties [2]. The collective findings suggest that radiation promotes the generation of CSCs from non-stem cancer cells and shed light on the novel interactions between cancer cells and radiotherapy, which pave the way for clarifying the precise mechanisms leading to cancer radioresistance.

4. Cellular Functions of LncRNAs in Radioresistance

With the advent of genome sequencing efforts [68,69], numerous RNA transcripts with similar properties to mRNAs that are not translated into proteins have been identified. These transcripts, collectively defined as long noncoding RNAs (lncRNAs), are generally primary non-protein coding sequences greater than 200 nucleotides in length [70]. Although the cellular function of the majority of lncRNAs is still unknown [70], a number of reports are suggested to be functional RNA molecules involved in the regulation of diverse biological processes [70]. LncRNAs can interact with DNA, RNA or proteins. Recent large-scale sequencing analyses have revealed that many transcripts of lncRNAs may, in fact, be translated into functional peptides [71]. Accumulating studies indicate that lncRNAs regulate the transcription of genes related to the DNA damage response via different regulatory modes, including signal, decoy, guide, and scaffold [72]. DNA damage response and repair capacity are closely related to sensitivity to radiotherapy. In addition, numerous lncRNAs are aberrantly expressed in cancer cells and have been implicated in development of the radioresistant phenotype of cancer cells. Thus, lncRNAs may present effective target molecules in combination with radiation treatment for cancer. Here, we have systematically reviewed documented literature focusing on the lncRNAs participating in resistance to radiotherapy.

4.1. LncRNAs Associated with Apoptosis

4.1.1. LincRNA-p21

LincRNA-p21 is an intergenic long noncoding RNA (3100 nucleotides) located on chromosome 17, ~15 kb upstream from the *Cdkn1a* (p21) gene [73]. *LincRNA-p21* has been identified as the downstream target of p53 modulating the expression of numerous genes involved in cell cycle control, DNA damage and repair pathways [73]. The RNA acts as a suppressor of p53-dependent transcriptional responses and its inhibition influences the expression patterns of genes that are generally repressed by p53. In the presence of DNA damage, *lincRNA-p21* is required to induce p53-dependent apoptosis via physical association with ribonucleoprotein K (hnRNP-K). This step leads to proper genomic localization of *lincRNA-p21*/hnRNP-K at the gene promoter region and consequently suppresses their expression in a p53-dependent manner [74]. Additionally, *lincRNA-p21* is implicated in cell cycle regulation. Specifically, *lincRNA-p21* is proposed to enforce the G1/S checkpoint and regulate cell proliferation via activating p21 expression in cis to promote Polycomb target genes expression [75]. Notably, expression of *lincRNA-p21* is downregulated in several cancer types, and recent reports have also demonstrated a role in radiation-mediated cell death [76,77]. *LincRNA-p21* is frequently reduced in colorectal cancer (CRC) cancer cell lines and human tissues and leads to elevation of the WNT/β-catenin signal pathway [77,78]. Furthermore, expression of *lincRNA-p21* is increased upon X-ray treatment. Higher levels of lincRNA enhance the sensitivity of CRC to radiotherapy via repression of β-catenin signals and induction of the proapoptotic gene, NOXA, consequently promoting apoptosis [77]. Silencing of *lincRNA-p21* causes β-catenin overexpression and leads to increased stemness and radioresistance of glioma stem cells [79]. Another study showed that *lincRNA-p21* is transcriptionally induced by ultraviolet B in a p53-dependent manner in keratinocytes in vitro or skin from mice in vivo. Ultraviolet B-mediated lincRNA-p21 triggered cell cycle arrest and apoptosis in keratinocytes, and conversely, its inhibition resulted in evasion of apoptosis caused by ultraviolet B [74].

4.1.2. LOC285194

The lncRNA *LOC285194*, also termed LSAMP antisense RNA, was first identified as a p53-regulated tumor suppressor that influences the cell cycle and apoptosis by regulating VEGF receptor 1 and miR-211 in osteosarcoma [80,81]. Recent evidence has shown decreased expression of *LOC285194* in esophageal squamous cell carcinoma in relation to larger tumor size, high-grade TNM stage, lymph node and distant metastasis. Additionally, low expression of *LOC285194* serves as an independent prognosis factor closely associated with preoperative chemoradiotherapy response and poorer disease-free and overall survival rates [82]. Thus, *LOC285194* may be considered a potential therapeutic marker for screening of patients to determine their suitability for chemoradiotherapy and estimate outcomes.

4.1.3. ANRIL

The lncRNA *ANRIL*, also designated *CDKN2B-AS* (CDKN2B antisense RNA 1), was initially identified from familial melanoma patients [83]. LncRNA *ANRIL* produces a 3834 nt RNA transcript in the antisense orientation of the *INK4B-ARF-INK4A* gene cluster. Previous studies have documented upregulation of ANRIL in various cancer types and its utility as a prognosis marker [84–86]. Upregulation of *ANRIL* in cancer cells has been shown to enhance resistance to radiotherapy via inhibition of apoptosis and induction of cell proliferation. Conversely, inhibition of *ANRIL* expression causes repression of cellular proliferation and radioresistance via induction of apoptosis. Further experiments revealed that oncogenic effects of *ANRIL* are mediated through negative regulation of miR-125a, a tumor suppressor implicated in apoptosis and metastasis [87]. Moreover, Silencing of ANRIL upregulates the expression of the pro-apoptotic genes, BAX and SMAC (second mitochondria-derived activator of caspases), but suppresses the anti-apoptotic gene, BCL-2 [88].

Thus, lncRNA *ANRIL* is considered an important suppressor of apoptosis that influences cancer cell sensitivity to radiotherapy.

4.1.4. *AK294004*

Recent microarray analyses by Wang et al. [89] investigated changes in the lncRNA profiles in nasopharyngeal carcinoma in response to radiation in combination with curcumin treatment, following reports that curcumin (Cur) could sensitize cancer cells to radiotherapy. Among the 116 radiation-induced and Cur-reversed differentially expressed lncRNAs, six (*AF086415*, *AK095147*, *RP1-179N16.3*, *MUDENG*, *AK056098*, and *AK294004*) were identified. Further functional studies indicated that lncRNA AK294004 directly targets Cyclin D1 and exerts a negative effect. In view of the finding that Cyclin D1 is an important mediator of the cellular DNA damage response and apoptosis after radiation treatment [90], *AK294004* may be a potential lncRNA participating in radioresistance of cancer [89].

4.1.5. *LncRNA-ROR*

LncRNA-ROR was initially identified in induced pluripotent stem cells and shown to play a key role in maintaining the properties of these cells by suppressing stress pathways such as the p53 response [91,92]. Further studies provided evidence that lncRNA-ROR serves as a suppressor of p53 in response to DNA damage [93] and contributes to cancer progression, recurrence and chemoresistance, in part, by negatively regulating p53 and miR-145 in various cancer types [92,94]. Expression of *lncRNA-ROR* is increased in several cancer types and serves as a prognosis marker including colorectal cancer [95–97], and silencing its expression in CRC cells enhances sensitivity to radiotherapy via negative regulation of the p53/miR-145 axis. Importantly, combination of radiotherapy with specific knockdown of *lncRNA-ROR* was shown to induce significant tumor reduction in a xenograft model [95]. Thus, *lncRNA-ROR* may present an effective potential therapeutic target in combination with radiotherapy.

4.1.6. *MALAT1*

Metastasis-associated lung adenocarcinoma transcript 1 (*MALAT1*) (also termed *NEAT2* or *nuclear-enriched abundant transcript 2*) was one of the first lncRNAs identified in relation to tumorigenesis and used as a prognostic marker for development of metastatic disease and poorer survival rate in early-stage lung adenocarcinoma [98]. *MALAT1* is overexpressed in various cancers and linked to promotion of radioresistance through triggering EMT, CSC activity, and anti-apoptosis ability [99–101]. For instance, *MALAT1* is significantly upregulated in nasopharyngeal carcinoma (NPC) specimens or cell lines. Silencing the expression of *MALAT1* sensitizes NPC cells to radiotherapy, both in vitro and in vivo. Further investigation revealed a negative regulation loop of *MALAT1* and miR-1. SLUG, a crucial regulator of EMT, was determined as a direct target of miR-1. The function of *MALAT1* in activating EMT and CSCs via modulating the miR-1/SLUG axis supports its utility as a therapeutic target for NPC patients [101]. *MALAT1* was upregulated in esophageal squamous cell carcinoma (ESCC) and cervical cancer tissues [99,102,103]. Following radiation treatment, expression of *MALAT1* was decreased in radiosensitive but increased in both radioresistant cancer cells and clinical cases. Ectopic expression of *MALAT1* induced an increase in CKS1 in ESCC cells and decrease in miR-145 in cervical cancer cells, and which is leading to inhibition of cancer cell apoptosis after radiation treatment [99,103]. These reports collectively support a critical role of *MALAT1* in radioresistance of cancers.

4.1.7. *NEAT1*

Nuclear paraspeckle assembly transcript 1 (*NEAT1*) has been identified as a transcriptional target of p53 involved in the cellular response to stress or DNA damage [104,105]. Upon activation of p53, formation of paraspeckles is stimulated in mouse and human cells. Silencing of *NEAT1* expression prevents paraspeckle formation and sensitizes preneoplastic cells to DNA damage-induced cell death, preventing chemical-induced skin tumorigenesis in mice and enhancing chemotherapy-induced cytotoxicity [105], consistent with the theory that increased DNA damage sensitizes cells to p53 reactivation therapy [106]. *NEAT1* overexpression has been reported in different types of solid tumors, such as lung cancer, esophageal cancer, CRC and HCC, whereby higher levels are associated with poor prognosis [107]. *NEAT1* targeting may therefore present a potential strategy to enhance the effectiveness of DNA-damaging chemotherapeutics and p53-reactivating molecules. Recent evidence suggested that the lncRNA *NEAT1* regulates EMT and radioresistance in NPC cells [108]. Specifically, *NEAT1* was significantly upregulated in NPC cell lines and tissues and its knockdown sensitized NPC cells to radiation in vitro. Further experiments revealed reciprocal suppression effects of *NEAT1* and miR-204. Upregulated *NEAT1* in NPC cells inhibited the targeting of miR-204 to ZEB1, an important modulator of EMT in cancer cells [10], resulting in radioresistance and EMT activation [108]. Thus, *NEAT1* is considered a potential target to enhance the effectiveness of radiotherapy.

4.2. LncRNAs Associated with DNA Repair

4.2.1. LINP1

DNA repair is a complex process in cells that occurs to identify and correct damaged DNA. This process is vital for maintaining genomic integrity and crucially involved in tumorigenesis and cancer radiotherapy. Non-homologous end joining (NHEJ) is one of the major mechanisms responsible for repairing damaged DNA in cancer cells [109]. Human triple-negative breast cancer (TNBC) is an aggressive subtype that presents poor prognosis and resistance to radiotherapy [110]. Recently, an lncRNA in the non-homologous end joining (NHEJ) pathway 1 (*LINP1*) was shown to be overexpressed in TNBC [111]. Upon EGFR (epidermal growth factor receptor) activation, *LINP1* is transcriptionally upregulated via RAS-MEK-ERK signaling and AP1 (activator protein 1) transcription factors. The increased level of *LINP1* acts as a scaffold to stabilize Ku80 and DNA-PKcs interactions and coordinates the NHEJ pathway to enhance DNA repair activity. RNA expression of *LINP1* is also downregulated through interactions with miR-29 in a p53-dependent manner. Importantly, p53-mediated inhibition of LINP1 increases the sensitivity of breast tumor cells to radiotherapy [111].

4.2.2. POU6F2-AS2

Recently, *POU6F2-AS2* was identified as a novel lncRNA involved in the DNA damage response that regulates the sensitivity of cancer cells to ionizing radiation in esophageal squamous cell carcinoma. Further experiments demonstrated that *POU6F2-AS2* interacts with YBX1 (Y-box binding protein) protein and regulates chromatin localization [112]. YBX1 has been characterized as a DNA and RNA binding protein involved in the regulation of DNA damage response, DNA repair regulation, pre-mRNA splicing and mRNA packaging. Moreover, YBX1 is highly overexpressed in multiple cancer types and may serve as a potential prognostic marker for poor outcomes and drug resistance in specific cancer types [113]. Thus, *POU6F2-AS2* may be a master regulator that participates in DNA or RNA synthesis and other processes [112].

4.3. LncRNAs Associated with both EMT and Radioresistance

4.3.1. TUG1

Taurine-upregulated gene 1 (*TUG1*) was initially reported to be induced following treatment with taurine in mouse retinal cells [114]. *TUG1* has been identified as a tumor suppressor or oncogene in various cancer types [115–119]. Recent studies also support an important role of *TUG1* in cancer cell invasion and resistance to radiotherapy. For instance, an earlier study demonstrated a significant increase in expression of *TUG1* in high-grade bladder cancer tissues while its silencing led to suppression of cell proliferation and metastasis. *TUG1* expression was markedly elevated upon radiation treatment [120]. Notably, *TUG1* expression promoted cancer cell invasion and radioresistance via triggering EMT. Further experiments disclosed that reciprocal repression of miR-145 mediates the effects of *TUG1*. Suppression of miR-145 by *TUG1* resulted in re-expression of ZEB2 (zinc finger E-box binding homeobox 2), a master inducer of EMT downregulated by miR-145, and consequently, enhanced EMT and radioresistance [119]. Additionally, silencing of TUG1 was shown to enhance sensitivity to radiotherapy via suppression of HMGB1 (high mobility group box 1) expression [120]. HMGB1 has been identified as a chromosome-binding protein that participates in DNA repair, transcription and nucleosome packaging [121]. The data collectively indicate that *TUG1* acts as a potential regulator of radioresistance in cancer through EMT induction and DNA repair regulation.

4.3.2. HOTAIR

Homeobox (HOX) transcript antisense RNA (*HOTAIR*) initially identified as a spliced and polyadenylated RNA participating in the promotion of carcinogenesis and cancer progression, is considered a prognosis marker for various cancer types [122–124]. In general, *HOTAIR* is a transacting lncRNA that interacts with Polycomb Repressive Complex 2 (PRC2) and lysine-specific demethylase 1 to negatively influence the expression of cancer-related genes [124,125]. PRC2 is a histone methyltransferase involved in epigenetic silencing during different processes, including cancer development [126]. In addition to promoting cancer progression and initiation, recent evidence indicates an important role of *HOTAIR* in radiotherapy for cancer. For instance, *HOTAIR* is upregulated in breast cancer [127], cervical cancer cells [128], CRC [129], pancreatic ductal adenocarcinoma (PDAC) and Lewis lung cancer [130,131]. Overexpression of *HOTAIR* in MDA-MB-231 causes radioresistance by promoting HOXD10 expression and activation of the PI3K/AKT-BAD signaling pathway [127]. Additionally, increased *HOTAIR* expression in cervical cancer cells is reported to enhance aggressive characteristics, such as invasion, proliferation, and radioresistance, via suppression of p21 [128]. Conversely, silencing of *HOTAIR* in CRC cells inhibits cell invasion and increases sensitivity to radiation by regulating apoptosis-related genes, such as BCL-2 and BAX [129]. In PDAC and Lewis lung cancer cells, radiation treatment was shown to repress cell viability and HOTAIR while enhancing WIF-1 (WNT inhibitory factor 1) expression. WIF-1 has been identified as an inhibitor of WNT/β-catenin signaling [132]. Silencing of HOTAIR expression promotes WIF-1 expression and inhibits the nuclear translocation of β-catenin. In contrast, upregulation of HOTAIR appears to enhance nuclear β-catenin expression via inhibiting WIF-1 expression, leading to radioresistance in both PDAC and Lewis lung cancer cells [130,131]. These findings collectively support the utility of HOTAIR as a valid therapeutic target for reversal of radioresistance in several types of cancer.

4.4. LncRNAs Associated with Epigenetic Regulation

PARTICLE

PARTICLE (*promoter of MAT2A-antisense radiation-induced circulating lncRNA*) was recently identified as a novel lncRNA participating in the regulation of cellular response to radiotherapy [133]. *PARTICLE* is located within the *MAT2A* gene and transcribed in an antisense orientation to the forward plus strand from the *MAT2A* promoter. *MAT2A* encodes the catalytic subunit of methionine adenosyltransferase (MAT), a crucial cellular enzyme contributing to production of s-adenosylmethionine (SAM), the principal methyl donor of cells [134,135]. *PARTICLE* is upregulated in both breast cancer cell lines and cells from head-and-neck cancer (HNC) patients after radiation treatment. Radiation-induced nuclear *PARTICLE* forms a DNA-lncRNA triplex at a CpG island upstream of the *MAT2A* promoter, which provides a recruitment platform for methyltransferase and subunits of polycomb repressor complex, including G9a (euchromatic histone lysine methyltransferase 2) and SUZ12 (SUZ12 polycomb repressive complex 2 subunit), leading to transcriptional repression of MAT2A. In addition, cytosolic *PARTICLE* serves as the scaffold for MAT2A. Colocalized *PARTICLE* and *MAT2A* cytosolic transcripts are exported via exosomes in response to radiation treatment in both cancer cells and clinical samples.

MAT2A is the key enzyme catalyzing the formation of SAM, the methyl donor for transmethylation, and plays an important role in DNA repair and protein methylation. Moreover, the level of epigenetic DNA methylation is increased through radiation-induced activation of MAT2A [136]. Thus, dysregulation of PARTICLE may be an important factor influencing the outcome of radiotherapy.

4.5. Plasma LncRNAs Associated with Radiotherapy

GAS5

Recently, Fayda et al. [18] evaluated the plasma levels of three lncRNAs (*GAS5*, *lincRNA-p21*, and *HOTAIR*) in the treatment response in 41 patients with HNC after chemoradiotherapy. The predictive values of these lncRNAs were investigated in patients with complete response (CR) versus those with partial response (PR)/progressive disease (PD). Data from the clinical analyses revealed significantly higher levels of post-treatment *GAS5* in patients with PR/PD, compared to patients with CR. Moreover, the pretreatment *GAS5* level was markedly increased in patients with PR/PD, compared to those with CR, in an MRI-based response evaluation. However, the levels of pre- or post-treatment *lincRNA-p21* and *HOTAIR* were not informative in terms of determining treatment response. Furthermore, *GAS5* has been reported to be down-regulated in multiple cancers and serve as a prognosis marker [137]. Thus, lncRNA *GAS5* may serve as an effective biomarker to predict treatment response in patients with HNC [18].

4.6. Identification of Novel LncRNAs That Potentially Participate in Resistance to Radiotherapy

5-FU-based concurrent chemoradiation is recommended as the standard treatment for colorectal cancer cells. A recent study established chemoradiation-resistant HCT116 cells to investigate the potential lncRNAs involved in treatment resistance. Following microarray expression analysis and further validation, three novel lncRNAs, *TCONS_00026506*, *ENST00000468960*, and *NR_038990*, were identified, which may serve as potential therapeutic targets for radioresistant cancer cells [138].

A recent comparison between the parental nasopharyngeal cancer (NPC) cell line, CNE-2, and radioresistant CNE-2 via next-generation deep sequencing led to the annotation of 2054 novel and 781 known lncRNAs [139]. Further validation via qRT-PCR in both established radioresistant CNE-2 and 6-10B cell lines showed that three novel lncRNAs (*n373932*, *n409627* and *n386034*) exhibit significant expression changes after radiation treatment. Further examination of the expression patterns of *n373932* and its associated gene, *SLITRK5*, in clinical specimens revealed a negative correlation between expression of *n373932* and *SLITRK5*. In view of the results, it is proposed that *n373932*, *n409627* and *n386034*, and interactions between *n373932* and *SLITRK5* are involved in radioresistance of cancer cells [139].

In another study, Zhou et al. [140] performed microarray analysis to identify changes in the lncRNA expression profiles during the time-period of development of radioresistant cells from parental hypopharyngeal squamous cell carcinoma (HSCC), FaDu, after radiation therapy. Among the consistently dysregulated lncRNAs, *TCONS_00018436* was identified as a potential lncRNA mediating resistance of HSCC cells to radiation. Further experiments demonstrated that *TCONS_00018436* exhibits anti-apoptotic activity following radiotherapy and its expression is dysregulated in recurrent HSCC clinical tissue samples [140].

5. Cellular Functions of LncRNAs in CSCs

Targeting of CSCs is considered a promising approach for improving radiotherapeutic outcomes and preventing tumor recurrence and metastasis. Several studies have demonstrated that the dysregulation of lncRNAs in malignant tumors is closely related to the function of CSCs. Investigations linking lncRNAs with CSCs are an increasing focus of cancer therapy. Here, we have reviewed documented studies in the literature regarding lncRNAs participating in CSC regulation.

5.1. LncRNAs Associated with Stemness and Self-Renew of CSCs

5.1.1. LincRNA-p21

Recent studies have demonstrated that *lincRNA-p21* is a potent suppressor of the stem-like traits of CSCs purified from both CRC and glioma cells. *LincRNA-p21* displays anti-EMT activity and is downregulated in CRC and glioma CSCs, compared to non-CSC cancer cells. The lncRNA suppresses β-catenin signaling, leading to decreased cell viability, self-renewal, and glycolysis of CSCs. Its overexpression is reported to dramatically decrease the self-renewal capacity and tumorigenicity of CSCs in xenograft mice. Based on the findings to date, *lincRNA-p21* is considered a promising therapeutic agent against CSCs in CRC [79,141].

5.1.2. LncTCF7

LncTCF7 is located near the TCF7 gene that is overexpressed in HCC and NSCLC [142,143]. TCF7 plays an important role in EMT induction in both HCC and NSCLC cells. The lncRNA is strongly induced in HCC cells via the IL-6/STAT3 signaling axis and appears important for promotion of EMT by IL-6 [142,143]. LncTCF7 is overexpressed in HCC and NSCLC stem cells and shown to be critical for self-renewal while its silencing leads to suppression of the CSC fraction and stem cell-related gene expression. Notably, *lncTCF7* regulates self-renewal of HCC stem cells, as confirmed by tumor sphere formation in vitro and tumor initiating frequency in vivo. Studies to date have shown that the lncRNA recruits the SWI/SNF complex to bind the TCF7 promoter and activate its expression, and TCF7 which could activate the WNT signaling pathways to accelerate self-renewal of HCC stem cells. [142].

5.1.3. HIF2PUT

The lncRNA *HIF2PUT* (hypoxia-inducible factor-2α promoter upstream transcript) has been identified as a promoter upstream transcript (PROMPT) of hypoxia-inducible factor-2α (HIF-2α) in CRC and osteosarcoma stem cells [144,145]. The function of PROMPTs is often associated with adjacent protein-coding transcripts [146] and HIF-2α is closely linked to stem cell properties [147]. *HIF2PUT* expression is positively correlated with HIF-2α levels in patients with osteosarcoma and CRC. Notably, combined higher expression of *HIF2PUT* and HIF-2α is predictive of poorer prognosis of patients with osteosarcoma. Knockdown of *HIF2PUT* has been shown to inhibit HIF-2α expression and CSC-related genes and properties as well as spheroid formation ability, colony formation and invasiveness in CRC cells. These studies support the potential utility of *HIF2PUT* as a novel therapeutic target for different cancers.

5.1.4. HOTAIR

HOTAIR has been investigated in relation to many cancer types [122–124]. In breast cancer, *HOTAIR* enhances metastasis [125]. Additionally, *HOTAIR* regulates breast CSCs, and microarray profiles and functional analyses have revealed that its overexpression induces genes related to stem cell activity and EMT, including CD44, STAT3, ALDH2, ZEB1, Vimentin and SOX2, at least partially through transcriptional suppression of miR-34a [148,149]. *HOTAIR* expression is necessary for maintenance of the CSC phenotype in colon and breast cancer cell lines [149]. Furthermore, this lncRNA suppresses miR-7 expression through inhibition of HoxD10 in breast CSCs. Conversely, overexpression of miR-7 reverses EMT and decreases the CSC population in breast cancer cells via suppressing the STAT3 signaling pathway [150].

HOTAIR has also been shown to participate in the maintenance of stemness in CRC. Its silencing in CD133+ CRC cells leads to decreased cellular proliferation, metastasis and colony-forming properties as well as decreased Vimentin with enhanced E-cadherin expression [151]. Additionally, CD133+ CRC cells with low *HOTAIR* expression show decreased capacities of tumor growth and lung metastasis in xenograft mouse models [151]. Therefore, *HOTAIR* may present a potential therapeutic target against cancers.

5.1.5. Lnc34a

The microRNA, miR-34a, is a downstream target of p53 involved in suppression of various cancer types [152]. Among its many functions, miR-34a has been shown to limit self-renewal of CSCs [153]. Recently, the lncRNA *Lnc34a*, which initiates asymmetric division of stem cells by directly targeting miR-34a and causing disruption of spatial balance, was shown to be overexpressed in CSCs of CRC [154]. *Lnc34a* recruits DNMT3A (DNA methyltransferase 3 α) via PHB2 (prohibitin 2) and HDAC1 (histone deacetylase 1) to simultaneously methylate and deacetylate the promoter region of miR-34a. The epigenetic regulation of miR-34a is independent of its upstream regulator, p53. Higher *Lnc34a* levels promote CSC self-renewal capacity and tumor growth of CRC cells in xenograft models. Moreover, *Lnc34a* is overexpressed in late-stage CRCs, leading to epigenetic silencing of miR-34a and regulation of CRC malignancy [154].

5.1.6. TUG1

TUG1 is cancer-related, binds to PRC1 or PRC2, and suppresses gene expression. Expression of TUG1 is closely associated with cancer progression and therapy [117,118,120,155]. Notch signaling has been shown to promote CSC self-renewal and activity and suppress differentiation [156]. Recent studies have reported that Notch-directed *TUG1* acts as an epigenetic modulator that regulates the glioma cancer stem cell population [155]. *TUG1* is upregulated in CSCs of gliomas and downregulated upon inhibition of Notch. Overexpressed *TUG1* promotes self-renewal of glioma cells by functioning as a molecular sponge for miR-145, an important CSC regulator [157], in the cytoplasm and recruiting Polycomb via YY1 binding activity to repress differentiation genes in the nucleus, such as BDNF(brain derived neurotrophic factor), NGF (nerve growth factor), and NTF3 (neurotrophin 3). *TUG1* presents another specific therapeutic target to eliminate the GSC population [155].

5.1.7. TALNEC2

TALNEC2 was identified as a novel E2F1-regulated lncRNA localizing to the cytosol [158]. *TALNEC2* is overexpressed in GBM from patients with poor prognosis and glioma stem cells. E2Fs serve as transcription factors involved in the regulation of cell cycle progression, in particular, G1/S transition [159,160]. Expression of *TALNEC2* is increased in synchronized cells progressing through the late G1 and early S phases. Silencing of this lncRNA in various cancer cell lines causes cell cycle arrest at the G1 phase and inhibits cellular proliferation. Further functional analyses have revealed that inhibition of *TALNEC2* triggers repression of miR-21 and miR-191, and consequently decreases the self-renewal and mesenchymal transformation of CSCs, increases radiosensitivity and prolongs the survival of xenograft mice bearing CSCs of glioma [158]. Therefore, *TALNEC2* is considered an attractive therapeutic target for GBM.

5.1.8. HOXA11-AS

Homeobox A11 antisense (*HOXA11-AS*) is an lncRNA located near the homeobox A11 (*HOXA11*) gene that is highly expressed in several cancer types [161]. A recent study demonstrated that *HOXA11-AS* expression is correlated with poor cervical cancer prognosis. Overexpression of *HOXA11-AS* in cervical cancer cells promotes proliferation, metastasis and the CD133$^+$/CD44$^+$ CSC subpopulation. Conversely, its knockdown suppresses these aggressive biologic features, accompanied by decreased EMT and CSC-related genes, including NANOG, OCT4, SOX2, and β-catenin. Accordingly, *HOXA11-AS* is under investigation as a potential novel target for cervical cancer treatment [162].

5.1.9. LncRNA-Hh

LncRNA-Hh was recently identified as a Notch, Hedgehog (Hh) pathway-associated lncRNA [163]. Expression of lncRNA-Hh is upregulated in TWIST-positive mammosphere cells and involved in modulation of the Hh pathway. Overexpression of *lncRNA-Hh* in breast cancer cells increases Hh signaling accompanied by elevated levels of SOX2 and OCT4 via targeting to GAS1 (growth arrest specific 1), and consequently contributes to activation of EMT, CSC maintenance and tumorigenesis of breast cancer cells. Conversely, its silencing reverses these oncogenic effects. The data suggest that the Twist-lncRNA-Hh pathway is an important link between EMT and the CSC phenotype of cancer [163].

5.1.10. Linc00617

The lncRNA *TUNA* is required for pluripotency of mouse embryonic stem cells (mESC) [164]. *TUNA* physically binds the promoters of NANOG, SOX2, and FGF4 (fibroblast growth factor 4), and activates transcription by recruiting the protein complex including PTBP1 (polypyrimidine tract binding protein 1), hnRNP-K, and NCL (nucleolin). Recently, the human ortholog of *TUNA*, *Linc00617*, was identified on chromosome 14 [165]. *Linc00617* is overexpressed in breast cancer cell lines and cancer specimens, and closely associated with poor prognosis. Overexpression of *Linc00617* promotes metastasis of breast cancer cells and enhances EMT, accompanied by the acquisition of CSC properties. Furthermore, linc00617 has been shown to physically bind the SOX2 promoter and activate its transcription by recruiting hnRNP-K. Conversely, silencing of *linc00617* suppresses tumor progression. *Linc00617* has therefore emerged as a novel therapeutic target for aggressive breast cancer.

5.1.11. HULC

The lncRNA, highly upregulated in liver cancer (*HULC*), is involved in HCC development and progression [166–168]. A recent report has shown that HULC affects the stemness of HCC cells by cooperating with *MALAT-1*, contributing to the promotion of liver cancer stem generation through binding and loading on the promoter region of telomere repeat-binding factor 2 (TRF2) to enhance telomerase activity [168]. *HULC* also regulates lipid metabolism of hepatoma via regulating miR-9-PPARA (peroxisome proliferator activated receptor α) axis [166]. The findings suggest that HULC, in combination with *MALAT1*, may contribute significantly to malignant growth of liver cancer stem cells through metabolism regulation.

5.1.12. UCA1 (CUDR)

Cancer-upregulated drug resistant (*CUDR*) or urothelial cancer-associated 1 (*UCA1*) is an independent prognostic biomarker highly expressing in various human tumors and involved in tumorigenesis [169,170]. Recent studies have shown that *CUDR* enhances the interactions of SET1A and phosphorylated RB1 (pRB1) in HCC, producing an activated pRB1-SET1A complex. This complex subsequently generates a high level of H3K4 trimethylation that loads on the TRF2 promoter region, causing overexpression of TRF2, which participates in the malignant transformation of HCC stem cells via inducing alterations in telomere length [169]. Concurrently, another report suggested that lncRNA CUDR functions as an oncogene via the *CUDR-HULC* and *CUDR*-β-catenin signaling pathways [171]. Mechanistically, *CUDR* upregulates HULC and β-catenin by inhibiting methylation at the HULC promoter and promoting the formation of a β-catenin promoter-enhancer chromatin loop through interactions with CTCF [171]. Furthermore, CUDR inhibits methylation of the promoter of the lncRNA *H19* by combining with Cyclin D1 to form a complex. CUDR-cyclinD1 upregulates *H19* and subsequently, TERT and C-MYC, to promote self-renewal and proliferation of HCC stem cells [172]. The results collectively suggest that *CUDR* plays a significant role in the self-renewal and proliferation of HCC stem cells through multiple signaling pathways.

5.1.13. *NEAT1*

The lncRNA *NEAT1* is required for maintenance of CSCs of glioma [173,174]. NEAT1 is overexpressed in CD133$^+$ human glioma primary and CD133$^+$ U87 cells. In an earlier study, its knockdown in CD133$^+$ glioma cells resulted in decreased colony formation, cell proliferation, metastasis and increased cell cycle arrest and apoptosis. These effects were accompanied by induction of miR-107 and inhibition of CDK6 (cyclin dependent kinase 6) protein and the microRNA let-7e. Further experiments revealed that restoration of let-7e suppresses proliferation and metastasis but promotes apoptosis in *NEAT1* knockdown CSCs of glioma, which may be attributable to repression of NRAS, a direct target of let-7e known to induce tumorigenesis and stemness [174,175]. The data support a critical role of NEAT1 in the maintenance of stemness of glioma cells via multiple pathways.

5.2. LncRNAs Associated with both EMT and CSCs Generation

5.2.1. LncRNA-ROR

LncRNA-ROR has been identified as a modulator of cell reprogramming and pluripotency. For instance, in breast cancer, linc-ROR appears to function as a ceRNA of miR-205 to prevent degradation of ZEB2, promoting EMT and generating cells with stem cell-like properties [94]. Moreover, linc-ROR serves as a sponge for miR-145 to inhibit its suppressive effect on OCT4, SOX2 and NANOG expression [176]. *LncRNA-ROR* is also considered a key inducer of stemness transcriptional factors (OCT4, SOX2, and NANOG) and affects the CSC population in gastric cancer [177].

5.2.2. H19

H19 is an imprinted oncofetal lncRNA aberrantly expressed in various cancer types with multifaceted roles throughout tumorigenesis [178]. *H19* is induced by signals involving the EMT process and stemness, such as TGF-β, hypoxia, and HGF, suggesting a pivotal role in enhancing stemness of cancer cells via EMT [179]. Overexpression of lncRNA *H19* promotes metastasis, angiogenesis, and stemness in glioblastoma and cholangiocarcinoma cells through effects on EMT [180] and is associated with poor prognosis [180,181]. Furthermore, knockdown of *H19* has been shown to downregulate the stem cell-related genes SOX2, OCT4, and NANOG, as well as other CSC markers in glioblastoma and embryonic carcinoma cell lines [182,183]. These results support the utility of *H19* as a therapeutic target for cancers.

5.2.3. FOXF1-AS1

FOXF1-AS1 has been identified as a novel lncRNA regulating NSCLC progression [184]. Expression of *FOXF1-AS1* is downregulated in tissues of lung cancer. Overexpression of this lncRNA suppresses the migration and invasion of lung cancer cells through regulating EMT while its silencing enhances the stem-like properties of lung cancer cells. Further experiments have revealed that *FOXF1-AS1* physically associates with the PRC2 component, EZH2 (enhancer of zeste 2 polycomb repressive complex 2 subunit), and its knockdown mediates metastasis and stemness of cancer cells in the EZH2-dependent manner. The collective data suggest that *FOXF1-AS1* may serve as an effective therapeutic target for treatment of NSCLC [184].

5.2.4. MALAT1

MALAT1 is reported to participate in the regulation of CSCs in various cancer types [185,186]. *MALAT1* is overexpressed in CSCs of pancreatic cancer and its elimination leads to a decrease in the pancreatic CSC fraction [186]. Knockdown of *MALAT-1* has been shown to inhibit expression of SOX2, suggesting that it contributes to the CSC phenotype via SOX2 regulation. *MALAT1* has been identified as a ceRNA for both miR-200c and miR-145, both of which target SOX2 [186–188]. Thus, the protein appears to regulate pancreatic CSCs through the miR-200c/miR-145/SOX2 signaling axis.

Additionally, loss of *MALAT-1* in the glioma stem cell line, SHG139S, is associated with suppression of stemness markers, such as SOX2 and Nestin [185].

6. Conclusions

Radiotherapy is one of the major treatment modes for patients with cancer and widely used for various malignant tumors [1]. Radiation treatment induces DNA damage via ionization or generation of reactive oxygen species (ROS), leading to elimination of tumor cells, but can concomitantly promote cancer cell metastasis through activation of EMT [3,8,12,13,42,44–47]. Metastasis is a major problem in cancer treatment and closely associated with the rates of morbidity and mortality [2,3,8,44]. Cancer cells with higher EMT activity have been shown to acquire stem cell-like activity [2,48]. Radiotherapy promotes the acquisition or activation of CSCs in cancer via inducing the expression of EMT-related genes [61,63]. CSCs represent a small subpopulation of tumor cells exhibiting radioresistant property within heterogeneous cancer masses. Notably, upon radiation treatment, a small number of non-stem cancer cells have been found to exhibit CSC characteristics. Radiation-induced CSC-like cells with intrinsic stem cell properties subsequently trigger relapse and metastasis of cancer (Figure 1A) [4,61,62].

Determination of CSC-related biomarkers for prediction of radiotherapy outcomes and the molecular mechanisms mediating CSCs and radioresistance remain an urgent requirement for the successful development of novel therapeutic strategies. LncRNAs have emerged as crucial players in the complex signaling network controlling the activation of CSCs and radioresistance. LncRNAs aberrantly expressed in CSCs are active participants in the major signaling pathways governing DNA damage response, DNA repair, apoptosis, and EMT [72,189].

Previous studies have suggested the crucial role of lncRNAs deregulation in cancer recurrence and prognosis [17,18]. Furthermore, advances in profiling of lncRNAs expressions in cancers have highlighted the potential roles as biomarkers in diagnosis and prognosis of the patients. Compared with protein-coding RNAs, lncRNAs are the functional molecules and which expressions are more closely associated with the real tumor status and biological function. In addition, the sensitivity and specificity of lncRNAs are higher than the conventional protein-based markers. Moreover, lncRNAs can be utilized in clinics as non-invasion and convenient biomarkers due to their presence in body fluids [190]. In the current article, several dysregulated lncRNAs involved in the regulation of radioresistance, metastasis and cancer stem cell properties, such as *ANRIL, TUG1, LOC285194, LncRNA-ROR, MALAT1, NEAT1, HOTAIR, POU6F2-AS2, GAS5, HIF2PUT, H19, TALNEC2, HOXA11-AS, Linc00617, HULC,* and *UCA1,* have been found to be associated with the outcomes of radiotherapy and act as valuable prognostic biomarkers (Table 1 and Figure 1B,C). Additionally, *HOTAIR, MALAT1, H9* and *GAS5* have been reported as prognostic markers in the plasma of cancer patients [190].

To date, two major mechanisms have emerged regarding lncRNA-mediated effects on CSC activity and radioresistance via regulation of EMT, DNA repair, apoptosis and stemness: (1) epigenetic regulation of genes, particularly via recruitment of the Polycomb repressor complex (PRC2); and (2) post-transcriptionally by acting as competing endogenous RNAs (ceRNAs) for miRNAs that target genes involved in stemness and radioresistance [100]. The potential lncRNAs influencing radioresistance through CSC generation and the molecular mechanisms involved in radioresistance and stemness are listed in Table 1. Moreover, radiotherapy has been shown to paradoxically induce metastasis of resistant cancer cells, and CSCs are proposed to have utility in predicting tumor recurrence and metastasis [2,48].

Table 1. Summary of the relevant long noncoding RNAs (lncRNAs) in radioresistance, epithelial–mesenchymal transition (EMT)/metastasis and cancer stem cells (CSCs) generation in cancer.

Gene Name	Physiological Functions			Molecules and Signaling Pathways Involved	Expression Status in Cancers	Prognostic Marker of Cancer	Reference
	Radioresistance	EMT and Metastasis	CSCs Generation				
LincRNA-p21	●		●	WNT/β-catenin and p21	Down		[73–79,141]
LOC285194	●	●		VEGF receptor 1 and miR-211	Down	●	[80–82]
ANRIL	●	●		miR-125a, Bax, Smac and Bcl-2	Up	●	[83–88]
AK294004	●			Cyclin D1	Up		[89,90]
LncRNA-ROR	●	●	●	p53, ZEB2, Oct4, SOX2, Nanog, miR-205 and miR-145	Up	●	[91–97,176,177]
MALAT1	●	●	●	Slug, SOX2, Cks1, miR-1, miR-145 and miR-200C	Up	●	[98–101]
NEAT1	●	●	●	miR-204 and ZEB1	Up	●	[104–108,174,175]
LINP1	●	●		Ku80 and DNA-PKcs	Up		[109–111]
POU6F2-AS2	●			YBX1	ND	●	[112,113]
TUG1	●	●	●	miR-145, BDNF, NGF, and NTF3	Up	●	[114–120,155]
HOTAIR	●	●	●	p21, Bcl-2, Bax, WIF-1, HOXD10, Bcl-2, PI3K/AKT-BAD, WNT/β-catenin, CD44, STAT3, ALDH2, ZEB1, Vimentin and SOX2	Up	●	[122–132,148–151]
PARTICLE	●			MAT2A	ND		[133]
GAS5	●			ND	Up	●	[18,137]
TCONS_00026506	●			ND	ND		[138]
ENST00000468960	●			ND	ND		[138]
NR_038990	●			ND	ND		[138]
n373932	●			SLITRK5	ND		[139]
n409627	●			ND	ND		[139]
n386034	●			ND	ND		[139]
TCONS_00018436	●			ND	Up regulation in recurrent cancers		[140]

Table 1. *Cont.*

Gene Name	Physiological Functions			Molecules and Signaling Pathways Involved	Expression Status in Cancers	Prognostic Marker of Cancer	Reference
	Radioresistance	EMT and Metastasis	CSCs Generation				
lncTCF7		●	●	TCF7	Up		[142,143]
HIF2PUT			●	HIF-2α	Up regulation in cancers	●	[144–147]
Lnc34a		●	●	miR-34a	Up		[152–154]
TALNEC2	●		●	miR-21 and miR-191	Up	●	[158–160]
HOXA11-AS		●	●	Nanog, Oct4, Sox2 and β-catenin	Up	●	[161,162]
LncRNA-Hh		●	●	Hh signaling, GAS1, SOX2 and Oct4	ND		[163]
Linc00617		●	●	Nanog, Sox2, and Fgf4	Up	●	[164,165]
HULC		●	●	TRF2, MALAT-1 and miR-9	Up	●	[166–168]
UCA1 (CUDR)		●	●	SET1A, pRB1, HULC, β-catenin, CTCF, C-Myc, cyclinD1, TERT and H19	Up	●	[169–172]
H19		●	●	SOX2, Oct4 and Nanog	Up	●	[178–183]
FOXF1-AS1		●	●	EZH2	Down		[184]

ND: not determined; ●: determined.

Recently, several studies utilizing large-scale genetic and molecular analyses have identified RNA-binding proteins (RBPs) as crucial regulators in genome stability after radiation treatment [191,192]. Upon DNA damage (e.g., ultraviolet and ionizing radiation), RBPs are activated to regulate DNA-damage response (DDR) involving DNA repair, cell cycle progression, and late responses involving genes regulation that influence cell fate. In addition to mRNAs, RBPs also bind lncRNAs, many of which are regulated in response to DNA damage and involved in the radioresistance. For instance, hnRNP-K RBP physically associates with *lincRNA-p21* and mediates in *trans* the transcriptional repression of a large set of genes in a p53-dependent manner [74]. Another study indicates that radiation-induced *LINP1* acts as a scaffold to stabilize Ku80 and DNA-PKcs interactions and coordinates the NHEJ pathway to enhance DNA repair activity [111]. Dysregulated *lincRNA-p21* and *LINP1* are shown to influence the radiosensitivity of cancer cells. Further studies on the lncRNAs and RBPs involved in CSCs and radioresistance should ultimately yield useful insights into the molecular mechanisms underlying radiation-induced CSC generation and cancer metastasis to facilitate the development of effective novel therapeutic strategies against cancer.

Acknowledgments: This work was supported by grants from Chang Gung Memorial Hospital, Taoyuan, Taiwan (CMRPD1D381, CMRPD1D382, CMRPD1D383, CRRPD1F0011, and CRRPD1F0012 to KHL) and from the Ministry of Science and Technology of the Republic of China (MOST 103-2320-B-182-018-MY3, 103-2320-B-182-017-MY3 to KHL; 105-2811-B-182-018, and 105-2321-B-182-002-MY3 to HCC).

Conflicts of Interest: The authors declare no conflict of interest.

References

1.   Delaney, G.; Jacob, S.; Featherstone, C.; Barton, M. The role of radiotherapy in cancer treatment: Estimating optimal utilization from a review of evidence-based clinical guidelines. *Cancer* **2005**, *104*, 1129–1137. [CrossRef] [PubMed]

2.   Lee, S.Y.; Jeong, E.K.; Ju, M.K.; Jeon, H.M.; Kim, M.Y.; Kim, C.H.; Park, H.G.; Han, S.I.; Kang, H.S. Induction of metastasis, cancer stem cell phenotype, and oncogenic metabolism in cancer cells by ionizing radiation. *Mol. Cancer* **2017**, *16*, 10. [CrossRef] [PubMed]

3.   Von Essen, C.F. Radiation enhancement of metastasis: A review. *Clin. Exp. Metastasis* **1991**, *9*, 77–104. [CrossRef] [PubMed]

4.   Phillips, T.M.; McBride, W.H.; Pajonk, F. The response of CD24(-/low)/CD44⁺ breast cancer-initiating cells to radiation. *J. Natl. Cancer Inst.* **2006**, *98*, 1777–1785. [CrossRef] [PubMed]

5.   Piao, L.S.; Hur, W.; Kim, T.K.; Hong, S.W.; Kim, S.W.; Choi, J.E.; Sung, P.S.; Song, M.J.; Lee, B.C.; Hwang, D.; et al. CD133⁺ liver cancer stem cells modulate radioresistance in human hepatocellular carcinoma. *Cancer Lett.* **2012**, *315*, 129–137. [CrossRef] [PubMed]

6.   Gomez-Casal, R.; Bhattacharya, C.; Ganesh, N.; Bailey, L.; Basse, P.; Gibson, M.; Epperly, M.; Levina, V. Non-small cell lung cancer cells survived ionizing radiation treatment display cancer stem cell and epithelial-mesenchymal transition phenotypes. *Mol. Cancer* **2013**, *12*, 94. [CrossRef] [PubMed]

7.   Diehn, M.; Clarke, M.F. Cancer stem cells and radiotherapy: New insights into tumor radioresistance. *J. Natl. Cancer Inst.* **2006**, *98*, 1755–1757. [CrossRef] [PubMed]

8.   Wild-Bode, C.; Weller, M.; Rimner, A.; Dichgans, J.; Wick, W. Sublethal irradiation promotes migration and invasiveness of glioma cells: Implications for radiotherapy of human glioblastoma. *Cancer Res.* **2001**, *61*, 2744–2750. [PubMed]

9.   Biswas, S.; Guix, M.; Rinehart, C.; Dugger, T.C.; Chytil, A.; Moses, H.L.; Freeman, M.L.; Arteaga, C.L. Inhibition of TGF-β with neutralizing antibodies prevents radiation-induced acceleration of metastatic cancer progression. *J. Clin. Investig.* **2007**, *117*, 1305–1313. [CrossRef] [PubMed]

10.   Tsai, J.H.; Yang, J. Epithelial-mesenchymal plasticity in carcinoma metastasis. *Genes Dev.* **2013**, *27*, 2192–2206. [CrossRef] [PubMed]

11.   De Craene, B.; Berx, G. Regulatory networks defining EMT during cancer initiation and progression. *Nat. Rev. Cancer* **2013**, *13*, 97–110. [CrossRef] [PubMed]

12. De Bacco, F.; Luraghi, P.; Medico, E.; Reato, G.; Girolami, F.; Perera, T.; Gabriele, P.; Comoglio, P.M.; Boccaccio, C. Induction of MET by ionizing radiation and its role in radioresistance and invasive growth of cancer. *J. Natl. Cancer Inst.* **2011**, *103*, 645–661. [CrossRef] [PubMed]

13. Zhang, X.; Li, X.; Zhang, N.; Yang, Q.; Moran, M.S. Low doses ionizing radiation enhances the invasiveness of breast cancer cells by inducing epithelial-mesenchymal transition. *Biochem. Biophys. Res. Commun.* **2011**, *412*, 188–192. [CrossRef] [PubMed]

14. Kurrey, N.K.; Jalgaonkar, S.P.; Joglekar, A.V.; Ghanate, A.D.; Chaskar, P.D.; Doiphode, R.Y.; Bapat, S.A. Snail and slug mediate radioresistance and chemoresistance by antagonizing p53-mediated apoptosis and acquiring a stem-like phenotype in ovarian cancer cells. *Stem Cells* **2009**, *27*, 2059–2068. [CrossRef] [PubMed]

15. Mani, S.A.; Guo, W.; Liao, M.J.; Eaton, E.N.; Ayyanan, A.; Zhou, A.Y.; Brooks, M.; Reinhard, F.; Zhang, C.C.; Shipitsin, M. The epithelial-mesenchymal transition generates cells with properties of stem cells. *Cell* **2008**, *133*, 704–715. [CrossRef] [PubMed]

16. Wang, K.C.; Chang, H.Y. Molecular mechanisms of long noncoding RNAs. *Mol. Cell* **2011**, *43*, 904–914. [CrossRef] [PubMed]

17. Schmitt, A.M.; Chang, H.Y. Long Noncoding RNAs in Cancer Pathways. *Cancer Cell* **2016**, *29*, 452–463. [CrossRef] [PubMed]

18. Fayda, M.; Isin, M.; Tambas, M.; Guveli, M.; Meral, R.; Altun, M.; Sahin, D.; Ozkan, G.; Sanli, Y.; Isin, H.; et al. Do circulating long non-coding RNAs (lncRNAs) (LincRNA-p21, GAS 5, HOTAIR) predict the treatment response in patients with head and neck cancer treated with chemoradiotherapy? *Tumour Biol.* **2016**, *37*, 3969–3978. [CrossRef] [PubMed]

19. Zielske, S.P.; Spalding, A.C.; Wicha, M.S.; Lawrence, T.S. Ablation of breast cancer stem cells with radiation. *Transl. Oncol.* **2011**, *4*, 227–233. [CrossRef] [PubMed]

20. Clarke, M.F.; Dick, J.E.; Dirks, P.B.; Eaves, C.J.; Jamieson, C.H.; Jones, D.L.; Visvader, J.; Weissman, I.L.; Wahl, G.M. Cancer stem cells-perspectives on current status and future directions: AACR workshop on cancer stem cells. *Cancer Res.* **2006**, *66*, 9339–9344. [CrossRef] [PubMed]

21. Lee, H.E.; Kim, J.H.; Kim, Y.J.; Choi, S.Y.; Kim, S.W.; Kang, E.; Chung, I.Y.; Kim, I.A.; Kim, E.J.; Choi, Y.; et al. An increase in cancer stem cell population after primary systemic therapy is a poor prognostic factor in breast cancer. *Br. J. Cancer* **2011**, *104*, 1730–1738. [CrossRef] [PubMed]

22. Lapidot, T.; Sirard, C.; Vormoor, J.; Murdoch, B.; Hoang, T.; Caceres-Cortes, J.; Minden, M.; Paterson, B.; Caligiuri, M.A.; Dick, J.E.; et al. A cell initiating human acute myeloid leukaemia after transplantation into SCID mice. *Nature* **1994**, *367*, 645–648. [CrossRef] [PubMed]

23. Al-Hajj, M.; Wicha, M.S.; Benito-Hernandez, A.; Morrison, S.J.; Clarke, M.F. Prospective identification of tumorigenic breast cancer cells. *Proc. Natl. Acad. Sci. USA* **2003**, *100*, 3983–3988. [CrossRef] [PubMed]

24. Kreso, A.; Dick, J.E. Evolution of the cancer stem cell model. *Cell Stem Cell* **2014**, *14*, 275–291. [CrossRef] [PubMed]

25. Wang, J.; Guo, L.P.; Chen, L.Z.; Zeng, Y.X.; Lu, S.H. Identification of cancer stem cell-like side population cells in human nasopharyngeal carcinoma cell line. *Cancer Res.* **2007**, *67*, 3716–3724. [CrossRef] [PubMed]

26. Hu, L.; McArthur, C.; Jaffe, R.B. Ovarian cancer stem-like side-population cells are tumourigenic and chemoresistant. *Br. J. Cancer* **2010**, *102*, 1276–1283. [CrossRef] [PubMed]

27. Kondo, T.; Setoguchi, T.; Taga, T. Persistence of a small subpopulation of cancer stem-like cells in the C6 glioma cell line. *Proc. Natl. Acad. Sci. USA* **2004**, *101*, 781–786. [CrossRef] [PubMed]

28. Ginestier, C.; Hur, M.H.; Charafe-Jauffret, E.; Monville, F.; Dutcher, J.; Brown, M.; Jacquemier, J.; Viens, P.; Kleer, C.G.; Liu, S.; et al. ALDH1 is a marker of normal and malignant human mammary stem cells and a predictor of poor clinical outcome. *Cell Stem Cell* **2007**, *1*, 555–567. [CrossRef] [PubMed]

29. Sullivan, J.P.; Spinola, M.; Dodge, M.; Raso, M.G.; Behrens, C.; Gao, B.; Schuster, K.; Shao, C.; Larsen, J.E.; Sullivan, L.A.; et al. Aldehyde dehydrogenase activity selects for lung adenocarcinoma stem cells dependent on notch signaling. *Cancer Res.* **2010**, *70*, 9937–9948. [CrossRef] [PubMed]

30. Kim, M.P.; Fleming, J.B.; Wang, H.; Abbruzzese, J.L.; Choi, W.; Kopetz, S.; McConkey, D.J.; Evans, D.B.; Gallick, G.E. ALDH activity selectively defines an enhanced tumor-initiating cell population relative to CD133 expression in human pancreatic adenocarcinoma. *PLoS ONE* **2011**, *6*, e20636. [CrossRef] [PubMed]

31. Pattabiraman, D.R.; Weinberg, R.A. Tackling the cancer stem cells—What challenges do they pose? *Nat. Rev. Drug Discov.* **2014**, *13*, 497–512. [CrossRef] [PubMed]

32. Blazek, E.R.; Foutch, J.L.; Maki, G. Daoy medulloblastoma cells that express CD133 are radioresistant relative to CD133⁻ cells, and the CD133⁺ sector is enlarged by hypoxia. *Int. J. Radiat. Oncol. Biol. Phys.* **2007**, *67*, 1–5. [CrossRef] [PubMed]

33. De Jong, M.C.; Pramana, J.; van der Wal, J.E.; Lacko, M.; Peutz-Kootstra, C.J.; de Jong, J.M.; Takes, R.P.; Kaanders, J.H.; van der Laan, B.F.; Wachters, J.; et al. CD44 expression predicts local recurrence after radiotherapy in larynx cancer. *Clin. Cancer Res.* **2010**, *16*, 5329–5338. [CrossRef] [PubMed]

34. Du, Z.; Qin, R.; Wei, C.; Wang, M.; Shi, C.; Tian, R.; Peng, C. Pancreatic cancer cells resistant to chemoradiotherapy rich in "stem-cell-like" tumor cells. *Dig. Dis. Sci.* **2011**, *56*, 741–750. [CrossRef] [PubMed]

35. Morrison, R.; Schleicher, S.M.; Sun, Y.; Niermann, K.J.; Kim, S.; Spratt, D.E.; Chung, C.H.; Lu, B. Targeting the mechanisms of resistance to chemotherapy and radiotherapy with the cancer stem cell hypothesis. *J. Oncol.* **2010**, *2011*. [CrossRef] [PubMed]

36. Signore, M.; Ricci-Vitiani, L.; de Maria, R. Targeting apoptosis pathways in cancer stem cells. *Cancer Lett.* **2013**, *332*, 374–382. [CrossRef] [PubMed]

37. Weber, G.F. Why does cancer therapy lack effective anti-metastasis drugs? *Cancer Lett.* **2013**, *328*, 207–211. [CrossRef] [PubMed]

38. Cui, Y.H.; Suh, Y.; Lee, H.J.; Yoo, K.C.; Uddin, N.; Jeong, Y.J.; Lee, J.S.; Hwang, S.G.; Nam, S.Y.; Kim, M.J.; et al. Radiation promotes invasiveness of non-small-cell lung cancer cells through granulocyte-colony-stimulating factor. *Oncogene* **2015**, *34*, 5372–5382. [CrossRef] [PubMed]

39. Zhao, Q.; Mao, A.; Guo, R.; Zhang, L.; Yan, J.; Sun, C.; Tang, J.; Ye, Y.; Zhang, Y.; Zhang, H.; et al. Suppression of radiation-induced migration of non-small cell lung cancer through inhibition of Nrf2-Notch Axis. *Oncotarget* **2017**, *8*, 36603–36613. [CrossRef] [PubMed]

40. Chen, Y.; Liu, W.; Wang, P.; Hou, H.; Liu, N.; Gong, L.; Wang, Y.; Ji, K.; Zhao, L.; Wang, P.; et al. Halofuginone inhibits radiotherapy-induced epithelial-mesenchymal transition in lung cancer. *Oncotarget* **2016**, *7*, 71341–71352. [CrossRef] [PubMed]

41. Liu, W.; Huang, Y.J.; Liu, C.; Yang, Y.Y.; Liu, H.; Cui, J.G.; Cheng, Y.; Gao, F.; Cai, J.M.; Li, B.L.; et al. Inhibition of TBK1 attenuates radiation-induced epithelial-mesenchymal transition of A549 human lung cancer cells via activation of GSK-3β and repression of ZEB1. *Lab. Investig.* **2014**, *94*, 362–370. [CrossRef] [PubMed]

42. Su, H.; Jin, X.; Zhang, X.; Zhao, L.; Lin, B.; Li, L.; Fei, Z.; Shen, L.; Fang, Y.; Pan, H.; et al. FH535 increases the radiosensitivity and reverses epithelial-to-mesenchymal transition of radioresistant esophageal cancer cell line KYSE-150R. *J. Transl. Med.* **2015**, *13*, 104. [CrossRef] [PubMed]

43. Zang, C.; Liu, X.; Li, B.; He, Y.; Jing, S.; He, Y.; Wu, W.; Zhang, B.; Ma, S.; Dai, W.; et al. IL-6/STAT3/TWIST inhibition reverses ionizing radiation-induced EMT and radioresistance in esophageal squamous carcinoma. *Oncotarget* **2017**, *8*, 11228–11238. [CrossRef] [PubMed]

44. Moncharmont, C.; Levy, A.; Guy, J.B.; Falk, A.T.; Guilbert, M.; Trone, J.C.; Alphonse, G.; Gilormini, M.; Ardail, D.; Toillon, R.A.; et al. Radiation-enhanced cell migration/invasion process: A review. *Crit. Rev. Oncol. Hematol.* **2014**, *92*, 133–142. [CrossRef] [PubMed]

45. Li, G.; Liu, Y.; Su, Z.W.; Ren, S.L.; Liu, C.; Tian, Y.Q.; Qiu, Y.Z. Irradiation induced epithelial-mesenchymal transition in nasopharyngeal carcinoma in vitro. *Chin. J. Otorhinolaryngol. Head Neck Surg.* **2013**, *48*, 662–667.

46. Kawamoto, A.; Yokoe, T.; Tanaka, K.; Saigusa, S.; Toiyama, Y.; Yasuda, H.; Inoue, Y.; Miki, C.; Kusunoki, M. Radiation induces epithelial-mesenchymal transition in colorectal cancer cells. *Oncol. Rep.* **2012**, *27*, 51–57. [CrossRef] [PubMed]

47. Park, J.K.; Jang, S.J.; Kang, S.W.; Park, S.; Hwang, S.G.; Kim, W.J.; Kang, J.H.; Um, H.D. Establishment of animal model for the analysis of cancer cell metastasis during radiotherapy. *Radiat. Oncol.* **2012**, *7*, 153. [CrossRef] [PubMed]

48. Li, F.; Zhou, K.; Gao, L.; Zhang, B.; Li, W.; Yan, W.; Song, X.; Yu, H.; Wang, S.; Yu, N. Radiation induces the generation of cancer stem cells: A novel mechanism for cancer radioresistance. *Oncol. Lett.* **2016**, *12*, 3059–3065. [PubMed]

49. Chang, L.; Graham, P.H.; Hao, J.; Bucci, J.; Cozzi, P.J.; Kearsley, J.H.; Li, Y. Emerging roles of radioresistance in prostate cancer metastasis and radiation therapy. *Cancer Metastasis Rev.* **2014**, *33*, 469–496. [CrossRef] [PubMed]

50. Bastos, L.G.; de Marcondes, P.G.; de-Freitas-Junior, J.C.; Leve, F.; Mencalha, A.L.; de Souza, W.F.; de Araujo, W.M.; Tanaka, M.N.; Abdelhay, E.S.; Morgado-Diaz, J.A. Progeny from irradiated colorectal cancer cells acquire an EMT-like phenotype and activate Wnt/β-catenin pathway. *J. Cell Biochem.* **2014**, *115*, 2175–2187. [CrossRef] [PubMed]
51. Zhang, P.; Wei, Y.; Wang, L.; Debeb, B.G.; Yuan, Y.; Zhang, J.; Yuan, J.; Wang, M.; Chen, D.; Sun, Y. ATM-mediated stabilization of ZEB1 promotes DNA damage response and radioresistance through CHK1. *Nat. Cell Biol.* **2014**, *16*, 864–875. [CrossRef] [PubMed]
52. Kim, E.; Youn, H.; Kwon, T.; Son, B.; Kang, J.; Yang, H.J.; Seong, K.M.; Kim, W.; Youn, B. PAK1 tyrosine phosphorylation is required to induce epithelial-mesenchymal transition and radioresistance in lung cancer cells. *Cancer Res.* **2014**, *74*, 5520–5531. [CrossRef] [PubMed]
53. Jiang, X.; Wang, J.; Zhang, K.; Tang, S.; Ren, C.; Chen, Y. The role of CD29-ILK-Akt signaling-mediated epithelial-mesenchymal transition of liver epithelial cells and chemoresistance and radioresistance in hepatocellular carcinoma cells. *Med. Oncol.* **2015**, *32*, 141. [CrossRef] [PubMed]
54. Zhang, X.; Zheng, L.; Sun, Y.; Wang, T.; Wang, B. Tangeretin enhances radiosensitivity and inhibits the radiation-induced epithelial-mesenchymal transition of gastric cancer cells. *Oncol. Rep.* **2015**, *34*, 302–310. [CrossRef] [PubMed]
55. Kajita, M.; McClinic, K.N.; Wade, P.A. Aberrant expression of the transcription factors snail and slug alters the response to genotoxic stress. *Mol. Cell Biol.* **2004**, *24*, 7559–7566. [CrossRef] [PubMed]
56. Wang, Z.; Li, Y.; Kong, D.; Banerjee, S.; Ahmad, A.; Azmi, A.S.; Ali, S.; Abbruzzese, J.L.; Gallick, G.E.; Sarkar, F.H. Acquisition of epithelial-mesenchymal transition phenotype of gemcitabine-resistant pancreatic cancer cells is linked with activation of the notch signaling pathway. *Cancer Res.* **2009**, *69*, 2400–2407. [CrossRef] [PubMed]
57. Dean, M.; Fojo, T.; Bates, S. Tumour stem cells and drug resistance. *Nat. Rev. Cancer* **2005**, *5*, 275–284. [CrossRef] [PubMed]
58. Diehn, M.; Cho, R.W.; Lobo, N.A.; Kalisky, T.; Dorie, M.J.; Kulp, A.N.; Qian, D.; Lam, J.S.; Ailles, L.E.; Wong, M.; et al. Association of reactive oxygen species levels and radioresistance in cancer stem cells. *Nature* **2009**, *458*, 780–783. [CrossRef] [PubMed]
59. Cho, Y.M.; Kim, Y.S.; Kang, M.J.; Farrar, W.L.; Hurt, E.M. Long-term recovery of irradiated prostate cancer increases cancer stem cells. *Prostate* **2012**, *72*, 1746–1756. [CrossRef] [PubMed]
60. Al-Assar, O.; Muschel, R.J.; Mantoni, T.S.; McKenna, W.G.; Brunner, T.B. Radiation response of cancer stem-like cells from established human cell lines after sorting for surface markers. *Int. J. Radiat. Oncol. Biol. Phys.* **2009**, *75*, 1216–1225. [CrossRef] [PubMed]
61. Lagadec, C.; Vlashi, E.; Della Donna, L.; Dekmezian, C.; Pajonk, F. Radiation-induced reprogramming of breast cancer cells. *Stem Cells* **2012**, *30*, 833–844. [CrossRef] [PubMed]
62. Wang, Y.; Li, W.; Patel, S.S.; Cong, J.; Zhang, N.; Sabbatino, F.; Liu, X.; Qi, Y.; Huang, P.; Lee, H. Blocking the formation of radiation-induced breast cancer stem cells. *Oncotarget* **2014**, *5*, 3743–3755. [CrossRef] [PubMed]
63. Ghisolfi, L.; Keates, A.C.; Hu, X.; Lee, D.K.; Li, C.J. Ionizing radiation induces stemness in cancer cells. *PLoS ONE* **2012**, *7*, e43628. [CrossRef] [PubMed]
64. Shuang, Z.Y.; Wu, W.C.; Xu, J.; Lin, G.; Liu, Y.C.; Lao, X.M.; Zheng, L.; Li, S. Transforming growth factor-β1-induced epithelial-mesenchymal transition generates ALDH-positive cells with stem cell properties in cholangiocarcinoma. *Cancer Lett.* **2014**, *354*, 320–328. [CrossRef] [PubMed]
65. Bessede, E.; Staedel, C.; Acuna Amador, L.A.; Nguyen, P.H.; Chambonnier, L.; Hatakeyama, M.; Belleannee, G.; Megraud, F.; Varon, C. Helicobacter pylori generates cells with cancer stem cell properties via epithelial-mesenchymal transition-like changes. *Oncogene* **2014**, *33*, 4123–4131. [CrossRef] [PubMed]
66. Kang, K.S.; Choi, Y.P.; Gao, M.Q.; Kang, S.; Kim, B.G.; Lee, J.H.; Kwon, M.J.; Shin, Y.K.; Cho, N.H. CD24(+) ovary cancer cells exhibit an invasive mesenchymal phenotype. *Biochem. Biophys. Res. Commun.* **2013**, *432*, 333–338. [CrossRef] [PubMed]
67. Zhi, Y.; Mou, Z.; Chen, J.; He, Y.; Dong, H.; Fu, X.; Wu, Y. B7H1 Expression and epithelial-to-mesenchymal transition phenotypes on colorectal cancer stem-like cells. *PLoS ONE* **2015**, *10*, e0135528. [CrossRef] [PubMed]
68. Mortazavi, A.; Williams, B.A.; McCue, K.; Schaeffer, L.; Wold, B. Mapping and quantifying mammalian transcriptomes by RNA-Seq. *Nat. Methods* **2008**, *5*, 621–628. [CrossRef] [PubMed]

69. Trapnell, C.; Williams, B.A.; Pertea, G.; Mortazavi, A.; Kwan, G.; van Baren, M.J.; Salzberg, S.L.; Wold, B.J.; Pachter, L. Transcript assembly and quantification by RNA-Seq reveals unannotated transcripts and isoform switching during cell differentiation. *Nat. Biotechnol.* **2010**, *28*, 511–515. [CrossRef] [PubMed]

70. Engreitz, J.M.; Ollikainen, N.; Guttman, M. Long non-coding RNAs: Spatial amplifiers that control nuclear structure and gene expression. *Nat. Rev. Mol. Cell Biol.* **2016**, *17*, 756–770. [CrossRef] [PubMed]

71. Matsumoto, A.; Pasut, A.; Matsumoto, M.; Yamashita, R.; Fung, J.; Monteleone, E.; Saghatelian, A.; Nakayama, K.I.; Clohessy, J.G.; Pandolfi, P.P. mTORC1 and muscle regeneration are regulated by the LINC00961-encoded SPAR polypeptide. *Nature* **2017**, *541*, 228–232. [CrossRef] [PubMed]

72. Ulitsky, I.; Bartel, D.P. LincRNAs: Genomics, evolution, and mechanisms. *Cell* **2013**, *154*, 26–46. [CrossRef] [PubMed]

73. Huarte, M.; Guttman, M.; Feldser, D.; Garber, M.; Koziol, M.J.; Kenzelmann-Broz, D.; Khalil, A.M.; Zuk, O.; Amit, I.; Rabani, M.A.; et al. large intergenic noncoding RNA induced by p53 mediates global gene repression in the p53 response. *Cell* **2010**, *142*, 409–419. [CrossRef] [PubMed]

74. Hall, J.R.; Messenger, Z.J.; Tam, H.W.; Phillips, S.L.; Recio, L.; Smart, R.C. Long noncoding RNA lincRNA-p21 is the major mediator of UVB-induced and p53-dependent apoptosis in keratinocytes. *Cell Death. Dis.* **2015**, *6*, e1700. [CrossRef] [PubMed]

75. Dimitrova, N.; Zamudio, J.R.; Jong, R.M.; Soukup, D.; Resnick, R.; Sarma, K.; Ward, A.J.; Raj, A.; Lee, J.T.; Sharp, P.A. LincRNA-p21 activates p21 in cis to promote Polycomb target gene expression and to enforce the G1/S checkpoint. *Mol. Cell* **2014**, *54*, 777–790. [CrossRef] [PubMed]

76. Zhai, H.; Fesler, A.; Schee, K.; Fodstad, O.; Flatmark, K.; Ju, J. Clinical significance of long intergenic noncoding RNA-p21 in colorectal cancer. *Clin. Colorectal. Cancer* **2013**, *12*, 261–266. [CrossRef] [PubMed]

77. Wang, G.; Li, Z.; Zhao, Q.; Zhu, Y.; Zhao, C.; Li, X.; Ma, Z.; Li, X.; Zhang, Y. LincRNA-p21 enhances the sensitivity of radiotherapy for human colorectal cancer by targeting the Wnt/β-catenin signaling pathway. *Oncol. Rep.* **2014**, *31*, 1839–1845. [CrossRef] [PubMed]

78. Yoon, J.H.; Abdelmohsen, K.; Srikantan, S.; Yang, X.; Martindale, J.L.; De, S.; Huarte, M.; Zhan, M.; Becker, K.G.; Gorospe, M.; et al. LincRNA-p21 suppresses target mRNA translation. *Mol. Cell* **2012**, *47*, 648–655. [CrossRef] [PubMed]

79. Yang, W.; Yu, H.; Shen, Y.; Liu, Y.; Yang, Z.; Sun, T. MiR-146b-5p overexpression attenuates stemness and radioresistance of glioma stem cells by targeting HuR/lincRNA-p21/β-catenin pathway. *Oncotarget* **2016**, *7*, 41505–41526. [CrossRef] [PubMed]

80. Pasic, I.; Shlien, A.; Durbin, A.D.; Stavropoulos, D.J.; Baskin, B.; Ray, P.N.; Novokmet, A.; Malkin, D. Recurrent focal copy-number changes and loss of heterozygosity implicate two noncoding RNAs and one tumor suppressor gene at chromosome 3q13. 31 in osteosarcoma. *Cancer Res.* **2010**, *70*, 160–171. [CrossRef] [PubMed]

81. Liu, Q.; Huang, J.; Zhou, N.; Zhang, Z.; Zhang, A.; Lu, Z.; Wu, F.; Mo, Y.Y. LncRNA loc285194 is a p53-regulated tumor suppressor. *Nucleic Acids Res.* **2013**, *41*, 4976–4987. [CrossRef] [PubMed]

82. Tong, Y.S.; Zhou, X.L.; Wang, X.W.; Wu, Q.Q.; Yang, T.X.; Lv, J.; Yang, J.S.; Zhu, B.; Cao, X.F. Association of decreased expression of long non-coding RNA LOC285194 with chemoradiotherapy resistance and poor prognosis in esophageal squamous cell carcinoma. *J. Transl. Med.* **2014**, *12*, 233. [CrossRef] [PubMed]

83. Pasmant, E.; Laurendeau, I.; Heron, D.; Vidaud, M.; Vidaud, D.; Bieche, I. Characterization of a germ-line deletion, including the entire INK4/ARF locus, in a melanoma-neural system tumor family: Identification of ANRIL, an antisense noncoding RNA whose expression coclusters with ARF. *Cancer Res.* **2007**, *67*, 3963–3969. [CrossRef] [PubMed]

84. Zhang, E.B.; Kong, R.; Yin, D.D.; You, L.H.; Sun, M.; Han, L.; Xu, T.P.; Xia, R.; Yang, J.S.; De, W.; et al. Long noncoding RNA ANRIL indicates a poor prognosis of gastric cancer and promotes tumor growth by epigenetically silencing of miR-99a/miR-449a. *Oncotarget* **2014**, *5*, 2276–2292. [CrossRef] [PubMed]

85. Iranpour, M.; Soudyab, M.; Geranpayeh, L.; Mirfakhraie, R.; Azargashb, E.; Movafagh, A.; Ghafouri-Fard, S. Expression analysis of four long noncoding RNAs in breast cancer. *J. Int. Soc. Oncodevelopm. Biol. Med.* **2016**, *37*, 2933–2940. [CrossRef] [PubMed]

86. Zhu, H.; Li, X.; Song, Y.; Zhang, P.; Xiao, Y.; Xing, Y. Long non-coding RNA ANRIL is up-regulated in bladder cancer and regulates bladder cancer cell proliferation and apoptosis through the intrinsic pathway. *Biochem. Biophys. Res. Commun.* **2015**, *467*, 223–228. [CrossRef] [PubMed]

87. Hu, X.; Jiang, H.; Jiang, X. Downregulation of lncRNA ANRIL inhibits proliferation, induces apoptosis, and enhances radiosensitivity in nasopharyngeal carcinoma cells through regulating miR-125a. *Cancer Biol. Ther.* **2017**, 1–8. [CrossRef] [PubMed]

88. Sun, Y.M.; Lin, K.Y.; Chen, Y.Q. Diverse functions of miR-125 family in different cell contexts. *J. Hematol. Oncol.* **2013**, *6*, 6. [CrossRef] [PubMed]

89. Wang, Q.; Fan, H.; Liu, Y.; Yin, Z.; Cai, H.; Liu, J.; Wang, Z.; Shao, M.; Sun, X.; Diao, J.; et al. Curcumin enhances the radiosensitivity in nasopharyngeal carcinoma cells involving the reversal of differentially expressed long non-coding RNAs. *Int. J. Oncol.* **2014**, *44*, 858–864. [CrossRef] [PubMed]

90. Musgrove, E.A.; Caldon, C.E.; Barraclough, J.; Stone, A.; Sutherland, R.L. Cyclin D as a therapeutic target in cancer. *Nat. Rev. Cancer* **2011**, *11*, 558–572. [CrossRef] [PubMed]

91. Loewer, S.; Cabili, M.N.; Guttman, M.; Loh, Y.H.; Thomas, K.; Park, I.H.; Garber, M.; Curran, M.; Onder, T.; Agarwal, S.; et al. Large intergenic non-coding RNA-RoR modulates reprogramming of human induced pluripotent stem cells. *Nat. Genet.* **2010**, *42*, 1113–1117. [CrossRef] [PubMed]

92. Cheng, E.C.; Lin, H. Repressing the repressor: A lincRNA as a MicroRNA sponge in embryonic stem cell self-renewal. *Dev. Cell* **2013**, *25*, 1–2. [CrossRef] [PubMed]

93. Zhang, A.; Zhou, N.; Huang, J.; Liu, Q.; Fukuda, K.; Ma, D.; Lu, Z.; Bai, C.; Watabe, K.; Mo, Y.Y.; et al. The human long non-coding RNA-RoR is a p53 repressor in response to DNA damage. *Cell Res.* **2013**, *23*, 340–350. [CrossRef] [PubMed]

94. Hou, P.; Zhao, Y.; Li, Z.; Yao, R.; Ma, M.; Gao, Y.; Zhao, L.; Zhang, Y.; Huang, B.; Lu, J. LincRNA-ROR induces epithelial-to-mesenchymal transition and contributes to breast cancer tumorigenesis and metastasis. *Cell Death Dis.* **2014**, *5*, e1287. [CrossRef] [PubMed]

95. Yang, P.; Yang, Y.; An, W.; Xu, J.; Zhang, G.; Jie, J.; Zhang, Q. The long noncoding RNA-ROR promotes the resistance of radiotherapy for human colorectal cancer cells by targeting the p53/miR-145 pathway. *J. Gastroenterol. Hepatol.* **2017**, *32*, 837–845. [CrossRef] [PubMed]

96. Pan, Y.; Li, C.; Chen, J.; Zhang, K.; Chu, X.; Wang, R.; Chen, L. The emerging roles of long noncoding RNA ROR (lincRNA-ROR) and its possible mechanisms in human cancers. *Cell Physiol. Biochem.* **2016**, *40*, 219–229. [CrossRef] [PubMed]

97. Wang, S.H.; Zhang, M.D.; Wu, X.C.; Weng, M.Z.; Zhou, D.; Quan, Z.W. Overexpression of LncRNA-ROR predicts a poor outcome in gallbladder cancer patients and promotes the tumor cells proliferation, migration, and invasion. *Tumour Biol.* **2016**, *37*, 12867–12875. [CrossRef] [PubMed]

98. Ji, P.; Diederichs, S.; Wang, W.; Boing, S.; Metzger, R.; Schneider, P.M.; Tidow, N.; Brandt, B.; Buerger, H.; Bulk, E. MALAT-1, a novel noncoding RNA, and thymosin β4 predict metastasis and survival in early-stage non-small cell lung cancer. *Oncogene* **2003**, *22*, 8031–8041. [CrossRef] [PubMed]

99. Li, Z.; Zhou, Y.; Tu, B.; Bu, Y.; Liu, A.; Xie, C. Long noncoding RNA MALAT1 affects the efficacy of radiotherapy for esophageal squamous cell carcinoma by regulating CKS1 expression. *J. Oral. Pathol. Med.* **2016**. [CrossRef] [PubMed]

100. Heery, R.; Finn, S.P.; Cuffe, S.; Gray, S.G. Long non-coding RNAs: Key regulators of epithelial-mesenchymal transition, tumour drug resistance and cancer stem cells. *Cancers* **2017**, *9*, 38. [CrossRef] [PubMed]

101. Jin, C.; Yan, B.; Lu, Q.; Lin, Y.; Ma, L. The role of MALAT1/miR-1/slug axis on radioresistance in nasopharyngeal carcinoma. *Tumour Biol.* **2016**, *37*, 4025–4033. [CrossRef] [PubMed]

102. Hu, L.; Wu, Y.; Tan, D.; Meng, H.; Wang, K.; Bai, Y.; Yang, K. Up-regulation of long noncoding RNA MALAT1 contributes to proliferation and metastasis in esophageal squamous cell carcinoma. *J. Exp. Clin. Cancer Res.* **2015**, *34*, 7. [CrossRef] [PubMed]

103. Lu, H.; He, Y.; Lin, L.; Qi, Z.; Ma, L.; Li, L.; Su, Y. Long non-coding RNA MALAT1 modulates radiosensitivity of HR-HPV+ cervical cancer via sponging miR-145. *Tumour Biol.* **2016**, *37*, 1683–1691. [CrossRef] [PubMed]

104. Blume, C.J.; Hotz-Wagenblatt, A.; Hullein, J.; Sellner, L.; Jethwa, A.; Stolz, T.; Slabicki, M.; Lee, K.; Sharathchandra, A.; Benner, A. P53-dependent non-coding RNA networks in chronic lymphocytic leukemia. *Leukemia* **2015**, *29*, 2015–2023. [CrossRef] [PubMed]

105. Adriaens, C.; Standaert, L.; Barra, J.; Latil, M.; Verfaillie, A.; Kalev, P.; Boeckx, B.; Wijnhoven, P.W.; Radaelli, E.; Vermi, W.; et al. P53 induces formation of NEAT1 lncRNA-containing paraspeckles that modulate replication stress response and chemosensitivity. *Nat. Med.* **2016**, *22*, 861–868. [CrossRef] [PubMed]

106. Dobbelstein, M.; Sorensen, C.S. Exploiting replicative stress to treat cancer. *Nat. Rev. Drug Discov.* **2015**, *14*, 405–423. [CrossRef] [PubMed]

107. Yu, X.; Li, Z.; Zheng, H.; Chan, M.T.; Wu, W.K. NEAT1: A novel cancer-related long non-coding RNA. *Cell Prolif.* **2017**. [CrossRef] [PubMed]

108. Lu, Y.; Li, T.; Wei, G.; Liu, L.; Chen, Q.; Xu, L.; Zhang, K.; Zeng, D.; Liao, R. The long non-coding RNA NEAT1 regulates epithelial to mesenchymal transition and radioresistance in through miR-204/ZEB1 axis in nasopharyngeal carcinoma. *Tumour Biol.* **2016**, *37*, 11733–11741. [CrossRef] [PubMed]

109. Goldstein, M.; Kastan, M.B. The DNA damage response: Implications for tumor responses to radiation and chemotherapy. *Annu. Rev. Med.* **2015**, *66*, 129–143. [CrossRef] [PubMed]

110. Cancer Genome Atlas Network. Comprehensive molecular portraits of human breast tumours. *Nature* **2012**, *490*, 61–70.

111. Zhang, Y.; He, Q.; Hu, Z.; Feng, Y.; Fan, L.; Tang, Z.; Yuan, J.; Shan, W.; Li, C.; Hu, X. Long noncoding RNA LINP1 regulates repair of DNA double-strand breaks in triple-negative breast cancer. *Nat. Struct. Mol. Biol.* **2016**, *23*, 522–530. [CrossRef] [PubMed]

112. Liu, J.; Sun, X.; Zhu, H.; Qin, Q.; Yang, X.; Sun, X. Long noncoding RNA POU6F2-AS2 is associated with oesophageal squamous cell carcinoma. *J. Biochem.* **2016**, *160*, 195–204. [CrossRef] [PubMed]

113. Matsumoto, K.; Bay, B.H. Significance of the Y-box proteins in human cancers. *J. Mol. Genet. Med.* **2005**, *1*, 11–17. [CrossRef] [PubMed]

114. Xu, Y.; Wang, J.; Qiu, M.; Xu, L.; Li, M.; Jiang, F.; Yin, R.; Xu, L. Upregulation of the long noncoding RNA TUG1 promotes proliferation and migration of esophageal squamous cell carcinoma. *Tumour Biol.* **2015**, *36*, 1643–1651. [CrossRef] [PubMed]

115. Zhang, Q.; Geng, P.L.; Yin, P.; Wang, X.L.; Jia, J.P.; Yao, J. Down-regulation of long non-coding RNA TUG1 inhibits osteosarcoma cell proliferation and promotes apoptosis. *Asian Pac. J. Cancer Prev.* **2013**, *14*, 2311–2315. [CrossRef] [PubMed]

116. Zhang, E.B.; Yin, D.D.; Sun, M.; Kong, R.; Liu, X.H.; You, L.H.; Han, L.; Xia, R.; Wang, K.M.; Yang, J.S.; et al. P53-regulated long non-coding RNA TUG1 affects cell proliferation in human non-small cell lung cancer, partly through epigenetically regulating HOXB7 expression. *Cell Death Dis.* **2014**, *5*, e1243. [CrossRef] [PubMed]

117. Han, Y.; Liu, Y.; Gui, Y.; Cai, Z. Long intergenic non-coding RNA TUG1 is overexpressed in urothelial carcinoma of the bladder. *J. Surg. Oncol.* **2013**, *107*, 555–559. [CrossRef] [PubMed]

118. Huang, M.D.; Chen, W.M.; Qi, F.Z.; Sun, M.; Xu, T.P.; Ma, P.; Shu, Y.Q. Long non-coding RNA TUG1 is up-regulated in hepatocellular carcinoma and promotes cell growth and apoptosis by epigenetically silencing of KLF2. *Mol. Cancer* **2015**, *14*, 165. [CrossRef] [PubMed]

119. Tan, J.; Qiu, K.; Li, M.; Liang, Y. Double-negative feedback loop between long non-coding RNA TUG1 and miR-145 promotes epithelial to mesenchymal transition and radioresistance in human bladder cancer cells. *FEBS Lett.* **2015**, *589*, 3175–3181. [CrossRef] [PubMed]

120. Jiang, H.; Hu, X.; Zhang, H.; Li, W. Down-regulation of LncRNA TUG1 enhances radiosensitivity in bladder cancer via suppressing HMGB1 expression. *Radiat. Oncol.* **2017**, *12*, 65. [CrossRef] [PubMed]

121. Zhang, Q.; Wang, Y. HMG modifications and nuclear function. *Biochim. Biophys. Acta* **2010**, *1799*, 28–36. [CrossRef] [PubMed]

122. Rinn, J.L.; Kertesz, M.; Wang, J.K.; Squazzo, S.L.; Xu, X.; Brugmann, S.A.; Goodnough, L.H.; Helms, J.A.; Farnham, P.J.; Segal, E. Functional demarcation of active and silent chromatin domains in human HOX loci by noncoding RNAs. *Cell* **2007**, *129*, 1311–1323. [CrossRef] [PubMed]

123. Hajjari, M.; Salavaty, A. HOTAIR: An oncogenic long non-coding RNA in different cancers. *Cancer Biol. Med.* **2015**, *12*, 1–9. [PubMed]

124. Kogo, R.; Shimamura, T.; Mimori, K.; Kawahara, K.; Imoto, S.; Sudo, T.; Tanaka, F.; Shibata, K.; Suzuki, A.; Komune, S. Long noncoding RNA HOTAIR regulates polycomb-dependent chromatin modification and is associated with poor prognosis in colorectal cancers. *Cancer Res.* **2011**, *71*, 6320–6326. [CrossRef] [PubMed]

125. Gupta, R.A.; Shah, N.; Wang, K.C.; Kim, J.; Horlings, H.M.; Wong, D.J.; Tsai, M.C.; Hung, T.; Argani, P.; Rinn, J.L.; et al. Long non-coding RNA HOTAIR reprograms chromatin state to promote cancer metastasis. *Nature* **2010**, *464*, 1071–1076. [CrossRef] [PubMed]

126. Davidovich, C.; Zheng, L.; Goodrich, K.J.; Cech, T.R. Promiscuous RNA binding by Polycomb repressive complex 2. *Nat. Struct. Mol. Biol.* **2013**, *20*, 1250–1257. [CrossRef] [PubMed]

127. Zhou, Y.; Wang, C.; Liu, X.; Wu, C.; Yin, H. Long non-coding RNA HOTAIR enhances radioresistance in MDA-MB231 breast cancer cells. *Oncol. Lett.* **2017**, *13*, 1143–1148. [CrossRef] [PubMed]

128. Jing, L.; Yuan, W.; Ruofan, D.; Jinjin, Y.; Haifeng, Q. HOTAIR enhanced aggressive biological behaviors and induced radio-resistance via inhibiting p21 in cervical cancer. *Tumour Biol.* **2015**, *36*, 3611–3619. [CrossRef] [PubMed]

129. Yang, X.D.; Xu, H.T.; Xu, X.H.; Ru, G.; Liu, W.; Zhu, J.J.; Wu, Y.Y.; Zhao, K.; Wu, Y.; Xing, C.G.; et al. Knockdown of long non-coding RNA HOTAIR inhibits proliferation and invasiveness and improves radiosensitivity in colorectal cancer. *Oncol. Rep.* **2016**, *35*, 479–487. [CrossRef] [PubMed]

130. Jiang, Y.; Li, Z.; Zheng, S.; Chen, H.; Zhao, X.; Gao, W.; Bi, Z.; You, K.; Wang, Y.; Li, W.; et al. The long non-coding RNA HOTAIR affects the radiosensitivity of pancreatic ductal adenocarcinoma by regulating the expression of Wnt inhibitory factor 1. *Tumour Biol.* **2016**, *37*, 3957–3967. [CrossRef] [PubMed]

131. Chen, J.; Shen, Z.; Zheng, Y.; Wang, S.; Mao, W. Radiotherapy induced Lewis lung cancer cell apoptosis via inactivating β-catenin mediated by upregulated HOTAIR. *Int. J. Clin. Exp. Pathol.* **2015**, *8*, 7878–7886. [PubMed]

132. Hsieh, J.C.; Kodjabachian, L.; Rebbert, M.L.; Rattner, A.; Smallwood, P.M.; Samos, C.H.; Nusse, R.; Dawid, I.B.; Nathans, J. A new secreted protein that binds to Wnt proteins and inhibits their activities. *Nature* **1999**, *398*, 431–436. [PubMed]

133. O'Leary, V.B.; Ovsepian, S.V.; Carrascosa, L.G.; Buske, F.A.; Radulovic, V.; Niyazi, M.; Moertl, S.; Trau, M.; Atkinson, M.J.; Anastasov, N. Particle, a triplex-forming long ncRNA, regulates locus-specific methylation in response to low-dose irradiation. *Cell Rep.* **2015**, *11*, 474–485. [CrossRef] [PubMed]

134. Alvarez, L.; Corrales, F.; Martin-Duce, A.; Mato, J.M. Characterization of a full-length cDNA encoding human liver S-adenosylmethionine synthetase: Tissue-specific gene expression and mRNA levels in hepatopathies. *Biochem. J.* **1993**, *293*, 481–486. [CrossRef] [PubMed]

135. Kotb, M.; Mudd, S.H.; Mato, J.M.; Geller, A.M.; Kredich, N.M.; Chou, J.Y.; Cantoni, G.L. Consensus nomenclature for the mammalian methionine adenosyltransferase genes and gene products. *Trends Genet.* **1997**, *13*, 51–52. [CrossRef]

136. Miousse, I.R.; Kutanzi, K.R.; Koturbash, I. Effects of ionizing radiation on DNA methylation: From experimental biology to clinical applications. *Int. J. Radiat. Biol.* **2017**, *93*, 457–469. [CrossRef] [PubMed]

137. Song, W.; Wang, K.; Zhang, R.J.; Dai, Q.X.; Zou, S.B. Long noncoding RNA GAS5 can predict metastasis and poor prognosis: A meta-analysis. *Minerva. Med.* **2016**, *107*, 70–76. [PubMed]

138. Xiong, W.; Jiang, Y.X.; Ai, Y.Q.; Liu, S.; Wu, X.R.; Cui, J.G.; Qin, J.Y.; Liu, Y.; Xia, Y.X.; Ju, Y.H.; et al. Microarray analysis of long non-coding RNA expression profile associated with 5-fluorouracil-based chemoradiation resistance in colorectal cancer cells. *Asian Pac. J. Cancer Prev.* **2015**, *16*, 3395–3402. [CrossRef] [PubMed]

139. Li, G.; Liu, Y.; Liu, C.; Su, Z.; Ren, S.; Wang, Y.; Deng, T.; Huang, D.; Tian, Y.; Qiu, Y. Genome-wide analyses of long noncoding RNA expression profiles correlated with radioresistance in nasopharyngeal carcinoma via next-generation deep sequencing. *BMC Cancer* **2016**, *16*, 719. [CrossRef] [PubMed]

140. Zhou, J.; Cao, S.; Li, W.; Wei, D.; Wang, Z.; Li, G.; Pan, X.; Lei, D. Time-course differential lncRNA and mRNA expressions in radioresistant hypopharyngeal cancer cells. *Oncotarget* **2017**, *8*, 40994. [CrossRef] [PubMed]

141. Wang, J.; Lei, Z.J.; Guo, Y.; Wang, T.; Qin, Z.Y.; Xiao, H.L.; Fan, L.L.; Chen, D.F.; Bian, X.W.; Liu, J.; et al. miRNA-regulated delivery of lincRNA-p21 suppresses beta-catenin signaling and tumorigenicity of colorectal cancer stem cells. *Oncotarget* **2015**, *6*, 37852–37870. [CrossRef] [PubMed]

142. Wang, Y.; He, L.; Du, Y.; Zhu, P.; Huang, G.; Luo, J.; Yan, X.; Ye, B.; Li, C.; Xia, P.; et al. The long noncoding RNA lncTCF7 promotes self-renewal of human liver cancer stem cells through activation of Wnt signaling. *Cell Stem Cell* **2015**, *16*, 413–425. [CrossRef] [PubMed]

143. Wu, J.; Wang, D. Long noncoding RNA TCF7 promotes invasiveness and self-renewal of human non-small cell lung cancer cells. *Hum. Cell* **2017**, *30*, 23–29. [CrossRef] [PubMed]

144. Wang, Y.; Yao, J.; Meng, H.; Yu, Z.; Wang, Z.; Yuan, X.; Chen, H.; Wang, A. A novel long non-coding RNA, hypoxia-inducible factor-2α promoter upstream transcript, functions as an inhibitor of osteosarcoma stem cells in vitro. *Mol. Med. Rep.* **2015**, *11*, 2534–2540. [CrossRef] [PubMed]

145. Yao, J.; Li, J.; Geng, P.; Li, Y.; Chen, H.; Zhu, Y. Knockdown of a HIF-2α promoter upstream long noncoding RNA impairs colorectal cancer stem cell properties in vitro through HIF-2α downregulation. *OncoTargets Ther.* **2015**, *8*, 3467–3474. [CrossRef] [PubMed]

146. Lloret-Llinares, M.; Mapendano, C.K.; Martlev, L.H.; Lykke-Andersen, S.; Jensen, T.H. Relationships between prompt and gene expression. *RNA Biol.* **2016**, *13*, 6–14. [CrossRef] [PubMed]

147. Myszczyszyn, A.; Czarnecka, A.M.; Matak, D.; Szymanski, L.; Lian, F.; Kornakiewicz, A.; Bartnik, E.; Kukwa, W.; Kieda, C.; Szczylik, C. The role of hypoxia and cancer stem cells in renal cell carcinoma pathogenesis. *Stem Cell Rev.* **2015**, *11*, 919–943. [CrossRef] [PubMed]

148. Padua Alves, C.; Fonseca, A.S.; Muys, B.R.; de Barros, E.L.B.R.; Burger, M.C.; de Souza, J.E.; Valente, V.; Zago, M.A.; Silva, W.A., Jr. Brief report: The lincRNA Hotair is required for epithelial-to-mesenchymal transition and stemness maintenance of cancer cell lines. *Stem Cells* **2013**, *31*, 2827–2832. [CrossRef] [PubMed]

149. Deng, J.; Yang, M.; Jiang, R.; An, N.; Wang, X.; Liu, B. Long non-coding RNA HOTAIR regulates the proliferation, self-renewal capacity, tumor formation and migration of the cancer stem-like cell (CSC) subpopulation enriched from breast cancer cells. *PLoS ONE* **2017**, *12*, e0170860. [CrossRef] [PubMed]

150. Zhang, H.; Cai, K.; Wang, J.; Wang, X.; Cheng, K.; Shi, F.; Jiang, L.; Zhang, Y.; Dou, J. MiR-7, inhibited indirectly by lincRNA HOTAIR, directly inhibits SETDB1 and reverses the EMT of breast cancer stem cells by downregulating the STAT3 pathway. *Stem Cells* **2014**, *32*, 2858–2868. [CrossRef] [PubMed]

151. Dou, J.; Ni, Y.; He, X.; Wu, D.; Li, M.; Wu, S.; Zhang, R.; Guo, M.; Zhao, F. Decreasing lncRNA HOTAIR expression inhibits human colorectal cancer stem cells. *Am. J. Transl. Res.* **2016**, *8*, 98–108. [PubMed]

152. Chang, T.C.; Wentzel, E.A.; Kent, O.A.; Ramachandran, K.; Mullendore, M.; Lee, K.H.; Feldmann, G.; Yamakuchi, M.; Ferlito, M.; Lowenstein, C.J.; et al. Transactivation of miR-34a by p53 broadly influences gene expression and promotes apoptosis. *Mol. Cell* **2007**, *26*, 745–752. [CrossRef] [PubMed]

153. Liu, C.; Kelnar, K.; Liu, B.; Chen, X.; Calhoun-Davis, T.; Li, H.; Patrawala, L.; Yan, H.; Jeter, C.; Honorio, S.; et al. The microRNA miR-34a inhibits prostate cancer stem cells and metastasis by directly repressing CD44. *Nat. Med.* **2011**, *17*, 211–215. [CrossRef] [PubMed]

154. Wang, L.; Bu, P.; Ai, Y.; Srinivasan, T.; Chen, H.J.; Xiang, K.; Lipkin, S.M.; Shen, X. A long non-coding RNA targets microRNA miR-34a to regulate colon cancer stem cell asymmetric division. *Elife* **2016**, *5*. [CrossRef] [PubMed]

155. Katsushima, K.; Natsume, A.; Ohka, F.; Shinjo, K.; Hatanaka, A.; Ichimura, N.; Sato, S.; Takahashi, S.; Kimura, H.; Totoki, Y.; et al. Targeting the notch-regulated non-coding RNA TUG1 for glioma treatment. *Nat. Commun.* **2016**, *7*, 13616. [CrossRef] [PubMed]

156. Wang, J.; Sullenger, B.A.; Rich, J.N. Notch signaling in cancer stem cells. *Adv. Exp. Med. Biol.* **2012**, *727*, 174–185. [PubMed]

157. Xu, N.; Papagiannakopoulos, T.; Pan, G.; Thomson, J.A.; Kosik, K.S. MicroRNA-145 regulates OCT4, SOX2, and KLF4 and represses pluripotency in human embryonic stem cells. *Cell* **2009**, *137*, 647–658. [CrossRef] [PubMed]

158. Brodie, S.; Lee, H.K.; Jiang, W.; Cazacu, S.; Xiang, C.; Poisson, L.M.; Datta, I.; Kalkanis, S.; Ginsberg, D.; Brodie, C. The novel long non-coding RNA TALNEC2, regulates tumor cell growth and the stemness and radiation response of glioma stem cells. *Oncotarget* **2017**, *8*, 31785–31801. [CrossRef] [PubMed]

159. Polager, S.; Ginsberg, D. E2F-at the crossroads of life and death. *Trends Cell Biol.* **2008**, *18*, 528–535. [CrossRef] [PubMed]

160. Wu, L.; Timmers, C.; Maiti, B.; Saavedra, H.I.; Sang, L.; Chong, G.T.; Nuckolls, F.; Giangrande, P.; Wright, F.A.; Field, S.J.; et al. The E2F1–3 transcription factors are essential for cellular proliferation. *Nature* **2001**, *414*, 457–462. [CrossRef] [PubMed]

161. Chen, J.; Fu, Z.; Ji, C.; Gu, P.; Xu, P.; Yu, N.; Kan, Y.; Wu, X.; Shen, R.; Shen, Y. Systematic gene microarray analysis of the lncRNA expression profiles in human uterine cervix carcinoma. *Biomed. Pharmacother.* **2015**, *72*, 83–90. [CrossRef] [PubMed]

162. Kim, H.J.; Eoh, K.J.; Kim, L.K.; Nam, E.J.; Yoon, S.O.; Kim, K.H.; Lee, J.K.; Kim, S.W.; Kim, Y.T. The long noncoding RNA HOXA11 antisense induces tumor progression and stemness maintenance in cervical cancer. *Oncotarget* **2016**, *7*, 83001–83016. [PubMed]

163. Zhou, M.; Hou, Y.; Yang, G.; Zhang, H.; Tu, G.; Du, Y.E.; Wen, S.; Xu, L.; Tang, X.; Tang, S.; et al. LncRNA-hh strengthen cancer stem cells generation in twist-positive breast cancer via activation of hedgehog signaling pathway. *Stem Cells* **2016**, *34*, 55–66. [CrossRef] [PubMed]

164. Lin, N.; Chang, K.Y.; Li, Z.; Gates, K.; Rana, Z.A.; Dang, J.; Zhang, D.; Han, T.; Yang, C.S.; Cunningham, T.J.; et al. An evolutionarily conserved long noncoding RNA TUNA controls pluripotency and neural lineage commitment. *Mol. Cell* **2014**, *53*, 1005–1019. [CrossRef] [PubMed]

165. Li, H.; Zhu, L.; Xu, L.; Qin, K.; Liu, C.; Yu, Y.; Su, D.; Wu, K.; Sheng, Y. Long noncoding RNA linc00617 exhibits oncogenic activity in breast cancer. *Mol. Carcinog.* **2017**, *56*, 3–17. [CrossRef] [PubMed]

166. Cui, M.; Xiao, Z.; Wang, Y.; Zheng, M.; Song, T.; Cai, X.; Sun, B.; Ye, L.; Zhang, X. Long noncoding RNA HULC modulates abnormal lipid metabolism in hepatoma cells through an miR-9-mediated RXRA signaling pathway. *Cancer Res.* **2015**, *75*, 846–857. [CrossRef] [PubMed]

167. Shi, F.; Xiao, F.; Ding, P.; Qin, H.; Huang, R. Long noncoding RNA highly up-regulated in liver cancer predicts unfavorable outcome and regulates metastasis by MMPS in triple-negative breast cancer. *Arch. Med. Res.* **2016**, *47*, 446–453. [CrossRef] [PubMed]

168. Wu, M.; Lin, Z.; Li, X.; Xin, X.; An, J.; Zheng, Q.; Yang, Y.; Lu, D. HULC cooperates with MALAT1 to aggravate liver cancer stem cells growth through telomere repeat-binding factor 2. *Sci. Rep.* **2016**, *6*, 36045. [CrossRef] [PubMed]

169. Wang, Y.; Chen, W.; Yang, C.; Wu, W.; Wu, S.; Qin, X.; Li, X. Long non-coding RNA UCA1a(CUDR) promotes proliferation and tumorigenesis of bladder cancer. *Int. J. Oncol.* **2012**, *41*, 276–284. [PubMed]

170. Wang, Z.; Wang, X.; Zhang, D.; Yu, Y.; Cai, L.; Zhang, C. Long non-coding RNA urothelial carcinoma-associated 1 as a tumor biomarker for the diagnosis of urinary bladder cancer. *Tumour Biol.* **2017**, *39*, 1010428317709990. [CrossRef] [PubMed]

171. Gui, X.; Li, H.; Li, T.; Pu, H.; Lu, D. Long noncoding RNA CUDR regulates HULC and β-catenin to govern human liver stem cell malignant differentiation. *Mol. Ther.* **2015**, *23*, 1843–1853. [CrossRef] [PubMed]

172. Pu, H.; Zheng, Q.; Li, H.; Wu, M.; An, J.; Gui, X.; Li, T.; Lu, D. CUDR promotes liver cancer stem cell growth through upregulating TERT and C-Myc. *Oncotarget* **2015**, *6*, 40775–40798. [CrossRef] [PubMed]

173. Yang, X.; Xiao, Z.; Du, X.; Huang, L.; Du, G. Silencing of the long non-coding RNA NEAT1 suppresses glioma stem-like properties through modulation of the miR-107/CDK6 pathway. *Oncol. Rep.* **2017**, *37*, 555–562. [CrossRef] [PubMed]

174. Gong, W.; Zheng, J.; Liu, X.; Ma, J.; Liu, Y.; Xue, Y. Knockdown of NEAT1 restrained the malignant progression of glioma stem cells by activating microRNA let-7e. *Oncotarget* **2016**, *7*, 62208–62223. [CrossRef] [PubMed]

175. Zhang, F.; Cheong, J.K. The renewed battle against RAS-mutant cancers. *Cell Mol. Life Sci.* **2016**, *73*, 1845–1858. [CrossRef] [PubMed]

176. Zhou, X.; Gao, Q.; Wang, J.; Zhang, X.; Liu, K.; Duan, Z. Linc-RNA-RoR acts as a "sponge" against mediation of the differentiation of endometrial cancer stem cells by microRNA-145. *Gynecol. Oncol.* **2014**, *133*, 333–339. [CrossRef] [PubMed]

177. Wang, S.; Liu, F.; Deng, J.; Cai, X.; Han, J.; Liu, Q. Long noncoding RNA ROR regulates proliferation, invasion, and stemness of gastric cancer stem cell. *Cell Reprogram.* **2016**, *18*, 319–326. [CrossRef] [PubMed]

178. Matouk, I.; Raveh, E.; Ohana, P.; Lail, R.A.; Gershtain, E.; Gilon, M.; De Groot, N.; Czerniak, A.; Hochberg, A. The increasing complexity of the oncofetal H19 gene locus: Functional dissection and therapeutic intervention. *Int. J. Mol. Sci.* **2013**, *14*, 4298–4316. [CrossRef] [PubMed]

179. Matouk, I.J.; Raveh, E.; Abu-lail, R.; Mezan, S.; Gilon, M.; Gershtain, E.; Birman, T.; Gallula, J.; Schneider, T.; Barkali, M.; et al. Oncofetal H19 RNA promotes tumor metastasis. *Biochim. Biophys. Acta* **2014**, *1843*, 1414–1426. [CrossRef] [PubMed]

180. Xu, Y.; Wang, Z.; Jiang, X.; Cui, Y. Overexpression of long noncoding RNA H19 indicates a poor prognosis for cholangiocarcinoma and promotes cell migration and invasion by affecting epithelial-mesenchymal transition. *Biomed. Pharmacother.* **2017**, *92*, 17–23. [CrossRef] [PubMed]

181. Jiang, X.; Yan, Y.; Hu, M.; Chen, X.; Wang, Y.; Dai, Y.; Wu, D.; Zhuang, Z.; Xia, H. Increased level of H19 long noncoding RNA promotes invasion, angiogenesis, and stemness of glioblastoma cells. *J. Neurosurg.* **2016**, *2016*, 129–136. [CrossRef] [PubMed]

182. Li, W.; Jiang, P.; Sun, X.; Xu, S.; Ma, X.; Zhan, R. Suppressing H19 modulates tumorigenicity and stemness in U251 and U87MG glioma cells. *Cell Mol. Neurobiol.* **2016**, *36*, 1219–1227. [CrossRef] [PubMed]

183. Zeira, E.; Abramovitch, R.; Meir, K.; Even Ram, S.; Gil, Y.; Bulvik, B.; Bromberg, Z.; Levkovitch, O.; Nahmansson, N.; Adar, R.; et al. The knockdown of H19 lncRNA reveals its regulatory role in pluripotency and tumorigenesis of human embryonic carcinoma cells. *Oncotarget* **2015**, *6*, 34691–34703. [PubMed]

184. Miao, L.; Huang, Z.; Zengli, Z.; Li, H.; Chen, Q.; Yao, C.; Cai, H.; Xiao, Y.; Xia, H.; Wang, Y. Loss of long noncoding RNA FOXF1-AS1 regulates epithelial-mesenchymal transition, stemness and metastasis of non-small cell lung cancer cells. *Oncotarget* **2016**, *7*, 68339–68349. [CrossRef] [PubMed]

185. Han, Y.; Zhou, L.; Wu, T.; Huang, Y.; Cheng, Z.; Li, X.; Sun, T.; Zhou, Y.; Du, Z. Downregulation of lncRNA-MALAT1 affects proliferation and the expression of stemness markers in glioma stem cell line SHG139S. *Cell Mol. Neurobiol.* **2016**, *36*, 1097–1107. [CrossRef] [PubMed]

186. Jiao, F.; Hu, H.; Han, T.; Yuan, C.; Wang, L.; Jin, Z.; Guo, Z.; Wang, L. Long noncoding RNA MALAT-1 enhances stem cell-like phenotypes in pancreatic cancer cells. *Int. J. Mol. Sci.* **2015**, *16*, 6677–6693. [CrossRef] [PubMed]

187. Xia, F.; Xiong, Y.; Li, Q. Interaction of lincRNA ROR and p53/miR-145 correlates with lung cancer stem cell signatures. *J. Cell Biochem.* **2017**. [CrossRef] [PubMed]

188. Singh, S.K.; Chen, N.M.; Hessmann, E.; Siveke, J.; Lahmann, M.; Singh, G.; Voelker, N.; Vogt, S.; Esposito, I.; Schmidt, A.; et al. Antithetical NFATc1-Sox2 and p53-miR200 signaling networks govern pancreatic cancer cell plasticity. *EMBO J.* **2015**, *34*, 517–530. [CrossRef] [PubMed]

189. He, Y.; Meng, X.M.; Huang, C.; Wu, B.M.; Zhang, L.; Lv, X.W.; Li, J. Long noncoding RNAs: Novel insights into hepatocelluar carcinoma. *Cancer Lett.* **2014**, *344*, 20–27. [CrossRef] [PubMed]

190. Shi, T.; Gao, G.; Cao, Y. Long noncoding RNAs as novel biomarkers have a promising future in cancer diagnostics. *Dis. Markers* **2016**, *2016*, 9085195. [CrossRef] [PubMed]

191. Dutertre, M.; Lambert, S.; Carreira, A.; Amor-Gueret, M.; Vagner, S. DNA damage: RNA-binding proteins protect from near and far. *Trends Biochem. Sci.* **2014**, *39*, 141–149. [CrossRef] [PubMed]

192. Dutertre, M.; Vagner, S. DNA-damage response RNA-binding proteins (DDRBPs): Perspectives from a new class of proteins and their rna targets. *J. Mol. Biol.* **2016**. [CrossRef] [PubMed]

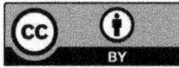

International Journal of
Molecular Sciences

MDPI

Article

Tumor-Stroma Crosstalk in Bone Tissue: The Osteoclastogenic Potential of a Breast Cancer Cell Line in a Co-Culture System and the Role of EGFR Inhibition

Laura Mercatali [1,*], Federico La Manna [1], Giacomo Miserocchi [1], Chiara Liverani [1], Alessandro De Vita [1] , Chiara Spadazzi [1], Alberto Bongiovanni [1], Federica Recine [1], Dino Amadori [1], Martina Ghetti [1,2] and Toni Ibrahim [1]

[1] Osteoncology and Rare Tumors Center, Istituto Scientifico Romagnolo per lo Studio e la Cura dei Tumori (IRST) IRCCS, 47014 Meldola, Italy; federico.lamanna@lumc.nl (F.L.M) giacomo.miserocchi@irst.emr.it (G.M.); chiara.liverani@irst.emr.it (C.L.); alessandro.devita@irst.emr.it (A.D.V.); chiara.spadazzi@irst.emr.it (C.S.); alberto.bongiovanni@irst.emr.it (A.B.); federica.recine@irst.emr.it (F.R.); editing@irst.emr.it (D.A.); martina.ghetti@irst.emr.it (M.G.); toni.ibrahim@irst.emr.it (T.I.)
[2] Biomedical and Neuromotor Sciences Department, University of Bologna, 40123 Bologna, Italy
* Correspondence: laura.mercatali@irst.emr.it; Tel.: +39-0543-739239

Received: 29 June 2017; Accepted: 25 July 2017; Published: 29 July 2017

Abstract: Although bone metastases represent a major challenge in the natural history of breast cancer (BC), the complex interactions involved have hindered the development of robust in vitro models. The aim of this work is the development of a preclinical model of cancer and bone stromal cells to mimic the bone microenvironment. We studied the effects on osteoclastogenesis of BC cells and Mesenchymal stem cells (MSC) cultured alone or in combination. We also analyzed: (a) whether the blockade of the Epithelial Growth Factor Receptor (EGFR) pathway modified their influence on monocytes towards differentiation, and (b) the efficacy of bone-targeted therapy on osteoclasts. We evaluated the osteoclastogenesis modulation of human peripheral blood monocytes (PBMC) indirectly induced by the conditioned medium (CM) of the human BC cell line SCP2, cultured singly or with MSC. Osteoclastogenesis was evaluated by TRAP analysis. The effect of the EGFR blockade was assessed by treating the cells with gefitinib, and analyzed with the 3-(4,5-dimethylthiazol-2-yl)-2,5-diphenyltetrazolium bromide (MTT) assay and Western Blot (WB). We observed that SCP2 co-cultured with MSC increased the differentiation of PBMC. This effect was underpinned upon pre-treatment of the co-culture with gefitinib. Co-culture of SCP2 with MSC increased the expression of both the bone-related marker Receptor Activator of Nuclear Factor κB (RANK) and EGFR in BC cells. These upregulations were not affected by the EGFR blockade. The effects of the CM obtained by the cells treated with gefitinib in combination with the treatment of the preosteoclasts with the bone-targeted agents and everolimus enhanced the inhibition of the osteoclastogenesis. Finally, we developed a fully human co-culture system of BC cells and bone progenitor cells. We observed that the interaction of MSC with cancer cells induced in the latter molecular changes and a higher power of inducing osteoclastogenesis. We found that blocking EGFR signaling could be an efficacious strategy for breaking the interactions between cancer and bone cells in order to inhibit bone metastasis.

Keywords: breast cancer; co-culture; osteoclasts; mesenchymal stromal cells; non-canonical osteoclastogenesis

1. Introduction

Bone metastases are a common event in breast cancer (BC) patients [1], often leading to severe symptoms such as pain, bone fractures, spinal cord compression and hypercalcemia [2]. The mechanisms underlying BC-derived bone metastases have been intensively investigated but the complex interactions involved have hindered both the development of comprehensive in vitro systems [3] and the generation of translational benefits [4,5].

Mesenchymal stromal cells (MSC) are multipotent stem cells precursors of tissue-specific cell lineages in many adult tissues [6]. Within the bone marrow, MSC give rise to both bone stromal cells, i.e., osteoblasts, osteocytes, adipocytes, and more specialized, niche-maintaining cells such as CAR cells, leptin-receptor-positive cells, and sinusoid-associated pericytes [7]. Together with osteoblasts, MSC express two essential factors for the maturation of osteoclasts, the giant, multinucleated, monocyte-derived cells responsible for bone resorption: the Receptor Activator of Nuclear Factor kappa-Bligand (RANKL) and the macrophage colony-stimulating factor (M-CSF) [8]. The inhibition of either the maturation or the activity of osteoclasts has already proven effective in treating bone metastases [1,9], and has led to the development of many osteoclast-targeted drugs [10,11]. These pharmacological agents, which constitute the bone-targeted therapy, are mainly represented by the anti-RANKL antibody denosumab (Den), and bisphosphonates, such as zoledronic acid (Zol). Everolimus (Eve) has been recently considered suitable for targeting bone metastases as it inhibits both cancer cells and osteoclasts. [12–14]. EGFR, also known as ErbB-1 or HER1, is one of the four members of the ErbB tyrosine kinases receptors family. EGFR is frequently amplified or overexpressed in many neoplastic lesions, including lung, breast, colorectal, head and neck, pancreatic and gastric cancers [15]. A higher expression of EGFR in "triple-negative" BC has been shown to correlate with a higher incidence of metastases [16]. This receptor is also expressed by MSC, and the activation of the EGFR pathway is involved with MSC in the regulation of RANKL and OPG secretion [16]. Thus, a deregulated EGFR signaling in MSC may alter the homeostatic ratio of RANKL/OPG of the bone microenvironment, initiating a "vicious cycle" that leads to the uncoupling of the physiological balance between bone erosion and bone deposition, driving it towards cancer cell metabolism [8,16,17]. Gefitinib (Gef), a selective, reversible inhibitor of EGFR, effective in treating locally advanced or metastatic non-small-cells lung cancer (NSCLC), has received FDA approval as a first-line treatment in NSCLC patients [18]. In spite of the antitumor activity shown by Gef both in vitro and xenograft models of breast and prostate cancers [19–22], phase-I/-II clinical trials on advanced BC patients treated with Gef yielded conflicting results, with little assessed clinical benefits for patients [8,23–27]. However, treatment of bone metastases with Gef has also been explored [28,29], based on the unexpected observation that treatment with this type of tyrosine kinase inhibitor (TKI) could relieve bone pain in BC patients [30,31]. Ultimately, the available data from both preclinical studies and clinical observations may pave the way for the use of Gef and other TKIs for the treatment of bone metastases.

The aim of this study was to develop a preclinical model for studying the effects of the crosstalk between stromal cells and cancer cells on osteoclastogenesis. Furthermore, we investigated if the blockade of the EGFR pathway in cancer and bone cells could have an effect on the bone microenvironment. We combined direct sharing medium and indirect co-cultures (COCOs) (Figure 1) in order to understand the molecular relation between cancer cells and MSC and their effect on osteoclasts. Firstly, we co-cultured cancer cells and MSC by direct sharing medium COCO. We then performed osteoclastogenesis assays in presence of the CM obtained from the cells previously mono- and co-cultured. These interactions were then challenged by treating the COCOs of stromal and cancer cells with Gef.

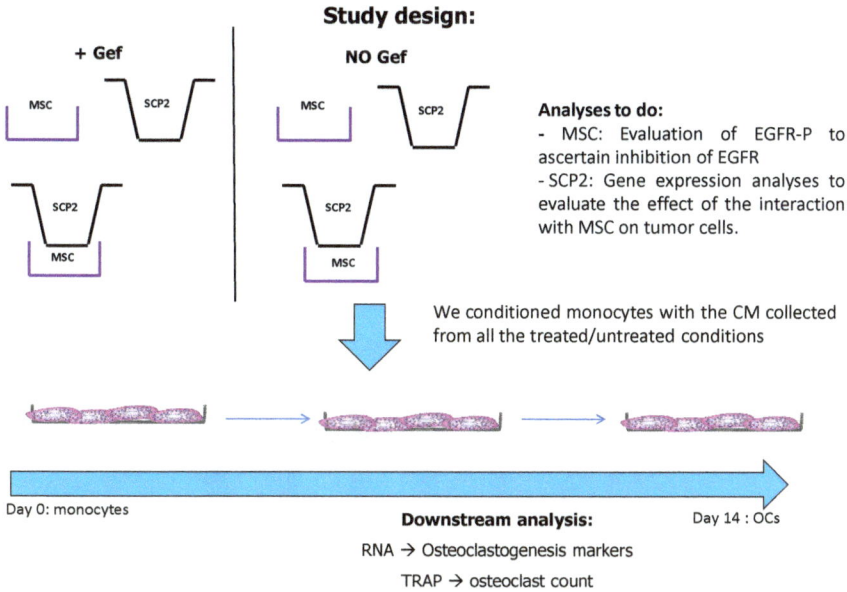

Figure 1. Experimental design: the preclinical model optimized in this paper includes a 2-phase cell culture; in the first phase cancer cells and Mesenchymal stem cells (MSC) were co-cultured sharing medium using transwell inserts. The media obtained from SCP2, MSC and the COCO were collected and used to condition the monocytes toward differentiation throughout the osteoclastogenic assay (CM changed every 2–3 days; assay total duration, 14 days). The conditioning of the monocyte with the CM derived from all the samples during the second phase of the experiment (indirect COCO).

2. Results

2.1. Mesenchymal stem cells (MSC) Induce the Expression of RANK and EGFR in Cancer Cells

We first investigated the effects of the COCO with MSC on the SCP2 gene expression in order to understand if cancer cells behave differently when in contact with bone microenvironment factors. We selected markers recapitulating different hallmarks of cancer progression, in particular bone metastasis. We selected 3 markers of osteomimicry: connexin 43 (cx43), osteopontin (spp1), and RANK. Osteomimicry is the capability of cancer cells to colonize the bone in order to form metastasis, and express the genes, that are usually expressed by bone cells, by adapting to the new microenvironment [32,33]. Marker cx43 is usually expressed on osteoblasts and osteocytes, and it is in charge of mechanotransduction and the control of body mass. Marker spp1 is a matrix protein involved in the attachment of osteoclasts to the bone matrix [34] RANK is a receptor of osteoclast precursors that, when binding to the RANK ligand, mediates their differentiation into mature osteoclasts. It has been shown that BC cells with high tropism to the bone often overexpress RANK [35,36]. We assayed the expression of TFF1, a marker expressed at higher levels in primary BC patients with relapse to the bone [37] and angiopoietin-1 (angpt1), which is involved in the angiogenic response of the osteomimicry-related markers [38,39]. We added EGFR to the panel, as one of the aims of this study was to understand the role of the EGFR pathway in the bone microenvironment. To this aim, the expression of markers related to cell–cell communication, invasion and bone marrow colonization was analyzed in SCP2 cells after co-culturing for 72 h with MSC. SCP2 cells were cultured with MSC, using the inserts cultured with cancer cells that had been laid on well plates where MSC had been previously seeded. This type of COCO allows for media sharing and interactions between cells seeded on different floors (Figure 1). Data on cancer cell gene expression were normalized using baseline SCP2 culture as reference. As shown in Figure 2, we found that the COCO with MSC showed a trend towards the upregulation of two genes involved in the bone vicious cycle: EGFR and RANK [36,40,41], the latter showing an increase by over 1.5 times the basal level.

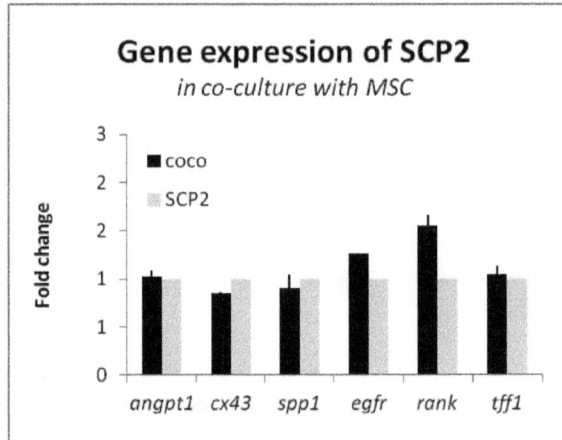

Figure 2. Co-culture with MSC upregulates EGFR and RANK expression in SCP2. Expression of *angpt1*, *cx43*, *spp1*, *egfr*, *rank* and *tff1* in SCP2 cells co-cultured with MSC. Fold change compared to SCP2 monoculture at baseline.

2.2. Cancer Cells and MSC Contribute to Osteoclastogenesis

In order to understand if cancer cells and MSC affect bone microenvironment contributing to osteoclastogenesis, we dissected the contribution of either SCP2 or MSC on osteoclastogenesis, by supplementing pre-osteoclasts with the CM of either the SCP2 or the MSC mono-cultures and the SCP2-MSC COCO. To achieve the COCO CM, we harvested the CM both after 24 h (Early-CM) and after 72 h (Late-CM) of COCO. In order to consider the osteoclastogenic power of CM with respect to the positive and negative control, we measured the average number of TRAP-positive osteoclast cell-like cells and their average surface area, given that a large surface area is one of the features of mature osteoclasts.

Cancer cells and COCO promote Osteoclastogenesis

At a molecular level, both CM from SCP2 and MSC induced osteoclastogenesis upregulating the osteoclast marker cathepsin k (*ctsk*), as shown in Figure 3A,B, with MSC-derived CM. We observed no upregulation of the early osteoclast-specific transcription factor Jun dimerization protein 2 (*jdp2*), probably because it had been already turned off on day 14 of differentiation [42]. Compared to undifferentiated pre-osteoclasts (negative control, i.e., monocytes cultured without GF supplementation), SCP2-derived CM showed a trend towards the induction of osteoclastogenesis, both as for the number of TRAP-positive osteoclasts (Figure 3C) and the surface area measurement (Figure 3D).

The CM from COCO induced a significant increase of the expression of *ctsk* in pre-osteoclast cultures, without affecting the expression of *jdp2*, and with no major differences between Early- and Late-CM (Figure 3B). Based on this result, we performed the TRAP assay on the osteoclasts cultured with Late-CM only (COCO), comparing data with both the positive and negative controls. The average surface area of the osteoclasts generated by the CM derived from the SCP2-MSC COCO was comparable to that of the osteoclasts cultured in the positive control, and was significantly higher than the negative control. It however did not affect the average number of osteoclasts (Figure 3C,D).

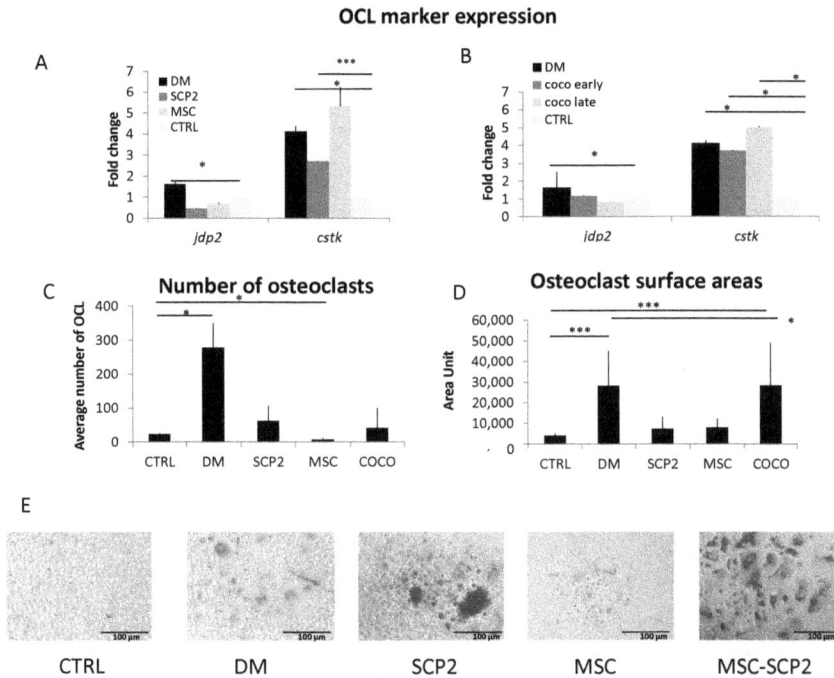

Figure 3. SCP2 and MSC mono-culture and COCO induce osteoclastogenesis. Expression of *jdp2* and *ctsk* in osteoclasts cultured either in DM or in pre-osteoclast medium supplemented with CM from: (**A**) SCP2 or MSC monoculture; (**B**) SCP2-MSC COCO after 24 h (Early-CM) or 72 h (Late-CM) of COCO. qPCR data refer to RNA from pre-osteoclasts. Data were normalized on pre-osteoclasts. *t*-test was performed comparing the gene expression of the different conditions with the control. * $p < 0.05$; *** $p < 0.01$. Average number (**C**) and average surface area (**D**) of TRAP-positive osteoclasts induced by culture in DM, pre-osteoclast medium (CTRL) or pre-osteoclast medium supplemented with SCP2-CM (SCP2), with MSC-CM (MSC) or with CM from SCP2-MSC COCO; *t*-test was performed for all conditions taking the negative control as control (CTRL). * $p < 0.05$; *** $p < 0.01$; (**E**) pictures of osteoclasts on day 14 obtained in the different experimental conditions performed at $10\times$ magnification.

Osteoclasts are not the only TRAP-positive polinucleated cells of a monocytic origin. In a previous work we confirmed that the osteoclast cell-like cells positive to TRAP are real osteoclasts, as we observed the presence of two specific osteoclast markers, i.e., Actin ring and calcitonin receptor (CTR), both in the negative control and in the differentiation medium (DM) condition [12].

2.3. Gef Induces RANK and EGFR mRNA Expression and Inhibits the EGFR Pathway at the Protein Level

To investigate the involvement of the EGFR pathway on the crosstalk of SCP2 cells and MSC, we treated both SCP2 and MSC monocultures and COCOs with Gef. As the first step, we tested the effect of different concentrations of Gef on SCP2 cells. As expected, the SCP2 cell line, like the parental cell line MDA-MB-231 [19], was not very sensitive to the EGFR blockade induced by Gef (Figure 4A). We then analyzed the expression of *angpt1*, *cx43*, *spp1*, *egfr*, *rank* and *tff1* after treating the SCP2 culture or the SCP2-MSC COCO with Gef at 1 μg/mL (plasmatic peak concentration) for 24 h (Figure 4B), after normalizing the gene expression on the SCP2 culture at baseline, to evaluate any molecular changes.

Gef-treated cells showed a modulation only of RANK and EGFR compared to the negative control (monocytes cultured without GF and CM). RANK increased both in SCP2 cultured singly (Figure 3B) and in COCO. We observed the same trend also for EGFR (Figure 3). The treatment with Gef induced a significant upregulation of *rank*, compared to untreated baseline SCP2 cells, once again showing a gene expression profile similar to untreated SCP2-MSC COCO.

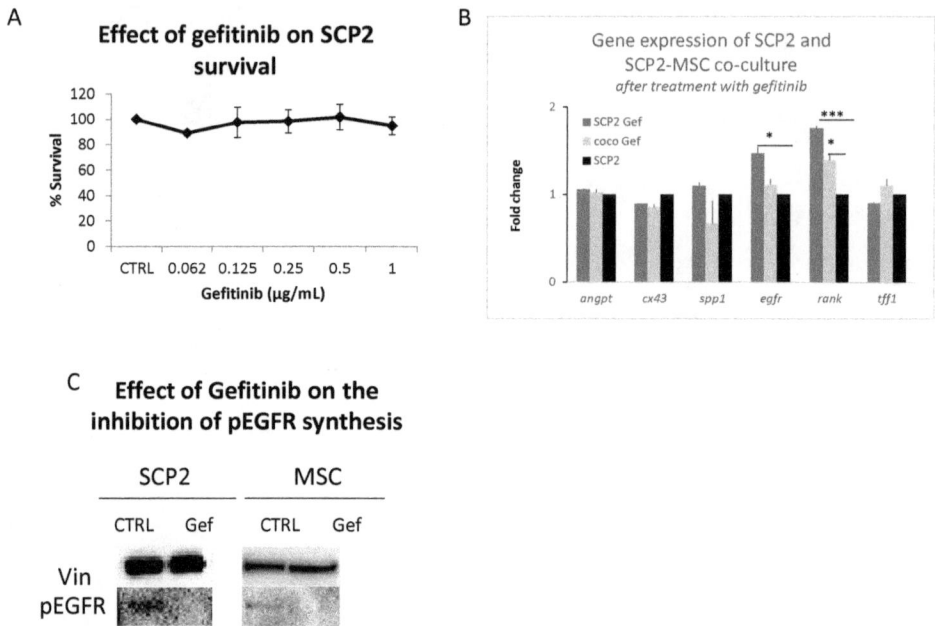

Figure 4. Gef inhibits the EGFR pathway and modulates cancer cell gene expression analyses. (**A**) Survival rate of SCP2 treated with Gef. Data were normalized to untreated sample (CTRL); (**B**) Expression of *angpt1*, *cx43*, *spp1*, *egfr*, *rank* and *tff1* in SCP2 cells (SCP2 Gef) or in SCP2-MSC COCO (TRW Gef) treated with Gef 1μg/mL. Fold change compared to SCP2 culture at baseline. * $p < 0.05$. *** $p < 0.01$; (**C**) Synthesis of phosphorylated-EGFR (pEGFR) in SCP2 and MSC in absence (CTRL) and treated with Gef. In each condition we added EGFR with an incubation step of 10 min (50 ng/mL).

To confirm that our observations depended on the blocking of EGFR, we tested the activation of the EGFR pathway at the protein level, both in SCP2 and MSC cultures. After the addition of EGF cytokine we detected the activation of the EGFR pathway, in terms of phospho-EGFR, in the cultures of SCP2 and MSC Gef treatment inhibited EGFR signaling, as we observed lack of phospho-EGFR in the treated cells (Figure 4C).

2.4. Gefitinib Impairs Osteoclastogenesis Induced by MSC-SCP2 COCO

We investigated the effect of *Gef* on the osteoclastogenic potential of CM from SCP2 and MSC mono- and co-cultures. We observed a statistically significant downregulation of *ctsk* in the CM from Gef-treated MSC and COCO (Figure 4A,B). The treatment did not inhibit the osteoclastogenic power of the CM obtained from SCP2. This could mean that the osteoclastogenic induction by MSC depends on the EGFR pathway; this trend was confirmed by the data obtained from counting the number of osteoclasts and quantifying the surface area, with statistical significance reached by the decreased mean surface area Figure 5C,D. No significant modulation of *jdp2* could be detected. At the cytological level, the CM of the *Gef*-treated cultures reduced the osteoclastogenic potential as shown in Figure 4B.

We observed no statistically different level of osteoclastogenesis from the negative control, neither in the number (Figure 5C) nor in the surface area (Figure 5D) of osteoclasts.

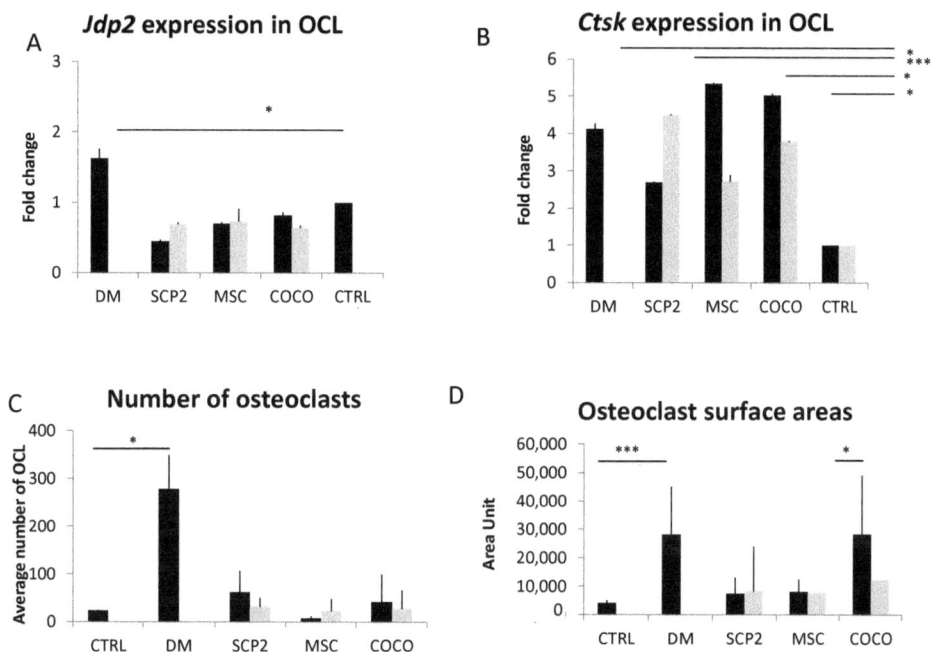

Figure 5. Gef impairs osteoclastogenesis induced by MSC-SCP2 COCO. Expression of *jdp2* (**A**) and *ctsk* (**B**) in osteoclasts cultured either in DM or with CM from SCP2, MSC or SCP2-MSC COCO previously treated (grey bars) or not (black bars) with Gef 1 µg/ml. Significance is compared to undifferentiated pre-osteoclasts (CTRL); Average number (**C**) and average surface area (**D**) of osteoclasts cultured in pre-osteoclast medium (CTRL), in DM or with CM from SCP2, MSC or SCP2-MSC COCO previously treated (grey bars) or not (black bars) with Gef 1µg/mL. * $p < 0.05$; *** $p < 0.01$. Gef was not added to CTRL and DM conditions in this context (absence of grey bars).

2.5. Bone-Targeted Therapy Empower Gef Inhibition of Osteoclastogenesis

As in clinical practice bone metastasis patients are usually treated with bone target therapy as Den and Zol, we treated the monocytes with these drugs to understand the impact of the inhibition of EGFR on standard treatment. We also tested the effect of Eve, as we previously had observed its strong effect on osteocolstogenesis inhibition. We employed CM from MSC, SCP2 and SCP2-MSC COCO for each treatment. At the end of the assay, the number of osteoclasts was considerably decreased in all the conditions. Compared to the control without treatment, all the drugs showed an important inhibitory effect on the percentage of differentiated osteoclasts, both in DM and CM conditions. Zol had the strongest effects on this reduction. We also evaluated the effects of the CM derived from the cells treated with Gef. All the combinations underpinned the development of mature osteoclasts (Figure 6B). The greatest effect on osteoclast development was performed by Zol, which showed a complete inhibition of the CM from MSC and SCP2 conditions (Figure 6B).

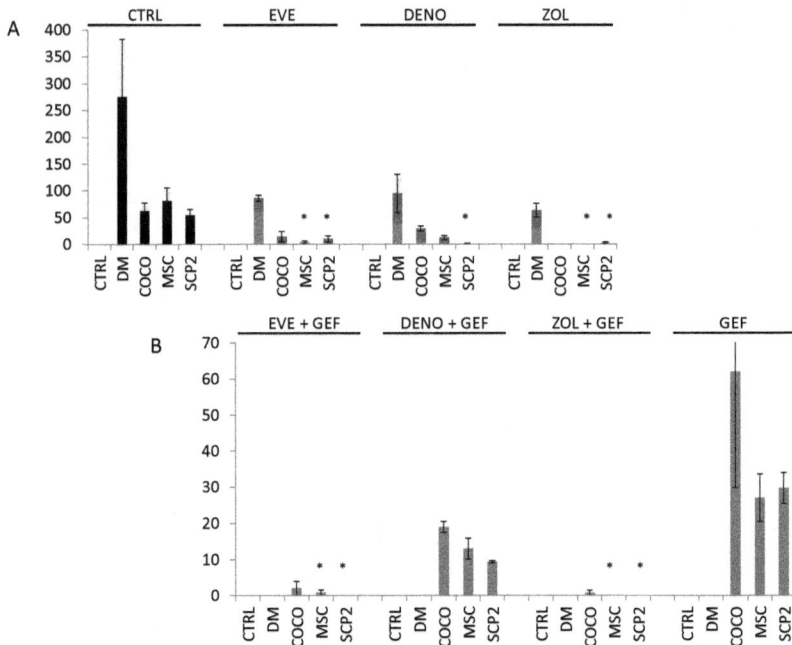

Figure 6. Eve and Zol on osteoclasts together with Gef treatment on MSC and SCP2 totally abrogated osteoclastogenesis. (**A**) Osteoclastogenesis assay from PBMC treated with bone-targeted therapy drugs (Den and Zol) and Eve. Osteoclastogenesis differentiation was evaluated in PBMC cultured with basal media with the addition of growth factors MCSF and RANKL, or with CM from MSC-SCP2 in COCO or mono-culture and treated with drugs; (**B**) Drug effects on osteoclastogenesis in combination with Gef. During the osteoclastogenic assay bone-targeted therapy drugs and Eve were added. Significance was compared to untreated osteoclasts; * $p < 0.05$.

3. Discussion

This study aimed to evaluate the crosstalk between BC cells and bone-derived stromal cells through the development of a fully human preclinical model useful for studying drug activity on the bone microenvironment. We used the SCP2 BC cell line, an MDA-MB-231-derived triple-negative cell line with an intrinsic bone metastatic signature [43], which constitutes a good candidate for investigating BC metastasis in vitro.

Several studies have investigated the interactions of BC cells with primary osteoblasts or with osteogenically differentiated [19–22,44] and undifferentiated [45,46] MSC.Since undifferentiated MSC represent a key mediator in the bone microenvironment crosstalk [44,47,48], we investigated their interactions with cancer cells. First, we allowed the MSC to interact through medium sharing with the SCP2 cells. Then, we assayed this dynamically generated CM to modulate osteoclastogenesis.

We challenged this optimized preclinical model with Gef and bone-targeted therapies and Eve to evaluate the contribution of the EGFR pathway to the interaction between MSC and SCP2 cells, as well as to the osteoclastogenic effect of the CM.

Lu et al. showed that Gef significantly reduced the development of metastasis after intracardic or intratibial inoculation of mice with SCP20 cells, a highly bone-metastatic clone of the MDA-MB-231 cells [19]. Normanno et al. extensively investigated the contribution of the EGFR pathway to the crosstalk of different stromal cell populations within the bone marrow, and of stromal cells with cancer cells. They showed relevant cytological effects of Gef in the setting assayed, including the direct cytotoxic effect of the drug and the inhibition of osteoclastogenesis [17,46,49].

Our results indicated that MSC induced the upregulation of RANK in SCP2 and, to a lesser extent, of the EGFR pathway, suggesting that the crosstalk with MSC promoted the stimulation of these two signaling pathways. Considering that RANK, as previously discussed, is related to osteomimicry, this remarkable observation supports that our experimental approach is informative of the molecular interactions occurring in vivo. On the other hand, EGFR is the target of Gef: its increase after COCO with bone cells endorses the biological rationale to use this drug for inhibiting cancer cells in the bone microenvironment.

Treatment of MSC-SCP2 COCO with Gef only partially altered this upregulation. This finding should undergo further investigation as recent studies have evidenced the interaction between these two signaling pathways, for example in bone metastasis from soft tissue sarcomas [50]. Interestingly, the CM from MSC-SCP2 COCO seemed to induce osteoclastogenesis more efficiently than the CM from either MSC or SCP2 monocultures. The treatment of MSC-SCP2 COCO with Gef, although not affecting the number of induced osteoclasts, significantly reduced their relative surface area, thus highlighting an interfering effect of this drug on the osteoclastogenesis process.

When the osteoclasts were treated with BTT and Eve, we observed that all drugs showed an inhibition effect on osteoclastogenesis. Zol and Eve performed the strongest inhibition on the development of mature osteoclasts in the MSC-sample, cultured singly or co-cultured with SCP2.

4. Materials and Methods

4.1. Cell Cultures and Reagents

The SCP2 cell line was kindly provided by Yibin Kang laboratory, where these cells had been initially isolated, as an osteotropic clone of the BC cell line MDA-MB-231 [38]. Human MSC where purchased from Lonza (Lonza, Basel, Switzerland). Cells were cultured as a monolayer in 75 cm^2 flasks at 37 °C in a 5% CO_2 atmosphere in DMEM medium (Euroclone, Milan, Italy) supplemented with 10% fetal bovine serum (Euroclone, Milan, Italy), 1% penicillin/streptomycin (PAA, Piscataway, NJ, USA) and 1% glutamine (PAA), referred as "complete medium".

4.2. Drug Sensitivity Assay

To assess SCP2 sensitivity to Gef, the 3-(4,5-dimethylthiazol-2-yl)-2,5-diphenyltetrazolium bromide (MTT) assay was performed (Sigma-Aldrich, Steinheim, Germany). Five thousand SCP2 cells were plated in a 96-well plate and treated for 24 h with Gef at the following concentrations: 0.0625, 0.125, 0.25, 0.5 and 1 μg/mL. After treatment, medium was discarded and cells were cultured with fresh DMEM for further 24 h, for washing out the drug. Then, a stock solution of MTT (5 mg/mL) was diluted 1:10 in fresh DMEM and 100 μL were dispensed in each well. Cells were incubated for 2 h at 37 °C in the dark. After incubation, the MTT solution was discarded and cells were incubated with 100 μL of an HCl isopropanol solution in order to solubilize formazan crystals. Absorbance was determined by spectrophotometric measurement at 550 nm.

4.3. MSC-SCP2 COCO Assay and Generation of CM

For COCO assays, 2×10^5 MSC were plated in 6-well plates and, separately, 1×10^5 SCP2 cells were plated in a 24 mm diameter transwell insert with 0.4 μm pores (Corning Ltd., Flintshire, UK). Cells were then allowed to adhere to their supports and, after 24 h, SCP2-seeded inserts were placed over the MSC cultures to start COCO. One SCP2-seeded insert was harvested for gene expression analysis at baseline. Cells were co-cultured in 4 mL complete DMEM for 24 h, then medium from COCOs was harvested to produce the Early-CM and replaced with 4 mL fresh complete DMEM, either or not supplemented with 1 μg/mL Gef. After 24 h of refreshment, media were completely discarded and cells were cultured in fresh complete DMEM, for washing out the drug. After further 24 h, COCOs were stopped to harvest the Late-CM from the cells not treated with Gef, and the Gef-CM from the cells treated with Gef. CM were harvested also from MSC and SCP2 cultured separately. CM were collected, centrifuged for 5 min at 1200 rpm and immediately stored at −20 °C. SCP2 and MSC were harvested for RNA and protein extraction, respectively.

4.4. Generation of Pre-Osteoclasts

Human pre-osteoclasts were generated from PBMC, following a previously established protocol with some modifications [12]. Briefly, PBMC of healthy donors who had given their written informed consent were separated by Ficoll density centrifugation (Lymphosep, Biowest, Nuaillé, France), counted and seeded in αMEM medium (Lonza) supplemented with 10% FBS, 1% penicillin/streptomycin, 1% glutamine (referred to as complete αMEM), in 24-well plates at a density of 750,000 cells/cm^2. After 2–3 h the medium was replaced with pre-osteoclast medium (complete αMEM supplemented with 20 ng/mL recombinant human M-CSF, Peprotech, Rocky Hill, NJ, USA). Pre-osteoclasts were cultured in pre-osteoclast medium, with medium refreshment every 3 days until cultures had reached about 80% confluency.

4.5. Osteoclastogenesis Assay with CM and Drugs

Pre-osteoclasts were cultured either in DM (complete αMEM supplemented with 20 ng/mL M-CSF and 20 ng/mL RANKL), or in pre-osteoclast medium (as a negative control for osteoclastogenesis) or in pre-osteoclast medium supplemented with 20% of CM collected in the COCO assay. Culture conditions for osteoclastogenesis assay are summarized in Table 1.

Table 1. Assay condition of the osteoclastogenesis assay.

Differentiation Medium	Pre-Osteoclast Medium	Pre-Osteoclast Medium		
		supplemented with Early-CM from:	supplemented with Late-CM from:	supplemented with Gef-CM from:
Alone (positive control)	Alone (negative control)	MSC culture	MSC culture	MSC culture
		SCP2 culture	SCP2 culture	SCP2 culture
		COCO	COCO	COCOC

After 14 days of the beginning of the experiment, cells were fixed by incubation in 3.7% PBS buffered formaldehyde (Polyscience, Niles, IL, USA) for 10 min at room temperature and then stained for tartrate-resistant acid phosphatase (TRAP kit, Sigma-Aldrich, Steinheim, Germany). Nuclei were counterstained with hematoxylin (TRAP kit). Multinucleated (>4 nuclei), TRAP-positive cells with at least 3 nuclei were marked as osteoclast cell-like cells. To measure the extent of osteoclastogenesis in the different experimental conditions, we measured the osteoclast surface area. Three pictures per well per culture condition were taken with AxioVision software (ZEISS, Oberkochen, Germany) and the surface area of osteoclasts was measured with ImageJ software (http://imagej.nih.gov/ij, NIH, Bethesda, MD, USA). The resulting total area was then divided by the number of measured osteoclasts, to obtain the average value. Experiments were done in triplicate.

Osteoclastogenesis assay was performed also in presence of drugs. Eve 0.1 μg/mL was added (Afinitor®, Novartis, East Hanover, NJ, USA) on day 3, and Zol 10 μmol (Zometa©, Novartis, East Hanover, NJ, USA) and Den (5 μg/mL) (XGEVA®, Thousand Oaks, CA, USA) on day 7. Each drug was added for 72 h. For each condition the CM of MSC, SCP2 and the COCO treated with and without Gef were added.

4.6. Western Blot

For phosphorylated-EGFR (pEGFR) evaluation in MSC and SCP2, proteins were isolated by direct cell lysis with a lysis buffer composed of 50 mM Tris-HCl (pH 8), 150 mM NaCl, 1% Triton

X-100 and 0.1% SDS, supplemented with 1 mM phenylmethylsulfonyl fluoride and 1:100 protease inhibitors (Sigma-Aldrich, Milan, Italy). For pEGFR positive controls, MSC and SCP2 cultures were treated with 50 ng/mL human recombinant EGF (Merck Millipore, Billerica, MA, USA) 15 min before cell lysis. The protein content was quantified using BCA protein assay kit (Thermo Fisher Scientific, Waltman, MA, USA). An equal amount of protein was separated from each sample on Bolt 4–12% Bis-Tris Plus 10 well (Novex, Life Technologies, Carlsbad, CA, USA) and transferred to Mini Format, 0.2 μm PVDF (Biorad, Hercules, CA, USA). The membranes were blocked for 2 h in 5% non-fat dry milk PBS with 0.1% Tween 20 (Sigma-Aldrich, Milan, Italy) at room temperature and incubated overnight at 4 °C with primary antibody. After washing, the membranes were incubated for 1 h at room temperature with goat anti-mouse IgG-HRP (1:5000, Santa Cruz Biotechnology, Dallas, TX, USA) and goat anti-rabbit IgG-HRP (1:5000, Santa Cruz Biotechnology) for anti-vinculin, and anti-pEGFR pretreated membranes, respectively. The acquisition was performed after 5 min of treatment with Clarity[TM] (Western ECL Substrate, Hercules, CA, USA). The following primary antibodies were used: anti-pEGFR (Tyr1173) (1:500, Upstate Cell Signaling Solution, Lake Placid, NY, USA), anti-vinculin (1:1000, Thermo Fisher Scientific).

4.7. RNA Extraction and Real-time Quantitative PCR (qPCR)

SCP2 and osteoclast cultures were directly lysed with 800 μL TRIzol® reagent (Life Technologies). RNA was then extracted according to the manufacturer's protocol, resuspended in molecular-grade bidistilled water and quantified with Nanodrop-1000 (Thermo Scientific). Five hundred ng of RNA for SCP2 and 250 ng of osteoclasts were then used for RT-PCR using iScript™ cDNA Synthesis Kit (Biorad, Hercules, CA, USA) according to the manufacturer's protocol. For qPCR, either SYBR® green or TaqMan® chemistry was used, according to the specific target gene assay (Table 2).

Table 2. Primers and probes.

SYBR™ Green Assays		
Gene symbol	Forward primer (5′–3′)	Reverse primer (5′–3′)
ACTB	GCACAGAGCCTCGCCTT	CCTTGCACATGCCGGAG
HPRT1	AGACTTTGCTTTCCTTGGTCAGG	GTCTGGCTTATATCCAACACTTCG
SPP1	AGATGGGTCAGGGTTTAGCC	CATCACCTGTGCCATACCAG
GJA1 (CX43)	TCTGAGTGCCTGAACTTGC	ACTGACAGCCACACCTTCC
ANGPT1	CCGACTTCATGTTTTCCACA	ACCGGATTTCTCTTCCCAGA
JDP2	CTTCTTCTTGTTCCGGCATC	CTTCCTGGAGGTGAAACTGG
CTSK	GCCAGACAACAGATTTCCATC	CAGAGCAAAGCTCACCAGAG
TaqMan® Assays		
Gene symbol	Assay identification number	
ACTB	Hs99999903_m1	
HPRT1	Hs02800695_m1	
EGFR	Hs01076078_m1	
TNFRSF11A (RANK)	Hs00921372_m1	
TFF1	Hs00907239_m1	

For SYBR® assays, SYBR® Select Master Mix (Life Technologies) was used with the following cycling conditions: 5 min at 50 °C and 5 min at 95 °C (hold), followed by 15 s at 95 °C and 60 s at 60 °C for 40 cycles, followed by melting curve stage. For TaqMan® assays, TaqMan® Universal PCR Master mix (Life Technologies) was used, with the same thermal profile as for intercalating dyes assays, excluding the melting curve stage. Gene expression was quantified by the Δ–Δ C_t method, normalizing samples first on the housekeeping genes *actb* and *hprt*, and then on the baseline reference samples.

4.8. Satistical Analysis

Each experiment was performed in triplicate. Data are presented as mean ± SD. Differences were assessed by a two-tailed Student's *t*-test and accepted as significant at $p < 0.05$.

5. Conclusions

We developed a fully human COCO system of BC cells and bone progenitor cells resembling some of the molecular interactions observed in vivo. We observed that MSC interaction with cancer cells induced molecular changes in the RANK pathway necessary for osteoclastogenesis and key to the formation of bone metastasis and the EGFR pathway. Our model also confirmed that the crosstalk between cancer and bone cells is crucial for bone metastasis.

The observation of the EGFR upregulation supports our idea of challenging the model with a TKI drug, as the EGFR inhibition caused a fault in the osteoclastogenesis process. This effect was enhanced by the osteoclast treatment with either Eve or Zol. These results open the way for further investigation on the combination of conventional therapy with EGFR-targeting drugs in patients with bone metastasis.

Acknowledgments: We would like to thank Cristiano Verna and Veronica Zanoni for editorial assistance, and Yibin Kang for providing the SCP2 cell line.

Author Contributions: Laura Mercatali and Toni Ibrahim conceived the idea for the study; Laura Mercatali, Federico La Manna, Chiara Spadazzi, Giacomo Miserocchi, Chiara Liverani, Alessandro De Vita, Martina Ghetti and Laura Mercatali performed the experiments; Toni Ibrahim, Laura Mercatali, Alberto Bongiovanni, Federica Recine and Dino Amadori interpreted the data; Federico La Manna and Giacomo Miserocchi wrote the paper. All the authors read and approved the final version of the manuscript for submission.

Conflicts of Interest: The authors declare no conflict of interest.

Abbreviations

COCO	MSC-SCP2 co-culture
CM	conditioned medium
DM	differentiation medium
Gef	gefitinib
EGFR	epidermal growth factor receptor
Eve	everolimus
MSC	mesenchymal stromal cells
GF	growth factors
M-CSF	macrophage colony-stimulating factor
MTT	(4,5-dimethylthiazol-2-yl)-2,5-diphenyltetrazolium bromide
NSCLC	non-small cell lung cancer
PBMC	human peripheral blood mononuclear cells
Den	denosumab
RANKL	receptor activator of nuclear factor kB ligand
TKI	tyrosine kinase inhibitor
TRAP	tartrate-resistant acid phosphatase
WB	western blot

References

1. Ibrahim, T.; Mercatali, L.; Amadori, D. A new emergency in oncology: Bone metastases in breast cancer patients (Review). *Oncol. Lett.* **2013**, *6*, 306–310. [CrossRef] [PubMed]
2. Coleman, R.E.; Rubens, R.D. The clinical course of bone metastases from breast cancer. *Br. J. Cancer* **1987**, *55*, 61–66. [CrossRef] [PubMed]
3. Liverani, C.; Mercatali, L.; Spadazzi, C.; La Manna, F.; De Vita, A.; Riva, N.; Calpona, S.; Ricci, M.; Bongiovanni, A.; Gunelli, E.; et al. CSF-1 blockade impairs breast cancer osteoclastogenic potential in co-culture systems. *Bone* **2014**, *66*, 214–222. [CrossRef] [PubMed]

4.   Stickeler, E.; Fehm, T. Targeted and osteo-oncologic treatment in early breast cancer: What is state-of-the-art and what might become so within the next 5 years? *Breast Care* **2014**, *9*, 161–167. [CrossRef] [PubMed]

5.   Weilbaecher, K.N.; Guise, T.A.; McCauley, L.K. Cancer to bone: A fatal attraction. *Nat. Rev. Cancer* **2011**, *11*, 411–425. [CrossRef] [PubMed]

6.   Phinney, D.G.; Sensebe, L. Mesenchymal stromal cells: Misconceptions and evolving concepts. *Cytotherapy* **2013**, *15*, 140–145. [CrossRef] [PubMed]

7.   Anthony, B.A.; Link, D.C. Regulation of hematopoietic stem cells by bone marrow stromal cells. *Trends Immunol.* **2014**, *35*, 32–37. [CrossRef] [PubMed]

8.   Lu, X.; Kang, Y. Epidermal growth factor signalling and bone metastasis. *Br. J. Cancer* **2010**, *102*, 457–461. [CrossRef] [PubMed]

9.   Coleman, R.E.; McCloskey, E.V. Bisphosphonates in oncology. *Bone* **2011**, *49*, 71–76. [CrossRef] [PubMed]

10.   Gnant, M.; Mlineritsch, B.; Stoeger, H.; Luschin-Ebengreuth, G.; Heck, D.; Menzel, C.; Jakesz, R.; Seifert, M.; Hubalek, M.; Pristauz, G.; et al. Adjuvant endocrine therapy plus zoledronic acid in premenopausal women with early-stage breast cancer: 62-Month follow-up from the ABCSG-12 randomised trial. *Lancet Oncol.* **2011**, *12*, 631–641. [CrossRef]

11.   Stopeck, A.T.; Lipton, A.; Body, J.J.; Steger, G.G.; Tonkin, K.; de Boer, R.H.; Lichinitser, M.; Fujiwara, Y.; Yardley, D.A.; Viniegra, M.; et al. Denosumab compared with zoledronic acid for the treatment of bone metastases in patients with advanced breast cancer: A randomized, double-blind study. *J. Clin. Oncol.* **2010**, *28*, 5132–5139. [CrossRef] [PubMed]

12.   Mercatali, L.; Spadazzi, C.; Miserocchi, G.; Liverani, C.; De Vita, A.; Bongiovanni, A.; Recine, F.; Amadori, D.; Ibrahim, T. The effect of everolimus in an in vitro model of triple negative breast cancer and osteoclasts. *Int. J. Mol. Sci.* **2016**, *17*, 1827. [CrossRef] [PubMed]

13.   Baselga, J.; Campone, M.; Piccart, M.; Rugo, H.S.; Sahmoud, T.; Noguchi, S.; Gnant, M.; Pritchard, K.I.; Lebrun, F.; Beck, J.; et al. Eve in postmenopausal hormone-receptor-positive advanced breast cancer. *N. Engl. J. Med.* **2012**, *366*, 520–529. [CrossRef] [PubMed]

14.   Gnant, M.; Baselga, J.; Rugo, H.S.; Noguchi, S.; Burris, H.A.; Piccart, M.; Hortobagyi, G.N.; Eakle, J.; Mukai, H.; Iwata, H.; et al. Effect of eve on bone marker levels and progressive disease in bone in BOLERO-2. *J. Natl. Cancer Inst.* **2013**, *105*, 654–663. [CrossRef] [PubMed]

15.   Roskoski, R., Jr. The ErbB/HER family of protein-tyrosine kinases and cancer. *Pharmacol. Res.* **2014**, *79*, 34–74. [CrossRef] [PubMed]

16.   Foley, J.; Nickerson, N.K.; Nam, S.; Allen, K.T.; Gilmore, J.L.; Nephew, K.P.; Riese, D.J. EGFR signaling in breast cancer: Bad to the bone. *Semin. Cell Dev. Biol.* **2010**, *21*, 951–960. [CrossRef] [PubMed]

17.   Normanno, N.; Gullick, W.J. Epidermal growth factor receptor tyrosine kinase inhibitors and bone metastases: Different mechanisms of action for a novel therapeutic application? *Endocr. Relat. Cancer* **2006**, *13*, 3–6. [CrossRef] [PubMed]

18.   National Comprehensive Care Network. NCCN Clinical Practice Guidelines in Oncology: Non-Small Cell Lung Cancer V4. 2016. Available online: https://www.nccn.org/ (accessed on 15 August 2016).

19.   Lu, X.; Wang, Q.; Hu, G.; Van Poznak, C.; Fleisher, M.; Reiss, M.; Massagué, J.; Kang, Y. ADAMTS1 and MMP1 proteolytically engage EGF-like ligands in an osteolytic signaling cascade for bone metastasis. *Genes Dev.* **2009**, *23*, 1882–1894. [CrossRef] [PubMed]

20.   Ciardiello, F.; Caputo, R.; Bianco, R.; Damiano, V.; Fontanini, G.; Cuccato, S.; De Placido, S.; Bianco, A.R.; Tortora, G. Inhibition of growth factor production and angiogenesis in human cancer cells by ZD1839 (Iressa), a selective epidermal growth factor receptor tyrosine kinase inhibitor. *Clin. Cancer Res.* **2001**, *7*, 1459–1465. [PubMed]

21.   Moasser, M.M.; Basso, A.; Averbuch, S.D.; Rosen, N. The tyrosine kinase inhibitor ZD1839 ("Iressa") inhibits HER2-driven signaling and suppresses the growth of ER2-overexpressing tumor cells. *Cancer Res.* **2001**, *61*, 7184–7188. [PubMed]

22.   Borghese, C.; Cattaruzza, L.; Pivetta, E.; Normanno, N.; de Luca, A.; Mazzucato, M.; Celegato, M.; Colombatti, A.; Aldinucci, D. Gefitinib inhibits the cross-talk between mesenchymal stem cells and prostate cancer cells leading to tumor cell proliferation and inhibition of docetaxel activity. *J. Cell. Biochem.* **2013**, *114*, 1135–1144. [CrossRef] [PubMed]

23. Baselga, J.; Albanell, J.; Ruiz, A.; Lluch, A.; Gascón, P.; Guillém, V.; González, S.; Sauleda, S.; Marimón, I.; Tabernero, J.M.; et al. Phase II and tumor pharmacodynamic study of gefitinib in patients with advanced breast cancer. *J. Clin. Oncol.* **2005**, *23*, 5323–5333. [CrossRef] [PubMed]

24. Lorusso, P.M. Phase I studies of ZD1839 in patients with common solid tumors. *Semin. Oncol.* **2003**, *30*, 21–29. [CrossRef] [PubMed]

25. Joensuu, G. A phase II trial of gefitinib in patients with rising PSA following radical prostatectomy or radiotherapy. *Acta Oncol.* **2012**, *51*, 130–133. [CrossRef] [PubMed]

26. Osborne, C.K.; Neven, P.; Dirix, L.Y.; Mackey, J.R.; Robert, J.; Underhill, C.; Schiff, R.; Gutierrez, C.; Migliaccio, I.; Anagnostou, V.K.; et al. Gefitinib or placebo in combination with tamoxifen in patients with hormone receptor-positive metastatic breast cancer: A randomized phase II study. *Clin. Cancer Res.* **2011**, *17*, 1147–1159. [CrossRef] [PubMed]

27. Somlo, G.; Martel, C.L.; Lau, S.K.; Frankel, P.; Ruel, C.; Gu, L.; Hurria, A.; Chung, C.; Luu, T.; Morgan, R., Jr.; et al. A phase I/II prospective, single arm trial of gefitinib, trastuzumab, and docetaxel in patients with stage IV HER-2 positive metastatic breast cancer. *Breast Cancer Res. Treat.* **2012**, *131*, 899–906. [CrossRef] [PubMed]

28. Zampa, G.; Moscato, M.; Brannigan, B.W.; Morabito, A.; Bell, D.W.; Normanno, N. Prolonged control of bone metastases in non-small-cell lung cancer patients treated with gefitinib. *Lung Cancer* **2008**, *60*, 452–454. [CrossRef] [PubMed]

29. Zukawa, M.; Nakano, M.; Hirano, N.; Mizuhashi, K.; Kanamori, M. The effectiveness of gefitinib on spinal metastases of lung cancer—Report of two cases. *Asian Spine J.* **2008**, *2*, 109–113. [CrossRef] [PubMed]

30. Von Minckwitz, G.; Jonat, W.; Fasching, P.; du Bois, A.; Kleeberg, U.; Lück, H.J.; Kettner, E.; Hilfrich, J.; Eiermann, W.; Torode, J.; et al. A multicentre phase II study on gefitinib in taxane- and anthracycline-pretreated metastatic breast cancer. *Breast Cancer Res. Treat.* **2005**, *89*, 165–172. [CrossRef] [PubMed]

31. Albain, K.S.; Gradishar, W.J.; Hayes, D.F.; Rowinsky, E.; Hudis, C.; Pusztai, L.; Tripathy, D.; Modi, S.; Rubi, S. Open-label, phase II, multicenter trial of ZD1839 ("Iressa") in patients with advanced breast cancer. *Breast Cancer Res. Treat.* **2002**, *76*, S33.

32. Ibrahim, T.; Flamini, E.; Mercatali, L.; Sacanna, E.; Serra, P.; Amadori, D. Pathogenesis of osteoblastic bone metastases from prostate cancer. *Cancer* **2010**, *116*, 1406–1418. [CrossRef] [PubMed]

33. Awolaran, O.; Brooks, S.A.; Lavender, V. Breast cancer osteomimicry and its role in bone specific metastasis; an integrative, systematic review of preclinical evidence. *Breast* **2016**, *30*, 156–171. [CrossRef] [PubMed]

34. Plotkin, L.; Speacht, T.L.; Donahue, H.J. Cx43 and mechanotransduction in bone. *Curr. Osteoporos. Rep.* **2015**, *13*, 67–72. [CrossRef] [PubMed]

35. Jones, D.H.; Nakashima, T.; Sanchez, O.H.; Kozieradzki, I.; Komarova, S.V.; Sarosi, I.; Morony, S.; Rubin, E.; Sarao, R.; Hojilla, C.V.; et al. Regulation of cancer cell migration and bone metastasis by RANKL. *Nature* **2006**, *440*, 692–696. [CrossRef] [PubMed]

36. Ibrahim, T.; Sacanna, E.; Gaudio, M.; Mercatali, L.; Scarpi, E.; Zoli, W.; Serra, P.; Ricci, R.; Serra, L.; Kang, Y.; et al. Role of RANK, RANKL, OPG, and CXCR4 tissue markers in predicting bone metastases in breast cancer patients. *Clin. Breast Cancer* **2011**, *11*, 369–375. [CrossRef] [PubMed]

37. Smid, M.; Wang, Y.; Klijn, J.G.; Sieuwerts, A.M.; Zhang, Y.; Atkins, D.; Martens, J.W.; Foekens, J.A. Genes associated with breast cancer metastatic to bone. *J. Clin. Oncol.* **2006**, *24*, 2261–2267. [CrossRef] [PubMed]

38. Bougen, N.M.; Amiry, N.; Yuan, Y.; Kong, X.J.; Pandey, V.; Vidal, L.J.; Perry, J.K.; Zhu, T.; Lobie, P.E. Trefoil factor 1 suppression of E-CADHERIN enhances prostate carcinoma cell invasiveness and metastasis. *Cancer Lett.* **2013**, *332*, 19–29. [CrossRef] [PubMed]

39. Markicevic, M.; Džodić, R.; Buta, M.; Kanjer, K.; Mandušić, V.; Nešković-Konstantinović, Z.; Nikolić-Vukosavljević, D. Trefoil factor 1 in early breast carcinoma: A potential indicator of clinical outcome during the first 3 years of follow-up. *Int. J. Med. Sci.* **2014**, *11*, 663–673. [CrossRef] [PubMed]

40. Santini, D.; Schiavon, G.; Vincenzi, B.; Gaeta, L.; Pantano, F.; Russo, A.; Ortega, C.; Porta, C.; Galluzzo, S.; Armento, G.; et al. Receptor activator of NF-κB (RANK) expression in primary tumors associates with bone metastasis occurrence in breast cancer patients. *PLoS ONE* **2011**, *6*, e19234. [CrossRef] [PubMed]

41. Blake, M.L.; Tometsko, M.; Miller, S.; Jones, J.C.; Dougall, W.C. RANK expression on breast cancer cells promotes skeletal metastasis. *Clin. Exp. Metastasis* **2014**, *31*, 233–245. [CrossRef] [PubMed]

42. Kawaida, R.; Ohtsuka, T.; Okutsu, J.; Takahashi, T.; Kadono, Y.; Oda, H.; Hikita, A.; Nakamura, K.; Tanaka, S.; Furukawa, H. Jun dimerization protein 2 (JDP2), a member of the AP-1 family of transcription factor, mediates osteoclast differentiation induced by RANKL. *J. Exp. Med.* **2003**, *197*, 1029–1035. [CrossRef] [PubMed]

43. Minn, A.J.; Kang, Y.; Serganova, I.; Gupta, G.P.; Giri, D.D.; Doubrovin, M.; Ponomarev, V.; Gerald, W.L.; Blasberg, R.; Massagué, J. Distinct organ-specific metastatic potential of individual breast cancer cells and primary tumors. *J. Clin. Investig.* **2005**, *115*, 44–55. [CrossRef] [PubMed]

44. Prockop, D.J.; Gregory, C.A.; Spees, J.L. One strategy for cell and gene therapy: Harnessing the power of adult stem cells to repair tissues. *Proc. Natl. Acad. Sci. USA* **2003**, *100*, 11917–11923. [CrossRef] [PubMed]

45. Normanno, N.; de Luca, A.; Aldinucci, D.; Maiello, M.R.; Mancino, M.; D'Antonio, A.; de Filippi, R.; Pinto, A. Gefitinib inhibits the ability of human bone marrow stromal cells to induce osteoclast differentiation: Implications for the pathogenesis and treatment of bone metastasis. *Endocr. Relat. Cancer* **2005**, *12*, 471–482. [CrossRef] [PubMed]

46. Chaturvedi, P.; Gilkes, D.M.; Wong, C.C.; Kshitiz, L.; Luo, W.; Zhang, H.; Wei, H.; Takano, N.; Schito, L.; Levchenko, A.; Semenza, G.L. Hypoxia-inducible factor-dependent breast cancer-mesenchymal stem cell bidirect sharing mediumional signaling promotes metastasis. *J. Clin. Investig.* **2013**, *123*, 189–205. [CrossRef] [PubMed]

47. Karnoub, A.E.; Dash, A.B.; Vo, A.P.; Sullivan, A.; Brooks, M.W.; Bell, G.W.; Richardson, A.L.; Polyak, K.; Tubo, R.; Weinberg, R.A. Mesenchymal stem cells within tumour stroma promote breast cancer metastasis. *Nature* **2007**, *449*, 557–563. [CrossRef] [PubMed]

48. Barcellos-de-Souza, P.; Gori, V.; Bambi, F.; Chiarugi, P. Tumor microenvironment: Bone marrow-mesenchymal stem cells as key players. *Biochim. Biophys. Acta* **2013**, *1836*, 321–335. [CrossRef] [PubMed]

49. Normanno, N.; de Luca, A.; Maiello, M.R.; Campiglio, M.; Napolitano, M.; Mancino, M.; Carotenuto, A.; Viglietto, G.; Menard, S. The MEK/MAPK pathway is involved in the resistance of breast cancer cells to the EGFR tyrosine kinase inhibitor gefitinib. *J. Cell. Physiol.* **2006**, *207*, 420–427. [CrossRef] [PubMed]

50. Conti, A.; Espina, V.; Chiechi, A.; Magagnoli, G.; Novello, C.; Pazzaglia, L.; Quattrini, I.; Picci, P.; Liotta, L.A.; Benassi, M.S. Mapping protein signal pathway interaction in sarcoma bone metastasis: Linkage between rank, metalloproteinases turnover and growth factor signaling pathways. *Clin. Exp. Metastasis* **2014**, *31*, 15–24. [CrossRef] [PubMed]

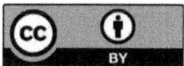

International Journal of
Molecular Sciences

MDPI

Review

Collateral Damage Intended—Cancer-Associated Fibroblasts and Vasculature Are Potential Targets in Cancer Therapy

Ana Cavaco, Maryam Rezaei, Stephan Niland * and Johannes A. Eble *

Institute of Physiological Chemistry and Pathobiochemistry, Münster University Hospital,
48149 Münster, Germany; acmcavaco@gmail.com (A.C.); mrezaei@uni-muenster.de (M.R.)
* Correspondence: nilands@uni-muenster.de (S.N.); Johannes.eble@uni-muenster.de (J.A.E.);
   Tel.: +49-251-835-5578 (S.N.); +49-251-835-5591 (J.A.E.)

Received: 28 September 2017; Accepted: 2 November 2017; Published: 7 November 2017

Abstract: After oncogenic transformation, tumor cells rewire their metabolism to obtain sufficient energy and biochemical building blocks for cell proliferation, even under hypoxic conditions. Glucose and glutamine become their major limiting nutritional demands. Instead of being autonomous, tumor cells change their immediate environment not only by their metabolites but also by mediators, such as juxtacrine cell contacts, chemokines and other cytokines. Thus, the tumor cells shape their microenvironment as well as induce resident cells, such as fibroblasts and endothelial cells (ECs), to support them. Fibroblasts differentiate into cancer-associated fibroblasts (CAFs), which produce a qualitatively and quantitatively different extracellular matrix (ECM). By their contractile power, they exert tensile forces onto this ECM, leading to increased intratumoral pressure. Moreover, along with enhanced cross-linkage of the ECM components, CAFs thus stiffen the ECM. Attracted by tumor cell- and CAF-secreted vascular endothelial growth factor (VEGF), ECs sprout from pre-existing blood vessels during tumor-induced angiogenesis. Tumor vessels are distinct from EC-lined vessels, because tumor cells integrate into the endothelium or even mimic and replace it in vasculogenic mimicry (VM) vessels. Not only the VM vessels but also the characteristically malformed EC-lined tumor vessels are typical for tumor tissue and may represent promising targets in cancer therapy.

Keywords: abnormal tumor vasculature; anti angiogenesis; cancer-associated fibroblasts; endothelial cell–tumor cell interaction; targeted tumor therapy; tumor neovascularization; tumor metabolism; tumor stroma; tumor vessel disruption; vasculogenic mimicry

1. Introduction

In the last few decades, tumor therapy has made appreciable progress. In addition to surgical intervention, radio- and chemotherapy have significantly increased survival of tumor patients. Most recently, immunotherapy directed against immune checkpoint inhibitors has been improved and advanced to first line therapy for different cancers [1,2].

While the oncogenically transformed tumor cell has been and will continue to be the focus of cancer therapy, an increasing number of publications in recent years has also shed light on cells in the vicinity of tumor cells and their role in tumor progression. Stromal fibroblasts, endothelial cells (ECs) and immune cells belong to this cellular environment. They are not unaffected bystanders, but their behavior changes in response to neighboring tumor cells. Thus, they may support growth and progression of cancer cells which eventually subvert the resident cells. This review highlights metabolic alterations and intercellular communication of tumor cells and their neighboring stromal fibroblasts and ECs. In addition, immune cells, such as macrophages, granulocytes, and leukocytes, are affected in a solid tumor and in turn affect tumor growth. These immunological aspects have been excellently reviewed elsewhere [3] and will not be covered here. This review focuses on fibrotic and vascular phenomena within growing solid tumor tissue.

2. Setting the Stage: Cancer Cells Determine the Tumor Microenvironment via Metabolites and Cytokines, via Cell–Matrix and Cell–Cell Contacts

2.1. Metabolic Reprogramming of Cancer Cells

Proliferating tumor cells lack oxygen due to a malfunction or even absence of a proper tumor vasculature. Lack of oxygen strongly contributes to a reprogramming of cancer cell metabolism and is typical of the tumor microenvironment (TME) [4]. Driven by the oxygen-dependent hypoxia-inducible transcription factor-1α (HIF-1α) [4] and by the transcription factor cellular Myelocytomatose (c-Myc) [5], expression of key enzymes which regulate fundamental metabolic pathways is controlled in an orchestrated and cancer cell-specific way [6–8]. Glycolysis and glutaminolysis are the most prominently activated pathways in cancer cells (Figure 1) which, together with hypoxia, belong to the metabolic hallmarks of cancer [9]. The prime carbon and energy source of proliferating tumor cells is glucose (Glc in Figure 1), which, after uptake by glucose transporter tye 2 (GLUT2), is utilized via glycolysis. Glycolytic key enzymes, such as hexokinase 2 and the pyruvate kinase isoform M2 (PK-M2), are upregulated [10]. Moreover, PK-M2 forms a less active dimer instead of the highly active tetramer found in normal cells [11,12]. Only high concentrations of fructose-1,6-bisphosphate triggers the formation of the enzymatically active tetramer of PK-M2 [11,12]. Reduced pyruvate kinase activity results in accumulation of upstream metabolites [7,8,13], such as phosphoenolpyruvate (PEP in Figure 1), prompts the synthesis of the amino acids serine (Ser) and glycine (Gly) and stimulates the flow of metabolites into the pentose phosphate pathway, which yields nicotinamide adenine dinucleotide phosphate (NADPH + H$^+$) and ribose-5-phosphate (R5P), the building block for nucleotides, RNA and DNA. Folate-bound C1 bodies (methylene, hydroxymethyl, formyl groups) for purine and pyrimidine synthesis are provided by the conversion of serine to glycine [6,12].

Instead of being transported into mitochondria, the end product of glycolysis, pyruvate, is cytosolically reduced to lactic acid, which dissociates into lactate and protons, and both are transported out of the cells. This explains the tumor-characteristic increase of extracellular lactate and the acidification of the tumor environment. Almost a century ago, Otto Warburg discovered that tumor cells prominently use glycolysis, even if sufficient oxygen is provided [14]. The lactic acid produced by aerobic glycolysis fails to feed the mitochondrial tricarboxylic acid (TCA) cycle [15]. To fuel the TCA cycle, glutamine (Gln in Figure 1) becomes another carbon source of the cancer cell metabolism. Glutamine utilization is mainly regulated by the glutaminase transporter and by mitochondrial glutaminase-1 in a c-Myc-dependent manner [16]. Its product, glutamate, not only replenishes the TCA cycle, but also serves as starting material for glutathione (GSH) synthesis in the cytosol. As GSH is part of the predominant intracellular redox buffer, the increased glutamine demand of tumor cells also affects redox homeostasis. The end product of glutaminolysis, α-KG, not only fuels the TCA cycle but can be converted by mutated isocitrate dehydrogenase isoforms to 2-hydroxyglutarate, whose concentration is elevated in several brain tumors [17].

This characteristic reprogramming of the metabolism allows to identify and to target tumor cells for diagnosis and therapy of cancer patients. Increased uptake and utilization of glucose and glutamine by cancer cells is diagnostically exploited by using 2-deoxy-2-(^{18}F)fluoro-D-glucose ([18]FDG) in positron emission tomography-computed tomography (PET-CT) and labeled glutamine derivatives [16]. Several transport proteins for glucose and glutamine, as well as key enzymes of the aberrantly activated glycolysis and glutaminolysis, have been identified as therapeutic targets in cancer therapy, such as GLUT2, hexokinase-2, pyruvate kinase type M2 [8,10], glutaminase-1 and glutamate dehydrogenase [16,18].

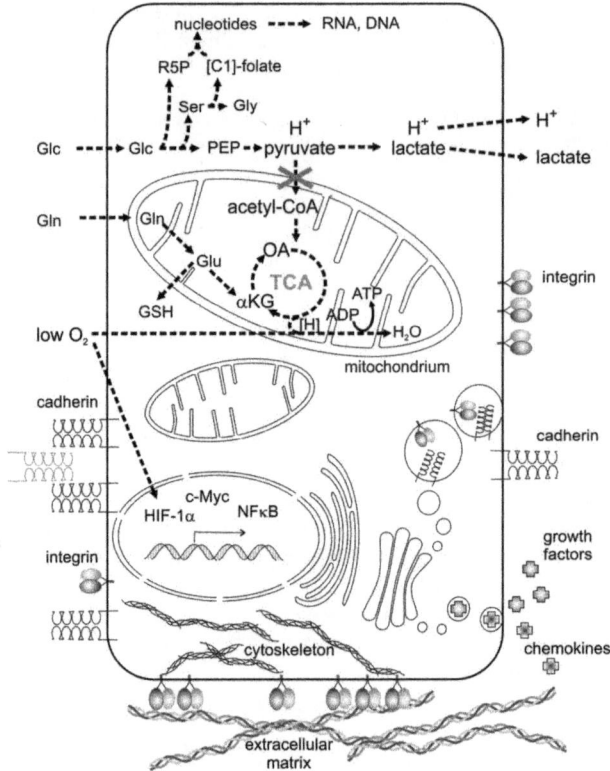

Figure 1. Metabolic reprogramming and an altered intercellular communication are hallmarks of cancer cells. Enhanced demands of glucose (Glc) and glutamine (Gln) as well as low supply of oxygen are characteristic features of cancer cell metabolism. They activate distinct transcription factors, such as hypoxia-inducible factor 1α (HIF-1α), cellular Myelocytomatose (c-Myc) and nuclear factor κ-light-chain-enhancer of activated B cells (NFκB), and upregulate expression of glycolytic and glutaminolytic key enzymes. Aerobic glycolysis leads to a high lactate concentration and a low pH of the tumor microenvironment (TME). Glycolytic metabolites stimulate the pentose phosphate pathway to produce ribose-5-phosphate (R5P) and the production of the amino acids serine (Ser) and glycine (Gly), thereby filling the tetrahydrofolate pool of C1-groups ([C1]-folate). The tricarboxylic acid (TCA) cycle is fueled by glutamine (Gln) via glutamate (Glu) and α-ketoglutarate (αKG). Glutamate is also converted to glutathione (GSH), an intracellular redox buffer. Metabolites, phosphoenolpyruvate and oxaloacetate are abbreviated to PEP and OA, respectively. Membrane-bound cell adhesion molecules (e.g., integrins) and cell–cell contact molecules (e.g., cadherin), as well as secreted and soluble growth factors and chemokines are other key communicator molecules between cancer cells and their neighboring stromal cells. Cell adhesion molecules bind to the extracellular matrix (ECM) and sense its rigidity and mechanical forces.

The metabolic reprogramming of tumor cells and secretion of metabolites also contribute to communication with stromal cells. In some cancer types, cancer-associated fibroblasts (CAFs) and cancer cells seem to establish a symbiotic relationship regarding their energy metabolism [19–21]. Lactate, produced and secreted by cancer cells is taken up by CAFs and utilized as an energy source for their pro-tumorigenic functions [22]. Conversely, cancer cells release reactive oxygen species (ROS) that induce aerobic glycolysis in CAFs, which leads to secretion of additional lactate and pyruvate. They may provide metabolic energy for cancer cells [22,23]. The direction in which the lactate/pyruvate flows depends on the conditions of the TME [19]. Caused by excess lactic acid production, the pH drop likely contributes to the acquisition of drug resistance in tumor cells [24]. Likewise, ECs near tumor cells adjust their metabolism and alter the glycolytic metabolism, a property that has recently been highlighted to be a potential therapeutic approach [25,26].

2.2. Cohesion, Adhesion and Soluble Mediators in the Communication between Tumor Cells

Cell–cell contacts (cohesion) between layer-forming epithelial and ECs are mediated by cadherins and other cell–cell contact molecules. Epithelial cell-derived carcinoma cells typically express E-cadherin, while VE-cadherin is the principal cadherin of ECs. Cadherins are transmembrane proteins consisting of five extracellular IgG-folds, a transmembrane part and a cytoplasmic tail, the latter of which is anchored via α-, β-, and γ-catenins to the actin cytoskeleton [27]. Two cadherin molecules of one cell form a homodimer which interacts with a cadherin homodimer of the same type on a neighboring cell in a Ca^{2+}-ion dependent manner, thus mediating cell-type specific cohesion and ruling out interactions with cells of other tissues which bear other cadherin types (Figure 1). While E-cadherin-expressing carcinoma cells cohere, loss of cadherin expression or function promotes contact loss to neighboring tumor cells. Thus, a carcinoma cell can disseminate from a tumor cell cluster, a hallmark of malignancy. A detached carcinoma cell changes its cellular morphology and increases its migratory potential, a process called epithelial–mesenchymal transition (EMT). EMT correlates with tumor cell scattering and metastasis [28]. E-Cadherin surface exposure is regulated at the transcriptional level by the key transcription factors, Snail family transcriptional repressor 1 (SNAI1) and TWIST1, and by epigenetic factors, such as DNA-hypermethylation, as well as by endocytosis and subsequent degradation [28]. Moreover, growth factor receptors, such as Epidermal growth factor receptor (EGFR) and hepatocyte growth factor receptor (HGFR, c-Met), may activate Src, which triggers phosphorylation and endocytosis of E-cadherin, leading to dissemination of tumor cells from the tumor mass. Even if not completely abolished, reduced E-cadherin levels have been observed in subgroups of carcinoma cells, which migrate collectively. Downregulation of E-cadherin during EMT may be accompanied by the upregulation of mesenchymal cadherins, such as N-cadherin and cadherin-11, which allow new interactions of tumor cells with stromal fibroblasts. Moreover, by expressing VE-cadherin, tumor cells may also mimic ECs and thus are able to establish unconventional interactions with ECs. Such heterotypic cohesion events may enable tumor cells to contact with stromal fibroblasts and ECs directly via cell–cell contacts [28].

Adhesion is the interaction of cells with their extracellular matrix (ECM). As a three-dimensional interstitial fibrillar meshwork, the ECM scaffolds the stromal tissue and as a two-dimensional basement membrane (BM), it supports epithelial or endothelial tissue layers. Integrins, heterodimeric transmembrane proteins consisting of an α subunit and a subgroup-determining β-subunit, are the corresponding adhesion receptors on adherent cells (Figure 1). Integrins with a β1, β3, and β4 subunit bind via their ectodomains to ECM proteins, which trigger integrin clustering and subsequent signaling. Lacking a kinase domain, integrins interact with several adaptor, signaling, and cytoskeletal proteins via their cytoplasmic domains, thereby transducing both environmental cues and mechanical forces between the ECM and the cytoskeleton [29,30]. It is of special interest that tumor cells generate mechanical forces via actin-associated motor proteins, such as myosin II. These intracellular forces are transmitted to the ECM network via integrins and build up tension in it. This mechanical tension is another key parameter which determines the TME and is sensed by resident cells, e.g., fibroblasts. Diagnostically, the BM plays a pivotal role in tumor metastasis. It is a sheet-like matrix structure containing characteristic proteins, such as type IV collagen, laminins, nidogens, and the principal BM proteoglycan perlecan. In addition to its physiological functions as morphogen, the BM acts as a cell barrier. Physiologically, it can only be penetrated by leukocytes during immune surveillance of tissues. Pathologically, oncogenically transformed tumor cells are able to breach the BM due to their altered integrin repertoire and expression of ECM degrading matrix metalloproteinases (MMPs), and thus they are considered malignant [31]. Breaching the BM defines malignancy and is another hallmark of cancer [9].

Growth factors and chemokines are other means of communication between tumor cells and within the TME (Figure 1). These soluble signaling molecules are produced by tumor cells or by resident cells. As a consequence of the TME, tumor cells may produce growth factors, such as Hepatocyte growth factor (HGF), Fibroblast growth factors (FGFs), Transforming growth factor β isoforms (TGFβs), Vascular endothelial growth factors isoforms(VEGFs), and cytokines, such as Receptor activator of nuclear factor kappa-B ligand (RANKL) and other members of the Tumor necrosis factor α (TNFα) superfamily [32,33]. This cocktail of growth factors and cytokines also contributes to the specific TME. The growth factors act in an autocrine and/or paracrine manner on tumor cells and/or resident cells, and stimulate their proliferation. Tumor cells alter the expression and activity of secreted cytokines as well as of various cytokine receptors. This alters their responsiveness to such factors. Several mutations in growth factor receptors, such as EGFR, hepatocyte growth factor receptor (cMET), and Fibroblast growth factor receptor isoforms (FGFRs), have been described to initiate uncontrolled cell proliferation of transformed cells [34,35]. Secreted by cancer cells, transforming growth factor-β (TGFβ) is a key driver in the differentiation of fibroblasts to Cancer-associated fibroblasts (CAFs). VEGF-A produced by tumor cells, under hypoxic conditions, attracts ECs to the tumor cell mass resulting in tumor-induced angiogenesis. Conversely, growth factors and cytokines produced by the resident cells may affect the cancer cells and may induce them to change their repertoire of integrins and cadherins [36–38]. For example, after stimulation by HGF, cMet triggers the internalization and subsequent degradation of E-cadherin in carcinoma cells, resulting in EMT and tumor cell dissemination [28].

In all body fluids, extracellular membrane vesicles (EVs) of different size, such as exosomes, microparticles or microvesicles, and apoptotic bodies, contain numerous signaling molecules dependent on their cellular origin. They are released from sender cells to be taken up by target cells. In this way, they convey intercellular signals in autocrine, paracrine, and even endocrine manners [39–41]. Thus, they crucially mediate intratumoral signaling, tumor progression, metastasis, and chemotherapy resistance. Exosomes with a diameter of 30–100 nm generally contain membrane fusion proteins (e.g., tetraspanins, lactadherin, and integrins), cytoskeletal proteins (e.g., actin and tubulin), membrane trafficking proteins (e.g., Rab proteins, ADP ribosylation factor (ARF) GTPases, and annexins), cytoplasmic enzymes (e.g., Glyceraldehyde 3-phosphate dehydrogenase (GAPDH), peroxidases, pyruvate kinases, and lactate dehydrogenase) and, signal transduction proteins (e.g., protein kinases and heterotrimeric G-proteins) [42,43].

Tumor cells communicate with neighboring resident cells via local metabolic parameters, such as lactic acid-mediated acidosis, low oxygen supply and increased ROS levels. Furthermore, secreted mediators, such as growth factors and chemokines, and the composition and mechanical tension of the ECM and integrin-mediated cell–matrix contacts, as well as cadherin-mediated cell–cell contacts are other means of communication in the TME (Figure 1). These factors determine the TME, in which the resident cells change their metabolism and behavior in support of the tumor cell. This niche supports cancer progression and can be compared to the "soil" in which, according to Stephen Paget's "seed and soil" theory (1889) [44], cancer cells thrive or metastasizing cells settle. The tumor cells prepare this "soil" either directly or by making neighboring cells, such as fibroblasts and ECs, change the "soil" in favor of the tumor.

3. Stromal Fibroblasts, the Immediate Neighbors of Tumor Cells

The TME constitutes a very complex niche, with extreme importance for the maintenance and progression of the tumor cells [45]. It consists of two components: cells and the ECM. The tumor stroma, or "reactive stroma" comprises three important cell groups [19,46]: CAFs (described in more detail in this section), angiogenic vascular cells (discussed in the next section) and infiltrating immune cells [3]. The pro-tumorigenic TME is characterized by an increased deposition and an altered composition of the ECM, by higher microvessel density, and by the activation of cancer-recruited stromal cells [46].

However, the TME differs between tumors, with diverse tumor stroma composition and different portions and activation states of stromal cells and it may alter during tumor progression, due to the evolving environmental conditions and oncogenic signals from growing tumors [47]. Differences in the TME are also observed within the same tumor, with disparities between the invasive edge and the tumor core, in line with the metabolic alterations, such as the availability of oxygen and nutrients [47]. Additionally, the presence of different cell types producing specific growth factors influences the tumor cells differently [48]. Finally, mechanical aspects of the tumor stroma, such as stiffness of the ECM and interstitial fluid pressure, play a crucial role in the TME [46,49]. As complex and diverse as it is, the TME dictates the fate of the tumor by providing survival and expansion signals, by setting the selection criteria of mutant subclones and by creating tumor cell heterogeneity, thereby posing an enormous challenge in cancer therapy [48].

3.1. CAFs Are Crucial for the Maintenance of a Pro-Tumorigenic TME

CAFs are the most prominent cell type in the tumor stromal compartment. They are crucial in forming and maintaining a pro-tumorigenic niche. Their presence in the tumor tissue has been associated with a poor prognosis in many cancer types as, e.g., gastric [50], colon [51], breast [52], and pancreatic cancers [53]. CAFs have been described as myofibroblasts, resembling the activated fibroblasts in wound healing. In some aspects, the tumor stroma is similar to granulation tissue, since the main cellular components are fibroblasts, together with immune, inflammatory and ECs [54]. Furthermore, in both tumor progression and wound healing, more ECM is deposited and cross-linked. As a consequence of this, the ECM scaffold is remarkably stiffened. In addition, more soluble cytokines, such as TGFβ1, are tethered to the ECM scaffold [54,55]. Dvorak even defined a tumor as "a wound that never heals" [54].

Normally, the ECM is sparsely populated by undifferentiated spindle-shaped fibroblasts [56]. When tissue injury takes place, these fibroblasts are activated. They start to express high levels of α-smooth muscle actin (αSMA), gain a stellate shape and produce more ECM [56]. Differentiating into myofibroblasts, they acquire contractile properties to close the wound. Moreover, they take on a secretory, migratory, and proliferatory phenotype. This further enhances activation and recruitment to the damaged tissue [56,57]. Once wound healing is accomplished, these cells revert to their normal phenotype or undergo apoptosis [56,58]. In a neoplastic lesion, this reversion or apoptosis does not happen. Instead, their proliferation, secretion of paracrine and autocrine cytokines [59], and ECM production and remodeling are enhanced [60]. Among the cytokines, TGFβ1, monocyte chemotactic protein (MCP1), platelet-derived growth factor (PDGF), and FGF, as well as secreted proteases have been implicated in CAFs activation [61,62]. Cancer cell-derived exosomes containing TGFβ and betaglycan have been reported to induce differentiation of fibroblasts to myofibroblasts by SMAD signaling and upregulation of basic FGF (bFGF, FGF2) production and α-smooth muscle actin expression [63]. While normal fibroblasts were reported to suppress tumor formation [64], CAFs emerge in the tumor as promoters of a pro-tumorigenic TME and thus lay an indispensable foundation for cancer progression. What is the origin of the CAFs present in the TME? There are several and controversial hypotheses about possible precursor cells and about different stimuli which ultimately induce formerly tumor-suppressing fibroblasts to express miscellaneous other marker proteins and change their phenotype into that of pro-tumorigenic CAFs. In accordance to these hypotheses is a description of CAFs as a heterogeneous cell population with numerous and different functions in the tumor. This heterogeneity complicates their investigation.

Specific markers for CAFs have not yet been identified, but diverse proteins are altered upon differentiation of fibroblasts into CAFs. αSMA, a component of cytoskeletal stress fibers, was one of the first proteins to be described as a marker for myofibroblasts in both fibrotic tissue and cancer [65]. In addition, a filament-associated, calcium-binding protein called fibroblast-specific protein 1 (FSP1) was typically expressed de novo in activated fibroblasts [66]. Platelet derived growth factor receptor-β (PDGFRβ) and NG2 chondroitin sulfate proteoglycan (NG2) were found in some populations of pancreatic CAFs, in co-localization with αSMA and FSP1, albeit in different percentages.

This may indicate different subpopulations of CAFs [67]. Fibroblast activation protein (FAP) is another marker, originally described as a cell surface glycoprotein of reactive stromal fibroblasts [68]. ECM protein tenascin C was also described to be a typical secretion product and hence potential marker of CAFs [69]. The lack of a universal CAFs marker is likely to be due to the diversity of CAFs. Depending on the tumor type and organ in which they differentiate, diverse CAF populations exist which possess different characteristics [51]. Herrera et al. showed that different subpopulations of colon CAFs, obtained from different patients, had distinct promigratory effects on colon cancer cells [51]. The diversity of tumor CAFs may be rooted in their origin [51]. CAFs can originate from several cell types, such as normal fibroblasts, myofibroblasts, adipocytes, smooth muscle cells, or bone marrow-derived progenitor cells [70,71]. Moreover, the differentiation pattern of CAFs may depend on environmental cues provided by different components of the TME, such as the ECM and the cytokine mixture. Local fibroblasts from the stroma where the neoplastic lesion develops can differentiate into CAF, as a result of stimulation by cytokines of the PDGF or TGFβ family produced by the cancer cells, macrophages and other stromal cells [72,73]. CAFs may also originate from ECs in a process called endothelial to mesenchymal transition, which ECs undergo when submitted to fibrotic conditions, e.g., under the influence of TGFβ1 [74]. By using two different tumor mouse models (pancreatic neuroendocrine tumor and melanoma), Zeisberg et al. demonstrated, that ECs acquire a mesenchymal phenotype and express markers such as FSP1, and to a smaller extent, αSMA [74]. This study showed that ECs are a possible source for CAFs in the microenvironment of angiogenic tumors.

Various functions are attributed to CAFs. Due to their acquired secretory phenotype, they play a central role in processes such as EMT, angiogenesis and immune cell recruitment. CAFs secrete TGFβ1 and thus induce EMT in many carcinomas by TGFβ1-mediated loss of adherens junctions and by increased motility of cancer cells which results in enhanced invasion and metastasis abilities [59,75]. Moreover, some of the first studies on the role of stromal cells in tumor angiogenesis used transgenic mice expressing green fluorescent protein (GFP) under the control of the vascular endothelial growth factor (VEGF) promoter. In spontaneous mammary tumors, as in wounds, the predominant GFP-positive cells were fibroblasts [76]. CAFs also have been reported to promote angiogenesis by different mechanisms: mouse cervical CAFs produce pro-angiogenic fibroblast growth factors FGF-2 and FGF-7 and, consequently interception of FGF impairs angiogenesis [77]. Another CAF-related mechanism to stimulate angiogenesis is to recruit endothelial progenitor cells (EPCs) into the carcinoma site by secretion of stromal cell-derived factor 1 (SDF-1), also known as C-X-C motif chemokine 12 (CXCL12) [78]. Moreover, Orimo et al. described that the interaction of CAF-secreted CXCL12 with its receptor C-X-C chemokine receptor type 4 (CXCR-4 (CXCR4), expressed by carcinoma cells, results in enhanced tumor growth [78]. This chemokine is also associated with an inflammatory response by recruiting leukocytes into the tumor stroma, where they contribute to angiogenesis by producing angiogenic factors, by remodeling the ECM via stimulated secretion of MMP-9, and by direct differentiation into ECs [79–81]. Moreover, immunosuppressive CAFs at the invasive front of a tumor interfere with dendritic cell differentiation [47]. CAFs also modulate the immune response by secreting cytokines and chemokines, such as interleukin-1 and MCP1, respectively [62]. In addition to cytokines, CAFs secrete exosomes, containing soluble factors that promote breast cancer cell migration. Such exosomes are yet another means of communication between cancer cells and stroma cells, but also between primary and secondary sites of a tumor [82].

3.2. ECM Is a Means of Communication in the TME and Signals via Distinct Parameters: Qualitative and Quantitative Composition, Cross-Linkage of Supramolecular Structures, Tensional Status and Degradation

The ECM forming the extracellular scaffold for fibroblasts is the characteristic component of connective tissue. Its border, the BM, forms the foundation to which cells of all other tissues, such as epithelial and ECs, muscle cells, neurons and adipocytes, are anchored. However, during carcinogenesis, the ECM is remodeled. This is mainly done by stromal cells, such as CAFs [83]. Moreover, breaching of the BM by tumor cells is a hallmark of malignancy.

The constitution of the ECM in different tumor types is highly heterogeneous. In addition, within the same tumor, differences can be noted, as ECM deposition may change depending on tumor staging [84]. Different types of collagens, laminins, proteoglycans, glycosaminoglycans, fibronectin, and vitronectin are among the most abundantly expressed ECM proteins in cancer stroma. They are deposited and remodeled by stromal cells, such as CAFs. The ECM in the TME is also functionally diverse, and the multiple interactions between the different constituents increase this diversity.

As major components of the BM, laminins are crucial in tumor angiogenesis and metastasis [85,86]. Usually laminin α4 chain is overexpressed in breast cancer and promotes cell detachment in vitro, and in vivo it stimulates tumor re-initiation in multiple organs, and disseminated metastatic cell proliferation [87].

Expression of fibronectin is upregulated in CAFs at metastatic sites, e.g., in the lung, and serves as a docking site for the hematopoietic progenitor cells and invading tumor cells [47]. Being part of the TME scaffold of aggressive tumors, it comes in two different splice variants which differ in the presence of the extra-domains (ED) A or B, called EDA and EDB [88–90]. Bordeleau et al. described the alternative splicing as an adaptation of the cells to their microenvironment [91]. The increased production of the EDB fibronectin isoform by ECs correlates with ECM stiffness [91]. Matrix stiffness-regulated splicing depends on the activation of various splice factors, on intracellular Rho/Rho-associated protein kinase (ROCK)-mediated contractility and on PI3K-AKT signaling [91]. Regulation of alternative splicing by ECM stiffness is likely to occur in other cell types, too [91]. In contrast, the alternatively spliced EDA fibronectin variant is deposited in regions of active fibrosis, e.g., in idiopathic pulmonary fibrosis [92,93]. In this context, EDA fibronectin plays a role in TGFβ-dependent differentiation of fibroblasts into myofibroblasts via autocrine/paracrine feedback loops and in metastasis, while EDB fibronectin is likely involved in EC proliferation and vascular morphogenesis, tumorigenesis and EMT [88,94].

Tenascin-C and periostin are matricellular proteins produced by CAFs. They collaboratively contribute to lung metastasis, in a process involving Wingless-related integration site (Wnt) and Notch signaling pathways [95]. Periostin recruits Wnt ligands and presents them to stem-like metastasis-initiating cells [96]. On the other hand, tenascin-C, produced by both CAFs and tumor cells, activates Wnt and Notch pathways, supporting the fitness of metastasis-initiating breast cancer cells and their "seeding" at the metastatic site [97]. Moreover, periostin also contributes to proper assembly and homeostasis of collagen. In addition, its deposition enables tenascin-C to bind to other ECM molecules such as collagen-I and fibronectin [98,99]. Tenascin-W, the fourth and newest member of the tenascin family, was discovered ten years ago. It is expressed in activated tumor stroma, facilitating tumorigenesis by supporting the migratory behavior of breast cancer cells [100]. Both tenascin-C and -W can be expressed in tumor stroma usually at similar percentages, being most likely produced by CAFs [101]. However, they do not necessarily coexist in a tumor, likely due to independent modulation mechanisms [101]. For example, tenascin-W is enriched in low-grade cancers, while tenascin-C expression is found irrespective of the tumor grade [100]. In addition, in colon cancer, tenascin-W, in contrast to tenascin-C, is ectopically expressed in tumor tissue and is considered as cancer biomarker of unfavorable disease progression, since it is not detectable in healthy colon stroma [102]. Moreover, tenascin-W is present in the stroma of mouse mammary tumor models developing metastasis, whereas tenascin-C is absent from both non-metastatic tumors and normal mammary tissue [103].

A fibrotic overexpression of collagenous ECM components contributes to a desmoplastic TME [83]. The mechanical robustness and stiffness of the ECM is strongly increased through inter- and intramolecular cross-linkages of fibrous collagen and elastin. They are catalyzed by members of the lysyl oxidase (LOX) gene family, such as lysyl oxidase-like protein-1 (LOXL1). The expression of this amine oxidase seems to correlate with increased tumor malignancy, since it is expressed in metastatic but not in non-metastatic cell lines [104,105]. Other experimental observations point out that LOXL1-expressing tumors are highly fibrotic and surrounded by many dense collagen fibers, [104].

Inhibition of LOX-dependent collagen crosslinking decreases tissue desmoplasia, tumor incidence and growth, and reduces mechanotransduction in the mammary epithelium [49].

The mechanical forces that increase ECM stiffening and intratumoral pressure are generated intracellularly by cytoskeletal motor proteins and transmitted via transmembrane integrins to ECM proteins such as collagens and laminins. The integrin repertoire of tumors alters during cancerogenesis [106]. Integrins are both mechanotransducers of tensile force and also elicit intracellular signaling pathways. Thereby, they regulate cell differentiation and fate [106]. Tumor cells express, e.g., β4 integrins which endow them with resistance to apoptosis [107]. In addition, β1-integrin expression has been described as critical for tumorigenesis initiation and for maintaining the proliferative capacity of late-stage tumor cells [108].

TGFβ stimulates CAFs by autocrine signaling to produce and deposit more collagens I and III and fibronectin, which then promote cell adhesion and strengthen mechanical signaling between CAFs and tumor cells [83]. Noteworthy, the ECM can also tether and store growth factors, e.g., latent TGFβ1 [109]. Integrin-mediated ECM contraction by CAFs releases TGFβ1 from ECM fibers under tension, especially in a fibrotic and stiffened matrix, and protease-independently activates TGFβ1 [109]. Excess production, remodeling, stiffening of the ECM and CAF differentiation mutually promote each other, resulting in increased release of TGFβ1 into the TME. Such self-sustaining growth signals promote cell activation, proliferation, and EMT, thereby reinforcing tumor progression [109].

Matrix stiffening and increased tensile forces modulate the cytoskeletal contractility in CAFs via the signaling molecules Yes-associated protein (YAP) and ROCK in a self-reinforcing positive feedback loop, by which CAFs maintain their differentiated phenotype [110]. Moreover, in vitro studies from our lab have shown that the stiffness of the ECM substrate influences not only the cytoskeletal αSMA-rich stress fibers but also the adhesion and proliferation of fibroblasts (Figure 2).

A stiff stroma and elevated Rho-dependent cytoskeletal tension promote focal adhesion formation, disruption of adherens junctions, and disturb tissue polarity [106,111,112]. In a striking study, Paszek et al. show that matrix stiffness is associated with integrin clustering, Extracellular signal–regulated kinase (ERK)-enhanced activation, and increased ROCK-generated contractility and formation of focal adhesions, in a mechanoregulatory circuit [106]. If this process becomes chronic, it promotes cell growth, disturbs tissue organization, and thus supports malignant transformation [106]. The desmoplastic response with enhanced matrix stiffening also influences the metastatic potential of epithelial cancer cells. Transformed cells often exert abnormally high forces, and these forces consequently disrupt cell–cell junctions, compromise tissue polarity, allow anchorage-independent survival, and ultimately increase invasion [49]. The cell-generated forces can also account for increased invadopodia, focal adhesion maturation and actomyosin contractility [49]. Tension-dependent matrix remodeling can also occur, as a consequence of increased contractility of tumor cells and CAFs, as it is observed in a reorientation of collagen fibrils surrounding the invasive front of the tumor [49]. Moreover, contraction of CAFs and tumor cells, and matrix stiffening cause high interstitial pressure which is another characteristic feature of the TME. Practically, the high tissue tension and high interstitial tension mechanically affects tumor vasculature by obliterating and provoking the collapse of blood and lymphatic vessels in the tumor [46,83].

Degradation of collagen and of other ECM molecules also contributes to tumor-induced ECM-remodeling and is another essential requirement for tumor invasion, where MMPs play a crucial role [113]. In mesenchymal cell migration, invading cells present focalized cell–matrix adhesions containing multi-molecular integrin clusters and increased proteolytic activity against ECM substrates [113]. Overexpression of MMPs-3, -11, -12, and -13 was detected in tumor stroma, along with MMP-2 in transformed mammary epithelial cells [49,114]. Furthermore, tumor cells recruit MMP-2- and MMP-9-producing neutrophils and macrophages [114]. Notably, immune cells tend to accumulate and migrate within dense collagen-enriched tumor stroma regions [115]. The activity of MMPs can be countered by both endogenous and pharmacological inhibitors. High expression of protease inhibitors (e.g., serpin family members) is associated with good prognosis, whilst tumors with high expression of integrins and MMPs correlate with poor prognosis and risk of recurrence [116].

Therapies employing pharmacological MMP inhibitors have been tested for various cancers with limited success so far [48].

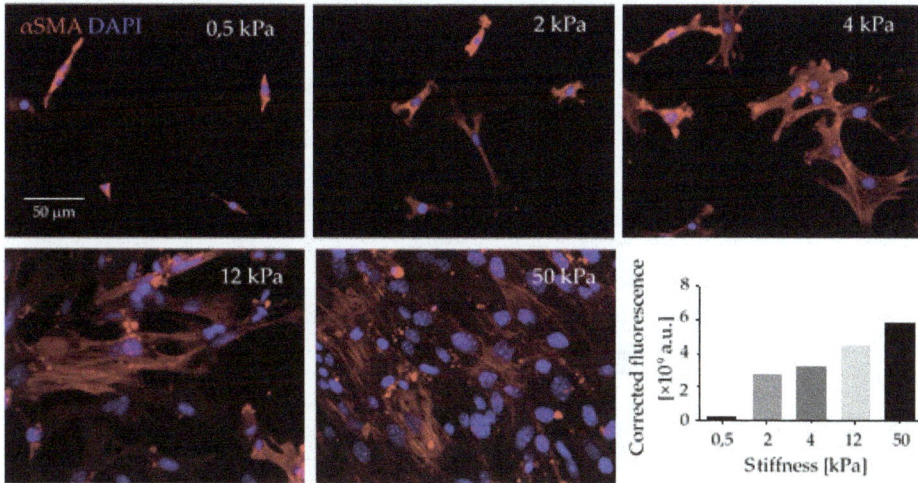

Figure 2. Mechanical stiffness of ECM is a crucial factor in CAF differentiation. Fibroblasts seeded in collagen-I coated polyacrylamide gels of defined stiffness (elastic modulus is given in kPa) exhibited increased adhesion and increased formation of α-Smooth muscle actin (αSMA)-rich stress fibers (red fluorescence). αSMA immunostaining was quantified as total corrected fluorescence. This experiment reflects in vivo conditions, where the stiff scaffold of desmoplastic ECM contributes to CAF differentiation, together with soluble factors such as TGFβ that are stored bound to ECM fibers and released when CAFs exert force on those fibers. Upon differentiation, CAFs change their morphology and express different biomarkers, such as αSMA stress fibers (red fluorescence). CAFs proliferate at higher rate, exhibit a secretory phenotype and enhanced contractibility; thus, they play an essential role in forming the TME. Scale Bar = 50 μm.

Proteolytic fragmentation of ECM proteins not only leads to remodeling or degradation of the ECM scaffold, but also release defined ECM protein fragments, so-called matrikines, which act as soluble mediators such as cytokines and influence both cancer and resident cells of the tumor tissue. Moreover, they have attracted special attention as potential new anti-cancer agents [117]. Matrikines can block pathways that are involved in proliferation and invasion of tumor cells, and they affect angiogenic and lymphangiogenic processes [117]. Collagen XVIII-derived endostatin [118] and perlecan-cleaved endorepellin [119], strongly inhibit tumor growth in many preclinical cancer models and show angiogenesis-blocking effects on sprouting ECs [117].

4. Interactions of Cancer Cells with Endothelial Cells

4.1. Tumor Vascularization

In the prevascular phase of tumor dormancy, there is a dynamic equilibrium between proliferation and hypoxia-induced apoptosis of cancer cells [120]. The oxygen diffusion limit in tissue is around 150 μm which restricts avascular tumor growth to just a few millimeters [121]. When a tumor grows beyond this size, it flips an angiogenic switch and triggers an angiogenic cascade to recruit its own vasculature and connect to the blood circuit [122,123]. The vasculature becomes permanently activated to form new vessels by sprouting from pre-existing vessels in order to supply the tumor with blood and sustain its growth [9]. This angiogenesis is driven by numerous pro-angiogenic cytokines, chemokines, and matrix-degrading enzymes during tumor development [124–127]. In addition to tumor cells themselves, infiltrating bone marrow-derived monocytes that differentiate into tumor-associated macrophages (TAMs) [128] are a further source of angiogenic factors [129–131] that recruit endothelial and mural cells, such as pericytes [132,133]. From the microscopic premalignant phase onwards, this neovascularization enables the tumor to grow exponentially [9,122,134,135].

Tumor blood vessels appear little differentiated, highly tortuous, disorganized, and chaotic. This is why blood flow is disturbed and drug delivery hampered. Tumor vasculature is unexpectedly complex and can be classified into at least six types [136]. Its specific organization and the underlying tumor vascularization mechanisms have been reviewed in [127,137–139]. A lack of mural cells, a poorly formed BM and a discontinuous endothelium, in which even tumor cells may be incorporated, render the tumor vasculature leaky and also promote metastasis, The tumor vasculature-surrounding ECM is anomalously rich in the oncofetal fibronectin ED-B splice variant, which is synthesized by neoplastic cells [140,141], and in tenascin-C and -W, which are synthesized by melanoma and glioblastoma cells and by CAFs of most carcinomas [101,142]. Tenascin-C promotes the survival of tumor stem cells, inhibits immune surveillance, stimulates angiogenesis, proliferation, invasiveness, and metastasis of tumor cells [101,142]. Furthermore, Tenascin-C expressing neuroblastoma cells can transdifferentiate into tumor cell-derived ECs [143]. Tenascin-W is exclusively detectable in tumor stroma and can be used as a tumor marker for breast and colon cancer [102,144]. In addition to preexisting vessels that can be co-opted by tumor cells (Figure 3A), neovessel formation can originate from quiescent vasculature in various ways, which are collectively called tumor angiogenesis. This general term includes EC sprouting, intussusceptive and glomeruloid angiogenesis (Figure 3B–D). Vasculogenesis, in contrast, is a process of tumor neovascularization in which bone marrow-derived cells are recruited and differentiate into EPCs (Figure 3E). Thus, tumor ECs are heterogeneous and can originate from multiple sources [145]. Furthermore, cancer stem-like cells can accomplish vasculogenesis [146], and tumor cells themselves may differentiate to take over EC functions and line partly or even completely plasma containing conduits [147]. Integration of tumor cells into an EC layer forms mosaic vessels (Figure 3F), and the complete lining of blood-filled tubes with tumor cells is a process called vasculogenic mimicry (VM) (Figure 3G–H) [148,149]. These heterogeneous formation mechanisms together with the persistent tumor vessel growth lead to a constantly shape-changing, tortuous, and highly irregular tumor vasculature of which about 30% comprise arteriovenous shunts that bypass capillaries [120]. The consequential poor perfusion causes hypoxia of ECs, which hereupon release more pro-angiogenic molecules and stimulate further tumor angiogenesis [120]. The highly irregular architecture of the tumor vasculature together with irregular direction of flow, turbulences, and pressure conditions renders the tumor vasculature intrinsically leaky [150–152]. This causes an increased interstitial pressure, which makes it difficult for chemotherapeutics that are administered via the bloodstream to reach their site of action [153].

The proliferation of tumor cells alongside of preexisting vessels is termed vessel co-option and occurs predominantly early in tumor growth, although there is evidence that hijacking vessels by co-option might persist during all stages of tumor growth [137,154,155]. With progressive tumor growth, tumor cells proliferate around constantly formed neovessels which markedly differ from normal vessels in morphology and molecular composition [156,157]. Angiogenic sprouting of ECs, which are pivotal in blood vessel growth [158], is usually involved in the formation of these vessels [159]. Triggered by an angiogenic stimulus, select ECs differentiate into tip cells that migrate along a stimulatory gradient into the avascular ECM. Other ECs start to proliferate and form cord-like structures behind the tip cells. These cords develop into endothelial tubes that finally anastomose; pericytes and smooth muscle cells are recruited, and a new BM is formed [160–162]. New tumor vessels can also arise via EC columns that move into the vessel lumen, and these transluminal pillars enlarge and form new vessel walls that split the pre-existing vessel into two in a process called intussusceptive angiogenesis [163–165]. Neovascularization by intussusceptive rather than sprouting angiogenesis is energy-saving and faster, and occurs inter alia in gliosarcoma multiforme, melanoma, breast and colon cancer [166]. Glomeruloid angiogenesis, found in many aggressive tumors, is another way of tumor angiogenesis in which several microvessels are ensheathed by a BM of varying thickness containing few pericytes to form complex vascular structures termed glomeruloid bodies [137,167,168]. Additionally, there is evidence for vasculogenesis by recruitment of bone marrow-derived EPCs that differentiate into ECs [120,169–171]. EPCs also promote the angiogenic switch and the transition from micro- to macro-metastasis [172]. Furthermore, in many cancers highly invasive and genetically dysregulated tumor cells have been reported to adopt an EC-like phenotype [173,174] and form partially non-EC-lined mosaic vessels and even completely non-EC-lined vascular-like channels to support their own blood supply by VM [148,149]. Such VM channels can arise either by tubular or patterned matrix type VM [175,176]. While VM networks of the tubular type morphologically resemble the pattern of embryonic vascular networks [137,177], the morphology and topology of the patterned matrix type strongly differs from EC-lined vessels. It displays an intricate meshwork of extravascular patterned depositions of matrix proteins such as laminins, collagens IV and VI, and heparan sulfate proteoglycans that wrap around interdigitating and branching cylinders of tumor cells and, unlike fibrovascular septa, form hollows that anastomose with blood vessels [175,178,179]. All these types of vessel formation can occur in parallel, and also gradual transitions are possible. All of them comprise numerous sequential steps which crucially depend on integrins [127] and MMPs [31,180–182] as well as on soluble growth factors [183].

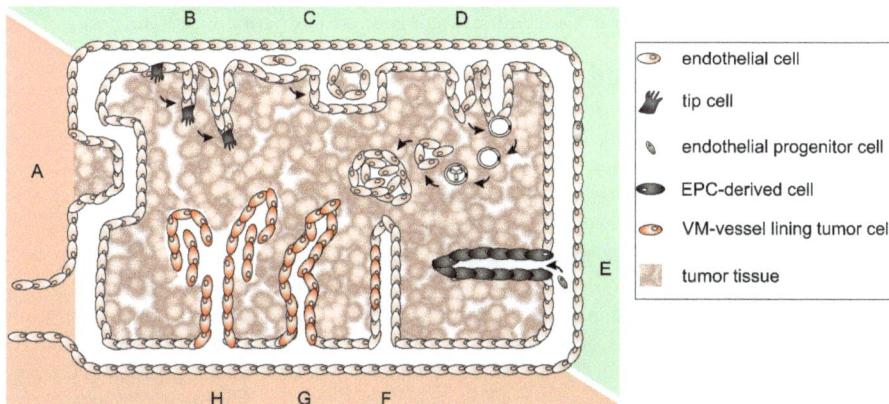

Figure 3. Different types of vascularization allow the blood supply of tumor tissue. Different types of vascularization can occur simultaneously and even merge: (**A**) co-option of preexisting vessels; (**B**) sprouting angiogenesis of endothelial cells; (**C**) intussusceptive angiogenesis; (**D**) glomeruloid angiogenesis; (**E**) vasculogenesis by recruitment of bone marrow-derived endothelial progenitor cells (EPCs); (**F**) in mosaic vessels, patches of tumor cells insert into the endothelium; (**G**) tubular type vasculogenic mimicry (VM) of tumor cells; and (**H**) patterned type VM of tumor cells. While angiogenesis (**B–D**), and vasculogenesis (**E**) depend on proliferation of ECs and bone marrow-derived EPCs, vessel co-option and VM (**F–H**) are EC proliferation-independent ways to support tumor growth. The recruitment of bone marrow-derived EPCs from distant parts of the body impairs radiation therapy, while vessel co-option and VM are unassailable to anti-angiogenic therapy. Vascularization mechanisms that are susceptible to anti-angiogenic therapy are highlighted in green, those that are insusceptible in red.

Once the tumor is connected to the vasculature, ECs become part of the tumor tissue and communicate with the other cells in the tumor tissue. Cancer progression is promoted when this communication goes awry [184,185]. At a later progression stage of a primary tumor, both angiogenetic and lymphangiogenic vessels allow tumor cells to disseminate and use the blood or lymph as a direct route of transportation to colonize distant organs. In this way, a cancer cell that successfully transmigrates through the endothelium into another tissue can form a metastasis. Regarding cancer invasion and metastasis, the endothelium acts rather as a launching site than as a barrier. ECs can affect the invasiveness of cancer cells by controlling their vascular dissemination [186] or by increasing their invasive capability [187].

Angiogenesis, vasculogenesis and vessel-based metastasis are controlled by cancer-endothelial cell (CEC) interactions. Different molecular modes of action underlying CEC interactions can be distinguished: (i) chemokine- and soluble factor-mediated interactions; (ii) tumor-endothelial communication via extracellular vesicles; and (iii) biomechanical (physical) interactions by, e.g., gap junctions and adheren junctions.

4.2. Soluble Factors Mediate CEC Interactions during Angiogenesis and Vasculogenesis

Tumor cell-secreted growth factors influence the TME and attract ECs. Such factors usually activate receptor kinases or ion channels to trigger an intracellular response. The most important endothelial growth and survival factors are the VEGFs. The VEGF family consists of five members (VEGF-A, -B, -C, and -D, and placental growth factor) that can bind to three tyrosine kinase receptors (VEGFR-1, -2, and -3) [188]. VEGF-A is the most significant inducer of local angiogenesis. Chronic VEGF stimulation in tumors promotes excessive sprouting and branching by tip cells leading to irregularities in the tumor endothelium and loss of its barrier function [189]. Almost all tumors express VEGF-A as essential growth factor in pathological angiogenesis. Furthermore, it is the prime elicitor of the angiogenic switch [190].

Originally identified as mediators of inflammatory diseases, chemokines link tumor and stromal cell communication networks to induce a proper microenvironment for tumor growth and metastasis [191]. Chemokines are a family of small cytokines secreted by cells. They bind to G protein-coupled chemokine receptors on target cells. CXCL12 is the most important CXC chemokine and is implicated in cancer cell extravasation and metastasis [192,193]. It is found in many tissues and in serum. Expressed by stromal cells of distant organs, CXCL12 promotes metastasis by attracting cancer cells and stimulating cancer cell extravasation, migration, and adhesion to ECM and to stromal cells. On cancer cells, it binds to and signals via CXC chemokine receptors type 4 (CXCR4) and 7 (CXCR7). A simultaneous and enhanced expression of CXCL12 and CXCR4 has been found in many cancers, such as breast [194], gastric [195], pancreatic [196,197], ovarian [198,199], cervical [200] and oral squamous cell carcinoma [191]. CXCL12 promotes the attachment of prostate cancer and breast cancer cells to ECs, and increases their transendothelial migration in vitro. Murakami et al. also demonstrated that ectopic expression of CXCR4 has similar effects on melanoma cells in vitro, and that it enhances lung metastasis in vivo [201].

Micro RNAs (miRNAs) are also significant regulators of angiogenesis and tumor metastasis. They are short (20–24 nucleotides) non-coding endogenous RNAs that occur in multicellular organisms and can influence the expression of many genes by post-transcriptional silencing or by causing the degradation of their mRNAs. miRNAs, which are frequently deregulated in many types of cancer, facilitate tumor growth, invasion, angiogenesis, and immune evasion through controlling translation of their target mRNAs [202,203]. For instance, in ECs co-cultured with hepatocellular carcinoma cells, three miRNAs, miR-146a, miR-181a*, and miR-140-5p, are upregulated, whereas miR-302c is downregulated [204]. Upregulation of miR-146a promotes EC migration and proliferation, as well as tumor growth and vascularization [204]. Furthermore, miRNAs can selectively be exported from cells in membrane-bound vesicles (exosomes and MPs), lipoproteins, and other ribonucleoprotein complexes. The content of these vesicles/particles varies with and corresponds to the (patho)physiological state distinct signature of the secreting cell. After the uptake of exosomal miRNAs by neighboring or distant cells, these miRNAs modulate the gene expression in the recipient cell [205]. Zhuang et al. have demonstrated that, via microvesicles, miR-9 transfers information from cancer to ECs. Thus, miR-9 supports angiogenesis and tumor growth [206].

4.3. Direct Tumor Cell–Endothelial Cell Interaction and Integration of Tumor Cells in Mosaic Vessels

Fifteen percent of vessels in xenografted and spontaneous human colon carcinomas have been reported to be of a mosaic type (Figure 3F) [207]. It is not yet clear whether these abnormal vessel structures are formed by cancer cells which integrate into the EC layer of the vessel wall or whether they arise by apoptosis of ECs and exposure of underlying cancer cells. Along with their incorporation into tumor blood vessels, cancer cells undergo epithelial–mesenchymal transition and acquire endothelial characteristics. The interaction between endothelial-like cancer cells (EndCC) and ECs, blood components, and inflammatory signals procures the differentiation of cancer cells into EndCCs. EndCCs interact with neighboring ECs, but they also possess migratory and invasive properties [208]. By biomechanical interaction of breast cancer cells with the endothelium, ECs stimulate proliferation, survival, and stemness of breast cancer cells and thus metastatic dissemination [209].

Gap junctions are special channels through the plasma membrane that directly connect the cytoplasms of neighboring cells and thus mediate short-range and direct intercellular communication which is necessary for proper tissue development and homeostasis [210]. They consist of transmembrane proteins of the connexin family [210] and allow free diffusion of small molecules and ions, and also the transport of miRNAs and small interfering RNA (siRNA) silencing signals [211,212] between cells. Altered expression of gap junction proteins is an important step in carcinogenesis [213]. Moreover, connexins play a crucial role in the direct cellular communication between cancer cells and ECs [214–217]. Extravasating breast cancer cells induce in ECs tyrosine phosphorylation of connexin 43 which facilitates further tumor cell extravasation [218]. The gap junction inhibitor, oleamide, significantly decreases homotypic communication between cancer cells and also heterotypic interaction between cancer cells and-ECs. Oleamide treatment in vitro attenuates the expression levels of several angiogenic factors, such as VEGF, HIF-1α, CXCR4, Cx26, Cx43, and MMP-9, presumably via an impaired connexin-mediated intercellular communication [219].

ECs are tightly connected via VE-cadherin-containing adherens junctions [220–222]. VE-cadherin's C-terminus is linked via β-catenin or plakoglobin to the actin cytoskeleton [223]. Blocking VE-cadherin by monoclonal antibodies inhibits angiogenesis, tumor growth, and metastasis [224]. Endothelial barrier integrity depends on differential phosphorylation of six out of nine tyrosine residues in the cytoplasmic tail of VE-cadherin [225,226]. Especially phosphorylation of Y658 and Y731 decreases vessel tightness [227]. Different cancer types vary with respect to VE-cadherin phosphorylation in neighboring ECs, which differentially affects cancer metastasis [228–230].

5. Tumor Cells Imitating Endothelial Cells in Vasculogenic Mimicry Vessels

Vasculogenic Mimicry and Its Molecular Phenotypes

Vasculogenic mimicry as one form of neovascularization was first described by Maniotis et al. [148]. Unlike angiogenesis and vasculogenesis, VM does not depend on ECs, but tumor cells themselves form vascular channels to support at least the supply with oxygen and nutrients. Since the first report of VM in 1999, its existence was controversially debated [231]. Notwithstanding, VM is clearly associated with tumor aggressiveness, and poor prognosis [232,233]. VM channels are typically characterized as an intricate meshwork of micro-channels of irregular diameter that anastomose with endothelium-lined blood vessels, but in contrast to them they are devoid of endothelial markers such as CD31. Simultaneously, they are covered by extravascular depositions of glycosylated matrix proteins, such as laminins, collagens IV and VI, and heparan sulfate proteoglycans that are positive for periodic acid Schiff (PAS) staining (Figure 4) [175,178,179,234]. Continuity and anastomosis with endothelium-lined normal vessels is a prerequisite for the functional significance of such VM channels [231], together with red blood cells in their lumen [148]. Moreover, it is conceivable that VM channels, which are too small to transport red blood cells, could also supply tumor tissue with nutrients and oxygen by hemoglobin from ruptured erythrocytes [147,235]. In a murine xenograft tumor model of inflammatory breast cancer, tumor cell lines that either do or do not show VM were used. Thus, VM channels could be discriminated from other tumor vasculature by three-dimensional contrast-enhanced dynamic micro-Magnetic resonance imaging (MRI) with G6-(1B4M-Gd)$_{256}$ dendrimer as contrast agent [236,237]. Meanwhile, VM has been observed in more than fifteen cancers, such as astrocytoma World Health Organization (WHO) grade II–III [238], glioblastoma (astrocytoma WHO grade IV) [177], melanoma [239,240], cancers of breast [237], gallbladder [241], pancreas [242], liver [243], esophageal [244], gastrointestinal [245], and colorectal tract [246], lung [247,248], ovaries [249,250], prostate [251], and various sarcomas [252,253]. In multiple myeloma, bone marrow macrophages and mast cells are additionally involved in VM of bone marrow vascularization [254,255].

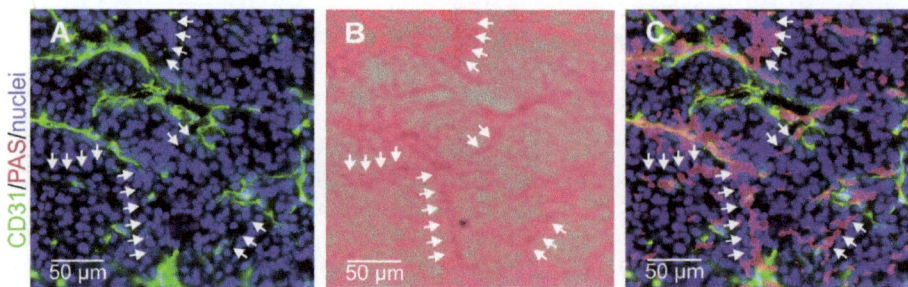

Figure 4. Vasculogenic mimicry of cancer cells lining tumor vessels. CD31-negative/PAS-positive VM channels in a HT1080 xenograft mouse tumor model were visualized by consecutive immunostaining and histochemical staining of the same cryosection: (**A,C**) normal CD31-positive blood vessels are labeled in green; and (**B,C**) CD31-negative VM channels are detectable by PAS staining. Nuclei are stained blue. (**A**) Cryosections were first immunostained and photographed; (**B**) subsequently, histochemically PAS-stained and photographed again; and (**C**) then the images were overlaid to demonstrate numerous CD31-negative/periodic acid Schiff (PAS)-positive VM channels (arrows). Representative images are shown.

Unlike the prediction based on numerous preclinical models, tumors are very likely to acquire an intrinsic resistance to angiostatic drugs [256,257]. Moreover, extrinsic mechanisms can contribute to resistance, demonstrating the important role that stromal cells play in the context of tumor neovascularization [258]. Tumor cells release many chemokines, inter alia the pro-angiogenic factors CCL2, CCL5, and CXCL12 [259] and cytokines, among them redundant pro-angiogenic cytokines, such as basic fibroblast growth factor (bFGF), interleukin-8 (IL-8), hepatocyte growth factor (HGF), PDGF, and VEGF [260], which are difficult to inhibit simultaneously. Furthermore, a tumor's blood supply by non-angiogenically originated vessels (Figure 3) is also not impaired by anti–angiogenic treatment [261]. The tumor stroma contains many different cells, among them ECs, mural cells, platelets, CAFs, and TAMs, whose roles in resistance to angiostatic therapy have been reviewed recently [258]. Similar to mesenchymal stem cells, which are capable of tubulogenesis in vitro [262], it appears that some aggressively growing tumor cells can phenotypically mimic or transdifferentiate into several of these cell types, e.g., they can adopt features of ECs [173,174], pericytes [263,264], and even platelets [265–267]. In initiation of VM, both EMT and tumor-initiating cancer stem-like cells (CSCs) play important roles [149,268,269]. In glioblastoma, a portion of the tumor vasculature arises from CSCs which have been reported to differentiate to tumor vessel pericytes upon CXCL12/CXCR4 and TGFβ signaling [263]. Macrophage migration inhibitory factor (MIF) also triggers via CXCR4 and AKT EMT in glioblastoma [270]. However, there are conflicting data whether CSCs transdifferentiate into ECs and/or pericytes [271].

To produce a functional tumor vasculature, many signaling molecules and pathways interact in a complex network, and the molecular regulation of tumor angiogenesis has been reviewed earlier to indicate therapeutic possibilities [272–274]. VM exhibits multiple molecular phenotypes, because several signaling pathways are interconnected here which are involved in vascular and embryonic/stem cell differentiation and in adaption to hypoxic conditions [174,275–277]. In adaption to the hypoxic conditions prevailing in tumor tissue, HIFs are crucially responsible. The HIF-driven pathways have been recently reviewed [278,279]. Hypoxia-response elements (HREs) are involved in regulating cell proliferation, cell death, angiogenesis, blood vessel co-option, cell adhesion molecules, secretion of MMPs, antigen presentation mechanisms and immunosuppressive factors, and additionally in vasculogenic mimicry [280]. Under normoxic conditions the α-subunit (HIF-1α, HIF-2α or HIF-3α) of the hypoxia-induced transcription factor HIF is rapidly degraded in the cytosol, whereas under hypoxic conditions it binds to the constitutively present β-subunit, thus forming an active heterodimer that translocates to the nucleus, where it controls gene expression by binding to HREs ([279] and references therein). While the transcription factor HIF-1α plays an important role in promoting sprouting angiogenesis [281], HIF-2α promotes EMT and thus VM in pancreatic cancer [282]. This is in line with the observation that VM is especially found in a hypoxic tumor core [283]. In a neuroblastoma model, an immunotherapy targeting tumor-derived ECs failed, because the treatment increased hypoxia, causing further EMT and tumor-derived EC trans-differentiation, and adaptation to the hypoxic microenvironment [284].

Hypoxia modulates the expression of many genes involved not only in angiogenesis, but also in VM, inter alia VEGF-A, VEGFR-1, Erythropoietin-producing human hepatocellular (EPH) receptor A2 (EphA2), TWIST, COX-2, and Nodal [285]. The transcription factor HIF-2α promotes EMT in pancreatic cancer by upregulating the transcription factors TWIST1 and TWIST2 in carcinoma cells which then upregulate VE-cadherin [282] and downregulate E-cadherin respectively [286]. Such VE-cadherin-expressing carcinoma cells may readily incorporate into the endothelium and give rise to composite vessels and eventually VM. Furthermore, under the selection pressure imposed by hypoxia, polyploid giant colorectal cancer cells have been reported to express EMT-related genes, to become pluripotent, and to give rise to erythroid cells expressing embryonic and fetal hemoglobin, and also to acquire EC-like features to form VM channels [287,288]. Furthermore, peroxiredoxin 2 (PRDX2), a major antioxidant enzyme, stimulates VM channel formation in colorectal cancer by keeping VEGFR-2 in its activated state [289]. The VM phenotype is thus associated with transdifferentiation of CSCs and cell plasticity [276,290], and VM channel-lining tumor cells phenotypically mimic ECs. However, they differ from ECs regarding their expression of TIE-1, VEGF-C, neuropilin.1 (NRP1), endoglin, Tissue factor pathway inhibitor (TFPI1), Laminin subunit γ2 (LAMC2), and EphA2, whereas they do not express Tyrosine kinase with immunoglobulin-like and EGF-like domains 2 (TIE-2), VEGFR-1, VEGFR-2, P-selectin, vascular adhesion protein-1 (VCAM-1), and CD31 [276].

Important transcription factors for the expression of VM-relevant genes are TWIST1 and BMI1, which are also relevant for EMT [291,292]. The EMT marker TWIST1 is activated by B-cell lymphoma 2 (Bcl-2) [293] and by metadherin (MTDH) [294], which drives CSC expansion and VM. Furthermore, CCL21/CXCR7 signaling activates the transcription factor SNAI2/Slug via ERK and Phosphatidylinositol-4,5-bisphosphate 3-kinase (PI3K)/AKT signaling in chondrosarcoma, and thus promotes EMT [295]. Together with TWIST1 and the Snail family transcription factors SNAI1/Snail and SNAI2/Slug, the Zinc finger E-box-binding homeobox 1 proteins ZEB1 and ZEB2 are pivotal EMT regulators with significant overlap in their signaling networks [296]. ZEB2, triggered by TGFβ1, promotes cell motility, invasiveness, expression of EC markers, and formation of VM vessels in hepatocellular carcinoma [296]. The paired-related homeobox transcription factor 1 (Prrx1) is also implicated in EMT, but although it is co-expressed and cooperates with TWIST1 in EMT, it suppresses stemness properties of cancer cells, and thus uncouples EMT and stemness [297]. In VM channel formation and differentiation, VE-cadherin [276], erythropoietin-producing hepatocellular receptor A2 (EphA2) [298], phosphatidyl inositol 3-kinase (PI3K) [298], MMPs [299], VEGFR-1, and HIF-1α are instrumental [174,300]. The migration inducting gene Mig-7 is expressed early in placenta development during maximal cytotrophoblast invasion and vascular remodeling, and also by carcinoma cells, where it is linked to VM [301,302]. Focal adhesion kinase (FAK) and Mig-7 induce upregulation of MMP-2 and MMP-9, which are involved in ECM degradation and VM [301,303–305].

The laminin binding lectin galectin-1 [306] is overexpressed on tumor-associated ECs and in their surrounding ECM [307]. It is also involved in the interaction of regulatory T (Treg) cells with dendritic or T cells, and it is upregulated in Treg cells upon T cell receptor activation [308]. In squamous cell carcinoma ECs, galectin-1 is overexpressed and binds directly to neuropilin-1 (NRP1), thereby enhancing phosphorylation of VEGF-R2 and triggering signaling via Mitogen-activated protein (MAP) kinases SAPK1/c-Jun N-terminal kinase (Jnk), which increases EC proliferation and adhesion, and in combination with VEGF-A it enhances cell migration [307]. The likewise laminin-binding galectin-3 [309] essentially promotes VM in melanoma by upregulating in melanoma cells the ectopic expression of genes that are otherwise typical for ECs, such as VE-cadherin, IL-8, fibronectin-1, endothelial differentiation sphingolipid G-protein receptor-1 (EDG-1), and MMP-2 [310]. While MMP-2 creates fragments from laminin-332 that increase EGFR and F-actin expression and promote VM in large cell lung cancer, MMP-13 counteracts VM by releasing different laminin-332 fragments that decrease expression of EGFR and F-actin [311]. Increased NRP1 expression upon upregulation of VEGFA, secretion of MMP-2 and -9, and activation of $\alpha v \beta 5$ integrin furthermore correlates with tumor cell invasiveness and VM [312,313]. Elevated NRP-1 expression levels are also implicated in development of resistance to anti–angiogenic therapy with VEGF-A blocking antibodies [314]. This may be due to the fact that NRP1 is not only a coreceptor of VEGFR-2 for VEGF-A but also signals upon binding of other growth factors such as class 3 semaphorins, TGFβ, HGF, FGF, and PDGF [315]. Upon PDGF-C stimulation, NRP-1 triggers invasion and VM of VEGFR-and PDGFR-deficient melanoma cells [313].

Nodal plays an essential role in VM such as in embryonic/stem cell differentiation as demonstrated by an impaired VM of aggressive melanoma cells upon downregulation of Nodal [174,316]. Notch 1 triggers EMT in hepatocellular carcinoma and promotes VM [317], while Notch4 is highly expressed in melanoma CSCs, where it promotes metastasis via the TWIST/VE-cadherin/E-cadherin pathway [269].

In addition to transcription factors, miRNAs are involved in post-transcriptional regulation of VM, thereby modulating tumor angiogenesis and cancer metastasis. TWIST1 upregulates 18 miRNAs in hepatocellular carcinoma cells, among them miR-27a-3p which targets VE-cadherin and suppresses EMT and VM [318]. Pointing in the same direction, miR-27a negatively regulates the expression of EphA2, SNAI1, and SNAi2 [319]. miR-27b binds to the 3′-untranslated region (3′-UTR) of VE-cadherin mRNA and inhibits ovarian cancer cell-mediated VM through suppression of VE-cadherin expression [320]. Loss of miR-26b promotes VM by increased EphA2 expression in glioma [321]. miR-124 regulates the expression of several EMT- and VM-relevant genes, such as CD151, ROCK1, integrin β1, Rac1, SNAI2, and angiomotin-like protein 1 (AMOTL1) [322–326]. TWIST1 downregulates miR-26b-5p in hepatocellular carcinoma by binding to its promotor region, thereby unchecking Smad1 expression and deregulating BMP4/Smad1 signaling, which promotes EMT [327]. miR-26-5p in hepatocellular carcinoma is a negative regulator of VE-cadherin, SNAI1, and MMP-2, and thus VM [328]. miR-186 downregulates the expression of TWIST1 in prostate cancer and thereby among other effects inhibits EMT and VM [329]. Loss of miR-4638-5p promotes VM in castration resistant prostate cancer by activating PI3K/AKT signaling via the kinase D-interacting substrate of 220 kDa (KIDINS220) scaffold protein [330]. KDKDM4b hypermethylates the miRNA-615-5p promotor in hepatocellular carcinoma, thereby epigenetically silencing this miRNA and consecutively increasing expression of the Ras-related protein RAB24, which activates the Rab-Ras-pathway and promotes adhesion, EMT, and VM [331].

Long non-coding RNAs (lncRNAs) are a recently discovered class of gene regulators in many physiological and pathological processes [332], and by their interaction with miRNAs [333] they are involved in metabolic reprogramming and EMT [334,335]. lncRNAs and their interaction with miRNAs in EMT have been reviewed recently [333]. The oncogenic lncRNA metastasis-associated lung adenocarcinoma transcript 1 (MALAT1) is implicated in tumor angiogenesis and also in VM by upregulating the expression of VE-cadherin, β-catenin, MMP-2, MMP-9, MMP-14, p-ERK, p-FAK, and p-paxillin [336], by upregulating N-cadherin and fibronectin, and by suppressing E-cadherin [113].

To maintain an anti-coagulatory milieu in VM vessels, channel lining tumor cells can upregulate the expression of tissue factor (TF), TF pathway inhibitor-1 (TFPI-1), and TFPI-2 [337]. VM channels not only supply the tumor with oxygen and nutrients but also might, to a limited extent, aid in some of the draining function of lymphatics [179,337,338].

Tumor growth and metastasis are promoted by angiogenic and vasculogenic pathways as well as by vessel co-option and VM. The latter two are notorious for conveying drug resistance. VM occurs in many, albeit not all, tumor tissues, but not in the healthy body, although some authors believe that hypoxic trophoblasts in placenta tissue are able to contribute to their own blood supply by VM [279]. VM correlates with a poor prognosis [247,339], because it promotes cancer growth and hematogenic dissemination of detaching tumor cells leading to metastasis [300,340–344]. In colorectal cancer, VM is positively associated with invasion depth, lymph node metastasis, distant metastasis and tumor-node-metastasis stages and negatively with patients' overall survival [345]. Likewise in ovarian carcinoma, VM is associated with tumor and lymph node metastasis grade, implantation, and stage, and with reduced patients' overall survival [346]. In ovarian carcinoma, VM correlates with the immunohistochemical detection of ALDH1, Kisspeptin (KiSS-1), and Metastasis associated in colon cancer-1 (MACC1), which are used to predict metastasis and prognosis, and VM proved to be a prognostic marker, as well as a potential target to treat epithelial ovarian carcinoma [346]. Similar data have been reported for colorectal carcinoma [345]. In addition, in non-small cell lung cancer, VM, promoted by Dickkopf-related protein 1 (DKK1) is associated with poor differentiation, advanced stage, and distant metastasis [347]. In hepatocellular carcinoma, both tubular and patterned type VM have been reported, and the latter has been ranked as an unfavorable prognostic marker [348].

6. Perspective: New Cancer Therapies Targeting Tumor Vasculature and CAFs

6.1. Anti-Angiogenesis and Normalization of the Tumor Vasculature

Cancer therapy comprises surgery, radio- and chemotherapy, targeted therapy, immunotherapy, hypothermia, hormone therapy, stem cell therapy and combinations of these methods [349]. Radiation therapy and chemotherapy target both cancer cells and tumor vasculature. Bone marrow-derived cells can restore radiation-damaged blood vessels, and they can support surviving tumor cells [272]. In addition, EPCs between the smooth muscle and adventitial layer of vessel walls, may trigger tumor neo-vascularization [156,272].

Endostatin and other anti–angiogenic inhibitors specifically target ECs rather than tumor cells to inhibit tumor angiogenesis. Such an anti–angiogenic therapy has four advantages over the usually applied cytotoxic chemotherapeutic drugs [272]: (i) angiogenesis is a homogeneous process, and therefore its inhibition should be effective in any solid tumor; (ii) an anti–angiogenic therapy approach is not impaired by tumor cells that become resistant to chemo- or radiation therapy; (iii) ECs can be directly targeted with blood-borne drugs without the need to counteract the usually high tumor interstitial pressure; and (iv) the tumor vasculature can be specifically targeted due to a differentially upregulated expression of receptors on tumor ECs versus normal EC. Therefore, anti–angiogenic therapies targeting VEGF family members, their receptors, or other pro-angiogenic factors raised high expectations [350]. However, they have not yet produced the clinical benefits initially envisioned [351].

In contrast to anti–angiogenesis, "vascular normalization" returns malformed and dysfunctional tumor vessels into vessels with a similar appearance and functionality as in normal tissues. It aims to overcome the serious problems arising from: (i) the physical barrier of tumor vessel walls; (ii) the high interstitial pressure in tumors; and (iii) the acquisition of drug resistance by genetic or epigenetic mechanisms [153]. However, delivery of chemotherapeutics may be impeded by an impervious endothelial layer [352]. Tumor-vascular disruptive agents induce a tumor-selective breakdown of the vessel wall barrier, and a combined targeting of both tumor vasculature and tumor cells may increase the efficacy of chemotherapeutics [250,353]. Until now, strategies to normalize tumor vasculature did not yet meet the initially high expectations [354], and other strategies are sought.

When anti-VEGF-induced vascular normalization ceases to be effective, the tumor becomes resistant to additional anti–angiogenic therapy and grows even more aggressive, for not yet understood mechanisms [355,356]. Various reasons may underlie this resistance to anti–angiogenic therapy and may occur simultaneously: Anti–angiogenic treatment-induced hypoxia may increase the production of other redundant angiogenic factors or the invasiveness of tumor cells. Tumor cells may also acquire mutations that render them tolerant to hypoxia. Moreover, some anti–angiogenic therapies lack specificity and have toxic side effects [273,274,357]. Such a development of drug resistance after initial success and even more aggressive tumor growth was not anticipated [358,359], and anti–angiogenic treatment turned out to have promised too much for various reasons [134,360–362]. Even if angiogenesis is curbed, neovascularization of tumor tissue may occur by other modes such as intussusceptive or glomeruloid angiogenesis, by CSC-promoted vasculogenesis, or even by VM of tumor cells [363]. In addition, vessel co-option confers resistance to anti–angiogenic therapy [155]. Moreover, many other tumor stromal cells, such as ECs, mural cells, platelets, CAFs, and TAMs, can contribute to the development of resistance to angiostatic therapy [258]. The balance between ECs on the one hand side and stromal fibroblasts and inflammatory cells, which release many cytokines and angiogenic factors other than VEGF, on the other hand could be disturbed by anti-VEGF therapy [123,261,364]. In this sense, CAFs even have been denounced Trojan horse-like mediators of resistance to anti-VEGF therapy [365].

6.2. VM Channels Are a Promising New Therapeutic Target

The so far little considered concept of VM as a new therapeutic target structure attracts increasing interest [276], because in VM channels tumor cells line the vasculature and hence are directly amenable to therapeutics from the bloodstream [276,366,367]. They have been suggested as targets for vascular disrupting agents, drug delivery, and antitumor therapy [136,353,368]. A combination of either VM inhibitors or VM disruptive agents with anti–angiogenic therapies may be promising, even if targeting VM channels, that show great diversity with respect to cellular phenotype in diverse tumors, is not as universally applicable as EC-targeting therapies, that aim at largely uniform ECs [300].

By now, numerous VM-characteristic molecular determinants and signaling pathways have already been delineated [276,278,366,369]. Tumor cells isolated from malignant pleural effusions, which develop in various malignancies due to impaired fluid drainage by blood or lymphatic vessels, inflammation and increased vascular permeability and are routinely drained for diagnosis, have been employed to test VM tube formation in vitro. Such cells may help to pinpoint drugable molecular targets (Figure 5) and to develop and optimize personalized therapy [370]. In addition, a standardized assay, which in vitro recreates the formation of fluid conducting VM channels by cancer cells surrounding a glycoprotein-rich inner layer, may be instrumental in finding and characterizing VM targeting drugs [371]. Potential molecular targets of special interest may be EMT-inducing transcription factors (EMT-TFs), such as TWIST1, SNAI1/2, and ZEB1/2 (Figure 5) [296], where ZEB2 is not only an EMT regulator but also involved in VM [372]. Expression of the transcription factor high mobility group box-1 (HMGB-1), that also interacts with nucleosomes and histones [373], is upregulated by anti–angiogenic treatment [284]. Hence, HMGB-1 has been proposed as a target for tumor therapy [374].

In addition, migration-inducting gene 7 (Mig-7), which is involved in VM by carcinoma cells, but not expressed in normal cells, may be a promising target in VM channels [302], and Mig-7-inhibitory agents together with anti–angiogenic or other conventional anti-cancer drugs might act synergistically [301,302]. The extracellular matrix metalloproteinase inducer (EMMPRIN, CD147) may also be a potential target for anti–angiogenic therapy in glioma [375]. The angiogenic factor YKL-40 (human cartilage glycoprotein HC-gp39, CHI3L1) is produced by cancer cells, inflammatory cells, and stem cells [376]. By transdifferentiation of glioma stem-like cells into vascular pericytes/smooth muscle cell- and EC-like cells, YKL-40 promotes both angiogenesis and VM [377], which in a xenograft tumor model is susceptible to treatment with a neutralizing monoclonal antibody against YKL-40 in combination with radiation therapy [378].

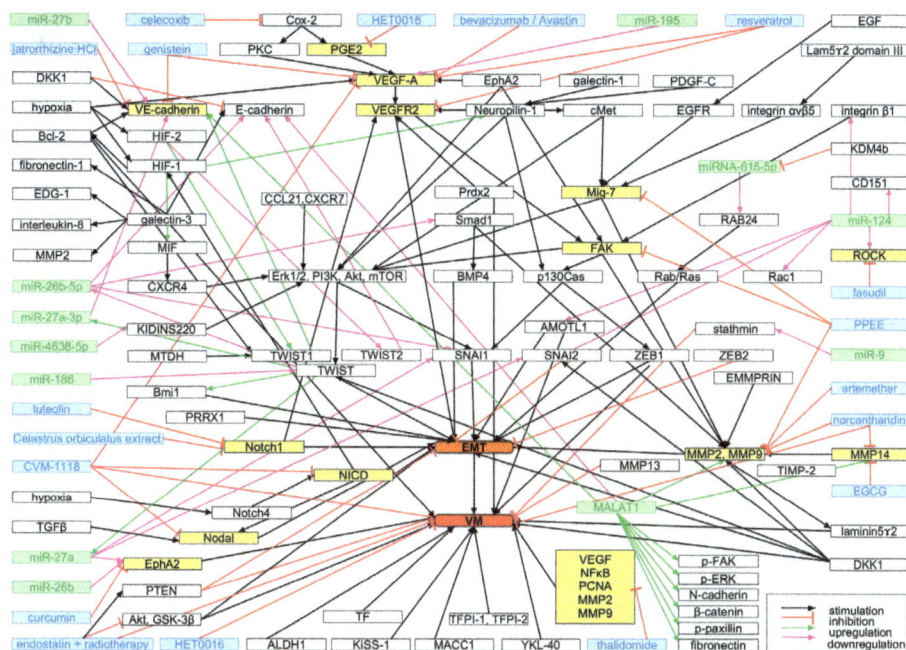

Figure 5. Molecular phenotype-defining signaling pathways in vasculogenic mimicry (VM). Signaling molecules that have been targeted to inhibit VM are highlighted in yellow and targeting compounds are marked in blue. Regulatory miRNAs are labeled green. EMT (highlighted in orange), which is pivotal for VM, and VM (highlighted in red) are the focal points in which all these signaling pathways converge. For details and references, see text.

More than ECs, cancer cells may be responsible for drug resistance to anti–angiogenic therapy [174]. Especially in VM developing tumors, VM channels lacking ECs are at least partially responsible for resistance to VEGF inhibition [379] or to anti-angiogenic agents, inter alia angiostatin and endostatin [367]. However, endostatin combined with radiotherapy suppresses VM formation through inhibition of EMT in esophageal cancer [380]. HET0016 (*N*-Hydroxy-*N*′-(4-butyl-2-methylphenyl)-formamidine), which was initially characterized as a selective inhibitor of 20-HETE (20-hydroxy-5,8,11,14-eicosatetraenoic acid) formation from arachidonic acid [381], can be used to target VM channels, whose formation is triggered by the small molecule proteinase kinase inhibitor vatalanib, which is used as anti–angiogenic therapeutic, [283]. Norcantharidin (3,6-endoxohexahydrophthalic anhydride), a demethylated derivative of cantharidin [382] downregulates MMP-9 via NFκB in hepatocellular carcinoma cells in vitro [383,384]. In vivo it also downregulates MMP-2 in a human melanoma mouse model [385], and MMPs-2 and -14 in gallbladder cancer, thereby enhancing the VM-inhibiting activity of TIMP-2 [386]. Mosaic vessel and VM channel formation in a B16F10 mouse melanoma model are reduced by thalidomide which inhibits expression of VEGF, NFκB, PCNA, MMP-2 and MMP-9 [387]. In addition, natural products with anti–angiogenic and anti-VM activity are very important for the development of new drugs. Such natural compounds and their molecular modes of action have been reviewed recently [388]. Genistein inhibits the expression of VEGF-A, PDGF, TF, urokinase-type plasminogen activator (uPA), and MMPs-2 and -9, whereas it stimulates expression of PAI-1, endostatin and angiostatin, as well as thrombospondin-1 [389]. In vivo, compounds such as genistein, jatrorrhizine hydrochloride, and curcumin inhibit VM in uveal and choroidal melanoma, respectively, via regulating VE-cadherin and EphA2 expression [390–392], whereas the antioxidant resveratrol has been reported to suppress VM in a murine melanoma model by decreasing the expression of VEGF and its receptors 1 and 2 [393]. The latter observation is in line with the finding that luteolin, likewise an antioxidant, inhibits Notch1-VEGF signaling and thus reduces VM formation in gastric cancer cells [394]. In addition, in a human hepatocellular carcinoma mouse model using GFP-labeled MHCC97-H cells, an ethnopharmacologically used *Celastrus orbiculatus* extract containing 11 terpenes, of which the effective component is not yet known, reduces VM formation by targeting Notch1 signaling [395]. An also not yet fully characterized ethanolic extract from *Paris polyphylla* has been reported to inhibit VM in a human osteosarcoma mouse model by downregulating the expression of FAK, Mig-7, and MMPs-2 and -9 [396]. Furthermore, inhibition of MMP-14 and tumor angiogenesis in two murine sarcoma and colon carcinoma models has been reported for the green tea ingredient (−)-epigallocatechin gallate (EGCG) [397].

Tumor vasculature targeting drug delivery systems have been reviewed recently, inter alia VM targeted approaches [398]. Targeting liposomes to endocytosis-prone surface receptors with ligand derivatives or antibodies improves the cellular internalization of encapsulated drugs. In combination therapy, liposomes and especially passive and active ligand-targeted liposomes have turned out to be efficient co-delivery systems for hydrophilic and lipophilic chemotherapeutic agents, such as drugs, anti-cancer metals, and gene agents [349]. Liposomes functionalized with a mannose-vitamin E derivative conjugate and a dequalinium lipid derivative to cross the blood brain barrier (BBB) and loaded with both the antimalarial drug artemether, as a regulator of apoptosis and VM channels, and the anticancer drug paclitaxel have been demonstrated in brain glioma-bearing rats to eliminate CSCs and tumor cells, and also to destroy VM channels [399]. In addition, aptamer-conjugated peptides allow delivering chemical drugs and gene drugs, e.g., antagomirs, simultaneously, as was demonstrated by co-delivery of the VM blocking ROCK inhibitor fasudil and VEGF inhibiting miR-195 [400].

6.3. Therapeutic Potential of Targeting CAFs

As CAFs are such central players in the tumor stroma, understanding the effect of CAFs on therapy and the development of a CAF-directed remedial treatment are of utmost importance as well. Indeed, CAFs affect irradiation therapy, as damaged or irradiated CAFs support tumor cell growth stronger than non-treated CAFs, possibly through up-regulation of cMet expression or its phosphorylation and MAP kinase activity in cancer cells [401]. Moreover, tumor stromal CAFs contribute to an increased intratumoral interstitial pressure, due to their potential to contract and to exert force on the ECM, thus compressing the interstitial space. This eventually results in attenuating therapeutic efficiency [46]. The interaction between cancer cells and CAFs can also reduce cytotoxic effects of chemotherapeutic drugs such as cisplatin by cell–cell adhesion through N-cadherin that activates the survival-promoting protein kinase B (PKB)/AKT and blocks pro-apoptotic Bad [402]. However, a clinical trial in which the Hedgehog signaling pathway was targeted and the tumor-induced mesenchyme activation was affected, did not show any therapeutic benefit [48].

7. Conclusions

As invasive cancer rates worldwide are continually increasing due to increased life expectancy, changes in lifestyle and nutrition, and environmental factors, cancer treatment is of prime importance. VM, albeit usually viewed as a negative prognostic marker, may constitute a potential new target for anti–angiogenic therapy [261,363]. VM and CAFs are not only passive bystanders but also active players within the tumor stroma, which contribute to tumor progression and dissemination. A better understanding of their molecular phenotypes and of their supportive roles for cancer cells are indispensable for pharmacological intervention, to resolve the burning issues of resistance to chemotherapeutic drugs and anti–angiogenic therapies, and to develop multimodal anti-angiogenic, anti-VM, and anti-proliferative strategies [138]. While tumors frequently develop resistance to anti–angiogenic drugs, new strategies that combine an anti–angiogenic therapy with a VM- or CAF-targeting approach may improve treatment success.

Acknowledgments: The authors thank the Deutsche Forschungsgemeinschaft (SFB1009, A09) and the Wilhelm Sander-Stiftung (grant 2016.113.1) for financial support. Moreover, this work was supported by financial funding from the People Programme (Marie Curie Actions) of the European Union's Seventh Framework Programme FP7/2007-2013/under REA grant agreement No. 316610 (Marie Curie-Initial Training Network CAFFEIN). The authors sincerely apologize to authors of important work not cited here for reasons of space limitation.

Conflicts of Interest: The authors declare no conflict of interest.

Abbreviations

Akt	Protein kinase B
AMOTL1	Angiomotin-like protein 1
ARF	ADP ribosylation factor
αSMA	α-Smooth muscle actin
Bcl-2	B-cell lymphoma 2
bFGF	Basic fibroblast growth factor
BM	Basement membrane
Bmi1	B lymphoma Mo-MLV insertion region 1 homolog
BMP	Bone morphogenetic protein
CAF	Cancer-associated fibroblast
CD	Cluster of differentiation
CEC	Cancer-endothelial cell interaction
CHI3L1	Chitinase-3-like protein 1
CSC	Cancer stem-like cell
cMET	Hepatocyte growth factor receptor
c-Myc	Cellular Myelocytomatose (transcription factor)
COX-2	Cyclooxygenase-2
CXC	Cysteine-any amino acid-cyteine motif
CXCL12	C-X-C motif chemokine 12 = stromal cell-derived factor 1 (SDF-1)
CXCR4	C-X-C chemokine receptor type 4
DKK1	Dickkopf-related protein 1
EC	Endothelial cell
ECM	Extracellular matrix
EDA	Extra-domain A fibronectin splice variant
EDB	Extra-domain B fibronectin splice variant
EDG-1	Endothelial differentiation sphingolipid G-protein receptor-1
EGCG	(−)-Epigallocatechin gallate
EGF(R)	Epidermal growth factor (receptor)
EMMPRIN	Extracellular matrix metalloproteinase inducer
EMT	Epithelial–mesenchymal transition
EndCC	Endothelial like cancer cell
EPC	Endothelial progenitor cell
EphA2	Erythropoietin-producing human hepatocellular (EPH) receptor A2
Erk	Extracellular signal–regulated kinase
FAK	Focal adhesion kinase
FGF(R)	Fibroblast growth factor (receptor)
GAPDH	Glyceraldehyde 3-phosphate dehydrogenase
Glc	Glucose
Gln	Glutamine
GLUT2	Glucose transporter type 2
GSH	Glutathione

HGF(R)	Hepatocyte growth factor (receptor), cMet
HIF	Hypoxia-inducible factor
HRE	Hypoxia-response element
IL	Interleukin
Jnk	c-Jun N-terminal kinase
KDM4b	Lysine-specific demethylase 4B
KIDINS220	Kinase D-interacting substrate of 220 kDa
KiSS-1	Kisspeptin
LAMC2	Laminin subunit γ2
Lam5g2	Laminin-332 γ2chain
LOX	lysyl oxidase
MACC1	Metastasis associated in colon cancer-1
MALAT1	Metastasis-associated lung adenocarcinoma transcript 1
MCP1	Monocyte chemotactic protein
Mig-7	Migration-inducing gene 7
miR	Micro RNA
MMP	Matrix metalloproteinase
MP	Microparticle
MRI	Magnetic resonance imaging
MTDH	Metadherin
NADPH + H$^+$	Nicotinamide adenine dinucleotide phosphate
NFκB	Nuclear factor κ-light-chain-enhancer of activated B cells
NICD	Notch intracellular domain
NRP1	Neuropilin-1
p130Cas	Cellular apoptosis susceptibility protein of 130 kDa
PAS	Periodic acid Schiff
PDGF	Platelet-derived growth factor
PEP	Phosphoenolpyruvate
PI3K	Phosphatidylinositol-4,5-bisphosphate 3-kinase
PK-M2	pyruvate kinase isoform M2
PPEE	*Paris polyphylla* ethanol extract
Prdx2	Peroxiredoxin-2
PRRX1	Paired-related homeobox transcription factor 1
ROCK	Rho-associated protein kinase
Rab	Ras superfamily of monomeric G protein
Rac1	Ras-related C3 botulinum toxin substrate
RANKL	Receptor activator of nuclear factor κ-B ligand
Ras	Rat sarcoma protein
ROCK	Rho-associated protein kinase
ROS	Reactive oxygen species
Smad	Small body size/mothers against decapentaplegic protein
SNAI	snail family transcriptional repressor
TAM	Tumor-associated macrophage
TCA	Tricarboxylic acid
TF	Tissue factor
TFPI1	Tissue factor pathway inhibitor
TGFβ1	Transforming growth factor-β1
TIE	Tyrosine kinase with immunoglobulin-like and EGF-like domains
TME	Tumor microenvironment
TNFα	Tumor necrosis factor α
VEGF(R)	Vascular endothelial growth factor (receptor)
VM	Vasculogenic mimicry
WHO	World Health Organization
Wnt	Wingless-related integration site

YAP	Yes-associated protein
YKL-40	Human cartilage glycoprotein HC-gp39, Chitinase-3-like protein 1, CHI3L1
ZEB	Zinc finger E-box-binding homeobox

References

1. Remon, J.; Pardo, N.; Martinez-Marti, A.; Cedres, S.; Navarro, A.; Martinez de Castro, A.M.; Felip, E. Immune-checkpoint inhibition in first-line treatment of advanced non-small cell lung cancer patients: Current status and future approaches. *Lung Cancer* **2017**, *106*, 70–75. [CrossRef] [PubMed]
2. Force, J.; Salama, A.K. First-line treatment of metastatic melanoma: Role of nivolumab. *Immunotargets Ther.* **2017**, *6*, 1–10. [CrossRef] [PubMed]
3. Gajewski, T.F.; Schreiber, H.; Fu, Y.X. Innate and adaptive immune cells in the tumor microenvironment. *Nat. Immunol.* **2013**, *14*, 1014–1022. [CrossRef] [PubMed]
4. Nakazawa, M.S.; Keith, B.; Simon, M.C. Oxygen availability and metabolic adaptations. *Nat. Rev. Cancer* **2016**, *16*, 663–673. [CrossRef] [PubMed]
5. Yeung, S.J.; Pan, J.; Lee, M.H. Roles of p53, MYC and HIF-1 in regulating glycolysis—The seventh hallmark of cancer. *Cell. Mol. Life Sci.* **2008**, *65*, 3981–3999. [CrossRef] [PubMed]
6. Li, Z.; Zhang, H. Reprogramming of glucose, fatty acid and amino acid metabolism for cancer progression. *Cell. Mol. Life Sci.* **2016**, *73*, 377–392. [CrossRef] [PubMed]
7. Lee, N.; Kim, D. Cancer metabolism: Fueling more than just growth. *Mol. Cells* **2016**, *39*, 847–854. [CrossRef] [PubMed]
8. Martinez-Outschoorn, U.E.; Peiris-Pages, M.; Pestell, R.G.; Sotgia, F.; Lisanti, M.P. Cancer metabolism: A therapeutic perspective. *Nat. Rev. Clin. Oncol.* **2017**, *14*, 11–31. [CrossRef] [PubMed]
9. Hanahan, D.; Weinberg, R.A. Hallmarks of cancer: The next generation. *Cell* **2011**, *144*, 646–674. [CrossRef] [PubMed]
10. Yu, L.; Chen, X.; Wang, L.; Chen, S. The sweet trap in tumors: Aerobic glycolysis and potential targets for therapy. *Oncotarget* **2016**, *7*, 38908–38926. [CrossRef] [PubMed]
11. Dayton, T.L.; Jacks, T.; Vander Heiden, M.G. PKM2, cancer metabolism, and the road ahead. *EMBO Rep.* **2016**, *17*, 1721–1730. [CrossRef] [PubMed]
12. Dong, G.; Mao, Q.; Xia, W.; Xu, Y.; Wang, J.; Xu, L.; Jiang, F. PKM2 and cancer: The function of PKM2 beyond glycolysis (Review). *Oncol. Lett.* **2016**, *11*, 1980–1986. [CrossRef] [PubMed]
13. Li, C.; Zhang, G.; Zhao, L.; Ma, Z.; Chen, H. Metabolic reprogramming in cancer cells: Glycolysis, glutaminolysis, and Bcl-2 proteins as novel therapeutic targets for cancer. *World J. Surg. Oncol.* **2016**, *14*, 15. [CrossRef] [PubMed]
14. Lee, M.; Yoon, J.H. Metabolic interplay between glycolysis and mitochondrial oxidation: The reverse Warburg effect and its therapeutic implication. *World J. Biol. Chem.* **2015**, *6*, 148–161. [CrossRef] [PubMed]
15. Corbet, C.; Feron, O. Cancer cell metabolism and mitochondria: Nutrient plasticity for TCA cycle fueling. *Biochim. Biophys. Acta* **2017**, *1868*, 7–15. [CrossRef] [PubMed]
16. De Vitto, H.; Perez-Valencia, J.; Radosevich, J.A. Glutamine at focus: Versatile roles in cancer. *Tumor Biol.* **2016**, *37*, 1541–1558. [CrossRef] [PubMed]
17. Dang, L.; White, D.W.; Gross, S.; Bennett, B.D.; Bittinger, M.A.; Driggers, E.M.; Fantin, V.R.; Jang, H.G.; Jin, S.; Keenan, M.C.; et al. Cancer-associated IDH1 mutations produce 2-hydroxyglutarate. *Nature* **2009**, *462*, 739–744. [CrossRef] [PubMed]
18. Jin, L.; Alesi, G.N.; Kang, S. Glutaminolysis as a target for cancer therapy. *Oncogene* **2016**, *35*, 3619–3625. [CrossRef] [PubMed]
19. Hanahan, D.; Coussens, L.M. Accessories to the crime: Functions of cells recruited to the tumor microenvironment. *Cancer Cell* **2012**, *21*, 309–322. [CrossRef] [PubMed]
20. Martinez-Outschoorn, U.E.; Lisanti, M.P.; Sotgia, F. Catabolic cancer-associated fibroblasts transfer energy and biomass to anabolic cancer cells, fueling tumor growth. *Semin. Cancer Biol.* **2014**, *25*, 47–60. [CrossRef] [PubMed]
21. Martinez-Outschoorn, U.E.; Sotgia, F.; Lisanti, M.P. Metabolic asymmetry in cancer: A "balancing act" that promotes tumor growth. *Cancer Cell* **2014**, *26*, 5–7. [CrossRef] [PubMed]

22. Rattigan, Y.I.; Patel, B.B.; Ackerstaff, E.; Sukenick, G.; Koutcher, J.A.; Glod, J.W.; Banerjee, D. Lactate is a mediator of metabolic cooperation between stromal carcinoma associated fibroblasts and glycolytic tumor cells in the tumor microenvironment. *Exp. Cell Res.* **2012**, *318*, 326–335. [CrossRef] [PubMed]

23. Sotgia, F.; Martinez-Outschoorn, U.E.; Howell, A.; Pestell, R.G.; Pavlides, S.; Lisanti, M.P. Caveolin-1 and cancer metabolism in the tumor microenvironment: Markers, models, and mechanisms. *Annu. Rev. Pathol.* **2012**, *7*, 423–467. [CrossRef] [PubMed]

24. Xing, Y.; Zhao, S.; Zhou, B.P.; Mi, J. Metabolic reprogramming of the tumour microenvironment. *FEBS J.* **2015**, *282*, 3892–3898. [CrossRef] [PubMed]

25. Potente, M.; Carmeliet, P. The Link Between Angiogenesis and Endothelial Metabolism. *Annu. Rev. Physiol.* **2017**, *79*, 43–66. [CrossRef] [PubMed]

26. Cantelmo, A.R.; Pircher, A.; Kalucka, J.; Carmeliet, P. Vessel pruning or healing: Endothelial metabolism as a novel target? *Expert Opin. Ther. Targets* **2017**, *21*, 239–247. [CrossRef] [PubMed]

27. Behrens, J. Cadherins and catenins: Role in signal transduction and tumor progression. *Cancer Metastasis Rev.* **1999**, *18*, 15–30. [CrossRef]

28. Le Bras, G.F.; Taubenslag, K.J.; Andl, C.D. The regulation of cell-cell adhesion during epithelial-mesenchymal transition, motility and tumor progression. *Cell Adhes. Migr.* **2012**, *6*, 365–373. [CrossRef] [PubMed]

29. Gehler, S.; Ponik, S.M.; Riching, K.M.; Keely, P.J. Bi-directional signaling: Extracellular matrix and integrin regulation of breast tumor progression. *Crit. Rev. Eukaryot. Gene Expr.* **2013**, *23*, 139–157. [CrossRef] [PubMed]

30. Xiong, J.; Balcioglu, H.E.; Danen, E.H. Integrin signaling in control of tumor growth and progression. *Int. J. Biochem. Cell Biol.* **2013**, *45*, 1012–1015. [CrossRef] [PubMed]

31. Murphy, G.; Nagase, H. Localizing matrix metalloproteinase activities in the pericellular environment. *FEBS J.* **2011**, *278*, 2–15. [CrossRef] [PubMed]

32. Papageorgis, P.; Stylianopoulos, T. Role of TGFβ in regulation of the tumor microenvironment and drug delivery (Review). *Int. J. Oncol.* **2015**, *46*, 933–943. [CrossRef] [PubMed]

33. Renema, N.; Navet, B.; Heymann, M.F.; Lezot, F.; Heymann, D. RANK-RANKL signalling in cancer. *Biosci. Rep.* **2016**, *36*. [CrossRef] [PubMed]

34. Matsumoto, K.; Umitsu, M.; De Silva, D.M.; Roy, A.; Bottaro, D.P. Hepatocyte growth factor/MET in cancer progression and biomarker discovery. *Cancer Sci.* **2017**, *108*, 296–307. [CrossRef] [PubMed]

35. Katoh, M. FGFR inhibitors: Effects on cancer cells, tumor microenvironment and whole-body homeostasis (Review). *Int. J. Mol. Med.* **2016**, *38*, 3–15. [CrossRef] [PubMed]

36. Khan, Z.; Marshall, J.F. The role of integrins in TGFβ activation in the tumour stroma. *Cell Tissue Res.* **2016**, *365*, 657–673. [CrossRef] [PubMed]

37. Goel, H.L.; Mercurio, A.M. Enhancing integrin function by VEGF/neuropilin signaling: Implications for tumor biology. *Cell Adhes. Migr.* **2012**, *6*, 554–560. [CrossRef] [PubMed]

38. Jeanes, A.; Gottardi, C.J.; Yap, A.S. Cadherins and cancer: How does cadherin dysfunction promote tumor progression? *Oncogene* **2008**, *27*, 6920–6929. [CrossRef] [PubMed]

39. Zhang, H.G.; Grizzle, W.E. Exosomes and cancer: A newly described pathway of immune suppression. *Clin. Cancer Res.* **2011**, *17*, 959–964. [CrossRef] [PubMed]

40. Henderson, M.C.; Azorsa, D.O. The genomic and proteomic content of cancer cell-derived exosomes. *Front. Oncol.* **2012**, *2*, 38. [CrossRef] [PubMed]

41. Dinger, M.E.; Mercer, T.R.; Mattick, J.S. RNAs as extracellular signaling molecules. *J. Mol. Endocrinol.* **2008**, *40*, 151–159. [CrossRef] [PubMed]

42. Rashed, M.H.; Bayraktar, E.; Helel, G.K.; Abd-Ellah, M.F.; Amero, P.; Chavez-Reyes, A.; Rodriguez-Aguayo, C. Exosomes: From garbage bins to promising therapeutic targets. *Int. J. Mol. Sci.* **2017**, *18*. [CrossRef] [PubMed]

43. Thery, C.; Ostrowski, M.; Segura, E. Membrane vesicles as conveyors of immune responses. *Nat. Rev. Immunol.* **2009**, *9*, 581–593. [CrossRef] [PubMed]

44. Paget, S. The distribution of secondary growths in cancer of the breast. *Cancer Metastasis Rev.* **1989**, *8*, 98–101. [CrossRef]

45. Pietila, M.; Ivaska, J.; Mani, S.A. Whom to blame for metastasis, the epithelial-mesenchymal transition or the tumor microenvironment? *Cancer Lett.* **2016**, *380*, 359–368. [CrossRef] [PubMed]

46. Heldin, C.H.; Rubin, K.; Pietras, K.; Ostman, A. High interstitial fluid pressure—An obstacle in cancer therapy. *Nat. Rev. Cancer* **2004**, *4*, 806–813. [CrossRef] [PubMed]

47. Quail, D.F.; Joyce, J.A. Microenvironmental regulation of tumor progression and metastasis. *Nat. Med.* **2013**, *19*, 1423–1437. [CrossRef] [PubMed]

48. Junttila, M.R.; de Sauvage, F.J. Influence of tumour micro-environment heterogeneity on therapeutic response. *Nature* **2013**, *501*, 346–354. [CrossRef] [PubMed]

49. Butcher, D.T.; Alliston, T.; Weaver, V.M. A tense situation: Forcing tumour progression. *Nat. Rev. Cancer* **2009**, *9*, 108–122. [CrossRef] [PubMed]

50. Fujii, S.; Fujihara, A.; Natori, K.; Abe, A.; Kuboki, Y.; Higuchi, Y.; Aizawa, M.; Kuwata, T.; Kinoshita, T.; Yasui, W.; et al. TEM1 expression in cancer-associated fibroblasts is correlated with a poor prognosis in patients with gastric cancer. *Cancer Med.* **2015**, *4*, 1667–1678. [CrossRef] [PubMed]

51. Herrera, M.; Islam, A.B.; Herrera, A.; Martin, P.; Garcia, V.; Silva, J.; Garcia, J.M.; Salas, C.; Casal, I.; de Herreros, A.G.; et al. Functional heterogeneity of cancer-associated fibroblasts from human colon tumors shows specific prognostic gene expression signature. *Clin. Cancer Res.* **2013**, *19*, 5914–5926. [CrossRef] [PubMed]

52. Yamashita, M.; Ogawa, T.; Zhang, X.; Hanamura, N.; Kashikura, Y.; Takamura, M.; Yoneda, M.; Shiraishi, T. Role of stromal myofibroblasts in invasive breast cancer: Stromal expression of alpha-smooth muscle actin correlates with worse clinical outcome. *Breast Cancer* **2012**, *19*, 170–176. [CrossRef] [PubMed]

53. Fujita, H.; Ohuchida, K.; Mizumoto, K.; Nakata, K.; Yu, J.; Kayashima, T.; Cui, L.; Manabe, T.; Ohtsuka, T.; Tanaka, M. alpha-Smooth muscle actin expressing stroma promotes an aggressive tumor biology in pancreatic ductal adenocarcinoma. *Pancreas* **2010**. [CrossRef] [PubMed]

54. Mueller, M.M.; Fusenig, N.E. Friends or foes—Bipolar effects of the tumour stroma in cancer. *Nat. Rev. Cancer* **2004**, *4*, 839–849. [CrossRef] [PubMed]

55. Mattey, D.L.; Dawes, P.T.; Nixon, N.B.; Slater, H. Transforming growth factor b1 and interleukin 4 induced a smooth muscle actin expression and myofibroblast-like differentiation in human synovial fibroblasts in vitro: Modulation by basic fibroblast growth factor. *Ann. Rheum. Dis.* **1997**, *56*, 426–431. [CrossRef] [PubMed]

56. Kalluri, R. The biology and function of fibroblasts in cancer. *Nat. Rev. Cancer* **2016**, *16*, 582–598. [CrossRef] [PubMed]

57. Micallef, L.; Vedrenne, N.; Billet, F.; Coulomb, B.; Darby, I.A.; Desmouliere, A. The myofibroblast, multiple origins for major roles in normal and pathological tissue repair. *Fibrogenes. Tissue Repair* **2012**, *5*, S5. [CrossRef]

58. Tomasek, J.J.; Gabbiani, G.; Hinz, B.; Chaponnier, C.; Brown, R.A. Myofibroblasts and mechano-regulation of connective tissue remodelling. *Nat. Rev. Mol. Cell Biol.* **2002**, *3*, 349–363. [CrossRef] [PubMed]

59. Bhowmick, N.A.; Neilson, E.G.; Moses, H.L. Stromal fibroblasts in cancer initiation and progression. *Nature* **2004**, *432*, 332–337. [CrossRef] [PubMed]

60. Polanska, U.M.; Orimo, A. Carcinoma-associated fibroblasts: Non-neoplastic tumour-promoting mesenchymal cells. *J. Cell Physiol.* **2013**, *228*, 1651–1657. [CrossRef] [PubMed]

61. Marsh, T.; Pietras, K.; McAllister, S.S. Fibroblasts as architects of cancer pathogenesis. *Biochim. Biophys. Acta* **2013**, *1832*, 1070–1078. [CrossRef] [PubMed]

62. Kalluri, R.; Zeisberg, M. Fibroblasts in cancer. *Nat. Rev. Cancer* **2006**, *6*, 392–401. [CrossRef] [PubMed]

63. Webber, J.; Steadman, R.; Mason, M.D.; Tabi, Z.; Clayton, A. Cancer exosomes trigger fibroblast to myofibroblast differentiation. *Cancer Res.* **2010**, *70*, 9621–9630. [CrossRef] [PubMed]

64. Dotto, G.P.; Weinberg, R.A.; Ariza, A. Malignant transformation of mouse primary keratinocytes by Harvey sarcoma virus and its modulation by surrounding normal cells. *Proc. Natl. Acad. Sci. USA* **1988**, *85*, 6389–6393. [CrossRef] [PubMed]

65. Serini, G.; Gabbiani, G. Mechanisms of myofibroblast activity and phenotypic modulation. *Exp. Cell Res.* **1999**, *250*, 273–283. [CrossRef] [PubMed]

66. Strutz, F.; Okada, H.; Lo, C.W.; Danoff, T.; Carone, R.L.; Tomaszewski, J.E.; Neilson, E.G. Identification and characterization of a fibroblast marker: FSP1. *J. Cell Biol.* **1995**, *130*, 393–405. [CrossRef] [PubMed]

67. Sugimoto, H.; Mundel, T.M.; Kieran, M.W.; Kalluri, R. Identification of fibroblast heterogeneity in the tumor microenvironment. *Cancer Biol. Ther.* **2006**, *5*, 1640–1646. [CrossRef] [PubMed]

68. Garin-Chesa, P.; Old, L.J.; Rettig, W.J. Cell surface glycoprotein of reactive stromal fibroblasts as a potential antibody target in human epithelial cancers. *Proc. Natl. Acad. Sci. USA* **1990**, *87*, 7235–7239. [CrossRef] [PubMed]

69. Ni, W.D.; Yang, Z.T.; Cui, C.A.; Cui, Y.; Fang, L.Y.; Xuan, Y.H. Tenascin-C is a potential cancer-associated fibroblasts marker and predicts poor prognosis in prostate cancer. *Biochem. Biophys. Res. Commun.* **2017**, *486*, 607–612. [CrossRef] [PubMed]

70. Orimo, A.; Weinberg, R.A. Stromal fibroblasts in cancer: A novel tumor-promoting cell type. *Cell Cycle* **2006**, *5*, 1597–1601. [CrossRef] [PubMed]

71. Paunescu, V.; Bojin, F.M.; Tatu, C.A.; Gavriliuc, O.I.; Rosca, A.; Gruia, A.T.; Tanasie, G.; Bunu, C.; Crisnic, D.; Gherghiceanu, M.; et al. Tumour-associated fibroblasts and mesenchymal stem cells: More similarities than differences. *J. Cell. Mol. Med.* **2011**, *15*, 635–646. [CrossRef] [PubMed]

72. Micke, P.; Ostman, A. Tumour-stroma interaction: Cancer-associated fibroblasts as novel targets in anti-cancer therapy? *Lung Cancer* **2004**, *45* (Suppl. 2), S163–S175. [CrossRef] [PubMed]

73. Mueller, L.; Goumas, F.A.; Affeldt, M.; Sandtner, S.; Gehling, U.M.; Brilloff, S.; Walter, J.; Karnatz, N.; Lamszus, K.; Rogiers, X.; et al. Stromal fibroblasts in colorectal liver metastases originate from resident fibroblasts and generate an inflammatory microenvironment. *Am. J. Pathol.* **2007**, *171*, 1608–1618. [CrossRef] [PubMed]

74. Zeisberg, E.M.; Potenta, S.; Xie, L.; Zeisberg, M.; Kalluri, R. Discovery of endothelial to mesenchymal transition as a source for carcinoma-associated fibroblasts. *Cancer Res.* **2007**, *67*, 10123–10128. [CrossRef] [PubMed]

75. Yu, Y.; Xiao, C.H.; Tan, L.D.; Wang, Q.S.; Li, X.Q.; Feng, Y.M. Cancer-associated fibroblasts induce epithelial-mesenchymal transition of breast cancer cells through paracrine TGF-β signalling. *Br. J. Cancer* **2014**, *110*, 724–732. [CrossRef] [PubMed]

76. Fukumura, D.; Xavier, R.; Sugiura, T.; Chen, Y.; Park, E.C.; Lu, N.; Selig, M.; Nielsen, G.; Taksir, T.; Jain, R.K.; et al. Tumor induction of VEGF promoter activity in stromal cells. *Cell* **1998**, *94*, 715–725. [CrossRef]

77. Pietras, K.; Pahler, J.; Bergers, G.; Hanahan, D. Functions of paracrine PDGF signaling in the proangiogenic tumor stroma revealed by pharmacological targeting. *PLoS Med.* **2008**, *5*, e19. [CrossRef] [PubMed]

78. Orimo, A.; Gupta, P.B.; Sgroi, D.C.; Arenzana-Seisdedos, F.; Delaunay, T.; Naeem, R.; Carey, V.J.; Richardson, A.L.; Weinberg, R.A. Stromal fibroblasts present in invasive human breast carcinomas promote tumor growth and angiogenesis through elevated SDF-1/CXCL12 secretion. *Cell* **2005**, *121*, 335–348. [CrossRef] [PubMed]

79. Suratt, B.T.; Petty, J.M.; Young, S.K.; Malcolm, K.C.; Lieber, J.G.; Nick, J.A.; Gonzalo, J.A.; Henson, P.M.; Worthen, G.S. Role of the CXCR4/SDF-1 chemokine axis in circulating neutrophil homeostasis. *Blood* **2004**, *104*, 565–571. [CrossRef] [PubMed]

80. Yang, L.; DeBusk, L.M.; Fukuda, K.; Fingleton, B.; Green-Jarvis, B.; Shyr, Y.; Matrisian, L.M.; Carbone, D.P.; Lin, P.C. Expansion of myeloid immune suppressor Gr+CD11b+ cells in tumor-bearing host directly promotes tumor angiogenesis. *Cancer Cell* **2004**, *6*, 409–421. [CrossRef] [PubMed]

81. Bergers, G.; Brekken, R.; McMahon, G.; Vu, T.H.; Itoh, T.; Tamaki, K.; Tanzawa, K.; Thorpe, P.; Itohara, S.; Werb, Z.; et al. Matrix metalloproteinase-9 triggers the angiogenic switch during carcinogenesis. *Nat. Cell Biol.* **2000**, *2*, 737–744. [CrossRef] [PubMed]

82. Luga, V.; Zhang, L.; Viloria-Petit, A.M.; Ogunjimi, A.A.; Inanlou, M.R.; Chiu, E.; Buchanan, M.; Hosein, A.N.; Basik, M.; Wrana, J.L. Exosomes mediate stromal mobilization of autocrine Wnt-PCP signaling in breast cancer cell migration. *Cell* **2012**, *151*, 1542–1556. [CrossRef] [PubMed]

83. Gkretsi, V.; Stylianou, A.; Papageorgis, P.; Polydorou, C.; Stylianopoulos, T. Remodeling components of the tumor microenvironment to enhance cancer therapy. *Front. Oncol.* **2015**, *5*, 214. [CrossRef] [PubMed]

84. Torimura, T.; Ueno, T.; Inuzuka, S.; Kin, M.; Ohira, H.; Kimura, Y.; Majima, Y.; Sata, M.; Abe, H.; Tanikawa, K. The extracellular matrix in hepatocellular carcinoma shows different localization patterns depending on the differentiation and the histological pattern of tumors: Immunohistochemical analysis. *J. Hepatol.* **1994**, *21*, 37–46. [CrossRef]

85. Miyazaki, K. Laminin-5 (laminin-332): Unique biological activity and role in tumor growth and invasion. *Cancer Sci.* **2006**, *97*, 91–98. [CrossRef] [PubMed]

86. Giannelli, G.; Bergamini, C.; Fransvea, E.; Sgarra, C.; Antonaci, S. Laminin-5 with transforming growth factor-beta1 induces epithelial to mesenchymal transition in hepatocellular carcinoma. *Gastroenterology* **2005**, *129*, 1375–1383. [CrossRef] [PubMed]

87. Ross, J.B.; Huh, D.; Noble, L.B.; Tavazoie, S.F. Identification of molecular determinants of primary and metastatic tumour re-initiation in breast cancer. *Nat. Cell Biol.* **2015**, *17*, 651–664. [CrossRef] [PubMed]

88. Ghigna, C.; Valacca, C.; Biamonti, G. Alternative splicing and tumor progression. *Curr. Genom.* **2008**, *9*, 556–570. [CrossRef] [PubMed]
89. Scarpino, S.; Stoppacciaro, A.; Pellegrini, C.; Marzullo, A.; Zardi, L.; Tartaglia, F.; Viale, G.; Ruco, L.P. Expression of EDA/EDB isoforms of fibronectin in papillary carcinoma of the thyroid. *J. Pathol.* **1999**, *188*, 163–167. [CrossRef]
90. Hauptmann, S.; Zardi, L.; Siri, A.; Carnemolla, B.; Borsi, L.; Castellucci, M.; Klosterhalfen, B.; Hartung, P.; Weis, J.; Stocker, G.; et al. Extracellular matrix proteins in colorectal carcinomas. Expression of tenascin and fibronectin isoforms. *Lab. Investig.* **1995**, *73*, 172–182. [PubMed]
91. Bordeleau, F.; Califano, J.P.; Negron Abril, Y.L.; Mason, B.N.; LaValley, D.J.; Shin, S.J.; Weiss, R.S.; Reinhart-King, C.A. Tissue stiffness regulates serine/arginine-rich protein-mediated splicing of the extra domain B-fibronectin isoform in tumors. *Proc. Natl. Acad. Sci. USA* **2015**, *112*, 8314–8319. [CrossRef] [PubMed]
92. Serini, G.; Bochaton-Piallat, M.L.; Ropraz, P.; Geinoz, A.; Borsi, L.; Zardi, L.; Gabbiani, G. The fibronectin domain ED-A is crucial for myofibroblastic phenotype induction by transforming growth factor-beta1. *J. Cell Biol.* **1998**, *142*, 873–881. [CrossRef] [PubMed]
93. Kuhn, C.; McDonald, J.A. The roles of the myofibroblast in idiopathic pulmonary fibrosis. Ultrastructural and immunohistochemical features of sites of active extracellular matrix synthesis. *Am. J. Pathol.* **1991**, *138*, 1257–1265. [PubMed]
94. Han, Z.; Zhou, Z.; Shi, X.; Wang, J.; Wu, X.; Sun, D.; Chen, Y.; Zhu, H.; Magi-Galluzzi, C.; Lu, Z.R. EDB Fibronectin specific peptide for prostate cancer targeting. *Bioconjug. Chem.* **2015**, *26*, 830–838. [CrossRef] [PubMed]
95. Oskarsson, T.; Massague, J. Extracellular matrix players in metastatic niches. *EMBO J.* **2012**, *31*, 254–256. [CrossRef] [PubMed]
96. Malanchi, I.; Santamaria-Martinez, A.; Susanto, E.; Peng, H.; Lehr, H.A.; Delaloye, J.F.; Huelsken, J. Interactions between cancer stem cells and their niche govern metastatic colonization. *Nature* **2011**, *481*, 85–89. [CrossRef] [PubMed]
97. Oskarsson, T.; Acharyya, S.; Zhang, X.H.; Vanharanta, S.; Tavazoie, S.F.; Morris, P.G.; Downey, R.J.; Manova-Todorova, K.; Brogi, E.; Massague, J. Breast cancer cells produce tenascin C as a metastatic niche component to colonize the lungs. *Nat. Med.* **2011**, *17*, 867–874. [CrossRef] [PubMed]
98. Egbert, M.; Ruetze, M.; Sattler, M.; Wenck, H.; Gallinat, S.; Lucius, R.; Weise, J.M. The matricellular protein periostin contributes to proper collagen function and is downregulated during skin aging. *J. Dermatol. Sci.* **2014**, *73*, 40–48. [CrossRef] [PubMed]
99. Kii, I.; Nishiyama, T.; Li, M.; Matsumoto, K.; Saito, M.; Amizuka, N.; Kudo, A. Incorporation of tenascin-C into the extracellular matrix by periostin underlies an extracellular meshwork architecture. *J. Biol. Chem.* **2010**, *285*, 2028–2039. [CrossRef] [PubMed]
100. Degen, M.; Brellier, F.; Kain, R.; Ruiz, C.; Terracciano, L.; Orend, G.; Chiquet-Ehrismann, R. Tenascin-W is a novel marker for activated tumor stroma in low-grade human breast cancer and influences cell behavior. *Cancer Res.* **2007**, *67*, 9169–9179. [CrossRef] [PubMed]
101. Brellier, F.; Tucker, R.P.; Chiquet-Ehrismann, R. Tenascins and their implications in diseases and tissue mechanics. *Scand. J. Med. Sci. Sports* **2009**, *19*, 511–519. [CrossRef] [PubMed]
102. Degen, M.; Brellier, F.; Schenk, S.; Driscoll, R.; Zaman, K.; Stupp, R.; Tornillo, L.; Terracciano, L.; Chiquet-Ehrismann, R.; Ruegg, C.; et al. Tenascin-W, a new marker of cancer stroma, is elevated in sera of colon and breast cancer patients. *Int. J. Cancer* **2008**, *122*, 2454–2461. [CrossRef] [PubMed]
103. Scherberich, A.; Tucker, R.P.; Degen, M.; Brown-Luedi, M.; Andres, A.C.; Chiquet-Ehrismann, R. Tenascin-W is found in malignant mammary tumors, promotes alpha8 integrin-dependent motility and requires p38MAPK activity for BMP-2 and TNF-alpha induced expression in vitro. *Oncogene* **2005**, *24*, 1525–1532. [CrossRef] [PubMed]
104. Akiri, G.; Sabo, E.; Dafni, H.; Vadasz, Z.; Kartvelishvily, Y.; Gan, N.; Kessler, O.; Cohen, T.; Resnick, M.; Neeman, M.; et al. Lysyl oxidase-related protein-1 promotes tumor fibrosis and tumor progression in vivo. *Cancer Res.* **2003**, *63*, 1657–1666. [PubMed]
105. Smith-Mungo, L.I.; Kagan, H.M. Lysyl oxidase: Properties, regulation and multiple functions in biology. *Matrix Biol.* **1998**, *16*, 387–398. [CrossRef]

106. Paszek, M.J.; Zahir, N.; Johnson, K.R.; Lakins, J.N.; Rozenberg, G.I.; Gefen, A.; Reinhart-King, C.A.; Margulies, S.S.; Dembo, M.; Boettiger, D.; et al. Tensional homeostasis and the malignant phenotype. *Cancer Cell* **2005**, *8*, 241–254. [CrossRef] [PubMed]

107. Weaver, V.M.; Lelievre, S.; Lakins, J.N.; Chrenek, M.A.; Jones, J.C.; Giancotti, F.; Werb, Z.; Bissell, M.J. b4 integrin-dependent formation of polarized three-dimensional architecture confers resistance to apoptosis in normal and malignant mammary epithelium. *Cancer Cell* **2002**, *2*, 205–216. [CrossRef]

108. White, D.E.; Kurpios, N.A.; Zuo, D.; Hassell, J.A.; Blaess, S.; Mueller, U.; Muller, W.J. Targeted disruption of b1-integrin in a transgenic mouse model of human breast cancer reveals an essential role in mammary tumor induction. *Cancer Cell* **2004**, *6*, 159–170. [CrossRef] [PubMed]

109. Wipff, P.J.; Rifkin, D.B.; Meister, J.J.; Hinz, B. Myofibroblast contraction activates latent TGF-β1 from the extracellular matrix. *J. Cell Biol.* **2007**, *179*, 1311–1323. [CrossRef] [PubMed]

110. Calvo, F.; Ege, N.; Grande-Garcia, A.; Hooper, S.; Jenkins, R.P.; Chaudhry, S.I.; Harrington, K.; Williamson, P.; Moeendarbary, E.; Charras, G.; et al. Mechanotransduction and YAP-dependent matrix remodelling is required for the generation and maintenance of cancer-associated fibroblasts. *Nat. Cell Biol.* **2013**, *15*, 637–646. [CrossRef] [PubMed]

111. Sahai, E.; Marshall, C.J. ROCK and Dia have opposing effects on adherens junctions downstream of Rho. *Nat. Cell Biol.* **2002**, *4*, 408–415. [CrossRef] [PubMed]

112. Burridge, K.; Wennerberg, K. Rho and Rac take center stage. *Cell* **2004**, *116*, 167–179. [CrossRef]

113. Fan, Y.; Shen, B.; Tan, M.; Mu, X.; Qin, Y.; Zhang, F.; Liu, Y. TGF-β-induced upregulation of malat1 promotes bladder cancer metastasis by associating with suz12. *Clin. Cancer Res.* **2014**, *20*, 1531–1541. [CrossRef] [PubMed]

114. Jodele, S.; Blavier, L.; Yoon, J.M.; DeClerck, Y.A. Modifying the soil to affect the seed: Role of stromal-derived matrix metalloproteinases in cancer progression. *Cancer Metastasis Rev.* **2006**, *25*, 35–43. [CrossRef] [PubMed]

115. Fang, M.; Yuan, J.; Peng, C.; Li, Y. Collagen as a double-edged sword in tumor progression. *Tumor Biol.* **2014**, *35*, 2871–2882. [CrossRef] [PubMed]

116. Bergamaschi, A.; Tagliabue, E.; Sorlie, T.; Naume, B.; Triulzi, T.; Orlandi, R.; Russnes, H.G.; Nesland, J.M.; Tammi, R.; Auvinen, P.; et al. Extracellular matrix signature identifies breast cancer subgroups with different clinical outcome. *J. Pathol.* **2008**, *214*, 357–367. [CrossRef] [PubMed]

117. Monboisse, J.C.; Oudart, J.B.; Ramont, L.; Brassart-Pasco, S.; Maquart, F.X. Matrikines from basement membrane collagens: A new anti-cancer strategy. *Biochim. Biophys. Acta* **2014**, *1840*, 2589–2598. [CrossRef] [PubMed]

118. Folkman, J. Antiangiogenesis in cancer therapy—Endostatin and its mechanisms of action. *Exp. Cell Res.* **2006**, *312*, 594–607. [CrossRef] [PubMed]

119. Willis, C.D.; Poluzzi, C.; Mongiat, M.; Iozzo, R.V. Endorepellin laminin-like globular 1/2 domains bind Ig3–5 of vascular endothelial growth factor (VEGF) receptor 2 and block pro-angiogenic signaling by VEGFA in endothelial cells. *FEBS J.* **2013**, *280*, 2271–2284. [CrossRef] [PubMed]

120. Billioux, A.; Modlich, U.; Bicknell, R. Angiogenesis. In *The Cancer Handbook*, 2nd ed.; Alison, M., Ed.; John Wiley & Sons: Hoboken, NJ, USA, 2007; Volume 1, pp. 144–154.

121. Folkman, J. Looking for a good endothelial address. *Cancer Cell* **2002**, *1*, 113–115. [CrossRef]

122. Hanahan, D.; Folkman, J. Patterns and emerging mechanisms of the angiogenic switch during tumorigenesis. *Cell* **1996**, *86*, 353–364. [CrossRef]

123. Blouw, B.; Song, H.; Tihan, T.; Bosze, J.; Ferrara, N.; Gerber, H.-P.; Johnson, R.S.; Bergers, G. The hypoxic response of tumors is dependent on their microenvironment. *Cancer Cell* **2003**, *4*, 133–146. [CrossRef]

124. Folkman, J.; Watson, K.; Ingber, D.; Hanahan, D. Induction of angiogenesis during the transition from hyperplasia to neoplasia. *Nature* **1989**, *339*, 58–61. [CrossRef] [PubMed]

125. Weidner, N.; Semple, J.P.; Welch, W.R.; Folkman, J. Tumor angiogenesis and metastasis—Correlation in invasive breast carcinoma. *N. Engl. J. Med.* **1991**, *324*, 1–8. [CrossRef] [PubMed]

126. Kandel, J.; Bossy-Wetzel, E.; Radvanyi, F.; Klagsbrun, M.; Folkman, J.; Hanahan, D. Neovascularization is associated with a switch to the export of bFGF in the multistep development of fibrosarcoma. *Cell* **1991**, *66*, 1095–1104. [CrossRef]

127. Niland, S.; Eble, J.A. Integrin-mediated cell-matrix interaction in physiological and pathological blood vessel formation. *J. Oncol.* **2012**, *2012*, 125278. [CrossRef] [PubMed]

128. Sica, A.; Schioppa, T.; Mantovani, A.; Allavena, P. Tumour-associated macrophages are a distinct M2 polarised population promoting tumour progression: Potential targets of anti-cancer therapy. *Eur. J. Cancer* **2006**, *42*, 717–727. [CrossRef] [PubMed]

129. Lin, E.Y.; Pollard, J.W. Tumor-associated macrophages press the angiogenic switch in breast cancer. *Cancer Res.* **2007**, *67*, 5064–5066. [CrossRef] [PubMed]

130. Schmid, M.C.; Varner, J.A. Myeloid cell trafficking and tumor angiogenesis. *Cancer Lett.* **2007**, *250*, 1–8. [CrossRef] [PubMed]

131. Aplin, A.C.; Fogel, E.; Nicosia, R.F. MCP-1 promotes mural cell recruitment during angiogenesis in the aortic ring model. *Angiogenesis* **2010**, *13*, 219–226. [CrossRef] [PubMed]

132. Hong, K.H.; Ryu, J.; Han, K.H. Monocyte chemoattractant protein-1-induced angiogenesis is mediated by vascular endothelial growth factor-A. *Blood* **2005**, *105*, 1405–1407. [CrossRef] [PubMed]

133. Niu, J.; Azfer, A.; Zhelyabovska, O.; Fatma, S.; Kolattukudy, P.E. Monocyte chemotactic protein (MCP)-1 promotes angiogenesis via a novel transcription factor, MCP-1-induced protein (MCPIP). *J. Biol. Chem.* **2008**, *283*, 14542–14551. [CrossRef] [PubMed]

134. Bergers, G.; Hanahan, D. Modes of resistance to anti-angiogenic therapy. *Nat. Rev. Cancer* **2008**, *8*, 592–603. [CrossRef] [PubMed]

135. Hanahan, D.; Weinberg, R.A. The hallmarks of cancer. *Cell* **2000**, *100*, 57–70. [CrossRef]

136. Nagy, J.A.; Chang, S.H.; Dvorak, A.M.; Dvorak, H.F. Why are tumour blood vessels abnormal and why is it important to know? *Br. J. Cancer* **2009**, *100*, 865–869. [CrossRef] [PubMed]

137. Dome, B.; Hendrix, M.J.; Paku, S.; Tovari, J.; Timar, J. Alternative vascularization mechanisms in cancer: Pathology and therapeutic implications. *Am. J. Pathol.* **2007**, *170*, 1–15. [CrossRef] [PubMed]

138. Hillen, F.; Griffioen, A.W. Tumour vascularization: Sprouting angiogenesis and beyond. *Cancer Metastasis Rev.* **2007**, *26*, 489–502. [CrossRef] [PubMed]

139. Nagy, J.A.; Dvorak, H.F. Heterogeneity of the tumor vasculature: The need for new tumor blood vessel type-specific targets. *Clin. Exp. Metastasis* **2012**, *29*, 657–662. [CrossRef] [PubMed]

140. Kaspar, M.; Zardi, L.; Neri, D. Fibronectin as target for tumor therapy. *Int. J. Cancer* **2006**, *118*, 1331–1339. [CrossRef] [PubMed]

141. Midulla, M.; Verma, R.; Pignatelli, M.; Ritter, M.A.; Courtenay-Luck, N.S.; George, A.J.T. Source of oncofetal ED-B-containing fibronectin: Implications of production by both tumor and endothelial cells. *Cancer Res.* **2000**, *60*, 164–169. [PubMed]

142. Midwood, K.S.; Orend, G. The role of tenascin-C in tissue injury and tumorigenesis. *J. Cell Commun. Signal.* **2009**, *3*, 287–310. [CrossRef] [PubMed]

143. Pezzolo, A.; Parodi, F.; Marimpietri, D.; Raffaghello, L.; Cocco, C.; Pistorio, A.; Mosconi, M.; Gambini, C.; Cilli, M.; Deaglio, S.; et al. Oct-4+/Tenascin C+ neuroblastoma cells serve as progenitors of tumor-derived endothelial cells. *Cell Res.* **2011**, *21*, 1470–1486. [CrossRef] [PubMed]

144. Martina, E.; Chiquet-Ehrismann, R.; Brellier, F. Tenascin-W: An extracellular matrix protein associated with osteogenesis and cancer. *Int. J. Biochem. Cell Biol.* **2010**, *42*, 1412–1415. [CrossRef] [PubMed]

145. Dudley, A.C. Tumor endothelial cells. *Cold Spring Harb. Perspect. Med.* **2012**, *2*, a006536. [CrossRef] [PubMed]

146. Benjamin, L.E.; Hemo, I.; Keshet, E. A plasticity window for blood vessel remodelling is defined by pericyte coverage of the preformed endothelial network and is regulated by PDGF-B and VEGF. *Development* **1998**, *125*, 1591–1598. [PubMed]

147. Burgers, A.C.; Lammert, E. Extraerythrocytic hemoglobin—A possible oxygen transporter in human malignant tumors. *Med. Hypotheses* **2011**, *77*, 580–583. [CrossRef] [PubMed]

148. Maniotis, A.J.; Folberg, R.; Hess, A.; Seftor, E.A.; Gardner, L.M.; Pe'er, J.; Trent, J.M.; Meltzer, P.S.; Hendrix, M.J. Vascular channel formation by human melanoma cells in vivo and in vitro: Vasculogenic mimicry. *Am. J. Pathol.* **1999**, *155*, 739–752. [CrossRef]

149. Sun, B.; Zhang, D.; Zhao, N.; Zhao, X. Epithelial-to-endothelial transition and cancer stem cells: Two cornerstones of vasculogenic mimicry in malignant tumors. *Oncotarget* **2017**, *8*, 30502–30510. [CrossRef] [PubMed]

150. Dvorak, H.F.; Senger, D.R.; Dvorak, A.M. Fibrin as a component of the tumor stroma: Origins and biological significance. *Cancer Metastasis Rev.* **1983**, *2*, 41–73. [CrossRef]

151. Dvorak, H.F. Tumors: Wounds that do not heal. Similarities between tumor stroma generation and wound healing. *N. Engl. J. Med.* **1986**, *315*, 1650–1659. [CrossRef] [PubMed]

152. Dvorak, H.F.; Brown, L.F.; Detmar, M.; Dvorak, A.M. Vascular permeability factor/vascular endothelial growth factor, microvascular hyperpermeability, and angiogenesis. *Am. J. Pathol.* **1995**, *146*, 1029–1039. [PubMed]

153. Jain, R.K. Normalizing tumor vasculature with anti-angiogenic therapy: A new paradigm for combination therapy. *Nat. Med.* **2001**, *7*, 987–989. [CrossRef] [PubMed]

154. Holash, J.; Maisonpierre, P.C.; Compton, D.; Boland, P.; Alexander, C.R.; Zagzag, D.; Yancopoulos, G.D.; Wiegand, S.J. Vessel cooption, regression, and growth in tumors mediated by angiopoietins and VEGF. *Science* **1999**, *284*, 1994–1998. [CrossRef] [PubMed]

155. Donnem, T.; Hu, J.; Ferguson, M.; Adighibe, O.; Snell, C.; Harris, A.L.; Gatter, K.C.; Pezzella, F. Vessel co-option in primary human tumors and metastases: An obstacle to effective anti-angiogenic treatment? *Cancer Med.* **2013**, *2*, 427–436. [CrossRef] [PubMed]

156. Asahara, T.; Murohara, T.; Sullivan, A.; Silver, M.; van der Zee, R.; Li, T.; Witzenbichler, B.; Schatteman, G.; Isner, J.M. Isolation of putative progenitor endothelial cells for angiogenesis. *Science* **1997**, *275*, 964–967. [CrossRef] [PubMed]

157. Ruoslahti, E. Specialization of tumour vasculature. *Nat. Rev. Cancer* **2002**, *2*, 83–90. [CrossRef] [PubMed]

158. Potente, M.; Gerhardt, H.; Carmeliet, P. Basic and therapeutic aspects of angiogenesis. *Cell* **2011**, *146*, 873–887. [CrossRef] [PubMed]

159. Carmeliet, P. Angiogenesis in health and disease. *Nat. Med.* **2003**, *9*, 653–660. [CrossRef] [PubMed]

160. Iruela-Arispe, M.L.; Davis, G.E. Cellular and molecular mechanisms of vascular lumen formation. *Dev. Cell* **2009**, *16*, 222–231. [CrossRef] [PubMed]

161. Strilic, B.; Kucera, T.; Eglinger, J.; Hughes, M.R.; McNagny, K.M.; Tsukita, S.; Dejana, E.; Ferrara, N.; Lammert, E. The molecular basis of vascular lumen formation in the developing mouse aorta. *Dev. Cell* **2009**, *17*, 505–515. [CrossRef] [PubMed]

162. Zovein, A.C.; Luque, A.; Turlo, K.A.; Hofmann, J.J.; Yee, K.M.; Becker, M.S.; Fassler, R.; Mellman, I.; Lane, T.F.; Iruela-Arispe, M.L. Beta1 integrin establishes endothelial cell polarity and arteriolar lumen formation via a Par3-dependent mechanism. *Dev. Cell* **2010**, *18*, 39–51. [CrossRef] [PubMed]

163. Djonov, V.; Schmid, M.; Tschanz, S.A.; Burri, P.H. Intussusceptive angiogenesis: Its role in embryonic vascular network formation. *Circ. Res.* **2000**, *86*, 286–292. [CrossRef] [PubMed]

164. Kurz, H.; Burri, P.H.; Djonov, V.G. Angiogenesis and vascular remodeling by intussusception: From form to function. *News Physiol. Sci.* **2003**, *18*, 65–70. [CrossRef] [PubMed]

165. Gianni-Barrera, R.; Trani, M.; Reginato, S.; Banfi, A. To sprout or to split? VEGF, Notch and vascular morphogenesis. *Biochem. Soc. Trans.* **2011**, *39*, 1644–1648. [CrossRef] [PubMed]

166. Nico, B.; Crivellato, E.; Guidolin, D.; Annese, T.; Longo, V.; Finato, N.; Vacca, A.; Ribatti, D. Intussusceptive microvascular growth in human glioma. *Clin. Exp. Med.* **2010**, *10*, 93–98. [CrossRef] [PubMed]

167. Brat, D.J.; Van Meir, E.G. Glomeruloid microvascular proliferation orchestrated by VPF/VEGF: A new world of angiogenesis research. *Am. J. Pathol.* **2001**, *158*, 789–796. [CrossRef]

168. Straume, O.; Chappuis, P.O.; Salvesen, H.B.; Halvorsen, O.J.; Haukaas, S.A.; Goffin, J.R.; Begin, L.R.; Foulkes, W.D.; Akslen, L.A. Prognostic importance of glomeruloid microvascular proliferation indicates an aggressive angiogenic phenotype in human cancers. *Cancer Res.* **2002**, *62*, 6808–6811. [PubMed]

169. Lyden, D.; Hattori, K.; Dias, S.; Costa, C.; Blaikie, P.; Butros, L.; Chadburn, A.; Heissig, B.; Marks, W.; Witte, L.; et al. Impaired recruitment of bone-marrow-derived endothelial and hematopoietic precursor cells blocks tumor angiogenesis and growth. *Nat. Med.* **2001**, *7*, 1194–1201. [CrossRef] [PubMed]

170. Reyes, M.; Dudek, A.; Jahagirdar, B.; Koodie, L.; Marker, P.H.; Verfaillie, C.M. Origin of endothelial progenitors in human postnatal bone marrow. *J. Clin. Investig.* **2002**, *109*, 337–346. [CrossRef] [PubMed]

171. Ribatti, D. The involvement of endothelial progenitor cells in tumor angiogenesis. *J. Cell. Mol. Med.* **2004**, *8*, 294–300. [CrossRef] [PubMed]

172. Moschetta, M.; Mishima, Y.; Sahin, I.; Manier, S.; Glavey, S.; Vacca, A.; Roccaro, A.M.; Ghobrial, I.M. Role of endothelial progenitor cells in cancer progression. *Biochim. Biophys. Acta* **2014**, *1846*, 26–39. [CrossRef] [PubMed]

173. Ricci-Vitiani, L.; Pallini, R.; Biffoni, M.; Todaro, M.; Invernici, G.; Cenci, T.; Maira, G.; Parati, E.A.; Stassi, G.; Larocca, L.M.; et al. Tumour vascularization via endothelial differentiation of glioblastoma stem-like cells. *Nature* **2010**, *468*, 824–828. [CrossRef] [PubMed]

174. Kirschmann, D.A.; Seftor, E.A.; Hardy, K.M.; Seftor, R.E.; Hendrix, M.J. Molecular pathways: Vasculogenic mimicry in tumor cells: Diagnostic and therapeutic implications. *Clin. Cancer Res.* **2012**, *18*, 2726–2732. [CrossRef] [PubMed]

175. Folberg, R.; Maniotis, A.J. Vasculogenic mimicry. *APMIS* **2004**, *112*, 508–525. [CrossRef] [PubMed]

176. Lin, A.Y.; Maniotis, A.J.; Valyi-Nagy, K.; Majumdar, D.; Setty, S.; Kadkol, S.; Leach, L.; Pe'er, J.; Folberg, R. Distinguishing Fibrovascular Septa From Vasculogenic Mimicry Patterns. *Arch. Pathol. Lab. Med.* **2005**, *129*, 884–892. [PubMed]

177. El Hallani, S.; Boisselier, B.; Peglion, F.; Rousseau, A.; Colin, C.; Idbaih, A.; Marie, Y.; Mokhtari, K.; Thomas, J.L.; Eichmann, A.; et al. A new alternative mechanism in glioblastoma vascularization: Tubular vasculogenic mimicry. *Brain* **2010**, *133*, 973–982. [CrossRef] [PubMed]

178. Bajcsy, P.; Lee, S.C.; Lin, A.; Folberg, R. Three-dimensional volume reconstruction of extracellular matrix proteins in uveal melanoma from fluorescent confocal laser scanning microscope images. *J. Microsc.* **2006**, *221*, 30–45. [CrossRef] [PubMed]

179. Clarijs, R.; Otte-Holler, I.; Ruiter, D.J.; de Waal, R.M. Presence of a fluid-conducting meshwork in xenografted cutaneous and primary human uveal melanoma. *Investig. Ophthalmol. Vis. Sci.* **2002**, *43*, 912–918.

180. Ahn, G.O.; Brown, J.M. Matrix metalloproteinase-9 is required for tumor vasculogenesis but not for angiogenesis: Role of bone marrow-derived myelomonocytic cells. *Cancer Cell* **2008**, *13*, 193–205. [CrossRef] [PubMed]

181. Iivanainen, E.; Kahari, V.M.; Heino, J.; Elenius, K. Endothelial cell-matrix interactions. *Microsc. Res. Tech.* **2003**, *60*, 13–22. [CrossRef] [PubMed]

182. Rundhaug, J.E. Matrix metalloproteinases and angiogenesis. *J. Cell. Mol. Med.* **2005**, *9*, 267–285. [CrossRef] [PubMed]

183. Eble, J.A.; Niland, S. The extracellular matrix of blood vessels. *Curr. Pharm. Des.* **2009**, *15*, 1385–1400. [CrossRef] [PubMed]

184. Andaloussi, S.E.L.; Mager, I.; Breakefield, X.O.; Wood, M.J. Extracellular vesicles: Biology and emerging therapeutic opportunities. *Nat. Rev. Drug Discov.* **2013**, *12*, 347–357. [CrossRef] [PubMed]

185. Tirziu, D.; Giordano, F.J.; Simons, M. Cell communications in the heart. *Circulation* **2010**, *122*, 928–937. [CrossRef] [PubMed]

186. Kedrin, D.; Gligorijevic, B.; Wyckoff, J.; Verkhusha, V.V.; Condeelis, J.; Segall, J.E.; van Rheenen, J. Intravital imaging of metastatic behavior through a mammary imaging window. *Nat. Methods* **2008**, *5*, 1019–1021. [CrossRef] [PubMed]

187. Mierke, C.T.; Zitterbart, D.P.; Kollmannsberger, P.; Raupach, C.; Schlotzer-Schrehardt, U.; Goecke, T.W.; Behrens, J.; Fabry, B. Breakdown of the endothelial barrier function in tumor cell transmigration. *Biophys. J.* **2008**, *94*, 2832–2846. [CrossRef] [PubMed]

188. Olsson, A.K.; Dimberg, A.; Kreuger, J.; Claesson-Welsh, L. VEGF receptor signalling—In control of vascular function. *Nat. Rev. Mol. Cell Biol.* **2006**, *7*, 359–371. [CrossRef] [PubMed]

189. Weis, S.M.; Cheresh, D.A. alphaV integrins in angiogenesis and cancer. *Cold Spring Harb. Perspect. Med.* **2011**, *1*, a006478. [CrossRef] [PubMed]

190. Dvorak, H.F. Vascular permeability factor/vascular endothelial growth factor: A critical cytokine in tumor angiogenesis and a potential target for diagnosis and therapy. *J. Clin. Oncol.* **2002**, *20*, 4368–4380. [CrossRef] [PubMed]

191. Guo, F.; Wang, Y.; Liu, J.; Mok, S.C.; Xue, F.; Zhang, W. CXCL12/CXCR4: A symbiotic bridge linking cancer cells and their stromal neighbors in oncogenic communication networks. *Oncogene* **2016**, *35*, 816–826. [CrossRef] [PubMed]

192. Teicher, B.A.; Fricker, S.P. CXCL12 (SDF-1)/CXCR4 pathway in cancer. *Clin. Cancer Res.* **2010**, *16*, 2927–2931. [CrossRef] [PubMed]

193. Reymond, N.; d'Agua, B.B.; Ridley, A.J. Crossing the endothelial barrier during metastasis. *Nat. Rev. Cancer* **2013**, *13*, 858–870. [CrossRef] [PubMed]

194. Liu, F.; Lang, R.; Wei, J.; Fan, Y.; Cui, L.; Gu, F.; Guo, X.; Pringle, G.A.; Zhang, X.; Fu, L. Increased expression of SDF-1/CXCR4 is associated with lymph node metastasis of invasive micropapillary carcinoma of the breast. *Histopathology* **2009**, *54*, 741–750. [CrossRef] [PubMed]

195. Iwasa, S.; Yanagawa, T.; Fan, J.; Katoh, R. Expression of CXCR4 and its ligand SDF-1 in intestinal-type gastric cancer is associated with lymph node and liver metastasis. *Anticancer Res.* **2009**, *29*, 4751–4758. [PubMed]

196. Liang, J.J.; Zhu, S.; Bruggeman, R.; Zaino, R.J.; Evans, D.B.; Fleming, J.B.; Gomez, H.F.; Zander, D.S.; Wang, H. High levels of expression of human stromal cell-derived factor-1 are associated with worse prognosis in patients with stage II pancreatic ductal adenocarcinoma. *Cancer Epidemiol. Biomark. Prev.* **2010**, *19*, 2598–2604. [CrossRef] [PubMed]

197. Thomas, R.M.; Kim, J.; Revelo-Penafiel, M.P.; Angel, R.; Dawson, D.W.; Lowy, A.M. The chemokine receptor CXCR4 is expressed in pancreatic intraepithelial neoplasia. *Gut* **2008**, *57*, 1555–1560. [CrossRef] [PubMed]

198. Guo, L.; Cui, Z.M.; Zhang, J.; Huang, Y. Chemokine axes CXCL12/CXCR4 and CXCL16/CXCR6 correlate with lymph node metastasis in epithelial ovarian carcinoma. *Chin. J. Cancer* **2011**, *30*, 336–343. [CrossRef] [PubMed]

199. Yu, Y.; Shi, X.; Shu, Z.; Xie, T.; Huang, K.; Wei, L.; Song, H.; Zhang, W.; Xue, X. Stromal cell-derived factor-1 (SDF-1)/CXCR4 axis enhances cellular invasion in ovarian carcinoma cells via integrin beta1 and beta3 expressions. *Oncol. Res.* **2013**, *21*, 217–225. [CrossRef] [PubMed]

200. Huang, Y.; Zhang, J.; Cui, Z.M.; Zhao, J.; Zheng, Y. Expression of the CXCL12/CXCR4 and CXCL16/CXCR6 axes in cervical intraepithelial neoplasia and cervical cancer. *Chin. J. Cancer* **2013**, *32*, 289–296. [CrossRef] [PubMed]

201. Murakami, T.; Maki, W.; Cardones, A.R.; Fang, H.; Tun Kyi, A.; Nestle, F.O.; Hwang, S.T. Expression of CXC chemokine receptor-4 enhances the pulmonary metastatic potential of murine B16 melanoma cells. *Cancer Res.* **2002**, *62*, 7328–7334. [PubMed]

202. Hayes, J.; Peruzzi, P.P.; Lawler, S. MicroRNAs in cancer: Biomarkers, functions and therapy. *Trends Mol. Med.* **2014**, *20*, 460–469. [CrossRef] [PubMed]

203. Kohlhapp, F.J.; Mitra, A.K.; Lengyel, E.; Peter, M.E. MicroRNAs as mediators and communicators between cancer cells and the tumor microenvironment. *Oncogene* **2015**, *34*, 5857–5868. [CrossRef] [PubMed]

204. Wurdinger, T.; Tannous, B.A.; Saydam, O.; Skog, J.; Grau, S.; Soutschek, J.; Weissleder, R.; Breakefield, X.O.; Krichevsky, A.M. miR-296 regulates growth factor receptor overexpression in angiogenic endothelial cells. *Cancer Cell* **2008**, *14*, 382–393. [CrossRef] [PubMed]

205. Boon, R.A.; Vickers, K.C. Intercellular transport of microRNAs. *Arterioscler Thromb Vasc. Biol.* **2013**, *33*, 186–192. [CrossRef] [PubMed]

206. Zhuang, G.; Wu, X.; Jiang, Z.; Kasman, I.; Yao, J.; Guan, Y.; Oeh, J.; Modrusan, Z.; Bais, C.; Sampath, D.; et al. Tumour-secreted miR-9 promotes endothelial cell migration and angiogenesis by activating the JAK-STAT pathway. *EMBO J.* **2012**, *31*, 3513–3523. [CrossRef] [PubMed]

207. Carmeliet, P.; Jain, R.K. Angiogenesis in cancer and other diseases. *Nature* **2000**, *407*, 249–257. [CrossRef] [PubMed]

208. Selek, L.; Dhobb, M.; van der Sanden, B.; Berger, F.; Wion, D. Existence of tumor-derived endothelial cells suggests an additional role for endothelial-to-mesenchymal transition in tumor progression. *Int. J. Cancer* **2011**, *128*, 1502–1503. [CrossRef] [PubMed]

209. Ghiabi, P.; Jiang, J.; Pasquier, J.; Maleki, M.; Abu-Kaoud, N.; Rafii, S.; Rafii, A. Endothelial cells provide a notch-dependent pro-tumoral niche for enhancing breast cancer survival, stemness and pro-metastatic properties. *PLoS ONE* **2014**, *9*, e112424. [CrossRef] [PubMed]

210. Gregory, L.A.; Ricart, R.A.; Patel, S.A.; Lim, P.K.; Rameshwar, P. microRNAs, Gap Junctional Intercellular Communication and Mesenchymal Stem Cells in Breast Cancer Metastasis. *Curr. Cancer Ther. Rev.* **2011**, *7*, 176–183. [CrossRef] [PubMed]

211. Valiunas, V.; Polosina, Y.Y.; Miller, H.; Potapova, I.A.; Valiuniene, L.; Doronin, S.; Mathias, R.T.; Robinson, R.B.; Rosen, M.R.; Cohen, I.S.; et al. Connexin-specific cell-to-cell transfer of short interfering RNA by gap junctions. *J. Physiol.* **2005**, *568*, 459–468. [CrossRef] [PubMed]

212. Kizana, E.; Cingolani, E.; Marban, E. Non-cell-autonomous effects of vector-expressed regulatory RNAs in mammalian heart cells. *Gene Ther.* **2009**, *16*, 1163–1168. [CrossRef] [PubMed]

213. Leithe, E.; Sirnes, S.; Omori, Y.; Rivedal, E. Downregulation of gap junctions in cancer cells. *Crit. Rev. Oncog.* **2006**, *12*, 225–256. [CrossRef] [PubMed]

214. Lopes-Bastos, B.M.; Jiang, W.G.; Cai, J. Tumour-Endothelial Cell Communications: Important and Indispensable Mediators of Tumour Angiogenesis. *Anticancer Res.* **2016**, *36*, 1119–1126. [PubMed]

215. Pollmann, M.A.; Shao, Q.; Laird, D.W.; Sandig, M. Connexin 43 mediated gap junctional communication enhances breast tumor cell diapedesis in culture. *Breast Cancer Res.* **2005**, *7*, R522–R534. [CrossRef] [PubMed]

216. Elzarrad, M.K.; Haroon, A.; Willecke, K.; Dobrowolski, R.; Gillespie, M.N.; Al-Mehdi, A.B. Connexin-43 upregulation in micrometastases and tumor vasculature and its role in tumor cell attachment to pulmonary endothelium. *BMC Med.* **2008**, *6*, 20. [CrossRef] [PubMed]
217. Ito, A.; Katoh, F.; Kataoka, T.R.; Okada, M.; Tsubota, N.; Asada, H.; Yoshikawa, K.; Maeda, S.; Kitamura, Y.; Yamasaki, H.; et al. A role for heterologous gap junctions between melanoma and endothelial cells in metastasis. *J. Clin. Investig.* **2000**, *105*, 1189–1197. [CrossRef] [PubMed]
218. Cai, J.; Jiang, W.G.; Mansel, R.E. Gap junctional communication and the tyrosine phosphorylation of connexin 43 in interaction between breast cancer and endothelial cells. *Int. J. Mol. Med.* **1998**, *1*, 273–278. [CrossRef] [PubMed]
219. Zibara, K.; Awada, Z.; Dib, L.; El-Saghir, J.; Al-Ghadban, S.; Ibrik, A.; El-Zein, N.; El-Sabban, M. Anti-angiogenesis therapy and gap junction inhibition reduce MDA-MB-231 breast cancer cell invasion and metastasis in vitro and in vivo. *Sci. Rep.* **2015**, *5*, 12598. [CrossRef] [PubMed]
220. Esser, S.; Lampugnani, M.G.; Corada, M.; Dejana, E.; Risau, W. Vascular endothelial growth factor induces VE-cadherin tyrosine phosphorylation in endothelial cells. *J. Cell Sci.* **1998**, *111 Pt 13*, 1853–1865. [PubMed]
221. Lampugnani, M.G.; Corada, M.; Caveda, L.; Breviario, F.; Ayalon, O.; Geiger, B.; Dejana, E. The molecular organization of endothelial cell to cell junctions: Differential association of plakoglobin, beta-catenin, and alpha-catenin with vascular endothelial cadherin (VE-cadherin). *J. Cell Biol.* **1995**, *129*, 203–217. [CrossRef] [PubMed]
222. Lampugnani, M.G.; Resnati, M.; Raiteri, M.; Pigott, R.; Pisacane, A.; Houen, G.; Ruco, L.P.; Dejana, E. A novel endothelial-specific membrane protein is a marker of cell-cell contacts. *J. Cell Biol.* **1992**, *118*, 1511–1522. [CrossRef] [PubMed]
223. Wallez, Y.; Vilgrain, I.; Huber, P. Angiogenesis: The VE-cadherin switch. *Trends Cardiovasc. Med.* **2006**, *16*, 55–59. [CrossRef] [PubMed]
224. Liao, F.; Li, Y.; O'Connor, W.; Zanetta, L.; Bassi, R.; Santiago, A.; Overholser, J.; Hooper, A.; Mignatti, P.; Dejana, E.; et al. Monoclonal antibody to vascular endothelial-cadherin is a potent inhibitor of angiogenesis, tumor growth, and metastasis. *Cancer Res.* **2000**, *60*, 6805–6810. [PubMed]
225. Wessel, F.; Winderlich, M.; Holm, M.; Frye, M.; Rivera-Galdos, R.; Vockel, M.; Linnepe, R.; Ipe, U.; Stadtmann, A.; Zarbock, A.; et al. Leukocyte extravasation and vascular permeability are each controlled in vivo by different tyrosine residues of VE-cadherin. *Nat. Immunol.* **2014**, *15*, 223–230. [CrossRef] [PubMed]
226. Gavard, J. Endothelial permeability and VE-cadherin: A wacky comradeship. *Cell Adhes. Migr.* **2014**, *8*, 158–164. [CrossRef]
227. Potter, M.D.; Barbero, S.; Cheresh, D.A. Tyrosine phosphorylation of VE-cadherin prevents binding of p120- and beta-catenin and maintains the cellular mesenchymal state. *J. Biol. Chem.* **2005**, *280*, 31906–31912. [CrossRef] [PubMed]
228. Peng, H.H.; Hodgson, L.; Henderson, A.J.; Dong, C. Involvement of phospholipase C signaling in melanoma cell-induced endothelial junction disassembly. *Front. Biosci.* **2005**, *10*, 1597–1606. [CrossRef] [PubMed]
229. Haidari, M.; Zhang, W.; Caivano, A.; Chen, Z.; Ganjehei, L.; Mortazavi, A.; Stroud, C.; Woodside, D.G.; Willerson, J.T.; Dixon, R.A. Integrin alpha2beta1 mediates tyrosine phosphorylation of vascular endothelial cadherin induced by invasive breast cancer cells. *J. Biol. Chem.* **2012**, *287*, 32981–32992. [CrossRef] [PubMed]
230. Aragon-Sanabria, V.; Pohler, S.E.; Eswar, V.J.; Bierowski, M.; Gomez, E.W.; Dong, C. VE-Cadherin Disassembly and Cell Contractility in the Endothelium are Necessary for Barrier Disruption Induced by Tumor Cells. *Sci. Rep.* **2017**, *7*, 45835. [CrossRef] [PubMed]
231. McDonald, D.M.; Munn, L.; Jain, R.K. Vasculogenic mimicry: How convincing, how novel, and how significant? *Am. J. Pathol.* **2000**, *156*, 383–388. [CrossRef]
232. Cao, Z.; Shang, B.; Zhang, G.; Miele, L.; Sarkar, F.H.; Wang, Z.; Zhou, Q. Tumor cell-mediated neovascularization and lymphangiogenesis contrive tumor progression and cancer metastasis. *Biochim. Biophys. Acta* **2013**, *1836*, 273–286. [CrossRef] [PubMed]
233. Murphy, G.F.; Wilson, B.J.; Girouard, S.D.; Frank, N.Y.; Frank, M.H. Stem cells and targeted approaches to melanoma cure. *Mol. Asp. Med.* **2014**, *39*, 33–49. [CrossRef] [PubMed]
234. Potgens, A.J.; van Altena, M.C.; Lubsen, N.H.; Ruiter, D.J.; de Waal, R.M. Analysis of the tumor vasculature and metastatic behavior of xenografts of human melanoma cell lines transfected with vascular permeability factor. *Am. J. Pathol.* **1996**, *148*, 1203–1217. [PubMed]

235. Lammert, E.; Axnick, J. Vascular lumen formation. *Cold Spring Harb. Perspect. Med.* **2012**, *2*, a006619. [CrossRef] [PubMed]

236. Kobayashi, H.; Shirakawa, K.; Kawamoto, S.; Saga, T.; Sato, N.; Hiraga, A.; Watanabe, I.; Heike, Y.; Togashi, K.; Konishi, J.; et al. Rapid accumulation and internalization of radiolabeled herceptin in an inflammatory breast cancer xenograft with vasculogenic mimicry predicted by the contrast-enhanced dynamic MRI with the macromolecular contrast agent G6-(1B4M-Gd)(256). *Cancer Res.* **2002**, *62*, 860–866. [PubMed]

237. Shirakawa, K.; Kobayashi, H.; Heike, Y.; Kawamoto, S.; Brechbiel, M.W.; Kasumi, F.; Iwanaga, T.; Konishi, F.; Terada, M.; Wakasugi, H. Hemodynamics in vasculogenic mimicry and angiogenesis of inflammatory breast cancer xenograft. *Cancer Res.* **2002**, *62*, 560–566. [PubMed]

238. Liu, Z.; Li, Y.; Zhao, W.; Ma, Y.; Yang, X. Demonstration of vasculogenic mimicry in astrocytomas and effects of Endostar on U251 cells. *Pathol. Res. Pract.* **2011**, *207*, 645–651. [CrossRef] [PubMed]

239. Thies, A.; Mangold, U.; Moll, I.; Schumacher, U. PAS-positive loops and networks as a prognostic indicator in cutaneous malignant melanoma. *J. Pathol.* **2001**, *195*, 537–542. [CrossRef] [PubMed]

240. Mihic-Probst, D.; Ikenberg, K.; Tinguely, M.; Schraml, P.; Behnke, S.; Seifert, B.; Civenni, G.; Sommer, L.; Moch, H.; Dummer, R. Tumor cell plasticity and angiogenesis in human melanomas. *PLoS ONE* **2012**, *7*, e33571. [CrossRef] [PubMed]

241. Sun, W.; Fan, Y.Z.; Zhang, W.Z.; Ge, C.Y. A pilot histomorphology and hemodynamic of vasculogenic mimicry in gallbladder carcinomas in vivo and in vitro. *J. Exp. Clin. Cancer Res.* **2011**, *30*, 46. [CrossRef] [PubMed]

242. Guo, J.Q.; Zheng, Q.H.; Chen, H.; Chen, L.; Xu, J.B.; Chen, M.Y.; Lu, D.; Wang, Z.H.; Tong, H.F.; Lin, S. Ginsenoside Rg3 inhibition of vasculogenic mimicry in pancreatic cancer through downregulation of VEcadherin/EphA2/MMP9/MMP2 expression. *Int. J. Oncol.* **2014**, *45*, 1065–1072. [CrossRef] [PubMed]

243. Sun, B.; Zhang, S.; Zhang, D.; Du, J.; Guo, H.; Zhao, X.; Zhang, W.; Hao, X. Vasculogenic mimicry is associated with high tumor grade, invasion and metastasis, and short survival in patients with hepatocellular carcinoma. *Oncol. Rep.* **2006**, *16*, 693–698. [CrossRef] [PubMed]

244. Tang, N.N.; Zhu, H.; Zhang, H.J.; Zhang, W.F.; Jin, H.L.; Wang, L.; Wang, P.; He, G.J.; Hao, B.; Shi, R.H. HIF-1alpha induces VE-cadherin expression and modulates vasculogenic mimicry in esophageal carcinoma cells. *World J. Gastroenterol.* **2014**, *20*, 17894–17904. [CrossRef] [PubMed]

245. Sun, B.; Qie, S.; Zhang, S.; Sun, T.; Zhao, X.; Gao, S.; Ni, C.; Wang, X.; Liu, Y.; Zhang, L. Role and mechanism of vasculogenic mimicry in gastrointestinal stromal tumors. *Hum. Pathol.* **2008**, *39*, 444–451. [CrossRef] [PubMed]

246. Baeten, C.I.; Hillen, F.; Pauwels, P.; de Bruine, A.P.; Baeten, C.G. Prognostic role of vasculogenic mimicry in colorectal cancer. *Dis. Colon Rectum* **2009**, *52*, 2028–2035. [CrossRef] [PubMed]

247. Williamson, S.C.; Metcalf, R.L.; Trapani, F.; Mohan, S.; Antonello, J.; Abbott, B.; Leong, H.S.; Chester, C.P.; Simms, N.; Polanski, R.; et al. Vasculogenic mimicry in small cell lung cancer. *Nat. Commun.* **2016**, *7*, 13322. [CrossRef] [PubMed]

248. Wu, S.; Yu, L.; Wang, D.; Zhou, L.; Cheng, Z.; Chai, D.; Ma, L.; Tao, Y. Aberrant expression of CD133 in non-small cell lung cancer and its relationship to vasculogenic mimicry. *BMC Cancer* **2012**, *12*, 535. [CrossRef] [PubMed]

249. Sood, A.K.; Seftor, E.A.; Fletcher, M.S.; Gardner, L.M.; Heidger, P.M.; Buller, R.E.; Seftor, R.E.; Hendrix, M.J. Molecular determinants of ovarian cancer plasticity. *Am. J. Pathol.* **2001**, *158*, 1279–1288. [CrossRef]

250. Tang, H.S.; Feng, Y.J.; Yao, L.Q. Angiogenesis, vasculogenesis, and vasculogenic mimicry in ovarian cancer. *Int. J. Gynecol. Cancer* **2009**, *19*, 605–610. [CrossRef] [PubMed]

251. Sharma, N.; Seftor, R.E.; Seftor, E.A.; Gruman, L.M.; Heidger, P.M., Jr.; Cohen, M.B.; Lubaroff, D.M.; Hendrix, M.J. Prostatic tumor cell plasticity involves cooperative interactions of distinct phenotypic subpopulations: Role in vasculogenic mimicry. *Prostate* **2002**, *50*, 189–201. [CrossRef] [PubMed]

252. Cai, X.S.; Jia, Y.W.; Mei, J.; Tang, R.Y. Tumor blood vessels formation in osteosarcoma: Vasculogenesis mimicry. *Chin. Med. J.* **2004**, *117*, 94–98. [PubMed]

253. Sun, B.; Zhang, S.; Zhao, X.; Zhang, W.; Hao, X. Vasculogenic mimicry is associated with poor survival in patients with mesothelial sarcomas and alveolar rhabdomyosarcomas. *Int. J. Oncol.* **2004**, *25*, 1609–1614. [CrossRef] [PubMed]

254. Ria, R.; Reale, A.; De Luisi, A.; Ferrucci, A.; Moschetta, M.; Vacca, A. Bone marrow angiogenesis and progression in multiple myeloma. *Am. J. Blood Res.* **2011**, *1*, 76–89. [PubMed]

255. Vacca, A.; Ria, R.; Reale, A.; Ribatti, D. Angiogenesis in multiple myeloma. *Chem. Immunol. Allergy* **2014**, *99*, 180–196. [CrossRef] [PubMed]

256. Ellis, L.M.; Fidler, I.J. Finding the tumor copycat. Therapy fails, patients don't. *Nat. Med.* **2010**, *16*, 974–975. [CrossRef] [PubMed]

257. Pinto, M.P.; Sotomayor, P.; Carrasco-Avino, G.; Corvalan, A.H.; Owen, G.I. Escaping Antiangiogenic Therapy: Strategies Employed by Cancer Cells. *Int. J. Mol. Sci.* **2016**, *17*. [CrossRef] [PubMed]

258. Huijbers, E.J.; van Beijnum, J.R.; Thijssen, V.L.; Sabrkhany, S.; Nowak-Sliwinska, P.; Griffioen, A.W. Role of the tumor stroma in resistance to anti-angiogenic therapy. *Drug Resist. Updat* **2016**, *25*, 26–37. [CrossRef] [PubMed]

259. Kotyza, J. Chemokines in tumor proximal fluids. *Biomed. Pap. Med. Fac. Univ. Palacky Olomouc. Czech Repub.* **2017**, *161*, 41–49. [CrossRef] [PubMed]

260. Pries, R.; Wollenberg, B. Cytokines in head and neck cancer. *Cytokine Growth Factor Rev.* **2006**, *17*, 141–146. [CrossRef] [PubMed]

261. Cao, Y. Future options of anti-angiogenic cancer therapy. *Chin. J. Cancer* **2016**, *35*, 21. [CrossRef] [PubMed]

262. Rytlewski, J.A.; Alejandra Aldon, M.; Lewis, E.W.; Suggs, L.J. Mechanisms of tubulogenesis and endothelial phenotype expression by MSCs. *Microvasc. Res.* **2015**, *99*, 26–35. [CrossRef] [PubMed]

263. Cheng, L.; Huang, Z.; Zhou, W.; Wu, Q.; Donnola, S.; Liu, J.K.; Fang, X.; Sloan, A.E.; Mao, Y.; Lathia, J.D.; et al. Glioblastoma stem cells generate vascular pericytes to support vessel function and tumor growth. *Cell* **2013**, *153*, 139–152. [CrossRef] [PubMed]

264. Shenoy, A.K.; Jin, Y.; Luo, H.C.; Tang, M.; Pampo, C.; Shao, R.; Siemann, D.W.; Wu, L.Z.; Heldermon, C.D.; Law, B.K.; et al. Epithelial-to-mesenchymal transition confers pericyte properties on cancer cells. *J. Clin. Investig.* **2016**, *126*, 4174–4186. [CrossRef] [PubMed]

265. Braeuer, R.R.; Watson, I.R.; Wu, C.J.; Mobley, A.K.; Kamiya, T.; Shoshan, E.; Bar-Eli, M. Why is melanoma so metastatic? *Pigm. Cell Melanoma Res.* **2014**, *27*. [CrossRef] [PubMed]

266. Chen, J.A.; Shi, M.; Li, J.Q.; Qian, C.N. Angiogenesis: Multiple masks in hepatocellular carcinoma and liver regeneration. *Hepatol. Int.* **2010**, *4*, 537–547. [CrossRef] [PubMed]

267. Timar, J.; Tovari, J.; Raso, E.; Meszaros, L.; Bereczky, B.; Lapis, K. Platelet-mimicry of cancer cells: Epiphenomenon with clinical significance. *Oncology* **2005**, *69*, 185–201. [CrossRef] [PubMed]

268. Kotiyal, S.; Bhattacharya, S. Epithelial Mesenchymal Transition and Vascular Mimicry in Breast Cancer Stem Cells. *Crit. Rev. Eukaryot. Gene Expr.* **2015**, *25*, 269–280. [CrossRef] [PubMed]

269. Lin, X.; Sun, B.C.; Zhu, D.W.; Zhao, X.L.; Sun, R.; Zhang, Y.H.; Zhang, D.F.; Dong, X.Y.; Gu, Q.; Li, Y.L.; et al. Notch4+cancer stem-like cells promote the metastatic and invasive ability of melanoma. *Cancer Sci.* **2016**, *107*, 1079–1091. [CrossRef] [PubMed]

270. Guo, X.; Xu, S.; Gao, X.; Wang, J.; Xue, H.; Chen, Z.; Zhang, J.; Guo, X.; Qian, M.; Qiu, W.; et al. Macrophage migration inhibitory factor promotes vasculogenic mimicry formation induced by hypoxia via CXCR4/AKT/EMT pathway in human glioblastoma cells. *Oncotarget* **2017**. [CrossRef]

271. Priya, S.K.; Nagare, R.P.; Sneha, V.S.; Sidhanth, C.; Bindhya, S.; Manasa, P.; Ganesan, T.S. Tumour angiogenesis-Origin of blood vessels. *Int. J. Cancer* **2016**, *139*, 729–735. [CrossRef] [PubMed]

272. Burrell, K.; Zadeh, G. Molecular Mechanisms of Tumor Angiogenesis. In *Tumor Angiogenesis*; Ran, S., Ed.; Intech Open: Rijeka, Croatia, 2012; pp. 275–296.

273. Shahneh, F.Z.; Baradaran, B.; Zamani, F.; Aghebati-Maleki, L. Tumor angiogenesis and anti-angiogenic therapies. *Hum. Antibodies* **2013**, *22*, 15–19. [CrossRef] [PubMed]

274. Plate, K.H.; Scholz, A.; Dumont, D.J. Tumor angiogenesis and anti-angiogenic therapy in malignant gliomas revisited. *Acta Neuropathol.* **2012**, *124*, 763–775. [CrossRef] [PubMed]

275. Paulis, Y.W.J.; Soetekouw, P.M.; Verheul, H.M.; Tjan-Heijnen, V.C.; Griffioen, A.W. Signalling pathways in vasculogenic mimicry. *Biochim. Biophys. Acta* **2010**, *1806*, 18–28. [CrossRef] [PubMed]

276. Delgado-Bellido, D.; Serrano-Saenz, S.; Fernandez-Cortes, M.; Oliver, F.J. Vasculogenic mimicry signaling revisited: Focus on non-vascular VE-cadherin. *Mol. Cancer* **2017**, *16*, 65. [CrossRef] [PubMed]

277. Seftor, E.A.; Meltzer, P.S.; Schatteman, G.C.; Gruman, L.M.; Hess, A.R.; Kirschmann, D.A.; Seftor, R.E.; Hendrix, M.J. Expression of multiple molecular phenotypes by aggressive melanoma tumor cells: Role in vasculogenic mimicry. *Crit. Rev. Oncol. Hematol.* **2002**, *44*, 17–27. [CrossRef]

278. Li, S.; Meng, W.; Guan, Z.; Guo, Y.; Han, X. The hypoxia-related signaling pathways of vasculogenic mimicry in tumor treatment. *Biomed. Pharmacother.* **2016**, *80*, 127–135. [CrossRef] [PubMed]

279. Macklin, P.S.; McAuliffe, J.; Pugh, C.W.; Yamamoto, A. Hypoxia and HIF pathway in cancer and the placenta. *Placenta* **2017**. [CrossRef] [PubMed]

280. Bordeleau, F.; Mason, B.N.; Lollis, E.M.; Mazzola, M.; Zanotelli, M.R.; Somasegar, S.; Califano, J.P.; Montague, C.; LaValley, D.J.; Huynh, J.; et al. Matrix stiffening promotes a tumor vasculature phenotype. *Proc. Natl. Acad. Sci. USA* **2017**, *114*, 492–497. [CrossRef] [PubMed]

281. Krock, B.L.; Skuli, N.; Simon, M.C. Hypoxia-induced angiogenesis: Good and evil. *Genes Cancer* **2011**, *2*, 1117–1133. [CrossRef] [PubMed]

282. Yang, J.; Zhu, D.M.; Zhou, X.G.; Yin, N.; Zhang, Y.; Zhang, Z.X.; Li, D.C.; Zhou, J. HIF-2alpha promotes the formation of vasculogenic mimicry in pancreatic cancer by regulating the binding of Twist1 to the VE-cadherin promoter. *Oncotarget* **2017**, *8*, 47801–47815. [CrossRef] [PubMed]

283. Angara, K.; Rashid, M.H.; Shankar, A.; Ara, R.; Iskander, A.; Borin, T.F.; Jain, M.; Achyut, B.R.; Arbab, A.S. Vascular mimicry in glioblastoma following anti-angiogenic and anti-20-HETE therapies. *Histol. Histopathol.* **2017**, *32*, 917–928. [CrossRef] [PubMed]

284. Pezzolo, A.; Marimpietri, D.; Raffaghello, L.; Cocco, C.; Pistorio, A.; Gambini, C.; Cilli, M.; Horenstein, A.; Malavasi, F.; Pistoia, V. Failure of anti tumor-derived endothelial cell immunotherapy depends on augmentation of tumor hypoxia. *Oncotarget* **2014**, *5*, 10368–10381. [CrossRef] [PubMed]

285. Fernandez-Barral, A.; Orgaz, J.L.; Gomez, V.; del Peso, L.; Calzada, M.J.; Jimenez, B. Hypoxia negatively regulates antimetastatic PEDF in melanoma cells by a hypoxia inducible factor-independent, autophagy dependent mechanism. *PLoS ONE* **2012**, *7*, e32989. [CrossRef] [PubMed]

286. Yang, J.; Zhang, X.; Zhang, Y.; Zhu, D.; Zhang, L.; Li, Y.; Zhu, Y.; Li, D.; Zhou, J. HIF-2alpha promotes epithelial-mesenchymal transition through regulating Twist2 binding to the promoter of E-cadherin in pancreatic cancer. *J. Exp. Clin. Cancer Res.* **2016**, *35*, 26. [CrossRef] [PubMed]

287. Alameddine, R.S.; Hamieh, L.; Shamseddine, A. From sprouting angiogenesis to erythrocytes generation by cancer stem cells: Evolving concepts in tumor microcirculation. *BioMed Res. Int.* **2014**, *2014*, 986768. [CrossRef] [PubMed]

288. Zhang, D.; Yang, X.; Yang, Z.; Fei, F.; Li, S.; Qu, J.; Zhang, M.; Li, Y.; Zhang, X.; Zhang, S. Daughter Cells and Erythroid Cells Budding from PGCCs and Their Clinicopathological Significances in Colorectal Cancer. *J. Cancer* **2017**, *8*, 469–478. [CrossRef] [PubMed]

289. Zhang, S.; Fu, Z.; Wei, J.; Guo, J.; Liu, M.; Du, K. Peroxiredoxin 2 is involved in vasculogenic mimicry formation by targeting VEGFR2 activation in colorectal cancer. *Med. Oncol.* **2015**, *32*, 414. [CrossRef] [PubMed]

290. Dong, J.; Zhao, Y.; Huang, Q.; Fei, X.; Diao, Y.; Shen, Y.; Xiao, H.; Zhang, T.; Lan, Q.; Gu, X. Glioma stem/progenitor cells contribute to neovascularization via transdifferentiation. *Stem Cell Rev.* **2011**, *7*, 141–152. [CrossRef] [PubMed]

291. Ren, H.; Du, P.; Ge, Z.; Jin, Y.; Ding, D.; Liu, X.; Zou, Q. TWIST1 and BMI1 in Cancer Metastasis and Chemoresistance. *J. Cancer* **2016**, *7*, 1074–1080. [CrossRef] [PubMed]

292. Liu, K.; Sun, B.; Zhao, X.; Wang, X.; Li, Y.; Qiu, Z.; Liu, T.; Gu, Q.; Dong, X.; Zhang, Y.; et al. Hypoxia promotes vasculogenic mimicry formation by the Twist1-Bmi1 connection in hepatocellular carcinoma. *Int. J. Mol. Med.* **2015**, *36*, 783–791. [CrossRef] [PubMed]

293. Sun, T.; Sun, B.C.; Zhao, X.L.; Zhao, N.; Dong, X.Y.; Che, N.; Yao, Z.; Ma, Y.M.; Gu, Q.; Zong, W.K.; et al. Promotion of tumor cell metastasis and vasculogenic mimicry by way of transcription coactivation by Bcl-2 and Twist1: A study of hepatocellular carcinoma. *Hepatology* **2011**, *54*, 1690–1706. [CrossRef] [PubMed]

294. Liang, Y.; Hu, J.; Li, J.; Liu, Y.; Yu, J.; Zhuang, X.; Mu, L.; Kong, X.; Hong, D.; Yang, Q.; et al. Epigenetic Activation of TWIST1 by MTDH Promotes Cancer Stem-like Cell Traits in Breast Cancer. *Cancer Res.* **2015**, *75*, 3672–3680. [CrossRef] [PubMed]

295. Li, G.; Yang, Y.; Xu, S.; Ma, L.; He, M.; Zhang, Z. Slug signaling is up-regulated by CCL21/CCR7 [corrected] to induce EMT in human chondrosarcoma. *Med. Oncol.* **2015**, *32*, 478. [CrossRef] [PubMed]

296. Yang, Z.; Sun, B.; Li, Y.; Zhao, X.; Zhao, X.; Gu, Q.; An, J.; Dong, X.; Liu, F.; Wang, Y. ZEB2 promotes vasculogenic mimicry by TGF-β1 induced epithelial-to-mesenchymal transition in hepatocellular carcinoma. *Exp. Mol. Pathol.* **2015**, *98*, 352–359. [CrossRef] [PubMed]

297. Puisieux, A.; Brabletz, T.; Caramel, J. Oncogenic roles of EMT-inducing transcription factors. *Nat. Cell Biol.* **2014**, *16*, 488–494. [CrossRef] [PubMed]

298. Wang, H.; Lin, H.; Pan, J.; Mo, C.; Zhang, F.; Huang, B.; Wang, Z.; Chen, X.; Zhuang, J.; Wang, D.; et al. Vasculogenic Mimicry in Prostate Cancer: The Roles of EphA2 and PI3K. *J. Cancer* **2016**, *7*, 1114–1124. [CrossRef] [PubMed]

299. Hess, A.R.; Seftor, E.A.; Seftor, R.E.B.; Hendrix, M.J.C. Phosphoinositide 3-kinase regulates membrane type 1-matrix metalloproteinase (MMP) and MMP-2 activity during melanoma cell vasculogenic mimicry. *Cancer Res.* **2003**, *63*, 4757–4762. [PubMed]

300. Zhang, J.; Qiao, L.; Liang, N.; Xie, J.; Luo, H.; Deng, G.; Zhang, J. Vasculogenic mimicry and tumor metastasis. *J. BUON* **2016**, *21*, 533–541. [PubMed]

301. Robertson, G.P. Mig-7 linked to vasculogenic mimicry. *Am. J. Pathol.* **2007**, *170*, 1454–1456. [CrossRef] [PubMed]

302. Petty, A.P.; Garman, K.L.; Winn, V.D.; Spidel, C.M.; Lindsey, J.S. Overexpression of carcinoma and embryonic cytotrophoblast cell-specific Mig-7 induces invasion and vessel-like structure formation. *Am. J. Pathol.* **2007**, *170*, 1763–1780. [CrossRef] [PubMed]

303. Hendrix, M.J.C.; Seftor, E.A.; Hess, A.R.; Seftor, R.E.B. Vasculogenic mimicry and tumour-cell plasticity: Lessons from melanoma. *Nat. Rev. Cancer* **2003**, *3*, 411–421. [CrossRef] [PubMed]

304. Petty, A.P.; Wright, S.E.; Rewers-Felkins, K.A.; Yenderrozos, M.A.; Vorderstrasse, B.A.; Lindsey, J.S. Targeting Migration inducting gene-7 inhibits carcinoma cell invasion, early primary tumor growth, and stimulates monocyte oncolytic activity. *Mol. Cancer Ther.* **2009**, *8*, 2412–2423. [CrossRef] [PubMed]

305. Sulzmaier, F.J.; Jean, C.; Schlaepfer, D.D. FAK in cancer: Mechanistic findings and clinical applications. *Nat. Rev. Cancer* **2014**, *14*, 598–610. [CrossRef] [PubMed]

306. Van den Brule, F.A.; Buicu, C.; Baldet, M.; Sobel, M.E.; Cooper, D.N.; Marschal, P.; Castronovo, V. Galectin-1 modulates human melanoma cell adhesion to laminin. *Biochem. Biophys. Res. Commun.* **1995**, *209*, 760–767. [CrossRef] [PubMed]

307. Hsieh, S.H.; Ying, N.W.; Wu, M.H.; Chiang, W.F.; Hsu, C.L.; Wong, T.Y.; Jin, Y.T.; Hong, T.M.; Chen, Y.L. Galectin-1, a novel ligand of neuropilin-1, activates VEGFR-2 signaling and modulates the migration of vascular endothelial cells. *Oncogene* **2008**, *27*, 3746–3753. [CrossRef] [PubMed]

308. Garin, M.I.; Chu, C.C.; Golshayan, D.; Cernuda-Morollon, E.; Wait, R.; Lechler, R.I. Galectin-1: A key effector of regulation mediated by CD4+CD25+ T cells. *Blood* **2007**, *109*, 2058–2065. [CrossRef] [PubMed]

309. Cooper, D.N.; Massa, S.M.; Barondes, S.H. Endogenous muscle lectin inhibits myoblast adhesion to laminin. *J. Cell Biol.* **1991**, *115*, 1437–1448. [CrossRef] [PubMed]

310. Mourad-Zeidan, A.A.; Melnikova, V.O.; Wang, H.; Raz, A.; Bar-Eli, M. Expression profiling of Galectin-3-depleted melanoma cells reveals its major role in melanoma cell plasticity and vasculogenic mimicry. *Am. J. Pathol.* **2008**, *173*, 1839–1852. [CrossRef] [PubMed]

311. Li, Y.; Sun, B.; Zhao, X.; Wang, X.; Zhang, D.; Gu, Q.; Liu, T. MMP-2 and MMP-13 affect vasculogenic mimicry formation in large cell lung cancer. *J. Cell. Mol. Med.* **2017**. [CrossRef] [PubMed]

312. Ruffini, F.; D'Atri, S.; Lacal, P.M. Neuropilin-1 expression promotes invasiveness of melanoma cells through vascular endothelial growth factor receptor-2-dependent and -independent mechanisms. *Int. J. Oncol.* **2013**, *43*, 297–306. [CrossRef] [PubMed]

313. Ruffini, F.; Levati, L.; Graziani, G.; Caporali, S.; Atzori, M.G.; D'Atri, S.; Lacal, P.M. Platelet-derived growth factor-C promotes human melanoma aggressiveness through activation of neuropilin-1. *Oncotarget* **2017**. [CrossRef] [PubMed]

314. Lambrechts, D.; Lenz, H.J.; de Haas, S.; Carmeliet, P.; Scherer, S.J. Markers of response for the antiangiogenic agent bevacizumab. *J. Clin. Oncol.* **2013**, *31*, 1219–1230. [CrossRef] [PubMed]

315. Graziani, G.; Lacal, P.M. Neuropilin-1 as Therapeutic Target for Malignant Melanoma. *Front. Oncol.* **2015**, *5*, 125. [CrossRef] [PubMed]

316. Hardy, K.M.; Kirschmann, D.A.; Seftor, E.A.; Margaryan, N.V.; Postovit, L.M.; Strizzi, L.; Hendrix, M.J. Regulation of the embryonic morphogen Nodal by Notch4 facilitates manifestation of the aggressive melanoma phenotype. *Cancer Res.* **2010**, *70*, 10340–10350. [CrossRef] [PubMed]

317. Jue, C.; Lin, C.; Zhisheng, Z.; Yayun, Q.; Feng, J.; Min, Z.; Haibo, W.; Youyang, S.; Hisamitsu, T.; Shintaro, I.; et al. Notch1 promotes vasculogenic mimicry in hepatocellular carcinoma by inducing EMT signaling. *Oncotarget* **2017**, *8*, 2501–2513. [CrossRef] [PubMed]

318. Zhao, N.; Sun, H.; Sun, B.; Zhu, D.; Zhao, X.; Wang, Y.; Gu, Q.; Dong, X.; Liu, F.; Zhang, Y.; et al. miR-27a-3p suppresses tumor metastasis and VM by down-regulating VE-cadherin expression and inhibiting EMT: An essential role for Twist-1 in HCC. *Sci. Rep.* **2016**, *6*, 23091. [CrossRef] [PubMed]

319. Zhao, N.; Sun, B.C.; Zhao, X.L.; Wang, Y.; Sun, H.Z.; Dong, X.Y.; Meng, J.; Gu, Q. Changes in microRNAs associated with Twist-1 and Bcl-2 overexpression identify signaling pathways. *Exp. Mol. Pathol.* **2015**, *99*, 524–532. [CrossRef] [PubMed]

320. Liu, W.; Lv, C.; Zhang, B.; Zhou, Q.; Cao, Z. MicroRNA-27b functions as a new inhibitor of ovarian cancer-mediated vasculogenic mimicry through suppression of VE-cadherin expression. *RNA* **2017**. [CrossRef] [PubMed]

321. Wu, N.; Zhao, X.; Liu, M.; Liu, H.; Yao, W.; Zhang, Y.; Cao, S.; Lin, X. Role of microRNA-26b in glioma development and its mediated regulation on EphA2. *PLoS ONE* **2011**, *6*, e16264. [CrossRef] [PubMed]

322. An, L.; Liu, Y.; Wu, A.; Guan, Y. microRNA-124 inhibits migration and invasion by down-regulating ROCK1 in glioma. *PLoS ONE* **2013**, *8*, e69478. [CrossRef] [PubMed]

323. Hunt, S.; Jones, A.V.; Hinsley, E.E.; Whawell, S.A.; Lambert, D.W. MicroRNA-124 suppresses oral squamous cell carcinoma motility by targeting ITGB1. *FEBS Lett.* **2011**, *585*, 187–192. [CrossRef] [PubMed]

324. Wang, P.; Chen, L.; Zhang, J.; Chen, H.; Fan, J.; Wang, K.; Luo, J.; Chen, Z.; Meng, Z.; Liu, L. Methylation-mediated silencing of the miR-124 genes facilitates pancreatic cancer progression and metastasis by targeting Rac1. *Oncogene* **2014**, *33*, 514–524. [CrossRef] [PubMed]

325. Liang, Y.J.; Wang, Q.Y.; Zhou, C.X.; Yin, Q.Q.; He, M.; Yu, X.T.; Cao, D.X.; Chen, G.Q.; He, J.R.; Zhao, Q. MiR-124 targets Slug to regulate epithelial-mesenchymal transition and metastasis of breast cancer. *Carcinogenesis* **2013**, *34*, 713–722. [CrossRef] [PubMed]

326. Wan, H.Y.; Li, Q.Q.; Zhang, Y.; Tian, W.; Li, Y.N.; Liu, M.; Li, X.; Tang, H. MiR-124 represses vasculogenic mimicry and cell motility by targeting amotL1 in cervical cancer cells. *Cancer Lett.* **2014**, *355*, 148–158. [CrossRef] [PubMed]

327. Wang, Y.; Sun, B.C.; Zhao, X.L.; Zhao, N.; Sun, R.; Zhu, D.W.; Zhang, Y.H.; Li, Y.L.; Gu, Q.; Dong, X.Y.; et al. Twist1-related miR-26b-5p suppresses epithelial-mesenchymal transition, migration and invasion by targeting SMAD1 in hepatocellular carcinoma. *Oncotarget* **2016**, *7*, 24383–24401. [CrossRef] [PubMed]

328. Wang, Y.; Sun, B.; Sun, H.; Zhao, X.; Wang, X.; Zhao, N.; Zhang, Y.; Li, Y.; Gu, Q.; Liu, F.; et al. Regulation of proliferation, angiogenesis and apoptosis in hepatocellular carcinoma by miR-26b-5p. *Tumor Biol.* **2016**, *37*, 10965–10979. [CrossRef] [PubMed]

329. Zhao, X.; Wang, Y.; Deng, R.; Zhang, H.; Dou, J.; Yuan, H.; Hou, G.; Du, Y.; Chen, Q.; Yu, J. miR186 suppresses prostate cancer progression by targeting Twist1. *Oncotarget* **2016**, *7*, 33136–33151. [CrossRef] [PubMed]

330. Wang, Y.; Shao, N.; Mao, X.Y.; Zhu, M.M.; Fan, W.F.; Shen, Z.X.; Xiao, R.; Wang, C.C.; Bao, W.P.; Xu, X.Y.; et al. MiR-4638–5p inhibits castration resistance of prostate cancer through repressing kidins220 expression and PI3K/AKT pathway activity. *Oncotarget* **2016**, *7*, 47444–47464. [CrossRef] [PubMed]

331. Chen, Z.; Wang, X.; Liu, R.; Chen, L.; Yi, J.; Qi, B.; Shuang, Z.; Liu, M.; Li, X.; Li, S.; et al. KDM4B-mediated epigenetic silencing of miRNA-615–5p augments RAB24 to facilitate malignancy of hepatoma cells. *Oncotarget* **2017**, *8*, 17712–17725. [CrossRef] [PubMed]

332. Gutschner, T.; Diederichs, S. The hallmarks of cancer: A long non-coding RNA point of view. *RNA Biol.* **2012**, *9*, 703–719. [CrossRef] [PubMed]

333. Cao, M.X.; Jiang, Y.P.; Tang, Y.L.; Liang, X.H. The crosstalk between lncRNA and microRNA in cancer metastasis: Orchestrating the epithelial-mesenchymal plasticity. *Oncotarget* **2017**, *8*, 12472–12483. [CrossRef] [PubMed]

334. Yu, C.; Xue, J.; Zhu, W.; Jiao, Y.; Zhang, S.; Cao, J. Warburg meets non-coding RNAs: The emerging role of ncRNA in regulating the glucose metabolism of cancer cells. *Tumor Biol.* **2015**, *36*, 81–94. [CrossRef] [PubMed]

335. Beltran-Anaya, F.O.; Cedro-Tanda, A.; Hidalgo-Miranda, A.; Romero-Cordoba, S.L. Insights into the Regulatory Role of Non-coding RNAs in Cancer Metabolism. *Front. Physiol.* **2016**, *7*, 342. [CrossRef] [PubMed]

336. Li, Y.; Wu, Z.; Yuan, J.; Sun, L.; Lin, L.; Huang, N.; Bin, J.; Liao, Y.; Liao, W. Long non-coding RNA MALAT1 promotes gastric cancer tumorigenicity and metastasis by regulating vasculogenic mimicry and angiogenesis. *Cancer Lett.* **2017**, *395*, 31–44. [CrossRef] [PubMed]

337. Ruf, W.; Seftor, E.A.; Petrovan, R.J.; Weiss, R.M.; Gruman, L.M.; Margaryan, N.V.; Seftor, R.E.; Miyagi, Y.; Hendrix, M.J.C. Differential role of tissue factor pathway inhibitors 1 and 2 in melanoma vasculogenic mimicry. *Cancer Res.* **2003**, *63*, 5381–5389. [PubMed]

338. Kucera, T.; Lammert, E. Ancestral vascular tube formation and its adoption by tumors. *Biol. Chem.* **2009**, *390*, 985–994. [CrossRef] [PubMed]

339. Qiao, L.; Liang, N.; Zhang, J.; Xie, J.; Liu, F.; Xu, D.; Yu, X.; Tian, Y. Advanced research on vasculogenic mimicry in cancer. *J. Cell. Mol. Med.* **2015**, *19*, 315–326. [CrossRef] [PubMed]

340. Cao, Z.; Bao, M.; Miele, L.; Sarkar, F.H.; Wang, Z.; Zhou, Q. Tumour vasculogenic mimicry is associated with poor prognosis of human cancer patients: A systemic review and meta-analysis. *Eur. J. Cancer* **2013**, *49*, 3914–3923. [CrossRef] [PubMed]

341. Guo, Q.; Yuan, Y.; Jin, Z.; Xu, T.; Gao, Y.; Wei, H.; Li, C.; Hou, W.; Hua, B. Association between tumor vasculogenic mimicry and the poor prognosis of gastric cancer in China: An updated systematic review and meta-analysis. *BioMed Res. Int.* **2016**, *2016*, 2408645. [CrossRef] [PubMed]

342. Liu, J.; Huang, J.; Yao, W.Y.; Ben, Q.W.; Chen, D.F.; He, X.Y.; Li, L.; Yuan, Y.Z. The origins of vacularization in tumors. *Front. Biosci. (Landmark Ed.)* **2012**, *17*, 2559–2565. [CrossRef] [PubMed]

343. Tan, L.Y.; Mintoff, C.; Johan, M.Z.; Ebert, B.W.; Fedele, C.; Zhang, Y.F.; Szeto, P.; Sheppard, K.E.; McArthur, G.A.; Foster-Smith, E.; et al. Desmoglein 2 promotes vasculogenic mimicry in melanoma and is associated with poor clinical outcome. *Oncotarget* **2016**. [CrossRef] [PubMed]

344. Yang, J.P.; Liao, Y.D.; Mai, D.M.; Xie, P.; Qiang, Y.Y.; Zheng, L.S.; Wang, M.Y.; Mei, Y.; Meng, D.F.; Xu, L.; et al. Tumor vasculogenic mimicry predicts poor prognosis in cancer patients: A meta-analysis. *Angiogenesis* **2016**, *19*, 191–200. [CrossRef] [PubMed]

345. Zhu, B.; Zhou, L.; Yu, L.; Wu, S.; Song, W.; Gong, X.; Wang, D. Evaluation of the correlation of vasculogenic mimicry, ALDH1, KAI1 and microvessel density in the prediction of metastasis and prognosis in colorectal carcinoma. *BMC Surg.* **2017**, *17*, 47. [CrossRef] [PubMed]

346. Yu, L.; Zhu, B.; Wu, S.; Zhou, L.; Song, W.; Gong, X.; Wang, D. Evaluation of the correlation of vasculogenic mimicry, ALDH1, KiSS-1, and MACC1 in the prediction of metastasis and prognosis in ovarian carcinoma. *Diagn. Pathol.* **2017**, *12*, 23. [CrossRef] [PubMed]

347. Yao, L.; Zhang, D.; Zhao, X.; Sun, B.; Liu, Y.; Gu, Q.; Zhang, Y.; Zhao, X.; Che, N.; Zheng, Y.; et al. Dickkopf-1-promoted vasculogenic mimicry in non-small cell lung cancer is associated with EMT and development of a cancer stem-like cell phenotype. *J. Cell. Mol. Med.* **2016**, *20*, 1673–1685. [CrossRef] [PubMed]

348. Liu, W.B.; Xu, G.L.; Jia, W.D.; Li, J.S.; Ma, J.L.; Chen, K.; Wang, Z.H.; Ge, Y.S.; Ren, W.H.; Yu, J.H.; et al. Prognostic significance and mechanisms of patterned matrix vasculogenic mimicry in hepatocellular carcinoma. *Med. Oncol.* **2011**, *28* (Suppl. 1), S228–S238. [CrossRef] [PubMed]

349. Zununi Vahed, S.; Salehi, R.; Davaran, S.; Sharifi, S. Liposome-based drug co-delivery systems in cancer cells. *Mater. Sci. Eng. C Mater. Biol. Appl.* **2017**, *71*, 1327–1341. [CrossRef] [PubMed]

350. Ferrara, N.; Gerber, H.P.; LeCouter, J. The biology of VEGF and its receptors. *Nat. Med.* **2003**, *9*, 669–676. [CrossRef] [PubMed]

351. Vredenburgh, J.J.; Desjardins, A.; Herndon, J.E., 2nd; Dowell, J.M.; Reardon, D.A.; Quinn, J.A.; Rich, J.N.; Sathornsumetee, S.; Gururangan, S.; Wagner, M.; et al. Phase II trial of bevacizumab and irinotecan in recurrent malignant glioma. *Clin. Cancer Res.* **2007**, *13*, 1253–1259. [CrossRef] [PubMed]

352. Van der Veldt, A.A.; Lubberink, M.; Bahce, I.; Walraven, M.; de Boer, M.P.; Greuter, H.N.; Hendrikse, N.H.; Eriksson, J.; Windhorst, A.D.; Postmus, P.E.; et al. Rapid decrease in delivery of chemotherapy to tumors after anti-VEGF therapy: Implications for scheduling of anti-angiogenic drugs. *Cancer Cell* **2012**, *21*, 82–91. [CrossRef] [PubMed]

353. Siemann, D.W. The unique characteristics of tumor vasculature and preclinical evidence for its selective disruption by tumor-vascular disrupting agents. *Cancer Treat. Rev.* **2011**, *37*, 63–74. [CrossRef] [PubMed]

354. Lin, Z.; Zhang, Q.; Luo, W. Angiogenesis inhibitors as therapeutic agents in cancer: Challenges and future directions. *Eur. J. Pharmacol.* **2016**, *793*, 76–81. [CrossRef] [PubMed]

355. Mahase, S.; Rattenni, R.N.; Wesseling, P.; Leenders, W.; Baldotto, C.; Jain, R.; Zagzag, D. Hypoxia-mediated mechanisms associated with antiangiogenic treatment resistance in glioblastomas. *Am. J. Pathol.* **2017**, *187*, 940–953. [CrossRef] [PubMed]

356. Pezzella, F.; Gatter, K.; Qian, C.N. Twenty years after: The beautiful hypothesis and the ugly facts. *Chin. J. Cancer* **2016**, *35*, 22. [CrossRef] [PubMed]

357. Jain, R.K. Antiangiogenesis strategies revisited: From starving tumors to alleviating hypoxia. *Cancer Cell* **2014**, *26*, 605–622. [CrossRef] [PubMed]

358. Folkman, J. Angiogenesis in cancer, vascular, rheumatoid and other disease. *Nat. Med.* **1995**, *1*, 27–31. [CrossRef] [PubMed]

359. Boehm, T.; Folkman, J.; Browder, T.; O'Reilly, M.S. Antiangiogenic therapy of experimental cancer does not induce acquired drug resistance. *Nature* **1997**, *390*, 404–407. [CrossRef] [PubMed]

360. Ribatti, D. The inefficacy of antiangiogenic therapies. *J. Angiogenes Res.* **2010**, *2*, 27. [CrossRef] [PubMed]

361. Sennino, B.; McDonald, D.M. Controlling escape from angiogenesis inhibitors. *Nat. Rev. Cancer* **2012**, *12*, 699–709. [CrossRef] [PubMed]

362. De Falco, S. Antiangiogenesis therapy: An update after the first decade. *Korean J. Intern. Med.* **2014**, *29*, 1–11. [CrossRef] [PubMed]

363. Jayson, G.C.; Kerbel, R.; Ellis, L.M.; Harris, A.L. Antiangiogenic therapy in oncology: Current status and future directions. *Lancet* **2016**, *388*, 518–529. [CrossRef]

364. Crawford, Y.; Ferrara, N. Tumor and stromal pathways mediating refractoriness/resistance to anti-angiogenic therapies. *Trends Pharmacol. Sci.* **2009**. [CrossRef] [PubMed]

365. Francia, G.; Emmenegger, U.; Kerbel, R.S. Tumor-associated fibroblasts as "Trojan Horse" mediators of resistance to anti-VEGF therapy. *Cancer Cell* **2009**, *15*, 3–5. [CrossRef] [PubMed]

366. Hendrix, M.J.; Seftor, E.A.; Seftor, R.E.; Chao, J.T.; Chien, D.S.; Chu, Y.W. Tumor cell vascular mimicry: Novel targeting opportunity in melanoma. *Pharmacol. Ther.* **2016**, *159*, 83–92. [CrossRef] [PubMed]

367. Seftor, R.E.; Hess, A.R.; Seftor, E.A.; Kirschmann, D.A.; Hardy, K.M.; Margaryan, N.V.; Hendrix, M.J. Tumor cell vasculogenic mimicry: From controversy to therapeutic promise. *Am. J. Pathol.* **2012**, *181*, 1115–1125. [CrossRef] [PubMed]

368. Chung, H.J.; Mahalingam, M. Angiogenesis, vasculogenic mimicry and vascular invasion in cutaneous malignant melanoma—Implications for therapeutic strategies and targeted therapies. *Expert Rev. Anticancer Ther.* **2014**, *14*, 621–639. [CrossRef] [PubMed]

369. Mao, J.M.; Liu, J.; Guo, G.; Mao, X.G.; Li, C.X. Glioblastoma vasculogenic mimicry: Signaling pathways progression and potential anti-angiogenesis targets. *Biomark. Res.* **2015**, *3*, 8. [CrossRef] [PubMed]

370. Sasanelli, F.; Hocking, A.; Pulford, E.; Irani, Y.; Klebe, S. Vasculogenic mimicry in vitro in tumour cells derived from metastatic malignant pleural effusions. *Pathology* **2017**. [CrossRef] [PubMed]

371. Racordon, D.; Valdivia, A.; Mingo, G.; Erices, R.; Aravena, R.; Santoro, F.; Bravo, M.L.; Ramirez, C.; Gonzalez, P.; Sandoval, A.; et al. Structural and functional identification of vasculogenic mimicry in vitro. *Sci. Rep.* **2017**, *7*, 6985. [CrossRef] [PubMed]

372. Xu, M.; Zhu, C.H.; Zhao, X.; Chen, C.; Zhang, H.L.; Yuan, H.H.; Deng, R.; Dou, J.Z.; Wang, Y.L.; Huang, J.; et al. Atypical ubiquitin E3 ligase complex Skp1-Pam-Fbxo45 controls the core epithelial-to-mesenchymal transition-inducing transcription factors. *Oncotarget* **2015**, *6*, 979–994. [CrossRef] [PubMed]

373. Bianchi, M.E.; Agresti, A. HMG proteins: Dynamic players in gene regulation and differentiation. *Curr. Opin. Genet. Dev.* **2005**, *15*, 496–506. [CrossRef] [PubMed]

374. Lotze, M.T.; DeMarco, R.A. Dealing with death: HMGB1 as a novel target for cancer therapy. *Curr. Opin. Investig. Drugs* **2003**, *4*, 1405–1409. [PubMed]

375. Yin, H.; Shao, Y.; Chen, X. The effects of CD147 on the cell proliferation, apoptosis, invasion, and angiogenesis in glioma. *Neurol. Sci.* **2017**, *38*, 129–136. [CrossRef] [PubMed]

376. Schultz, N.A.; Johansen, J.S. YKL-40-A Protein in the Field of Translational Medicine: A Role as a Biomarker in Cancer Patients? *Cancers (Basel)* **2010**, *2*, 1453–1491. [CrossRef] [PubMed]

377. Shao, R.; Taylor, S.L.; Oh, D.S.; Schwartz, L.M. Vascular heterogeneity and targeting: The role of YKL-40 in glioblastoma vascularization. *Oncotarget* **2015**, *6*, 40507–40518. [CrossRef] [PubMed]

378. Shao, R.; Francescone, R.; Ngernyuang, N.; Bentley, B.; Taylor, S.L.; Moral, L.; Yan, W. Anti-YKL-40 antibody and ionizing irradiation synergistically inhibit tumor vascularization and malignancy in glioblastoma. *Carcinogenesis* **2014**, *35*, 373–382. [CrossRef] [PubMed]

379. Ribatti, D. Tumor refractoriness to anti-VEGF therapy. *Oncotarget* **2016**, *7*, 46668–46677. [CrossRef] [PubMed]

380. Chen, X.; Zhang, H.; Zhu, H.; Yang, X.; Yang, Y.; Yang, Y.; Min, H.; Chen, G.; Liu, J.; Lu, J.; et al. Endostatin combined with radiotherapy suppresses vasculogenic mimicry formation through inhibition of epithelial-mesenchymal transition in esophageal cancer. *Tumor Biol.* **2016**, *37*, 4679–4688. [CrossRef] [PubMed]

381. Miyata, N.; Taniguchi, K.; Seki, T.; Ishimoto, T.; Sato-Watanabe, M.; Yasuda, Y.; Doi, M.; Kametani, S.; Tomishima, Y.; Ueki, T.; et al. HET0016, a potent and selective inhibitor of 20-HETE synthesizing enzyme. *Br. J. Pharmacol.* **2001**, *133*, 325–329. [CrossRef] [PubMed]

382. Lv, H.; Li, Y.; Du, H.; Fang, J.; Song, X.; Zhang, J. The synthetic compound norcantharidiniInduced apoptosis in mantle cell lymphoma in vivo and in vitro through the PI3K-Akt-NF- kappa B signaling pathway. *Evid. Based Complement. Alternat. Med.* **2013**, *2013*, 461487. [CrossRef] [PubMed]

383. Yeh, C.B.; Hsieh, M.J.; Hsieh, Y.H.; Chien, M.H.; Chiou, H.L.; Yang, S.F. Antimetastatic effects of norcantharidin on hepatocellular carcinoma by transcriptional inhibition of MMP-9 through modulation of NF-kB activity. *PLoS ONE* **2012**, *7*, e31055. [CrossRef] [PubMed]

384. Yeh, C.B.; Hsieh, M.J.; Hsieh, Y.H.; Chien, M.H.; Chiou, H.L.; Yang, S.F. Correction: Antimetastatic effects of norcantharidin on hepatocellular carcinoma by transcriptional inhibition of MMP-9 through modulation of NF-kB activity. *PLoS ONE* **2017**, *12*, e0171900. [CrossRef] [PubMed]

385. Wang, Z.; You, D.; Lu, M.; He, Y.; Yan, S. Inhibitory effect of norcantharidin on melanoma tumor growth and vasculogenic mimicry by suppressing MMP-2 expression. *Oncol. Lett.* **2017**, *13*, 1660–1664. [CrossRef] [PubMed]

386. Zhu, W.; Sun, W.; Zhang, J.T.; Liu, Z.Y.; Li, X.P.; Fan, Y.Z. Norcantharidin enhances TIMP-2 anti-vasculogenic mimicry activity for human gallbladder cancers through downregulating MMP-2 and MT1-MMP. *Int. J. Oncol.* **2015**, *46*, 627–640. [CrossRef] [PubMed]

387. Zhang, S.; Li, M.; Gu, Y.; Liu, Z.; Xu, S.; Cui, Y.; Sun, B. Thalidomide influences growth and vasculogenic mimicry channel formation in melanoma. *J. Exp. Clin. Cancer Res.* **2008**, *27*, 60. [CrossRef] [PubMed]

388. Guan, Y.Y.; Luan, X.; Lu, Q.; Liu, Y.R.; Sun, P.; Zhao, M.; Chen, H.Z.; Fang, C. Natural products with antiangiogenic and antivasculogenic mimicry activity. *Mini. Rev. Med. Chem.* **2016**, *16*, 1290–1302. [CrossRef] [PubMed]

389. Su, S.J.; Yeh, T.M.; Chuang, W.J.; Ho, C.L.; Chang, K.L.; Cheng, H.L.; Liu, H.S.; Cheng, H.L.; Hsu, P.Y.; Chow, N.H. The novel targets for anti-angiogenesis of genistein on human cancer cells. *Biochem. Pharmacol.* **2005**, *69*, 307–318. [CrossRef] [PubMed]

390. Cong, R.; Sun, Q.; Yang, L.; Gu, H.; Zeng, Y.; Wang, B. Effect of Genistein on vasculogenic mimicry formation by human uveal melanoma cells. *J. Exp. Clin. Cancer Res.* **2009**, *28*, 124. [CrossRef] [PubMed]

391. Liu, R.; Cao, Z.; Pan, Y.; Zhang, G.; Yang, P.; Guo, P.; Zhou, Q. Jatrorrhizine hydrochloride inhibits the proliferation and neovascularization of C8161 metastatic melanoma cells. *Anticancer Drugs* **2013**, *24*, 667–676. [CrossRef] [PubMed]

392. Chen, L.X.; He, Y.J.; Zhao, S.Z.; Wu, J.G.; Wang, J.T.; Zhu, L.M.; Lin, T.T.; Sun, B.C.; Li, X.R. Inhibition of tumor growth and vasculogenic mimicry by curcumin through down-regulation of the EphA2/PI3K/MMP pathway in a murine choroidal melanoma model. *Cancer Biol. Ther.* **2011**, *11*, 229–235. [CrossRef] [PubMed]

393. Vartanian, A.A.; Burova, O.S.; Stepanova, E.V.; Baryshnikov, A.Y.; Lichinitser, M.R. Melanoma vasculogenic mimicry is strongly related to reactive oxygen species level. *Melanoma Res.* **2007**, *17*, 370–379. [CrossRef] [PubMed]

394. Zang, M.; Hu, L.; Zhang, B.; Zhu, Z.; Li, J.; Zhu, Z.; Yan, M.; Liu, B. Luteolin suppresses angiogenesis and vasculogenic mimicry formation through inhibiting Notch1-VEGF signaling in gastric cancer. *Biochem. Biophys. Res. Commun.* **2017**. [CrossRef] [PubMed]

395. Jue, C.; Min, Z.; Zhisheng, Z.; Lin, C.; Yayun, Q.; Xuanyi, W.; Feng, J.; Haibo, W.; Youyang, S.; Tadashi, H.; et al. COE inhibits vasculogenic mimicry in hepatocellular carcinoma via suppressing Notch1 signaling. *J. Ethnopharmacol.* **2017**. [CrossRef] [PubMed]

396. Yao, N.; Ren, K.; Wang, Y.; Jin, Q.; Lu, X.; Lu, Y.; Jiang, C.; Zhang, D.; Lu, J.; Wang, C.; et al. Paris polyphylla suppresses proliferation and vsculogenic mimicry of human osteosarcoma cells and inhibits tumor growth in vivo. *Am. J. Chin. Med.* **2017**, 1–24. [CrossRef]

397. Yamakawa, S.; Asai, T.; Uchida, T.; Matsukawa, M.; Akizawa, T.; Oku, N. (−)-Epigallocatechin gallate inhibits membrane-type 1 matrix metalloproteinase, MT1-MMP, and tumor angiogenesis. *Cancer Lett.* **2004**, *210*, 47–55. [CrossRef] [PubMed]

398. Ying, M.; Chen, G.; Lu, W. Recent advances and strategies in tumor vasculature targeted nano-drug delivery systems. *Curr. Pharm. Des.* **2015**, *21*, 3066–3075. [CrossRef] [PubMed]

399. Li, X.Y.; Zhao, Y.; Sun, M.G.; Shi, J.F.; Ju, R.J.; Zhang, C.X.; Li, X.T.; Zhao, W.Y.; Mu, L.M.; Zeng, F.; et al. Multifunctional liposomes loaded with paclitaxel and artemether for treatment of invasive brain glioma. *Biomaterials* **2014**, *35*, 5591–5604. [CrossRef] [PubMed]

400. Liu, Y.; Wu, X.; Gao, Y.; Zhang, J.; Zhang, D.; Gu, S.; Zhu, G.; Liu, G.; Li, X. Aptamer-functionalized peptide H3CR5C as a novel nanovehicle for codelivery of fasudil and miRNA-195 targeting hepatocellular carcinoma. *Int. J. Nanomed.* **2016**, *11*, 3891–3905. [CrossRef] [PubMed]

401. Ohuchida, K.; Mizumoto, K.; Murakami, M.; Qian, L.W.; Sato, N.; Nagai, E.; Matsumoto, K.; Nakamura, T.; Tanaka, M. Radiation to stromal fibroblasts increases invasiveness of pancreatic cancer cells through tumor-stromal interactions. *Cancer Res.* **2004**, *64*, 3215–3222. [CrossRef] [PubMed]

402. Li, G.; Satyamoorthy, K.; Herlyn, M. N-cadherin-mediated intercellular interactions promote survival and migration of melanoma cells. *Cancer Res.* **2001**, *61*, 3819–3825. [PubMed]

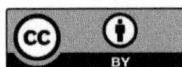

International Journal of
Molecular Sciences

MDPI

Article

Tanshinone IIA Inhibits Epithelial-Mesenchymal Transition in Bladder Cancer Cells via Modulation of STAT3-CCL2 Signaling

Sung-Ying Huang [1], Shu-Fang Chang [2], Kuan-Fu Liao [3,4] and Sheng-Chun Chiu [2,5,6,*]

[1] Department of Ophthalmology, Hsinchu Mackay Memorial Hospital, No. 690, Sec. 2, Guangfu Rd., East Dist, Hsinchu City 30071, Taiwan; hopes929@gmail.com
[2] Department of Research, Taichung Tzu Chi Hospital, Buddhist Tzu Chi Medical Foundation, No. 88, Section 1, Fengxing Road, Tanzi Dist., Taichung City 427, Taiwan; fantac10@gmail.com
[3] Graduate Institute of Integrated Medicine, China Medical University, No. 91, Hsueh-Shih Road, Taichung City 427, Taiwan; kuanfuliaog@gmail.com
[4] Department of Internal Medicine, Taichung Tzu Chi Hospital, Buddhist Tzu Chi Medical Foundation, No. 88, Section 1, Fengxing Road, Tanzi Dist., Taichung City 427, Taiwan
[5] Department of Laboratory Medicine, Taichung Tzu Chi Hospital, Buddhist Tzu Chi Medical Foundation, No. 88, Section 1, Fengxing Road, Tanzi Dist., Taichung City 427, Taiwan
[6] General Education Center, Tzu Chi University of Science and Technology, No. 880, Section 2, Chien-kuo Road, Hualien City 970, Taiwan
* Correspondence: tc1271201@tzuchi.com.tw; Tel.: +886-4-3606-0666 (ext. 3430)

Received: 29 June 2017; Accepted: 21 July 2017; Published: 25 July 2017

Abstract: Tanshinone IIA (Tan-IIA) is an extract from the widely used traditional Chinese medicine (TCM) Danshen (*Salvia miltiorrhiza*), and has been found to attenuate the proliferation of bladder cancer (BCa) cells (The IC_{50} were: 5637, 2.6 µg/mL; BFTC, 2 µg/mL; T24, 2.7 µg/mL, respectively.). However, the mechanism of the effect of Tan-IIA on migration inhibition of BCa cells remains unclear. This study investigates the anti-metastatic effect of Tan-IIA in human BCa cells and clarifies its molecular mechanism. Three human BCa cell lines, 5637, BFTC and T24, were used for subsequent experiments. Cell migration and invasion were evaluated by transwell assays. Real-time RT-PCR and western blotting were performed to detect epithelial-mesenchymal transition (EMT)-related gene expression. The enzymatic activity of matrix metalloproteinases (MMP) was evaluated by zymography assay. Tan-IIA inhibited the migration and invasion of human BCa cells. Tan-IIA suppressed both the protein expression and enzymatic activity of MMP-9/-2 in human BCa cells. Tan-IIA up-regulated the epithelial marker E-cadherin and down-regulated mesenchymal markers such as N-cadherin and Vimentin, along with transcription regulators such as Snail and Slug in BCa cells in a time- and dose-dependent manner. Mechanism dissection revealed that Tan-IIA-inhibited BCa cell invasion could function via suppressed chemokine (C-C motif) ligand 2 (CCL2) expression, which could be reversed by the addition of CCL2 recombinant protein. Furthermore, Tan-IIA could inhibit the phosphorylation of the signal transducer and activator of transcription 3 (STAT3) (Tyr705), which cannot be restored by the CCL2 recombinant protein addition. These data implicated that Tan-IIA might suppress EMT on BCa cells through STAT3-CCL2 signaling inhibition. Tan-IIA inhibits EMT of BCa cells via modulation of STAT3-CCL2 signaling. Our findings suggest that Tan-IIA can serve as a potential anti-metastatic agent in BCa therapy.

Keywords: bladder cancer; chemokine (C-C motif) ligand 2; epithelial-mesenchymal transition; signal transducer and activator of transcription 3; tanshinone IIA

1. Introduction

Bladder cancer (BCa) is one of the most prevalent types of cancer and is the leading cause of death among patients with urinary tract disease [1]. In 2016, the United States alone recorded more than 76,000 new cases of BCa and 16,000 deaths [2]. Most BCa cases are diagnosed as non-muscle invasive tumors; however, 50–70% of these tumors recur frequently and approximately 15% eventually develop into muscle-invasive or metastatic BCa [3,4]. Current treatment methods including radical cystectomy and systemic chemotherapy are effective in some muscle-invasive BCa patients, but 95% of metastatic BCa patients die within 5-years diagnosis, indicating the need for new therapeutic strategies [5].

Tan-IIA ($C_{19}H_{18}O_3$) is one of the major lipophilic compounds extracted from the root of a traditional Chinese medicine, Danshen (*Salvia miltiorrhiza*) [6,7], and has been used for the treatment of cardiovascular disease via its anti-oxidant and anti-inflammatory activity [8,9]. In addition, Tan-IIA has been found to exert antitumor activity in various types of cancer including osteosarcoma [10], gastric [11], lung [12], esophageal [13], and prostate cancers [14]. The antitumor activity of Tan-IIA mainly occurs through proliferation inhibition, apoptosis induction, and metastasis inhibition [15–18]. For instance, Tan-IIA increased CCAAT/enhancer-binding protein homologous protein (CHOP) and caspase-4 expression, and induced apoptosis of human esophageal Ec-109 cells via the endoplasmic reticulum (ER) stress pathway [19]. Tan-IIA induced cytochrome c-mediated caspase cascade apoptosis in A549 human lung cancer cells via the JNK pathway [20]. Tan-IIA caused apoptosis in human oral cancer KB cells through a mitochondria-dependent pathway [21]. However, Tan-IIA did not show significant cytotoxicity on human normal prostate epithelial cells (PrEC) and normal mammary epithelial cells (HMEC) at the concentrations high as 50 µM [22,23]. Also, the toxicity in normal tissues was not observed in Tan-IIA treated mice [24]. In our previous study, Tan-IIA was found to induce mitochondria-dependent apoptosis and suppress migration in BCa cells [25]. However, the mechanism by which Tan-IIA inhibits the migration and invasion of BCa cells remains undetermined.

Previous reports found a correlation of urinary CCL2 levels with tumor stage, grade and metastasis in patients with BCa [26,27], and patients with stages T2–T4 BCa were found to have a higher mean CCL2 concentration in their urine as compared to those with T1 stage tumors [27]. Previous studies also showed that CCL2 can regulate tumor progression and metastasis by altering the tumor microenvironment [28–30]. CCL2 induced epithelial mesenchymal transition (EMT) in order to promote tumor metastasis in various cancer types [31–33]. Down-regulation of CCL2 expression by inhibiting phosphorylation of STAT3 led to the suppression of metastasis in breast and lung cancer [34]. STAT3 signaling is an important pathway which is frequently activated in many tumors including BCa [35,36]. The transcriptional activity of STAT3 is required for the phosphorylation at the tyrosine residue 705 (Tyr705) and has been demonstrated to be critical for BCa cell growth and survival [36,37]. In addition, activation of STAT3 promoted migration and invasion of BCa cells [38]. Thus, we seek to elucidate the role of STAT3-CCL2 signaling in Tan-IIA-induced EMT inhibition in BCa cells.

The results of the present study demonstrate that Tan-IIA inhibited the migration and invasion of human BCa cells. Tan-IIA inhibited EMT in BCa cells via the suppression of CCL2 expression which cannot be reversed by addition of CCL2 recombinant protein. In addition, Tan-IIA suppressed the phosphorylation of STAT3 (Tyr705), which cannot be restored by addition of CCL2 recombinant protein. Our data suggests that Tan-IIA might inhibit EMT in BCa cells through the STAT3-CCL2 signaling inhibition.

2. Results

2.1. Tan-IIA Inhibits the Migration and Invasion of Human BCa Cells

Human BCa cells were treated with 4 µg/mL Tan-IIA for 24 h and then subjected to migration (24 h) and invasion (48 h) assay (Figure 1A). In the migration assay, Tan-IIA decreased the number of migrating cells to 25.6 ± 4.7% (5637), 32 ± 2.9% (BFTC), and 70.5 ± 9.7% (T24) as compared to the control group. In the invasion assay, Tan-IIA decreased the number of migrating cells to $11 \pm 2.9\%$ (5637), $51.8 \pm 4.4\%$ (BFTC), and $22.8 \pm 9.8\%$ (T24) as compared to the control group.

A

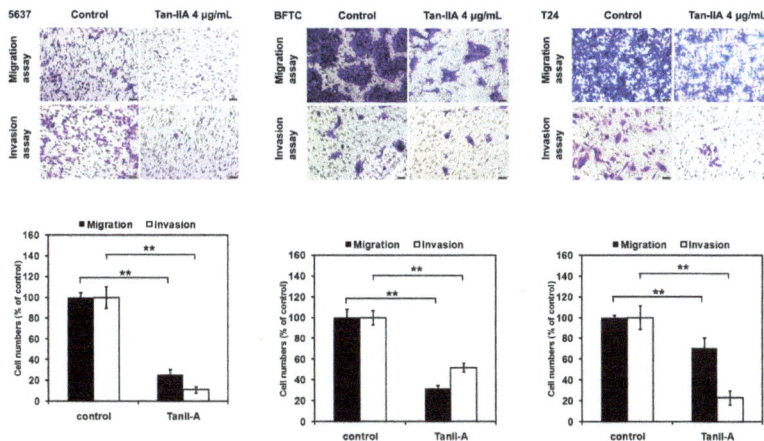

B

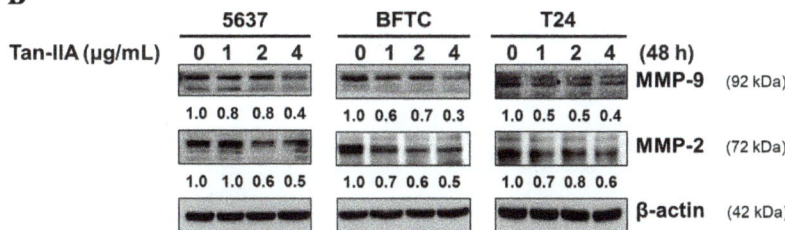

C

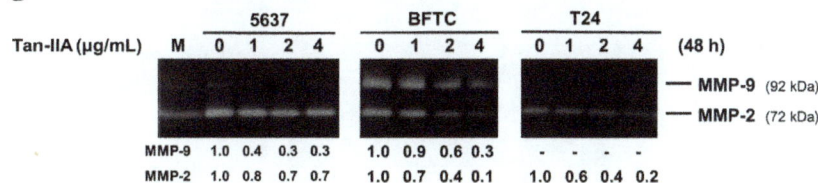

Figure 1. Tan-IIA inhibited migratory and invasive ability in human BCa cells. (**A**) Human BCa cells were treated with 0.2% DMSO as a vehicle control or 4 µg/mL Tan-IIA for 24 h and then seeded onto the transwell hanging insert for migration (24 h) and invasion (48 h) assays. Images were captured using an inverted microscope with 200× magnification; Scale bar: 50 µm. The migration and invasion of BCa cells were quantified by counting the stained cells that migrated into the underside of the hanging insert membrane; (**B**) human BCa cells were treated with different concentrations of Tan-IIA (1, 2 and 4 µg/mL) for 48 h. The protein of total cell lysates were then used to detect MMP-9/-2 protein expression using western blot, and the (**C**) supernatant was used to detect the enzymatic activity using zymography analysis. M: marker. Data are presented as means $\pm$ S.D. from three different experiments. ** $p < 0.01$ versus vehicle.

Western blot results indicated Tan-IIA down-regulated the protein expression of MMP-9/-2 in a dose-dependent manner (Figure 1B). Zymography analysis also showed that Tan-IIA attenuated the enzymatic activity of MMP-9/-2 in a dose-dependent manner (Figure 1C). Taken together, these results suggested that Tan-IIA might be an effective inhibitor of cell migration and invasion of BCa cells.

2.2. Tan-IIA Inhibits EMT in Human BCa Cells

EMT is a crucial step for the invasion and metastasis of BCa cells. We first show that Tan-IIA could inhibit cellular migration and invasion in BCa cells, and this is accompanied by the up-regulation of epithelial marker E-cadherin, the down-regulation of mesenchymal markers N-cadherin and Vimentin, and the down-regulation of transcription factor Snail and Slug, at both the mRNA and protein level as evidenced by quantitative RT-PCR (qRT-PCR) (Figure 2A) and western blot (Figure 2B,C).

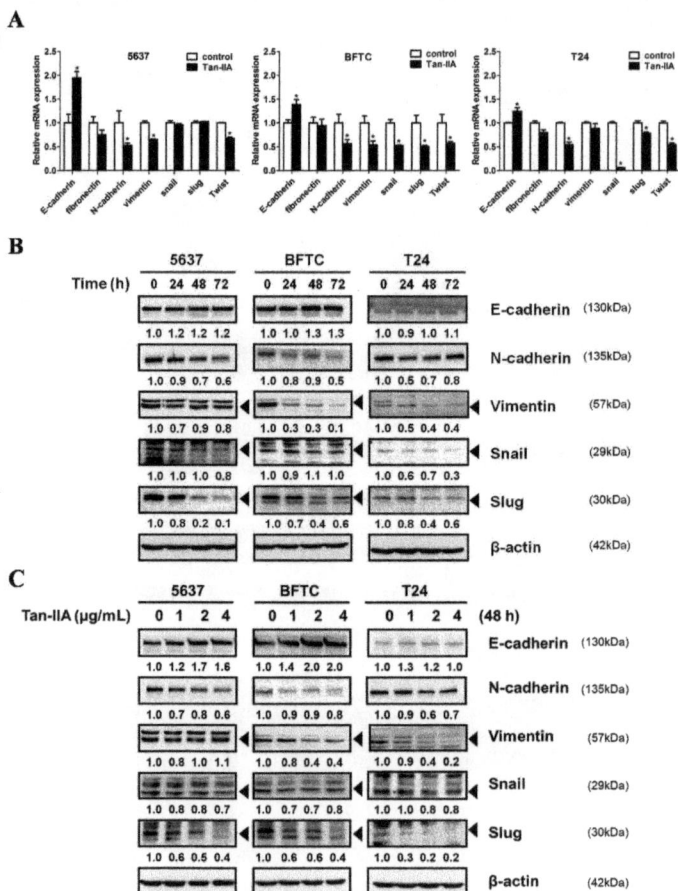

Figure 2. Tan-IIA inhibited EMT on human BCa cells. (**A**) Human BCa cells were treated with 4 µg/mL Tan-IIA for 24 h. The expression of EMT-related genes was detected by qRT-PCR analysis; (**B**) human BCa cells were treated with 4 µg/mL Tan-IIA for 24 to 72 h. The expressions of EMT-related genes were detected by western blot. (**C**) Human BCa cells were treated with increasing concentrations of Tan-IIA (1, 2 and 4 µg/mL) for 48 h. The expressions of EMT-related genes were detected by western blot. Data are presented as means ± S.D. from three different experiments. * $p < 0.05$ versus vehicle.

2.3. Tan-IIA Inhibits EMT via Down-Regulated CCL2 Expression in Human BCa Cells

Previous reports suggested that high levels of CCL2 expression play a key role in BCa progression and metastasis in vitro and in vivo [27,32,39]. Thus, we analyzed the CCL2 expression in the culture medium of human BCa cells treated with or without Tan-IIA. As shown in Figure 3A, Tan-IIA inhibited the CCL2 expression in all BCa cell lines detected by PCR and qRT-PCR. Furthermore, ELISA tests confirmed that the protein level of CCL2 secreted by BCa cells was inhibited by Tan-IIA treatment in a dose-dependent manner (Figure 3B). These results showed that Tan-IIA down-regulated CCL2 expression in BCa cells.

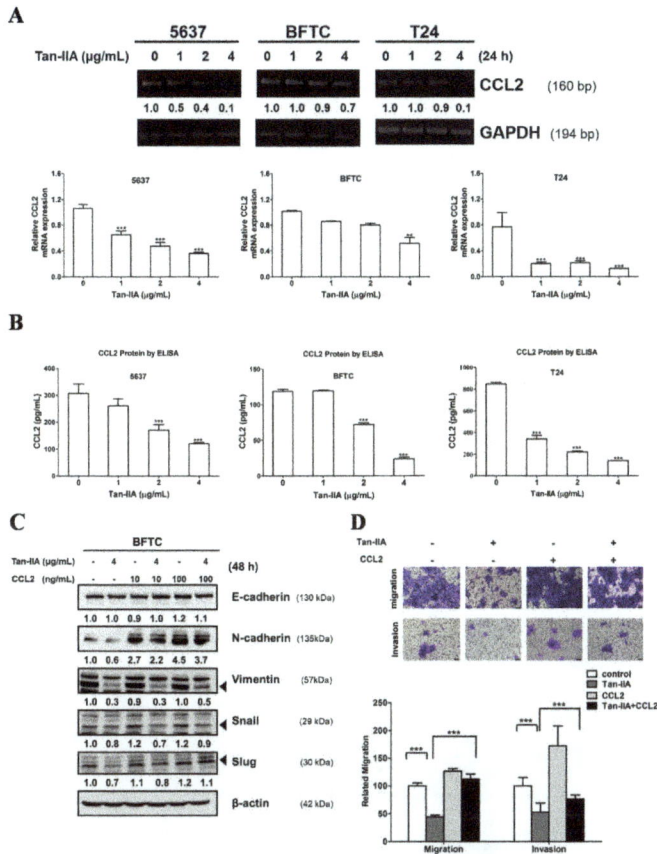

Figure 3. Tan-IIA inhibited the CCL2 expression and reversed the EMT in human BCa cells. (**A**) Human BCa cells were treated with increasing concentrations of Tan-IIA for 24 h. The expression of CCL2 was detected by PCR and qRT-PCR; (**B**) Human BCa cells were treated with increasing concentrations of Tan-IIA for 48 h. The supernatant was collected for CCL2 protein detection using ELISA assay; (**C**) BFTC cells were treated with or without 4 μg/mL Tan-IIA in the presence or absence of CCL2 recombinant protein for 48 h. The EMT-related gene expression was detected by western blot; (**D**) BFTC cells were treated with or without 4 μg/mL Tan-IIA in the presence or absence of 100 ng/mL human CCL2 recombinant protein for 24 h, followed by migration (24 h) or invasion (48 h) assays and analyzed as previous described. Data are presented as means ± S.D. from three different experiments. *** $p < 0.001$ versus vehicle.

To investigate the mechanism by which Tan-IIA inhibits CCL2 resulting in metastatic inhibition, BFTC cells were treated with or without human CCL2 recombinant protein (10 or 100 ng/mL) in the presence or absence of 4 μg/mL Tan-IIA for 48 h to examine the EMT-related genes expression. As shown in Figure 3C, treatment with CCL2 recombinant protein increased the expression of mesenchymal marker N-cadherin and Vimentin, along with transcription factor Snail and Slug, which were down-regulated by Tan-IIA treatment. In addition, treatment with CCL2 recombinant protein attenuated the inhibitory effect on migration and invasion induced by Tan-IIA treatment (Figure 3D). Together, these findings indicate that Tan-IIA inhibited EMT in BCa cells via the down-regulation of CCL2.

2.4. Tan-IIA Inhibits STAT3-CCL2 Signaling in Human BCa Cells

Recent studies indicated that CCL2 signaling plays a pivotal role in regulating STAT3 activation and EMT [40], and the inhibition of STAT3 signaling may reduce the invasiveness of BCa [41]. We further examined whether Tan-IIA could inhibit the activation of STAT3 on BCa cells. Human BCa cells were treated with Tan-IIA for indicated time points and p-STAT3 (Tyr705) was analyzed by western blot. As shown in Figure 4A,B, Tan-IIA inhibited the activation of STAT3 by decreasing the phosphorylation of STAT3 at Tyr705 in all BCa cell lines in a time- and dose-dependent manner. To elucidate the mechanism by which Tan-IIA inhibits CCL2 through regulating STAT3, BFTC cells were transfected with the STAT3 siRNA and the expression of STAT3 and CCL2 were examined by western blot. Silencing the expression of STAT3 leads to the inhibition of CCL2 expression (Figure 4C). However, treatment with human CCL2 recombinant protein (10 or 100 ng/mL) cannot restore the regulation of STAT3 via phosphorylation of Tyr705, and this was inhibited by Tan-IIA treatment. These results suggested that Tan-IIA down-regulated the CCL2 expression via inhibition of the STAT3 pathway in human BCa cells.

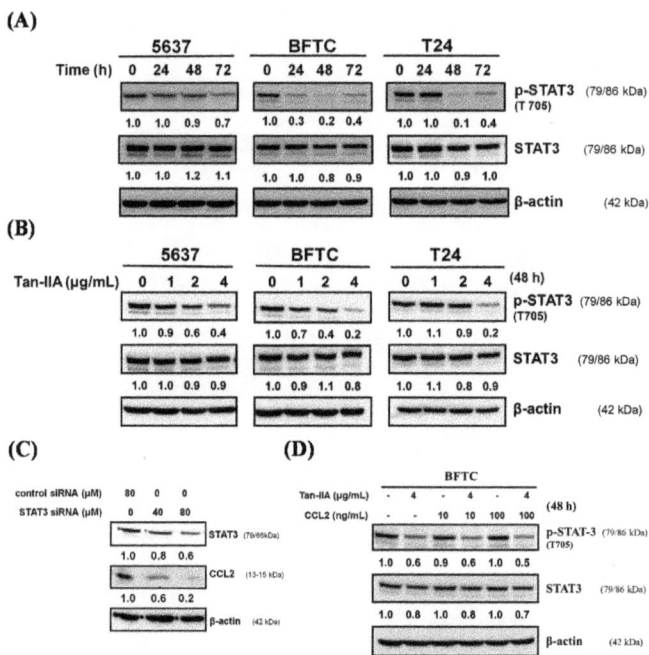

Figure 4. Tan-IIA inhibited STAT3-CCL2 signaling in human BCa cells. (**A**) Human BCa cells were treated with 4 μg/mL Tan-IIA for indicated time points, and the expression of phospho-STAT3 (T705) was detected by western blot; (**B**) human BCa cells were treated with increasing concentrations of Tan-IIA for 48 h, the expression of phospho-STAT3 (T705) were detected by western blot; (**C**) BFTC cells were transfected with control or STAT3 siRNA for 24 h, and the expression of STAT3 and CCL2 was detected by western blot; (**D**) BFTC cells were treated with or without 4 μg/mL Tan-IIA in the presence or absence of human CCL2 recombinant protein for 48 h. The expression of phospho-STAT3 (T705) and STAT3 was detected by western blot.

3. Discussion

Our previous study reported that Tan-IIA could inhibit the proliferation and migration of human BCa cells [25], but the underlying mechanism of Tan-IIA attenuating the migration and invasion of BCa cells remains unclear. EMT is a process by which epithelial cells gradually transform into mesenchymal-like cells to promote the migration and invasiveness of cancer cells [42]. Our results showed that Tan-IIA treatment could inhibit the process of EMT as evidenced by increased level of the epithelial marker E-cadherin and decreased level of mesenchymal markers (N-cadherin and Vimentin). Activation of MMP proteins leads to cell migration and penetration to the basement membrane, playing an important role in EMT processes [43]. In previous studies, Tan-IIA decreased migration or invasion through inhibiting MMP-9/-2 secretion in gastric cancer and osteosarcoma [11,18]. Similar results observed in our study showed that Tan-IIA suppressed both the protein expression and enzymatic activity of MMP-9/-2 on human BCa cells (Figure 1B). Together, these findings suggest that Tan-IIA inhibits EMT in human BCa cells.

Several reports have demonstrated the importance of CCL2 and EMT signals in BCa progression. Chiu et al. reported that blocking the CCL2/CCR2 pathway could decrease the migration and invasion of BCa cells [39]. Additional reports show that CCL2 signals promote EMT in various tumors including BCa [32,40,44,45]. The present study provides evidence that Tan-IIA decreased CCL2 expression in a dose-dependent manner by qRT-PCR and ELISA analysis (Figure 3). The addition of CCL2 recombinant protein resulted in a partial reversal of EMT markers, and attenuated the Tan-IIA-induced migration and invasion inhibition in BCa cells. Our results show that Tan-IIA inhibits the EMT in BCa cells via the suppression of CCL2 expression.

Additional reported data suggested that CCL2 induced EMT through the activation of STAT3 signals [33,40] and inhibited STAT3 signaling to reduce the invasiveness of tumor cells [41,46]. Our data showed that Tan-IIA could inhibit the p-STAT3 (Tyr705) in a time- and dose-dependent manner. Besides, inhibition of STAT3 expression by STAT3 siRNA transfection attenuated the expression of CCL2. The phosphorylation of STAT3, inhibited by Tan-IIA, cannot be restored by CCL2 recombinant protein addition. These data suggested that Tan-IIA inhibits EMT of human BCa cells via modulation of STAT3-CCL2 signaling (Figure 5). Several effects of Tan-IIA on human cancer were also integrated to get a better view of possible anti-cancerogenic effects of Tan-IIA [47–50]. In addition, since the results from this study were based on in vitro assays of human BCa cells, the in vivo experiments are necessary for future study.

EMT is orchestrated by several signaling pathways, including JAK/STAT3 and TGF-β/Smad signaling. Recent studies have demonstrated that TGF-β-mediated cancer metastasis was associated with the activation of STAT3 pathway in colorectal and lung cancer [51,52]. STAT3 activation can increase smad7 expression and form an inhibitory complex with smad3 which eventually suppress EMT [53]. Recent study elucidated the mechanisms behind the tumoricidal activity of TCM clinical prescription Jianpi Huayu Decoction (JHD) in Hepatocellular carcinoma (HCC) treatment. Their results indicated that Tan-IIA might be the one of crucial components of the JHD that targets on the TGF-β/Smad3 pathway and inhibits EMT [50]. Taken together, the targeted blockade of the STAT3/smad3 axis in tumor cells may be an effective therapeutic strategy against tumor metastatic progression and worth for further investigation.

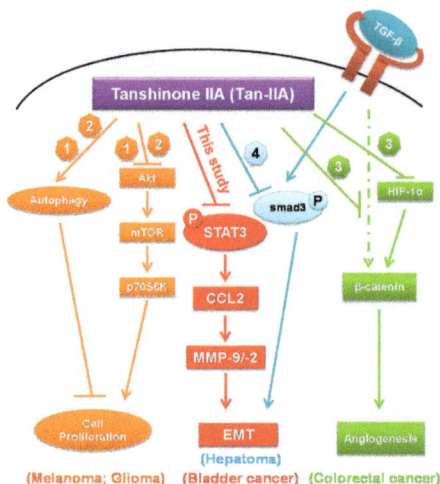

Figure 5. Schematic representation the anti-cancerogenic roles of Tan-IIA. CCL2: Chemokine (C-C motif) ligand 2; EMT: Epithelial-Mesenchymal Transition; HIF-1α: Hypoxia-inducible factor-1α; MMP: Matrix MetalloProteinases; mTOR: mammalian target of rapamycin; P: phosphorylation; p70S6K: p70 ribosomal protein S6 kinase; STAT3: signal transducer and activator of transcription 3; Tan-IIA: Tanshinone IIA; TGF-β: transforming growth factor β. ↓: stimulatory modification; ⊥: inhibitory modification; Dashed arrow: putative stimulatory modification [47–50].

4. Materials and Methods

4.1. Chemicals and Antibodies

Tanshinone IIA ($C_{19}H_{18}O_3$, >97% HPLC), Dimethyl sulfoxide (DMSO), [3-(4,5-dimethyl thizol-2-yl)-2,5-diphenyl tetrazolium bromide] (MTT), Tween-20, methanol, and horseradish peroxidase-conjugated secondary antibodies were purchased from Sigma Chemical Co. (St. Louis, MO, USA). The antibodies against p-STAT3 (Tyr705), STAT3, E-cadherin, N-cadherin, Vimentin, Slug, Snail, MMP-2, MMP-9 and β-actin were all purchased from Cell Signaling Technology, Inc., (Danvers, MA, USA). The human CCL2 recombinant protein was purchased from Santa Cruz Biotechnology, Inc. (Dallas, TX, USA). Polyvinyldenefluoride (PVDF) membranes, BSA protein assay kit and western blot chemiluminescence reagent were purchased from Amersham Biosciences (Arlington Heights, IL, USA).

4.2. Cell Culture

The human BCa cell lines 5637 (grade II carcinoma), BFTC (BFTC 905, papillary transitional cell carcinoma), and T24 (transitional cell carcinoma) were purchased from BCRC (Bioresource Collection and Research Center, Hsinchu, Taiwan). Cells were cultured in appropriate medium supplemented with 10% FBS, 100 U/mL penicillin and 100 U/mL streptomycin (all from Invitrogen, Carlsbad, CA, USA) at 37 °C in a humidified atmosphere with 5% CO_2.

4.3. Western Blot Analysis

Five hundred thousand cells per 6-cm plate were lysed with 200 μL M-PER mammalian protein extraction reagent containing protease inhibitor cocktail (Thermo Scientific, Rockford, IL, USA) and centrifuged at 13,000× *g* at 4 °C for 10 min. The protein concentration in the supernatants was quantified using a BSA Protein Assay Kit. Electrophoresis was performed on a NuPAGE Bis-Tris Electrophoresis System using 20 μg of reduced protein extract per lane. Resolved proteins were transferred to PVDF membranes, blocked with 5% skim milk for 1 h at room temperature, finally probed with the specific primary antibodies at 4 °C overnight. After the PVDF membrane was washed three times with TBS/0.2% Tween-20 at room temperature, it was incubated with appropriate secondary antibody labeled with horseradish peroxidase (Sigma Chemical, St. Louis, MO, USA) for 1 h at room temperature. All resolved proteins bands were detected using Western Lightning™ Chemiluminescence Reagent Plus (Amersham Biosciences, Arlington Heights, IL, USA).

4.4. Cell Migration and Invasion Assay

The trans-well assay was performed using Hanging inserts (Millipore Co., Billerica, MA, USA) with 8 μm polycarbonate membrane in a 24-well plate. Cells were seeded in 6 well plates and treated without or with 4 μg/mL Tan-IIA with or without CCL2 for 24 h. Cells were then detached and seeded (5×10^4) to the upper chamber of the transwell plates. Upper chambers were filled with serum free medium and lower chambers were filled with cultured medium containing 10% FBS as a chemo-attractant. Incubation was carried out at 37 °C for the indicated 24 h. The hanging inserts were washed with PBS, and cells on the upper filter surface were wiped away with a cotton swab. The inserts were subsequently fixed with 10% formalin for 10 min at room temperature, stained with 0.2% *w/v* crystal violet, washed with PBS, the remaining cells were counted on the opposite site of the filter under a light microscope operating at 200× magnification. The migration cell numbers of control group were considered as 100%. For the invasion assay, a Matrigel basement membrane matrix (BD Biosciences, San Jose, CA, USA) was coated to the upper side of the hanging inserts at a concentration of 2 mg/mL. Cells were seeded onto the coated hanging inserts and followed by migration assay protocol.

4.5. RNA Extraction and Real-Time RT-PCR

Total RNA was extracted from cell lines using RNeasy Mini Kit® (Qiagen, Valencia, CA, USA) and reverse transcribed at 37 °C for 60 min with Omniscript RT Kit® (Qiagen) according to the manufacturer's instructions. Real-time RT-PCR analysis was performed in triplicate in a Step One Plus Real-Time PCR system (Applied Biosystems, Foster City, CA, USA) with Power SYBR® Green PCR Master Mix (Applied Biosystems) in a final volume of 20 μL/reaction. Threshold cycle (C_t) value of each tested gene was normalized to the C_t value of the GAPDH control from the same RNA preparation. The ratio of transcription of each gene was calculated as $2^{-(\Delta Ct)}$, where ΔC_t is the difference C_t(test gene)$-C_t$(GAPDH). Real-time RT-PCR primer sequences used in this study are listed in Table 1.

Table 1. The gene-specific primers used in this study.

Gene	Primers
CCL2	sense: 5'-GATCTCAGTGCAGAGGCTCG-3' antisense: 5'-TGCTTGTCCAGGTGGTCCAT-3'
E-cadherin	sense: 5'-ACGTCGTAATCACCACACTGA-3' antisense: 5'-TTCGTCACTGCTACGTGTAGAA-3'
N-cadherin	sense: 5'-ACAGTGGCCACCTACAAAGG-3' antisense: 5'-CCGAGATGGGGTTGATAATG-3'
Fibronectin	sense: 5'-CCCACCGTCTCAACATGCTTAG-3' antisense: 5'-CTCGGCTTCCTCCATAACAAGTAC-3'
Vimentin	sense: 5'-CTTCGCCAACTACATCGACA-3' antisense: 5'-GCTTCAACGGCAAAGTTCTC-3'
Snail	sense: 5'-TCGTCCTTCTCCTCTACTTC-3' antisense: 5'-TTCCTTGTTGCAGTATTTGC-3'
Slug	sense: 5'-TGTTGCAGTGAGGGCAAGAA-3' antisense: 5'-GACCCTGGTTGCTTCAAGGA-3'
GAPDH	sense: 5'-CCATGGAGAAGGCTGGGG-3' antisense: 5'-CAAAGTTGTCATGGATGACC-3'

4.6. Enzyme-Linked Immunosorbent Assay (ELISA)

Human MCP-1/CCL2 ELISA kit was purchased from R&D Systems. BCa cells were cultured in serum-free medium with or without Tan-IIA for 72 h. The medium were collected (400 µL/sample in 96-well) for ELISA assay according to manufacturer's instructions.

4.7. Gelatin Zymography

The BCa cells were cultured in serum-free medium containing Tan-IIA (0, 1, 2, 4 µg/mL) for 48 h and the supernatant was collected. The supernatant was mixed with non-reducing SDS gel sample buffer. Electrophoresis was carried out using 10% native polyacrylamide gel containing 0.1% gelatin (Sigma, St. Louis, MO, USA) on a NuPAGE Bis-Tris Electrophoresis System. After electrophoresis, the gels were washed in wash buffer containing 2.5% Triton X-100 at room temperature, and then incubated with the reaction buffer containing 1 M $CaCl_2$, 2% NaN_3, 1 M Tris-HCl (pH 8.0) at 37 °C overnight. Gels were stained by Coomassie Brilliant Blue R-250 solution and gelatinolytic activity was shown as clear areas in the gel.

4.8. Small Interfering RNA (siRNA) Transfection

STAT3 siRNA (#6582) was purchased from Cell Signaling Technology, Inc., (Danvers, MA, USA). Non-targeting siRNA (ON-TARGET plus non-targeting pool) were purchased from Dharmacon RNAi Technologies (Lafayette, CO, USA). Non-targeting control sequences were not provided. BFTC cells at 50–60% confluence were transfected with siRNA (40 or 80 nM) using the DharmaFECT 4 transfection reagents (GE Healthcare Dharmacon, Lafayette, CO, USA) according to the manufacturer's protocol. Cells were cultured for 24 h, and then treated with Tan-IIA or vehicle for an additional 48 h. Proteins were then isolated for western blotting.

4.9. Statistical Analysis

All data were shown as mean ± S.D. Statistical differences were analyzed using the Student's *t*-test for normally distributed values.

5. Conclusions

In conclusion, our study demonstrated that Tan-IIA inhibits EMT in human BCa cells. The anti-metastatic effects of Tan-IIA in human BCa cells were shown by migration and invasion assay. Tan-IIA is shown to regulate EMT-related gene expression via the suppression of CCL2. The inhibition of CCL2 might be linked to the phosphorylation inhibition at Tyr705 of STAT3 by Tan-IIA. Tan-IIA has been shown to inhibit EMT in human BCa cells, and the mechanism involved was mediated through the modulation of STAT3-CCL2 signaling. Thus, our findings suggest a novel role of Tan-IIA in controlling BCa, suggesting that Tan-IIA might be a potential option for treating BCa metastasis.

Acknowledgments: This work was supported by grants from the Taichung Tzu Chi Hospital, Buddhist Tzu Chi Medical Foundation, Taichung, Taiwan (TTCRD104-10, TTCRD104-19, TTCRD105-17, TTCRD105-20). The funders had no role in study design, data collection and analysis, decision to publish, or preparation of the manuscript.

Author Contributions: Sung-Ying Huang and Sheng-Chun Chiu conceived and designed the experiments; Sung-Ying Huang, Sheng-Chun Chiu and Shu-Fang Chang performed the experiments; Sheng-Chun Chiu and Shu-Fang Chang analyzed the data; Sung-Ying Huang, Sheng-Chun Chiu and Kuan-Fu Liao contributed reagents/materials/analysis tools; Sung-Ying Huang, Sheng-Chun Chiu, Shu-Fang Chang and Kuan-Fu Liao wrote the paper.

Conflicts of Interest: The authors declare no conflict interests.

Int. J. Mol. Sci. **2017**, *18*, 1616

Abbreviations

CCL2	Chemokine (C-C motif) ligand 2
EMT	Epithelial-mesenchymal transition
MMP	Matrix metalloproteinases
STAT3	Signal transducer and activator of transcription 3
Tan-IIA	Tanshinone IIA

References

1. Siegel, R.L.; Miller, K.D.; Jemal, A. Cancer statistics, 2016. *CA Cancer J. Clin.* **2016**, *66*, 7–30. [CrossRef] [PubMed]
2. Antoni, S.; Ferlay, J.; Soerjomataram, I.; Znaor, A.; Jemal, A.; Bray, F. Bladder cancer incidence and mortality: A global overview and recent trends. *Eur. Urol.* **2017**, *71*, 96–108. [CrossRef] [PubMed]
3. Jemal, A.; Siegel, R.; Ward, E.; Hao, Y.; Xu, J.; Murray, T.; Thun, M.J. Cancer statistics, 2008. *CA Cancer J. Clin.* **2008**, *58*, 71–96. [CrossRef] [PubMed]
4. Lutzeyer, W.; Rubben, H.; Dahm, H. Prognostic parameters in superficial bladder cancer: An analysis of 315 cases. *J. Urol.* **1982**, *127*, 250–252. [CrossRef]
5. Wu, X.R. Urothelial tumorigenesis: a tale of divergent pathways. *Nat. Rev. Cancer* **2005**, *5*, 713–725. [CrossRef] [PubMed]
6. Che, A.J.; Zhang, J.Y.; Li, C.H.; Chen, X.F.; Hu, Z.D.; Chen, X.G. Separation and determination of active components in Radix Salviae miltiorrhizae and its medicinal preparations by nonaqueous capillary electrophoresis. *J. Sep. Sci.* **2004**, *27*, 569–575. [PubMed]
7. Zhou, L.; Zuo, Z.; Chow, M.S. Danshen: An overview of its chemistry, pharmacology, pharmacokinetics, and clinical use. *J. Clin. Pharmacol.* **2005**, *45*, 1345–1359. [CrossRef] [PubMed]
8. Wei, B.; You, M.G.; Ling, J.J.; Wei, L.L.; Wang, K.; Li, W.W.; Chen, T.; Du, Q.M.; Ji, H. Regulation of antioxidant system, lipids and fatty acid β-oxidation contributes to the cardioprotective effect of sodium tanshinone IIA sulphonate in isoproterenol-induced myocardial infarction in rats. *Atherosclerosis* **2013**, *230*, 148–156. [CrossRef] [PubMed]
9. Fan, G.; Jiang, X.; Wu, X.; Fordjour, P.A.; Miao, L.; Zhang, H.; Zhu, Y.; Gao, X. Anti-Inflammatory Activity of Tanshinone IIA in LPS-Stimulated RAW264.7 Macrophages via miRNAs and TLR4-NF-κB Pathway. *Inflammation* **2016**, *39*, 375–384. [CrossRef] [PubMed]
10. Huang, S.T.; Huang, C.C.; Huang, W.L.; Lin, T.K.; Liao, P.L.; Wang, P.W.; Liou, C.W.; Chuang, J.H. Tanshinone IIA induces intrinsic apoptosis in osteosarcoma cells both in vivo and in vitro associated with mitochondrial dysfunction. *Sci. Rep.* **2017**, *7*, 40382. [CrossRef] [PubMed]
11. Su, C.C. Tanshinone IIA decreases the migratory ability of AGS cells by decreasing the protein expression of matrix metalloproteinases, nuclear factor κB-p65 and cyclooxygenase-2. *Mol. Med. Rep.* **2016**, *13*, 1263–1268. [PubMed]
12. Xie, J.; Liu, J.; Liu, H.; Liang, S.; Lin, M.; Gu, Y.; Liu, T.; Wang, D.; Ge, H.; Mo, S.L. The antitumor effect of tanshinone IIA on anti-proliferation and decreasing VEGF/VEGFR2 expression on the human non-small cell lung cancer A549 cell line. *Acta Pharm. Sin. B* **2015**, *5*, 554–563. [CrossRef] [PubMed]
13. Wang, J.F.; Feng, J.G.; Han, J.; Zhang, B.B.; Mao, W.M. The molecular mechanisms of Tanshinone IIA on the apoptosis and arrest of human esophageal carcinoma cells. *BioMed Res. Int.* **2014**, *2014*. [CrossRef] [PubMed]
14. Chiu, S.C.; Huang, S.Y.; Chen, S.P.; Su, C.C.; Chiu, T.L.; Pang, C.Y. Tanshinone IIA inhibits human prostate cancer cells growth by induction of endoplasmic reticulum stress in vitro and in vivo. *Prostate Cancer Prostatic Dis.* **2013**, *16*, 315–322. [CrossRef] [PubMed]
15. Tsai, M.Y.; Yang, R.C.; Wu, H.T.; Pang, J.H.; Huang, S.T. Anti-angiogenic effect of Tanshinone IIA involves inhibition of matrix invasion and modification of MMP-2/TIMP-2 secretion in vascular endothelial cells. *Cancer Lett.* **2011**, *310*, 198–206. [CrossRef] [PubMed]
16. Wu, W.Y.; Yan, H.; Wang, X.B.; Gui, Y.Z.; Gao, F.; Tang, X.L.; Qin, Y.L.; Su, M.; Chen, T.; Wang, Y.P. Sodium tanshinone IIA silate inhibits high glucose-induced vascular smooth muscle cell proliferation and migration through activation of AMP-activated protein kinase. *PLoS ONE* **2014**, *9*, e94957. [CrossRef] [PubMed]

17. Yun, S.M.; Jung, J.H.; Jeong, S.J.; Sohn, E.J.; Kim, B.; Kim, S.H. Tanshinone IIA induces autophagic cell death via activation of AMPK and ERK and inhibition of mTOR and p70 S6K in KBM-5 leukemia cells. *Phytother. Res.* **2014**, *28*, 458–464. [CrossRef] [PubMed]

18. Zhang, Y.; Wei, R.X.; Zhu, X.B.; Cai, L.; Jin, W.; Hu, H. Tanshinone IIA induces apoptosis and inhibits the proliferation, migration, and invasion of the osteosarcoma MG-63 cell line in vitro. *Anticancer Drugs* **2012**, *23*, 212–219. [CrossRef] [PubMed]

19. Zhu, Y.Q.; Wang, B.Y.; Wu, F.; An, Y.K.; Zhou, X.Q. Influence of tanshinone IIA on the apoptosis of human esophageal Ec-109 cells. *Nat. Prod. Commun.* **2016**, *11*, 17–19. [PubMed]

20. Zhang, J.; Wang, J.; Jiang, J.Y.; Liu, S.D.; Fu, K.; Liu, H.Y. Tanshinone IIA induces cytochrome c-mediated caspase cascade apoptosis in A549 human lung cancer cells via the JNK pathway. *Int. J. Oncol.* **2014**, *45*, 683–690. [PubMed]

21. Tseng, P.Y.; Lu, W.C.; Hsieh, M.J.; Chien, S.Y.; Chen, M.K. Tanshinone IIA induces apoptosis in human oral cancer KB cells through a mitochondria-dependent pathway. *BioMed Res. Int.* **2014**, *2014*, 540516. [CrossRef] [PubMed]

22. Gong, Y.; Li, Y.; Lu, Y.; Li, L.; Abdolmaleky, H.; Blackburn, G.L.; Zhou, J.R. Bioactive tanshinones in Salvia miltiorrhiza inhibit the growth of prostate cancer cells in vitro and in mice. *Int. J. Cancer* **2011**, *129*, 1042–1052. [CrossRef] [PubMed]

23. Gong, Y.; Li, Y.; Abdolmaleky, H.M.; Li, L.; Zhou, J.R. Tanshinones inhibit the growth of breast cancer cells through epigenetic modification of aurora a expression and function. *PLoS ONE* **2012**, *7*, e33656. [CrossRef] [PubMed]

24. Liu, F.; Yu, G.; Wang, G.; Liu, H.; Wu, X.; Wang, Q.; Liu, M.; Liao, K.; Wu, M.; Cheng, X.; et al. An NQO1-initiated and p53-independent apoptotic pathway determines the anti-tumor effect of tanshinone IIA against non-small cell lung cancer. *PLoS ONE* **2012**, *7*, e42138. [CrossRef] [PubMed]

25. Chiu, S.C.; Huang, S.Y.; Chang, S.F.; Chen, S.P.; Chen, C.C.; Lin, T.H.; Liu, H.H.; Tsai, T.H.; Lee, S.S.; Pang, C.Y.; et al. Potential therapeutic roles of tanshinone IIA in human bladder cancer cells. *Int. J. Mol. Sci.* **2014**, *15*, 15622–15637. [CrossRef] [PubMed]

26. Vazquez-Lavista, L.G.; Lima, G.; Gabilondo, F.; Llorente, L. Genetic association of monocyte chemoattractant protein 1 (MCP-1)-2518 polymorphism in Mexican patients with transitional cell carcinoma of the bladder. *Urology* **2009**, *74*, 414–418. [CrossRef] [PubMed]

27. Amann, B.; Perabo, F.G.; Wirger, A.; Hugenschmidt, H.; Schultze-Seemann, W. Urinary levels of monocyte chemo-attractant protein-1 correlate with tumour stage and grade in patients with bladder cancer. *Br. J. Urol.* **1998**, *82*, 118–121. [CrossRef] [PubMed]

28. Brana, I.; Calles, A.; LoRusso, P.M.; Yee, L.K.; Puchalski, T.A.; Seetharam, S.; Zhong, B.; de Boer, C.J.; Tabernero, J.; Calvo, E. Carlumab, an anti-C-C chemokine ligand 2 monoclonal antibody, in combination with four chemotherapy regimens for the treatment of patients with solid tumors: An open-label, multicenter phase 1b study. *Target Oncol.* **2015**, *10*, 111–123. [CrossRef] [PubMed]

29. Mitchem, J.B.; Brennan, D.J.; Knolhoff, B.L.; Belt, B.A.; Zhu, Y.; Sanford, D.E.; Belaygorod, L.; Carpenter, D.; Collins, L.; Piwnica-Worms, D.; et al. Targeting tumor-infiltrating macrophages decreases tumor-initiating cells, relieves immunosuppression, and improves chemotherapeutic responses. *Cancer Res.* **2013**, *73*, 1128–1141. [CrossRef] [PubMed]

30. Mitchem, J.B.; DeNardo, D.G. Battle over CCL2 for control of the metastatic niche: neutrophils versus monocytes. *Breast Cancer Res.* **2012**, *14*, 315. [CrossRef] [PubMed]

31. Lee, C.C.; Ho, H.C.; Su, Y.C.; Lee, M.S.; Hung, S.K.; Lin, C.H. MCP1-Induced Epithelial-Mesenchymal Transition in Head and Neck Cancer by AKT Activation. *Anticancer Res.* **2015**, *35*, 3299–3306. [PubMed]

32. Rao, Q.; Chen, Y.; Yeh, C.R.; Ding, J.; Li, L.; Chang, C.; Yeh, S. Recruited mast cells in the tumor microenvironment enhance bladder cancer metastasis via modulation of ERβ/CCL2/CCR2 EMT/MMP9 signals. *Oncotarget* **2016**, *7*, 7842–7855. [CrossRef] [PubMed]

33. Chen, W.; Gao, Q.; Han, S.; Pan, F.; Fan, W. The CCL2/CCR2 axis enhances IL-6-induced epithelial-mesenchymal transition by cooperatively activating STAT3-Twist signaling. *Tumor Biol.* **2015**, *36*, 973–981. [CrossRef] [PubMed]

34. Hsu, Y.L.; Hung, J.Y.; Tsai, Y.M.; Tsai, E.M.; Huang, M.S.; Hou, M.F.; Kuo, P.L. 6-shogaol, an active constituent of dietary ginger, impairs cancer development and lung metastasis by inhibiting the secretion of CC-chemokine ligand 2 (CCL2) in tumor-associated dendritic cells. *J. Agric. Food Chem.* **2015**, *63*, 1730–1738. [CrossRef] [PubMed]

35. Kortylewski, M.; Yu, H. Stat3 as a potential target for cancer immunotherapy. *J. Immunother.* **2007**, *30*, 131–139. [CrossRef] [PubMed]

36. Yu, H.; Pardoll, D.; Jove, R. STATs in cancer inflammation and immunity: A leading role for STAT3. *Nat. Rev. Cancer* **2009**, *9*, 798–809. [CrossRef] [PubMed]

37. Chen, C.L.; Cen, L.; Kohout, J.; Hutzen, B.; Chan, C.; Hsieh, F.C.; Loy, A.; Huang, V.; Cheng, G.; Lin, J. Signal transducer and activator of transcription 3 activation is associated with bladder cancer cell growth and survival. *Mol. Cancer* **2008**, *7*, 78. [CrossRef] [PubMed]

38. Yang, C.; Zhang, W.; Wang, L.; Kazobinka, G.; Han, X.; Li, B.; Hou, T. Musashi-2 promotes migration and invasion in bladder cancer via activation of the JAK2/STAT3 pathway. *Lab. Investig.* **2016**, *96*, 950–958. [CrossRef] [PubMed]

39. Chiu, H.Y.; Sun, K.H.; Chen, S.Y.; Wang, H.H.; Lee, M.Y.; Tsou, Y.C.; Jwo, S.C.; Sun, G.H.; Tang, S.J. Autocrine CCL2 promotes cell migration and invasion via PKC activation and tyrosine phosphorylation of paxillin in bladder cancer cells. *Cytokine* **2012**, *59*, 423–432. [CrossRef] [PubMed]

40. Izumi, K.; Fang, L.Y.; Mizokami, A.; Namiki, M.; Li, L.; Lin, W.J.; Chang, C. Targeting the androgen receptor with siRNA promotes prostate cancer metastasis through enhanced macrophage recruitment via CCL2/CCR2-induced STAT3 activation. *EMBO Mol. Med.* **2013**, *5*, 1383–1401. [CrossRef] [PubMed]

41. Sun, Y.; Cheng, M.K.; Griffiths, T.R.; Mellon, J.K.; Kai, B.; Kriajevska, M.; Manson, M.M. Inhibition of STAT signalling in bladder cancer by diindolylmethane: Relevance to cell adhesion, migration and proliferation. *Curr. Cancer Drug Targets* **2013**, *13*, 57–68. [CrossRef] [PubMed]

42. Sung, W.J.; Kim, H.; Park, K.K. The biological role of epithelial-mesenchymal transition in lung cancer (Review). *Oncol. Rep.* **2016**, *36*, 1199–1206. [CrossRef] [PubMed]

43. Horejs, C.M. Basement membrane fragments in the context of the epithelial-to-mesenchymal transition. *Eur. J. Cell Biol.* **2016**, *95*, 427–440. [CrossRef] [PubMed]

44. Deshmane, S.L.; Kremlev, S.; Amini, S.; Sawaya, B.E. Monocyte chemoattractant protein-1 (MCP-1): An overview. *J. Interferon Cytokine Res.* **2009**, *29*, 313–326. [CrossRef] [PubMed]

45. Raman, D.; Baugher, P.J.; Thu, Y.M.; Richmond, A. Role of chemokines in tumor growth. *Cancer Lett.* **2007**, *256*, 137–165. [CrossRef] [PubMed]

46. Arabzadeh, A.; Dupaul-Chicoine, J.; Breton, V.; Haftchenary, S.; Yumeen, S.; Turbide, C.; Saleh, M.; McGregor, K.; Greenwood, C.M.; Akavia, U.D.; et al. Carcinoembryonic Antigen Cell Adhesion Molecule 1 long isoform modulates malignancy of poorly differentiated colon cancer cells. *Gut* **2016**, *65*, 821–829. [CrossRef] [PubMed]

47. Ding, L.; Wang, S.; Wang, W.; Lv, P.; Zhao, D.; Chen, F.; Meng, T.; Dong, L.; Qi, L. Tanshinone IIA affects autophagy and apoptosis of glioma cells by inhibiting phosphatidylinositol 3-Kinase/Akt/Mammalian target of rapamycin signaling pathway. *Pharmacology* **2017**, *99*, 188–195. [CrossRef] [PubMed]

48. Li, X.; Li, Z.; Li, X.; Liu, B.; Liu, Z. Mechanisms of tanshinone II a inhibits malignant melanoma development through blocking autophagy signal transduction in A375 cell. *BMC Cancer* **2017**, *17*, 357. [CrossRef] [PubMed]

49. Sui, H.; Zhao, J.; Zhou, L.; Wen, H.; Deng, W.; Li, C.; Ji, Q.; Liu, X.; Feng, Y.; Chai, N.; et al. Tanshinone IIA inhibits β-catenin/VEGF-mediated angiogenesis by targeting TGF-β1 in normoxic and HIF-1α in hypoxic microenvironments in human colorectal cancer. *Cancer Lett.* **2017**, *403*, 86–97. [CrossRef] [PubMed]

50. Zhong, C.; Zhang, Y.F.; Huang, J.H.; Wang, Z.Y.; Chen, Q.Y.; Su, L.T.; Liu, Z.T.; Xiong, C.M.; Tao, Z.; Guo, R.P. The Chinese medicine, Jianpi Huayu Decoction, inhibits the epithelial mesenchymal transition via the regulation of the Smad3/Smad7 cascade. *Am. J. Transl. Res.* **2017**, *9*, 2694–2711. [PubMed]

51. Calon, A.; Espinet, E.; Palomo-Ponce, S.; Tauriello, D.V.; Iglesias, M.; Cespedes, M.V.; Sevillano, M.; Nadal, C.; Jung, P.; Zhang, X.H.; et al. Dependency of colorectal cancer on a TGF-β-driven program in stromal cells for metastasis initiation. *Cancer Cell* **2012**, *22*, 571–584. [CrossRef] [PubMed]

52. Liu, R.Y.; Zeng, Y.; Lei, Z.; Wang, L.; Yang, H.; Liu, Z.; Zhao, J.; Zhang, H.T. JAK/STAT3 signaling is required for TGF-β-induced epithelial-mesenchymal transition in lung cancer cells. *Int. J. Oncol.* **2014**, *44*, 1643–1651. [CrossRef] [PubMed]

53. Luwor, R.B.; Baradaran, B.; Taylor, L.E.; Iaria, J.; Nheu, T.V.; Amiry, N.; Hovens, C.M.; Wang, B.; Kaye, A.H.; Zhu, H.J. Targeting Stat3 and Smad7 to restore TGF-β cytostatic regulation of tumor cells in vitro and in vivo. *Oncogene* **2013**, *32*, 2433–2441. [CrossRef] [PubMed]

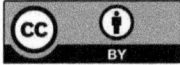

International Journal of
Molecular Sciences

MDPI

Article

Metformin Inhibits TGF-β1-Induced Epithelial-to-Mesenchymal Transition via PKM2 Relative-mTOR/p70s6k Signaling Pathway in Cervical Carcinoma Cells

Keyan Cheng and Min Hao *

Department of Obstetrics and Gynecology, The Second Hospital of Shanxi Medical University, Taiyuan 030000, China; chengkey@126.com
* Correspondence: eryuanhaomin@126.com; Tel./Fax: +86-35-1336-5114

Academic Editors: Gianni Sava and Alberta Bergamo
Received: 10 September 2016; Accepted: 22 November 2016; Published: 30 November 2016

Abstract: Background: Epithelial-to-mesenchymal transition (EMT) plays a prominent role in tumorigenesis. Metformin exerts antitumorigenic effects in various cancers. This study investigated the mechanisms of metformin in TGF-β1-induced Epithelial-to-mesenchymal transition (EMT) in cervical carcinoma cells. Methods: cells were cultured with 10 ng/mL TGF-β1 to induce EMT and treated with or without metformin. Cell viability was evaluated by CCK-8 (Cell Counting Kit 8, CCK-8) assay; apoptosis were analyzed by flow cytometry; cell migration was evaluated by wound-healing assay. Western blotting was performed to detect E-cadherin, vimentin, signal transducer and activator of transcription 3 (STAT3), snail family transcriptional repressor 2 (SNAIL2), phosphorylation of p70s6k (p-p70s6k) and -Pyruvate kinase M2 (PKM2) Results: TGF-β1 promoted proliferation and migration, and it attenuated apoptosis compared with cells treated with metformin with or without TGF-β1 in cervical carcinoma cells. Moreover, metformin partially abolished TGF-β1-induced EMT cell proliferation and reversed TGF-β1-induced EMT. In addition, the anti-EMT effects of metformin could be partially in accord with rapamycin, a specific mTOR inhibitor. Metformin decreased the p-p70s6k expression and the blockade of mTOR/p70s6k signaling decreased PKM2 expression. Conclusion: Metformin abolishes TGF-β1-induced EMT in cervical carcinoma cells by inhibiting mTOR/p70s6k signaling to down-regulate PKM2 expression. Our study provides a novel mechanistic insight into the anti-tumor effects of metformin.

Keywords: metformin; mammalian target of rapamycin; epithelial-mesenchymal transition; PKM2

1. Introduction

Cervical carcinoma is the second common gynecological carcinoma worldwide with more than 0.52 million new cases and 0.27 million deaths globally each year. Approximately 30% of cervical carcinoma patients will ultimately fail after surgery, radiotherapy, or chemotherapy treatment [1]. There is increasing evidence that Epithelial-to-mesenchymal transition (EMT) plays a prominent role in carcinoma tumorigenesis. The EMT enables carcinoma to invade and metastasize [2,3], induces cancer chemoresistance [4], and radioresistance [5,6], and has an immunoprotective effect [7]. Therefore, the EMT constitutes a major malignant propensity to cancer development and is a major obstacle to cure cancer.

During the EMT, epithelial cells undergo extensive genetic alterations, resulting in the loss of apical-basal polarity, the severing of cell-cell adhesion structures, and the degradation of basement membrane components [8]. The loss of E-cadherin is generally accepted as a hallmark of the EMT [9], which reduces cell-cell adhesion and destabilizes the epithelial architecture. This process is accompanied by increased expression of vimentin, which bestows a motile phenotype on cancer cells through changes in cellular architecture and cell-matrix interactions [10,11]. Snail, a transcription factor, acts as repressor of E-cadherin in response to TGF-β signaling [12], and has been linked to the induction of the EMT under different cellular contexts. A signal transducer and activator of transcription 3 (STAT3) is also involved in EMT by regulating the transcriptional regulators of E-cadherin [13]. Large studies indicated that alterations of EMT-related markers have been associated with metastatic disease and reduced survival, including cervical carcinoma [14,15].

Recent studies showed overexpression of pyruvate kinase M2 (PKM2) induced the epithelial-to-mesenchymal transition (EMT) and increased the metastatic potential of cancer cells [16]. PKM2 is an alternatively-spliced variant of the pyruvate kinase gene that is preferentially expressed during embryonic development and in cancer cells [17,18]. PKM2 regulates in the cancer-specific Warburg effect, which is responsible for the final rate-limiting step of glycolysis. Moreover, in cancer cells, PKM2 expression is associated with attenuated pyruvate kinase activity to meet the biosynthetic demands, which allows the diversion of glycolytic flux into the pentose phosphate pathway [18].

Metformin exerts its antitumorigenic effects through indirect mechanisms by increasing insulin sensitivity, inhibiting liver gluconeogenesis [19], and direct mechanisms involving activating AMP-activated protein kinase (AMPK), followed by inhibition of the mammalian target of the rapamycin (mTOR) pathway [20,21]. Moreover, metformin also plays a crucial role in modulating cell energy metabolism [22], and repressed the EMT through the mTOR signaling pathway [23]. Hosono et al. report that the mechanisms underlying the suppression on aberrant crypt foci formation of metformin are associated with the inhibition of the mTOR pathway [24]. Dann et al. reported that mTOR Complex1-S6K1 signaling is at the crossroads of obesity, diabetes, and cancer [25].

These mechanisms of metformin indicated that there likely is an antitumorigenic effect relationship between the mTOR pathway and PKM2 in various cancers. Moreover, the potential role of metformin in treating gynecologic oncology has been explored in a number of studies. A study reported that metformin inhibits βKlotho-related ERK1/2 signaling and AMPKα signaling to reverse the EMT in endometrial adenocarcinoma [26]. However, none of research involves the relationship of mTOR pathway and PKM2.

In this study, we investigate the role of metformin on inhibited TGF-β1-induced EMT in cervical carcinoma cells and explore the mechanisms that might be involved in tumorigenesis. Our data showed that the metformin reversed EMT. Metformin as the same anti-tumor effects as rapamycin, which decreased p-p70s6k and PKM2 expression. We infer that metformin is involved in mTOR/p70s6k/PKM2 signaling to promote cervical carcinoma resistance.

2. Results

2.1. Transforming Growth Factor Beta 1 (TGF-β1) Induces Epithelial-to-Mesenchymal Transition (EMT) in Cerivical Cancer Cells

In order to determine whether TGF-β1 induced EMT, HeLa, and SiHa cells were incubated with 10 ng/mL TGF-β1 for 48 h based on Hamabe' study [16]. The results obtained indicate that cells displayed an altered morphology, with flattened, stretched, and scattered fibroblast-like shapes. As shown in Figure 1, almost all HeLa (A) and SiHa (B) cells acquired spindle and fibroblastoid shapes with increased cell gaps. Moreover, protein levels of E-cadherin were abundantly expressed in the absence of TGF-β1 (pre-EMT). After these cells were stimulated by 10 ng/mL TGF-β1, E-cadherin expression was significantly decreased (post-EMT). In contrast, compared with the pre-EMT state, vimentin was increased (post-EMT), stimulated by TGF-β1 (Figure 1). In view of the changes in cell morphology and marker protein expression, these data indicated that EMT was induced when cervical carcinoma cells were stimulated with 10 ng/mL TGF-β1.

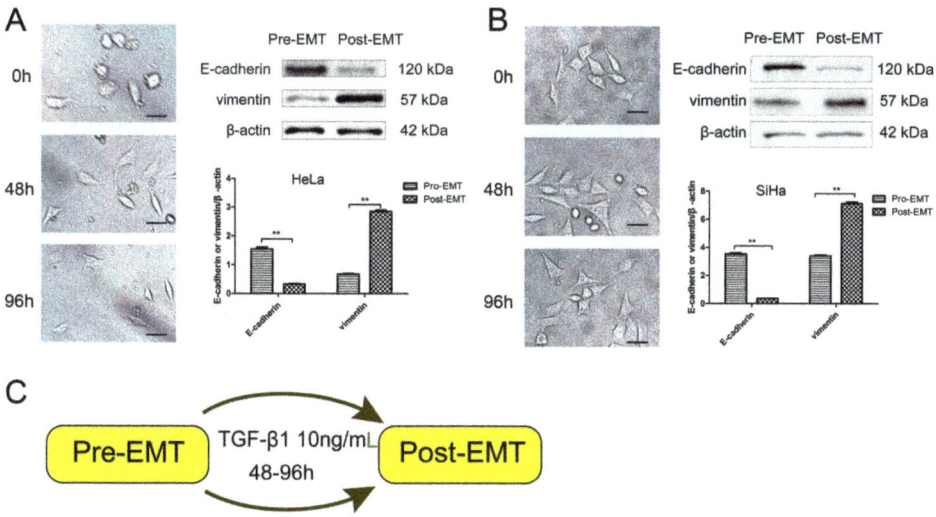

Figure 1. TGF-β1 induces EMT in cerivical cancer cells. (**A,B**) Photomicrographs of the morphological change in HeLa (**A**) and SiHa (**B**) cells. The number of hours indicates the period since EMT induction was initiated (scale bar, 50 μm). Western blot assays of E-cadherion, vimentin, and β-actin are shown in comparison with those in the pre-EMT condition; and (**C**) schematic representation of the procedure for EMT induction. The cells incubated for 48 h after seeding are defined as pre-EMT, and the cells cultured with 10 ng/mL TGF-β1 are defined as post-EMT. ** $p < 0.01$.

2.2. Metformin Inhibits the TGF-β1-Induced Proliferation, Migration, and Induces Apoptosis

To evaluate the potential anti-proliferative effect of metformin in cervical carcinoma cells, Cells were treated with 0, 1, 2.5, 5, 10, and 15 mM metformin, or 10 mM metformin with or without 10 ng/mL TGF-β1. The Cell Counting Kit-8 (CCK-8, Dojindo, Tokyo, Japan) assays were performed to determine the proliferation of cells. As shown in Figures 2A and 3A, metformin led to a significant decrease in proliferation compared with untreated (control) cells, which inhibited the proliferation of HeLa (Figure 2A) and SiHa (Figure 3A) cell lines in a dose-dependent manner. In addition, treatment with TGF-β1 significantly increased the proliferation of both cell lines in comparison with treated metformin with or without TGF-β1 at 72 h, which was abolished by the addition of metformin. When comparing the metformin plus TGF group with the metformin group, cells treated with metformin plus TGF significantly proliferated faster than the metformin cells in SiHa cells, but not HeLa. It appears from the data in Figures 2 and 3 that metformin only partially reversed the changes seen with TGF-β1.

The migration of cells were evaluated using wound-healing assays. Cells were treated with 10 mM metformin and with or without 10 ng/mL TGF-β1. Metformin significantly decreased the migration of cells compared with untreated (control) cells, and TGF-β1 significantly increased cell migration compared with untreated (control) cells in HeLa (Figure 2B) and SiHa (Figure 3B) cell lines at 24 h, which was abolished by the addition of metformin It was found that there is a statistical significance between the metformin group and the metformin with TGF-β1 group in HeLa cells (Figure 2B), but not in SiHa cells (Figure 3B). These data indicated that metformin could inhibit the migration ability of cells and reverse TGF-β1-induced EMT's migration ability of cells.

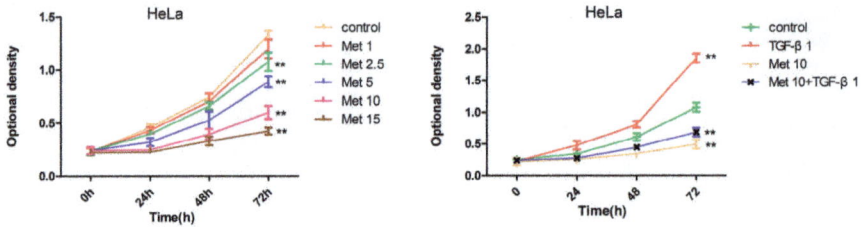

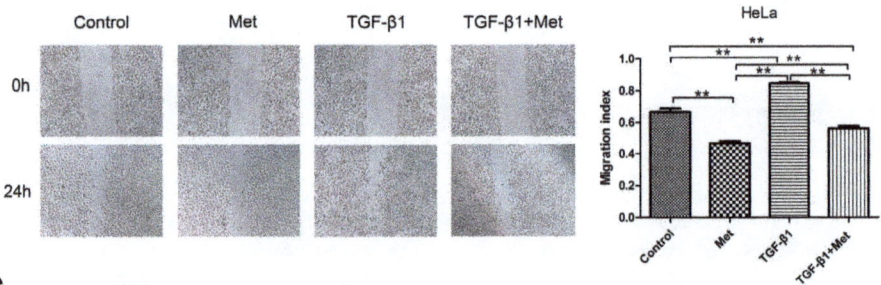

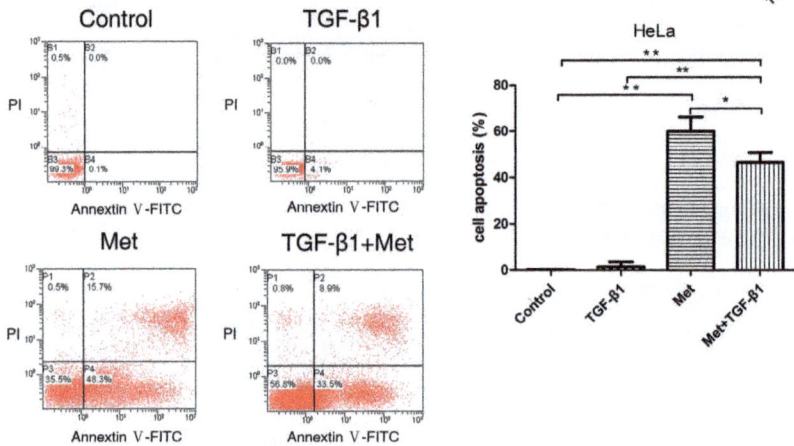

Figure 2. Metformin inhibits TGF-β1-induced proliferation, migration, and induces apoptosis in HeLa cells. (**A**) HeLa cells were treated with metformin (0, 1, 2.5, 5, 10 and 15 mM) or TGF-β1 with or without 10 mM metformin. Cell numbers were measured by CCK-8 assays at indicated times; (**B**) wound-healing assays. Representative images were obtained at 40× magnification. Graphs show the relative migration distance after 24 h incubation; (**C**) annexin V-FITC apoptosis assay. Cells were harvested and stained with Annexin V-FITC/PI (propidium iodide, PI), and cell apoptosis was analyzed using flow cytometry. Representative images are shown. TGF-β1: transforming growth factor β1; Met: metformin. * $p < 0.05$, ** $p < 0.01$.

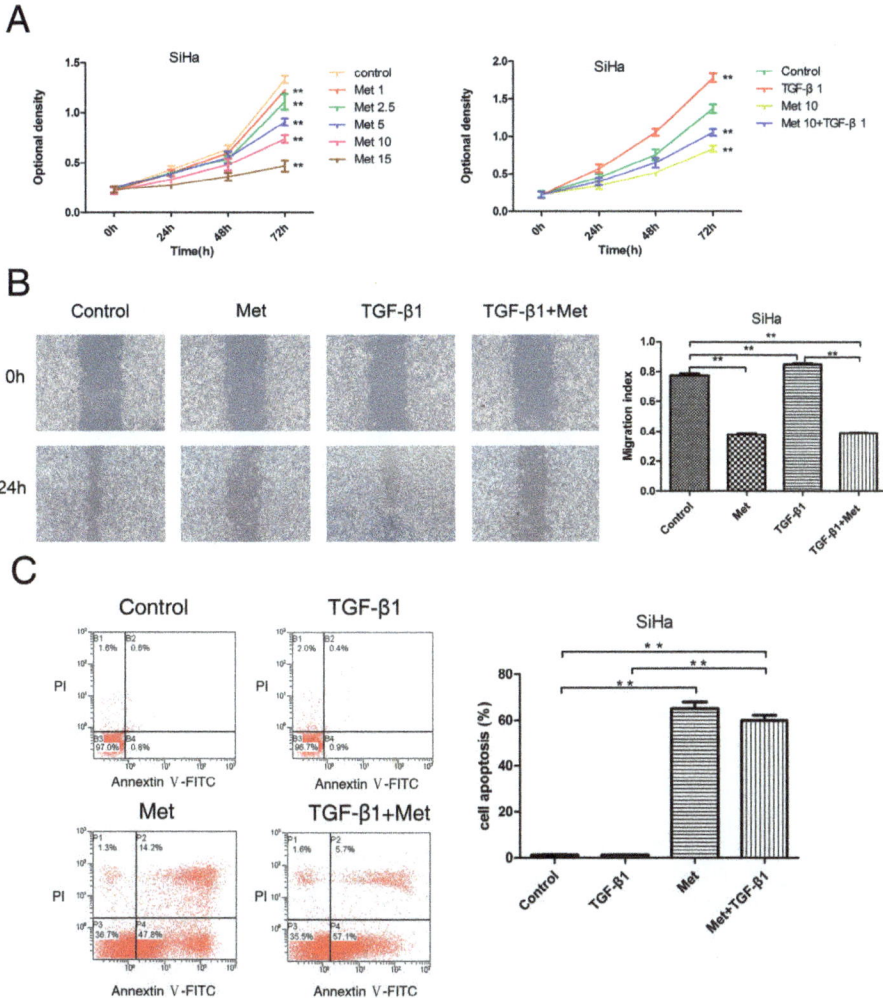

Figure 3. Metformin inhibits TGF-β1-induced proliferation, migration, and induces apoptosis in SiHa cells. (**A**) SiHa cells were treated with metformin (0, 1, 2.5, 5, 10, and 15 mM) or TGF-β1 with or without 10 mM metformin. Cell numbers were measured by CCK-8 assays at indicated times; (**B**) wound-healing assays. Representative images were obtained at 40× magnification. Graphs show the relative migration distance after 24 h incubation; (**C**) annexin V-FITC apoptosis assay. Cells were harvested and stained with Annexin V-FITC/PI (propidium iodide, PI), and cell apoptosis was analyzed using flow cytometry. Representative images are shown. TGF-β1: transforming growth factor β1; Met: metformin. ** *p* < 0.01.

To explore the potential effect of metformin for antagonzing the anti-apoptosis effect of TGF-β1 on cervical carcinoma cells by Annexin V-FITC and propidium iodide (PI) staining, we detected the effect of metformin with and without TGF-β1 on the apoptosis of HeLa (Figure 2C) and SiHa (Figure 3C) cells. The results obtained indicated that TGF-β1 induced a slight increase apoptosis compared with untreated cells in Hela cells (Figure 2C), but there was no statistical significance. Meanwhile, In SiHa (Figure 3C) cells treated with TGF-β1, the total apoptotic cells (early apoptotic + apoptotic) showed no effect compared to untreated cells. However, the apoptosis rate was increased by the addition of metformin in both cell lines. In addition, metformin with or without TGF-β1 exhibited a marked increase in apoptosis levels in both cell lines (Figures 2C and 3C). These data indicated that the addition of metformin significantly abolished the TGF-β1-induced anti-apoptosis effects in both cell lines.

2.3. PKM2 Expression Is Required to Induce EMT

Hamabe et al. reported that they used TGF-β1 to induce EMT in colorectal cancer cells. Then, siRNAs targeting PKM2 were designed to knockdown PKM2 in EMT conditions. They found that PKM2 knockdown failed to induce spindle-shaped morphological changes, and Western blot showed that PKM2 knockdown hindered E-cadherin loss and vimentin gain compared with the control [16]. To determine whether the EMT condition stimulates an increase in PKM2 compared with levels in the pre-EMT state. HeLa and SiHa cells were grown in a medium with 10 ng/mL TGF-β1. Consistent with this report, our results obtained showed that HeLa (Figure 1A) and SiHa (Figure 1B) cells changed morphology from epithelial to fibroblastic-like and spindle-shaped. E-cadherin expression was suppressed, whereas vimentin, and snail family zinc finger 2 (SNAIL2) expression were increased in the post-EMT condition (Figure 4). Moreover, PKM2 gene expression was induced in the EMT condition (Figure 4). The data indicated that the induction of EMT resulted in decreased E-cadherin expression, increased vimentin expression, and up-regulated PKM2 (Figure 4). These results confirmed that PKM2 expression was induced in the EMT condition.

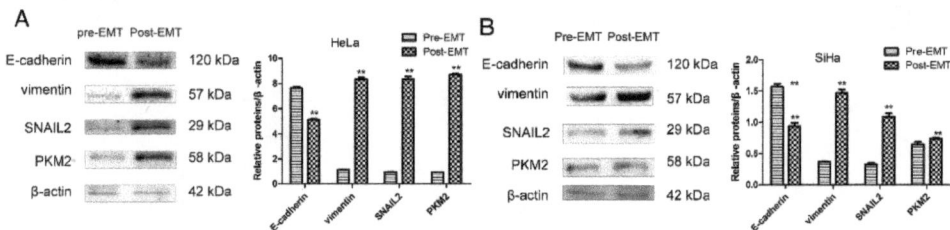

Figure 4. EMT condition stimulates an increase in PKM2. (**A**) HeLa and (**B**) SiHa cells were detected E-cadherin, vimentin, SNAIL2, and PKM2 expression by Western blot between pre-EMT and post-EMT state. Columns represent the average of at least three independent experiments; error bars represent the SD of the mean from triplicate results. ** $p < 0.01$.

2.4. mTOR/p70s6k Signaling Involved in Regulating PKM2 Expression in the EMT Condition

To investigate whether the mTOR pathway affects PKM2 expression in the EMT condition, the mTOR pathway was inhibited by rapamycin (an mTOR inhibtior) to evaluate PKM2 (a critical glycolytic enzyme), and p70s6k (S6K1, a downstream effector of mTOR) expression. HeLa and SiHa cells were induced by TGF-β1 for 48 h, then were treated with or without 50 nM rapamycin for 24 h, respectively. Rapamycin was dissolved in dimethylsulfoxide (DMSO) and the same dose of DMSO was used as a control. As shown in Figure 5, TGF-β1 significantly increased the expression of PKM2 and phosphorylation of p70s6k. While, rapamycin, a specific mTOR inhibitor, inhibited the phosphorylation of p70s6k expression, ribosomal p70S6 kinase (S6K1) is one of main downstream mTOR effectors. Moreover, to investigate whether inhibition of mTOR/p70s6k signaling decreased PKM2 expression, which is one of the main downstream S6K1 effectors, rapamycin was added to cell cultures to inhibit the mTOR pathway. The results obtained indicate that inhibition of the mTOR pathway significantly decreased the expression of PKM2 and phosphorylation of p70s6k in HeLa (Figure 5A) and SiHa cells (Figure 5B). In addition, at a concentration of 50 nM rapamycin reversed TGF-β1-induced EMT expression by repressing PKM2 and p-p70s6k expressions in HeLa (Figure 5A) and SiHa cells (Figure 5B). These data indicated that the inhibition of EMT was through the PKM2 relative-mTOR/p70s6k signaling pathway in cervical carcinoma cells.

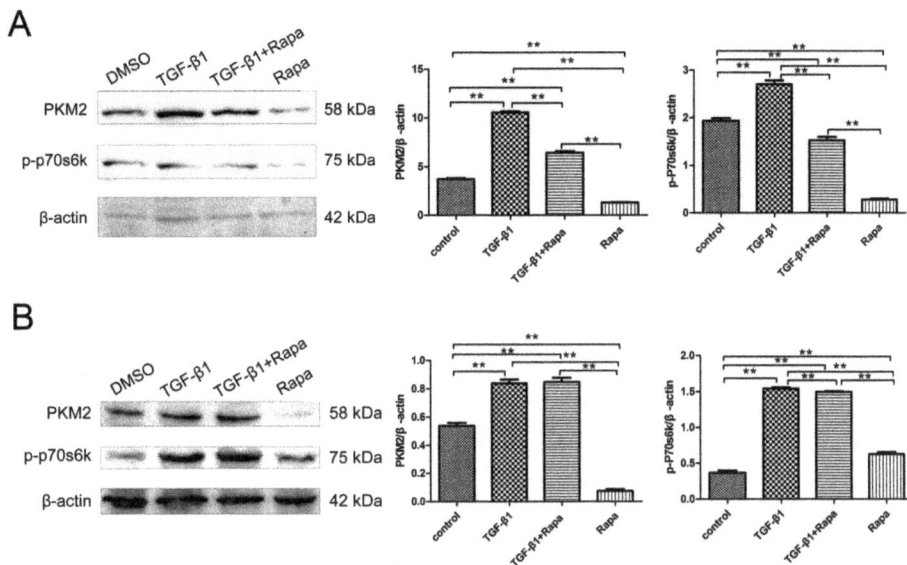

Figure 5. mTOR/p70s6k signaling involved in regulating PKM2 in the EMT condition. HeLa (**A**) and SiHa (**B**) cells were treated with TGF-β1, with or without rapamycin. Rapamycin was dissolved in DMSO and the same dose of DMSO was used as a control, and the p-p70s6k and PKM2 expressions were detected by Western blot. DMSO: dimethylsulfoxide; Rapa:rapamycin. ** $p < 0.01$.

2.5. Metformin Reverses TGF-β1-Induced EMT Involved in mTOR/p70s6k/PKM2 Signaling Pathways in Cervical Carcinoma Cells

To determine the mechanism of metformin involved the regulation of EMT in cervical carcinoma, the expression of EMT-related markers were examined by Western blot. The results obtained revealed that 10 mM metformin caused an accumulation of E-cadherin, and decreased vimentin, STAT3, and SNAIL2 expression in HeLa (Figure 6A) and SiHa cells (Figure 7A). Moreover, TGF-β1 significantly decreased the expression of E-cadherin and increased the expressions of vimentin, STAT3, and SNAIL2 in HeLa (Figure 6A) and SiHa cells (Figure 7A). In addition, concentration of metformin reversed TGF-β1-induced EMT marker expression by repressing vimentin, STAT3, and SNAIL2 expressions and restoring E-cadherin expression in HeLa (Figure 6A) and SiHa cells (Figure 7A).

Next, we explored the possible signaling pathways that may be involved. As shown in Figures 6 and 7, Western blots showed that metformin decreased the phosphorylation of p70s6k and down-regulated PKM2 levels in Hela (Figure 6A) and SiHa (Figure 7A) cells. TGF-β1 significantly increased the phosphorylation of p70s6k, which is the main downstream signaling intermediate of mTOR signaling. Simultaneously, TGF-β1 significantly up-regulated the expression of PKM2 in HeLa (Figure 6A) and SiHa cells (Figure 7A). While metformin reversed TGF-β1-induced EMT by repressing phosphorylation of p70s6k and PKM2 in HeLa (Figure 6A) and SiHa cells (Figure 7A). These results suggested that metformin reverses TGF-β1-induced EMT via the mTOR/p70s6k/PKM2 pathway.

Next, we examined the effect of metformin with or without TGF-β1 on the morphology of HeLa and SiHa cell lines. Metformin led to a significant decrease in proliferation in the both cells. Moreover, after stimulation with 10 ng/mL TGF-β1 for 48 h, both HeLa (Figure 6B) and SiHa cells (Figure 7B) cells became scattered, acquired a spindle-shaped morphology, and lost cell-cell contacts, which are characteristics of a mesenchymal-like morphology. Treatment with 10 mM metformin for 48 h abolished the TGF-β1-induced EMT morphological changes in HeLa and SiHa cells. The cells tended to aggregate and lose the spindle-shaped morphology.

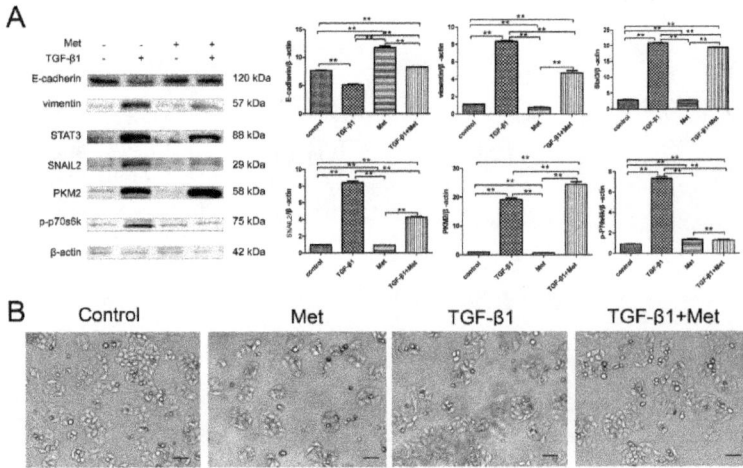

Figure 6. Metformin reverses TGF-β1-induced EMT in HeLa cells involving mTOR/p70s6k/PKM2 signaling pathways. (**A**) Cells were treated with TGF-β1, metformin, or both agents for 48 h. The protein expression levels of E-cadherin, vimentin, SNAIL2, STAT3, PKM2, p-p70s6k, and β-actin were detected by Western blot. β-actin was used as a loading control; and (**B**) the morphology of HeLa cells were treated with TGF-β1 and with or without metformin for 48 h. The cells were observed using phase contrast microscopy at 200× magnification. Scale bar: 50 μm. The data are presented as the mean ± SD of three replicates per group. TGF-β1: transforming growth factor β1; Met: metformin. ** $p < 0.01$.

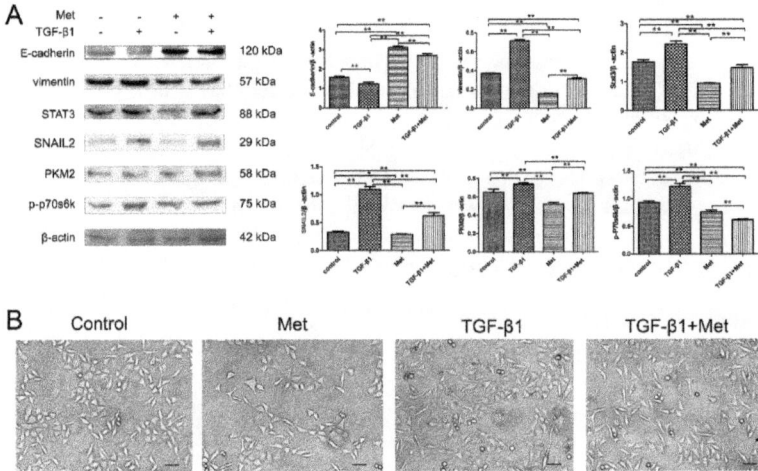

Figure 7. Metformin reverses TGF-β1-induced EMT in SiHa cells involving mTOR/p70s6k/PKM2 signaling pathways. (**A**) Cells were treated with TGF-β1, metformin, or both agents for 48 h. The protein expression levels of E-cadherin, vimentin, SNAIL2, STAT3, PKM2, p-p70s6k, and β-actin were presented by Western blot. β-actin was used as a loading control; and (**B**) the morphology of SiHa cells were treated with TGF-β1 with or without metformin for 48 h. The cells were observed using phase contrast microscopy at 200× magnification. Scale bar: 50 μm. The data are presented as the mean ± SD of three replicates per group. TGF-β1: transforming growth factor β1; Met: metformin. ** $p < 0.01$, * $p < 0.05$.

3. Discussion

In this study, we demonstrated that metformin inhibited TGF-β1-induced EMT in proliferation, migration, and induced apoptosis. Our result suggested that metformin inhibits TGF-β1-induced EMT via the mTOR/p70s6k/PKM2 signaling pathway in cervical carcinoma cells.

Metformin is an anti-diabetic drug with potential anti-neoplastic action, which decreases the incidence and progression of multiple human cancers [27,28], and improves patients' overall survival rate [29]. For example, in one study, ovarian or endometrial cancer patients with diabetes mellitus, who were being treated with metformin at the time of diagnosis, exhibited half the risk of mortality than that of the non-metformin-treated patients [29]. Moreover, metformin decreases hepatocellular carcinoma risk in a dose-dependent manner [30]. Several studies have also shown that metformin decreases cancer cell viability by inducing apoptosis in various cancer. Griss et al. reported that metformin inhibited cancer cell proliferation by suppressing mitochondrial-dependent biosynthetic activity [31], and metformin could induce breast cancer cell apoptosis [32]. In our study, we observed that metformin not only induced apoptosis and decreases cancer cell viability, but also reversed the anti-apoptosis effect of TGF-β1-induced EMT in cervical carcinoma cells. These data suggested the potential therapeutic implication of metformin for cervical carcinomas.

Recent studies indicated that metformin was a novel TGF-β suppressor with therapeutic potential for numerous diseases [33]. In our study, we used TGF-β1 to induce EMT and explore the possible mechanism of metformin that inhibited TGF-β1-induced EMT in cervical cancer. Moreover, metformin has been reported to inhibit EMT in lung adenocarcinoma [34], hepatocellular carcinoma [35], and inhibit mTOR signaling. PKM2 involved in tumorigenesis and affected the EMT situation. Silvestri et al. [36] reported that metformin induced apoptosis and down-regulated PKM2 in breast cancer cells. These studies showed that the mechanism of metformin may be associated with the following observations: (1) metformin inhibits mTOR activation by AMPK-dependence in different cancers [37–39]; (2) mTOR signaling regulates P70S6K signaling in cervical carcinoma cells [40]; (3) metformin induce intrinsic apoptosis via the inhibition of the HIF1α/PKM2 signaling pathway [41]; and (4) metformin is also a poisoner of mitochondria by impairing the function of complex I [42], leading to the increased aerobic glycolysis as compensation.

The mTOR pathway is a central regulator of glucose metabolism and glycolysis, and is important in the transcriptional program of glucose transporters and multiple rate-limiting glycolytic enzymes [43,44]. Meanwhile, the phosphorylation of p70 ribosomal S6 kinase 1 (S6K1), a downstream effector of mTOR, is modulated by the mTOR pathway [45]. Nobukini et al. reported that the activities of dS6k and S6K1 are regulated by the mammalian target of rapamycin (mTOR). They found the mechanisms regulating the mTOR/S6K1 signaling pathway will be fundamental in determining the mechanisms which control cell growth [46]. Montagne et al. reported that the deactivation of dS6K, the orthologue of mammalian S6K, is involved in slow overall growth rate and decreased cell size [47]. Consistent with these reports, in our study, we observed that metformin not only induced apoptosis and decreased cancer cell viability, but also abolished the TGF-β1 induced morphological changes through the mTOR/p70sk signaling pathway in cervical carcinoma cells.

Next, Hamabe et al. found that PKM2 plays a crucial role in the EMT development of cancer [16]. Recent studies also showed that PKM2 was an important glycolytic enzyme in the oncogenic mTOR-induced Warburg effect, in which hypoxia inducible factor-1α (HIF-1α) and c-Myc-hnRNP cascades are the transducers of mTOR regulation of PKM2 [48]. Sun et al. reported that mTOR up-regulation of pyruvate kinase isoenzyme type M2 plays a crucial role in aerobic glycolysis and tumor growth. PKM2 expression was augmented in mouse kidney tumors and consequent mTOR activation, and was reduced by mTOR suppression [48]. These studies illustrated that there was a correlation between mTOR/p70s6k/PKM2 signaling and EMT. Our data showed that TGF-β1 significantly increased the expression of PKM2 and phosphorylation of p70s6k, which means PKM2 and p70s6k are involved in EMT. Rapamycin, a mTOR inhibitor, inhibits the mTOR pathway, while p-p70sk6 and PKM2 were decreased. We prove that mTOR/p70s6k/PKM2 signaling is involved in EMT development.

Based on these studies, we propose that metformin exerts its antitumorigenic effects and abolished TGF-β1-induced EMT through mTOR/p70s6k/PKM2 signaling in cervical carcinoma cells. In the present study, we showed that metformin significantly decreased cell proliferation and migration and reverses EMT in cervical carcinoma cells. More importantly, we demonstrated that mTOR/p70s6k/PKM2 signaling is the target of metformin. This claim is supported by the observation that mTOR activity is inhibited by addition of metformin in vitro. Moreover, we found that the role of metformin inhibit phosphorylation of p70s6k when cervical carcinoma was treated with metformin. In addition, our results indicated that metformin attenuates the phosphorylation of p70s6k and PKM2. Metformin reversed TGF-β1-induced epithelial-to-mesenchymal transition via the mTOR/p70s6k/PKM2 signaling pathway (Figure 8).

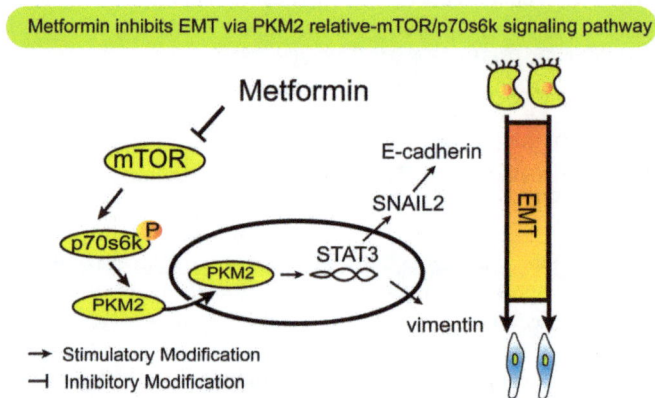

Figure 8. Schematic representation of metformin roles in TGF-β1-induced epithelial-to-mesenchymal transition in cervical carcinoma cells. EMT: Epithelial-to-Mesenchymal Transition; PKM2: Pyruvate kinase M2; P: STAT3: signal transducer and activator of transcription 3; SNAIL2: snail family transcriptional repressor 2; P: phosphorylation.

4. Materials and Methods

4.1. Cell Cultures and Treatments

The human cervical carcinoma cell lines HeLa (ATCC® CRM-CCL-2™) and SiHa (ATCC® HTB-35™) (ATCC, Rockville, MD, USA) were maintained in dulbecco's modified eagle medium (DMEM)medium, supplemented with 10% fetal bovine serum (FBS) and 1% penicillin/streptomycin at 37 °C in a humidified environment with 95% air and 5% CO_2. Rapamycin (PeproTech, Rocky Hill, NJ, USA), a specific mTOR inhibitor, was dissolved in dimethylsulfoxide (DMSO) at a stock concentration of 6.25 mM, and metformin (PeproTech, Rocky Hill, NJ, USA) was dissolved in phosphate-buffered saline (PBS) at a stock concentration of 50 mM. Both were stored at 4 °C. The cells were treated with 10 ng/mL TGF-β1 (PeproTech, Rocky Hill, NJ, USA) and with or without 10 mM metformin. The cells were collected for migration assay, CCK8 (CCK-8, Dojindo, Tokyo, Japan), and Western blot. The morphological changes of cells were observed under an inverted microscope.

4.2. Cell Viability Assay

Cell viability was detected by cell counting kit-8 (CCK-8, Dojindo, Tokyo, Japan) assay. Cells were seeded into 96-well plates at 1×10^4 cells/well and cultured overnight at 37 °C. At 24 h after seeding, the indicated concentrations of metformin, with or without TGF-β1, were added to each well and the cells were cultured for an additional 24, 48, and 72 h, respectively. At harvest time 10 μL of CCK-8 was added into each well and after one hour's incubation, cell viability was determined by measuring the absorbance of the converted dye at 450 nm. The experiments were performed in triplicate.

4.3. Wound Healing Assay

A wound healing assay was performed to test cell migration. The cells were plated in six-well culture plates in complete culture medium and allowed to grow to 90% confluence. An injury line was made using a 2-mm-wide plastic pipette tip. After washing three times with PBS, the cells were cultured with fresh serum-free medium containing 10 ng/mL TGF-β1 with or without the indicated concentration of metformin for 24 h. Subsequently, the ability of the cells to migrate into the cleared section was observed using a microscope. The migration rate was quantified by (scratch distance at 0 h—scratch distance at 24 h)/scratch distance at 0 h. Representative images were obtained at 40× magnification. All experiments were repeated at least three times.

4.4. Annexin V-FITC Apoptosis Assay

Cells were seeded in six-well plates at 4×10^5 cells/well and then treated with different concentrations of metformin, with or without 10 ng/mL TGF-β1 for 24 h. Apoptotic cells were detected by flow cytometry using an Annexin V-FITC kit according to the instructions.

4.5. Western Blot Analysis

The cells were harvested by centrifugation and washed with PBS. The cells were lysed in RIPA buffer containing protease inhibitors. Equal amounts of protein were separated by 10% sodium dodecyl sulfate-polyacrylamide gel electrophoresis and then transferred to Polyvinylidene Fluoride (PVDF) membranes by electroblotting. The membranes were blocked with 5% nonfat milk in Tris-buffered saline/0.1% Tween 20 for 1 h at room temperature and then incubated overnight at 4 °C with the primary antibodies. The anti-human E-cadherin, anti-human vimentin, anti-human SNAIL12, anti-human STAT3, and anti-human phospho-p70s6k primary antibodies were purchased from Cell Signaling Technology (Danvers, MA, USA). The anti-human β-actin primary antibodies and Horseradish Peroxidase (HRP)-conjugated goat anti-rabbit and HRP-conjugated goat anti-mouse secondary antibodies were purchased from ZSGB-BIO (Beijing, China). After incubation with the secondary antibody for 1 h at room temperature, the protein bands were detected using the ECL detection system (BD Biosciences, New York, NY, USA).

4.6. Statistical Analysis

The statistical analyses were performed using SPSS 19.0 (SPSS Inc., Chicago, IL, USA). The values are expressed as the means ± SD. Significant differences among groups were analyzed by one-way analysis of variance (ANOVA). An appropriate post-test has been applied for internal comparisons.

5. Conclusions

To our knowledge, this is the first study showing that metformin could reverse TGF-β1-induced EMT in tumor cells through mTOR/p70s6k/PKM2 pathways. Collectively, our data showed that TGF-β1induced proliferation and EMT, and metformin inhibited cell proliferation and reverseed EMT. The mechanism involved in the suppression of PKM2 activation was mediated by inhibiting mTOR/p70s6k signaling. Our data provides novel mechanistic insights into the antitumor effects of metformin.

Acknowledgments: There is no funding support for this study.

Author Contributions: Keyan Cheng and Min Hao conceived and designed the experiments; Keyan Cheng performed the experiments; Keyan Cheng analyzed the data; Keyan Cheng contributed reagents/materials/ analysis tools; Keyan Cheng wrote the paper.

Conflicts of Interest: The authors declare no conflict of interest.

Abbreviations

TGF-β1	Recombinant transforming growth factor-β1
mTOR	Mammalian target of rapamycin
S6K1	Ribosomal p70 S6 kinase
PKM2	Pyruvate kinase M2

References

1. Colombo, N.; Carinelli, S.; Colombo, A.; Marini, C.; Rollo, D.; Sessa, C.; ESMO guidelines working group. Cervical cancer: Esmo clinical practice guidelines for diagnosis, treatment and follow-up. *Ann. Oncol.* **2012**, *23*, 27–32. [CrossRef] [PubMed]
2. Prall, F. Tumour budding in colorectal carcinoma. *Histopathology* **2007**, *50*, 151–162. [CrossRef] [PubMed]
3. Thiery, J.P.; Acloque, H.; Huang, R.Y.; Nieto, M.A. Epithelial-mesenchymal transitions in development and disease. *Cell* **2009**, *139*, 871–890. [CrossRef] [PubMed]
4. Thomson, S.; Buck, E.; Petti, F.; Griffin, G.; Brown, E.; Ramnarine, N.; Iwata, K.K.; Gibson, N.; Haley, J.D. Epithelial to mesenchymal transition is a determinant of sensitivity of non-small-cell lung carcinoma cell lines and xenografts to epidermal growth factor receptor inhibition. *Cancer Res.* **2005**, *65*, 9455–9462. [CrossRef] [PubMed]
5. Kurrey, N.K.; Jalgaonkar, S.P.; Joglekar, A.V.; Ghanate, A.D.; Chaskar, P.D.; Doiphode, R.Y.; Bapat, S.A. Snail and slug mediate radioresistance and chemoresistance by antagonizing P53-mediated apoptosis and acquiring a stem-like phenotype in ovarian cancer cells. *Stem Cells* **2009**, *27*, 2059–2068. [CrossRef] [PubMed]
6. Lee, J.K.; Joo, K.M.; Lee, J.; Yoon, Y.; Nam, D.H. Targeting the epithelial to mesenchymal transition in glioblastoma: The emerging role of Met signaling. *Oncol. Targets Ther.* **2014**, *7*, 1933–1944.
7. Kudo-Saito, C.; Shirako, H.; Takeuchi, T.; Kawakami, Y. Cancer metastasis is accelerated through immunosuppression during snail-induced EMT of cancer cells. *Cancer Cell* **2009**, *15*, 195–206. [CrossRef] [PubMed]
8. Lee, J.M.; Dedhar, S.; Kalluri, R.; Thompson, E.W. The epithelial-mesenchymal transition: New insights in signaling, development, and disease. *J. Cell Biol.* **2006**, *172*, 973–981. [CrossRef] [PubMed]
9. Maeda, M.; Johnson, K.R.; Wheelock, M.J. Cadherin switching: Essential for behavioral but not morphological changes during an epithelium-to-mesenchyme transition. *J. Cell Sci.* **2005**, *118*, 873–887. [CrossRef] [PubMed]
10. Voulgari, A.; Pintzas, A. Epithelial-mesenchymal transition in cancer metastasis: Mechanisms, markers and strategies to overcome drug resistance in the clinic. *Biochim. Biophys. Acta* **2009**, *1796*, 75–90. [CrossRef] [PubMed]
11. Zeisberg, M.; Neilson, E.G. Biomarkers for epithelial-mesenchymal transitions. *J. Clin. Investig.* **2009**, *119*, 1429–1437. [CrossRef] [PubMed]
12. Peinado, H.; Quintanilla, M.; Cano, A. Transforming growth factor β-1 induces snail transcription factor in epithelial cell lines: Mechanisms for epithelial mesenchymal transitions. *J. Biol. Chem.* **2003**, *278*, 21113–21123. [CrossRef] [PubMed]
13. Zhao, S.; Venkatasubbarao, K.; Lazor, J.W.; Sperry, J.; Jin, C.; Cao, L.; Freeman, J.W. Inhibition of STAT3 Tyr705 phosphorylation by Smad4 suppresses transforming growth factor β-mediated invasion and metastasis in pancreatic cancer cells. *Cancer Res.* **2008**, *68*, 4221–4228. [CrossRef] [PubMed]
14. Mell, L.K.; Meyer, J.J.; Tretiakova, M.; Khramtsov, A.; Gong, C.; Yamada, S.D.; Montag, A.G.; Mundt, A.J. Prognostic significance of E-cadherin protein expression in pathological stage I–III endometrial cancer. *Clin. Cancer Res.* **2004**, *10*, 5546–5553. [CrossRef] [PubMed]
15. Li, B.; Shi, H.; Wang, F.; Hong, D.; Lv, W.; Xie, X.; Cheng, X. Expression of E-, P- and N-Cadherin and its clinical significance in cervical squamous cell carcinoma and precancerous lesions. *PLoS ONE* **2016**, *11*, e0155910. [CrossRef] [PubMed]
16. Hamabe, A.; Konno, M.; Tanuma, N.; Shima, H.; Tsunekuni, K.; Kawamoto, K.; Nishida, N.; Koseki, J.; Mimori, K.; Gotoh, N.; et al. Role of pyruvate kinase M2 in transcriptional regulation leading to epithelial-mesenchymal transition. *Proc. Natl. Acad. Sci. USA* **2014**, *111*, 15526–15531. [CrossRef] [PubMed]

17. Warburg, O. Origin of cancer cells. *Oncologia* **1956**, *9*, 75–83. [CrossRef] [PubMed]
18. Vander Heiden, M.G.; Cantley, L.C.; Thompson, C.B. Understanding the warburg effect: The metabolic requirements of cell proliferation. *Science* **2009**, *324*, 1029–1033. [CrossRef] [PubMed]
19. Giovannucci, E.; Harlan, D.M.; Archer, M.C.; Bergenstal, R.M.; Gapstur, S.M.; Habel, L.A.; Pollak, M.; Regensteiner, J.G.; Yee, D. Diabetes and cancer: A consensus report. *Diabetes Care* **2010**, *33*, 1674–1685. [CrossRef] [PubMed]
20. Viollet, B.; Guigas, B.; Garcia, N.S.; Leclerc, J.; Foretz, M.; Andreelli, F. Cellular and molecular mechanisms of metformin: An overview. *Clin. Sci.* **2012**, *122*, 253–270. [CrossRef] [PubMed]
21. Zakikhani, M.; Dowling, R.; Fantus, I.G.; Sonenberg, N.; Pollak, M. Metformin is an AMP kinase-dependent growth inhibitor for breast cancer cells. *Cancer Res.* **2006**, *66*, 10269–10273. [CrossRef] [PubMed]
22. Xing, Y.; Meng, Q.; Chen, X.; Zhao, Y.; Liu, W.; Hu, J.; Xue, F.; Wang, X.; Cai, L. TRIM44 promotes proliferation and metastasis in nonsmall cell lung cancer via mTOR signaling pathway. *Oncotarget* **2016**, *7*, 30479–30491. [PubMed]
23. Li, L.; Han, R.; Xiao, H.; Lin, C.; Wang, Y.; Liu, H.; Li, K.; Chen, H.; Sun, F.; Yang, Z.; et al. Metformin sensitizes EGFR-TKI-resistant human lung cancer cells in vitro and in vivo through Inhibition of IL-6 signaling and EMT reversal. *Clin. Cancer Res.* **2014**, *20*, 2714–2726. [CrossRef] [PubMed]
24. Hosono, K.; Endo, H.; Takahashi, H.; Sugiyama, M.; Uchiyama, T.; Suzuki, K.; Nozaki, Y.; Yoneda, K.; Fujita, K.; Yoneda, M.; et al. Metformin suppresses azoxymethane-induced colorectal aberrant crypt foci by activating AMP-activated protein kinase. *Mol. Carcinog.* **2010**, *49*, 662–671. [CrossRef] [PubMed]
25. Dann, S.G.; Selvaraj, A.; Thomas, G. mTOR complex1-S6K1 Signaling: At the crossroads of obesity, diabetes and cancer. *Trends Mol. Med.* **2007**, *13*, 252–259. [CrossRef] [PubMed]
26. Liu, Z.; Qi, S.; Zhao, X.; Li, M.; Ding, S.; Lu, J.; Zhang, H. Metformin inhibits 17β-estradiol-induced epithelial-to-mesenchymal transition via βklotho-related ERK1/2 signaling and AMPKα signaling in endometrial adenocarcinoma cells. *Oncotarget* **2016**, *7*, 21315–21331. [PubMed]
27. Wurth, R.; Pattarozzi, A.; Gatti, M.; Bajetto, A.; Corsaro, A.; Parodi, A.; Sirito, R.; Massollo, M.; Marini, C.; Zona, G.; et al. Metformin selectively affects human glioblastoma tumor-initiating cell viability: A role for metformin-induced inhibition of Akt. *Cell Cycle* **2013**, *12*, 145–156. [CrossRef] [PubMed]
28. Janzer, A.; German, N.J.; Gonzalez-Herrera, K.N.; Asara, J.M.; Haigis, M.C.; Struhl, K. Metformin and phenformin deplete tricarboxylic acid cycle and glycolytic intermediates during cell transformation and NTPs in cancer stem cells. *Proc. Natl. Acad. Sci. USA* **2014**, *111*, 10574–10579. [CrossRef] [PubMed]
29. Currie, C.J.; Poole, C.D.; Jenkins-Jones, S.; Gale, E.A.; Johnson, J.A.; Morgan, C.L. Mortality after incident cancer in people with and without Type 2 diabetes: Impact of metformin on survival. *Diabetes Care* **2012**, *35*, 299–304. [CrossRef] [PubMed]
30. Cauchy, F.; Mebarki, M.; Albuquerque, M.; Laouirem, S.; Rautou, P.E.; Soubrane, O.; Raymond, E.; Bedossa, P.; Paradis, V. Anti-angiogenic effect of metformin in human liver carcinogenesis related to metabolic syndrome. *Gut* **2015**, *64*, 1498–1500. [CrossRef] [PubMed]
31. Griss, T.; Vincent, E.E.; Egnatchik, R.; Chen, J.; Ma, E.H.; Faubert, B.; Viollet, B.; DeBerardinis, R.J.; Jones, R.G. Metformin antagonizes cancer cell proliferation by suppressing mitochondrial-dependent biosynthesis. *PLoS Biol.* **2015**, *13*, e1002309. [CrossRef] [PubMed]
32. Cabello, P.; Pineda, B.; Tormo, E.; Lluch, A.; Eroles, P. The Antitumor effect of metformin is mediated by miR-26a in breast cancer. *Int. J. Mol. Sci.* **2016**. [CrossRef] [PubMed]
33. Xiao, H.; Zhang, J.; Xu, Z.; Feng, Y.; Zhang, M.; Liu, J.; Chen, R.; Shen, J.; Wu, J.; Lu, Z.; et al. Metformin is a novel suppressor for transforming growth factor (TGF)-β1. *Sci. Rep.* **2016**, *6*, 28597. [CrossRef] [PubMed]
34. Kurimoto, R.; Iwasawa, S.; Ebata, T.; Ishiwata, T.; Sekine, I.; Tada, Y.; Tatsumi, K.; Koide, S.; Iwama, A.; Takiguchi, Y. Drug resistance originating from a TGF-β/FGF-2-driven epithelial-to-mesenchymal transition and its reversion in human lung adenocarcinoma cell lines harboring an EGFR mutation. *Int. J. Oncol.* **2016**, *48*, 1825–1836. [CrossRef] [PubMed]
35. You, A.; Cao, M.; Guo, Z.; Zuo, B.; Gao, J.; Zhou, H.; Li, H.; Cui, Y.; Fang, F.; Zhang, W.; et al. Metformin sensitizes sorafenib to inhibit postoperative recurrence and metastasis of hepatocellular carcinoma in orthotopic mouse models. *J. Hematol. Oncol.* **2016**. [CrossRef] [PubMed]
36. Silvestri, A.; Palumbo, F.; Rasi, I.; Posca, D.; Pavlidou, T.; Paoluzi, S.; Castagnoli, L.; Cesareni, G. Metformin induces apoptosis and downregulates pyruvate kinase M2 in breast cancer cells only when grown in nutrient-poor conditions. *PLoS ONE* **2015**, *10*, e0136250. [CrossRef] [PubMed]

37. Kalender, A.; Selvaraj, A.; Kim, S.Y.; Gulati, P.; Brule, S.; Viollet, B.; Kemp, B.E.; Bardeesy, N.; Dennis, P.; Schlager, J.J.; et al. Metformin, independent of AMPK, inhibits mTORC1 in a rag GTPase-dependent manner. *Cell Metab.* **2010**, *11*, 390–401. [CrossRef] [PubMed]

38. Ben Sahra, I.; Regazzetti, C.; Robert, G.; Laurent, K.; le Marchand-Brustel, Y.; Auberger, P.; Tanti, J.F.; Giorgetti-Peraldi, S.; Bost, F. Metformin, independent of AMPK, induces mTOR inhibition and cell-cycle arrest through REDD1. *Cancer Res.* **2011**, *71*, 4366–4372. [CrossRef] [PubMed]

39. Han, G.; Gong, H.; Wang, Y.; Guo, S.; Liu, K. AMPK/mTOR-Mediated inhibition of survivin partly contributes to metformin-induced apoptosis in human gastric cancer cell. *Cancer Biol. Ther.* **2015**, *16*, 77–87. [CrossRef] [PubMed]

40. Garcia-Martinez, J.M.; Moran, J.; Clarke, R.G.; Gray, A.; Cosulich, S.C.; Chresta, C.M.; Alessi, D.R. Ku-0063794 is a specific inhibitor of the mammalian target of Rapamycin (mTOR). *Biochem. J.* **2009**, *421*, 29–42. [CrossRef] [PubMed]

41. Chen, G.; Feng, W.; Zhang, S.; Bian, K.; Yang, Y.; Fang, C.; Chen, M.; Yang, J.; Zou, X. Metformin inhibits gastric cancer via the inhibition of HIF1α/PKM2 signaling. *Am. J. Cancer Res.* **2015**, *5*, 1423–1434. [PubMed]

42. Bridges, H.R.; Jones, A.J.; Pollak, M.N.; Hirst, J. Effects of metformin and other biguanides on oxidative phosphorylation in mitochondria. *Biochem. J.* **2014**, *462*, 475–487. [CrossRef] [PubMed]

43. Finlay, D.K.; Rosenzweig, E.; Sinclair, L.V.; Feijoo-Carnero, C.; Hukelmann, J.L.; Rolf, J.; Panteleyev, A.A.; Okkenhaug, K.; Cantrell, D.A. PDK1 regulation of mTOR and hypoxia-inducible factor 1 integrate metabolism and migration of CD8+ T cells. *J. Exp. Med.* **2012**, *209*, 2441–2453. [CrossRef] [PubMed]

44. Fingar, D.C.; Blenis, J. Target of Rapamycin (TOR): An integrator of nutrient and growth factor signals and coordinator of cell growth and cell cycle progression. *Oncogene* **2004**, *23*, 3151–3171. [CrossRef] [PubMed]

45. Khaleghpour, K.; Pyronnet, S.; Gingras, A.C.; Sonenberg, N. Translational homeostasis: Eukaryotic translation initiation factor 4E control of 4E-binding protein 1 and P70 S6 kinase activities. *Mol. Cell. Biol.* **1999**, *19*, 4302–4310. [CrossRef] [PubMed]

46. Nobukini, T.; Thomas, G. The mTOR/S6k signalling pathway: The role of the TSC1/2 tumour suppressor complex and the proto-oncogene Rheb. *Novartis Found. Symp.* **2005**, *262*, 148–154.

47. Montagne, J.; Stewart, M.J.; Stocker, H.; Hafen, E.; Kozma, S.C.; Thomas, G. Drosophila S6 kinase: A regulator of cell size. *Science* **1999**, *285*, 2126–2129. [CrossRef] [PubMed]

48. Sun, Q.; Chen, X.; Ma, J.; Peng, H.; Wang, F.; Zha, X.; Wang, Y.; Jing, Y.; Yang, H.; Chen, R.; et al. Mammalian target of rapamycin up-regulation of pyruvate kinase isoenzyme type M2 is critical for aerobic glycolysis and tumor growth. *Proc. Natl. Acad. Sci. USA* **2011**, *108*, 4129–4134. [CrossRef] [PubMed]

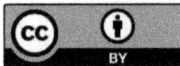

International Journal of
Molecular Sciences

MDPI

Article

3,3′-Diindolylmethane Suppressed Cyprodinil-Induced Epithelial-Mesenchymal Transition and Metastatic-Related Behaviors of Human Endometrial Ishikawa Cells via an Estrogen Receptor-Dependent Pathway

Bo-Gyoung Kim [†], **Jin-Wook Kim** [†], **Soo-Min Kim, Ryeo-Eun Go, Kyung-A Hwang** *
and **Kyung-Chul Choi** *

Laboratory of Biochemistry and Immunology, College of Veterinary Medicine, Chungbuk National University,
Cheongju 28644, Chungbuk, Korea; snubbomed@naver.com (B.-G.K.); kimjinewook@gmail.com (J.-W.K.);
tnals1613@gmail.com (S.-M.K.); gmyich@naver.com (R.-E.G.)
* Correspondence: hka9400@naver.com (K.-A.H.); kchoi@cbu.ac.kr (K.-C.C.); Tel.: +82-43-249-1745 (K.-AH.);
   +82-43-261-3664 (K.-C.C.); Fax: +82-43-267-3150 (K.-A.H. & K.-C.C.)
† These authors contributed equally to this work.

Received: 11 November 2017; Accepted: 5 January 2018; Published: 8 January 2018

Abstract: Cyprodinil (CYP) is a pyrimidine amine fungicide that has been extensively used in agricultural areas. 3,3′-Diindolylmethane (DIM) is a derivative of the dietary phytoestrogen, indole-3-carbinol (I3C), which is derived from cruciferous vegetables and considered to be a cancer-preventive phytonutrient agent. In this study, the effects of CYP and DIM were examined on the cell viability, invasion, and metastasis of human endometrial cancer cells, Ishikawa, via epithelial mesenchymal transition (EMT). CYP increased the level of cell viability of Ishikawa cells compared to DMSO as a control, as did E2. Ishikawa cells lost cell-to-cell contact and obtained a spindle-shaped or fibroblast-like morphology in response to the application of E2 or CYP by the cell morphology assay. In the cell migration and invasion assay, CYP enhanced the ability of migration and invasion of Ishikawa cells, as did E2. E2 and CYP increased the expressions of N-cadherin and Snail proteins, while decreasing the expression of E-cadherin protein as EMT-related markers. In addition, E2 and CYP increased the protein expressions of cathepsin D and MMP-9, metastasis-related markers. Conversely, CYP-induced EMT, cell migration, and invasion were reversed by fulvestrant (ICI 182,780) as an estrogen receptor (ER) antagonist, indicating that CYP exerts estrogenic activity by mediating these processes via an ER-dependent pathway. Similar to ICI 182,780, DIM significantly suppressed E2 and CYP-induced proliferation, EMT, migration, and invasion of Ishikawa cancer cells. Overall, the present study revealed that DIM has an antiestrogenic chemopreventive effect to withdraw the cancer-enhancing effect of E2 and CYP, while CYP has the capacity to enhance the metastatic potential of estrogen-responsive endometrial cancer.

Keywords: cyprodinil (CYP); 3,3′-diindolylmethane (DIM); epithelial-mesenchymal transition (EMT); metastasis

---

1. Introduction

Phytoestrogens of plant origin, such as plant polyphenols, are xenoestrogens that show structural similarity to 17β-estradiol (E2), the mammalian steroid hormone [1]. Phytoestrogens are generally categorized according to four main classes. The first group is isoflavones, such as daidzein, kaempherol, and genistein, while the second group consists of lignans, such as lariciresinol, matairesinol, pinoresinol, and secoisolariciresinol. The third group consists of coumestans, such as coumestrol, and the last comprises stilbenes, such as resveratrol [2]. Among plant-derived xenoestrogens, phytoestrogens are primarily found in fruits, soy, and vegetables. Phytoestrogens are also regarded as sources of cancer-preventive phytonutrient complex because they inhibit the growth and advance of many types of cancer [3–5]. For example, genistein, a major soy isoflavone, and 3,3'-diindolylmethane (DIM), a derivative of the dietary phytochemical complex, indole-3-carbinol (I3C), which is derived from cruciferous vegetables, are phytoestrogens known for reducing the risk of prostate and breast cancer [6,7]. 3,3'-diindolylmethane has been reported to influence the prevention of estrogen-dependent cancers similar to fulvestrant (ICI 182,780), an estrogen receptor (ER) antagonist [8]. Moreover, the in vitro effects of DIM were shown to inhibit epithelial-mesenchymal transition (EMT) and metastasis via the estrogen receptor (ER)-dependent pathway [9]. Previous studies have shown that anti-estrogenic effects of phytoestrogens are implicated in their chemoprevention activity against estrogen-dependent cancers via the ER-dependent pathway [10–12].

The EMT is an adjusted process that drives epithelial cells to lose their cell-cell and cell-extracellular matrix (ECM) interactions and to become mesenchymal cells through genetic reprogramming and cytoskeletal restructuration [13]. The EMT has potential driving forces in the initiation and development of cancer cells [14]. Moreover, the EMT phenotype has advanced migratory capacity, invasiveness, and increasing resistance to apoptosis [15]. Cancer cells that undergo EMT augment the extent of expression of cell motility-related proteins and present improved invasion and migration to other parts of the whole body, resulting in cancer metastasis [16].

It is generally agreed that estrogen plays a significant role in cancer metastasis. For example, estrogens and endocrine disrupting chemicals (EDCs) such as benzophenon-1 and nonylphenol spur metastasis through overexpression of cathepsin D in MCF-7 breast cancer cells via the ER-dependent signaling pathway [17,18]. As a lysosomal aspartyl protease, cathepsin D is related to the metastasis of estrogen-dependent cancer cells [19]. In other examples, BP-1 and octylphenol have been found to induce EMT of BG-1 ovarian cancer cells expressing ERs [20]. In addition, bisphenol compounds can give rise to EMT of BG1Luc4E2 ovarian cancer cells expressing ERs [21].

Cyprodinil (CYP) is an extensive pyrimidine amine fungicide that is utilized worldwide to protect fruit plants and vegetables from many types of pathogens [22]. In fungi, this reagent prevents the biosynthesis of methionine and amino acids of thionic types [23]. CYP gives rise to phosphorylation of the extracellular signal-regulated kinase (ERK) by which growth factors and transcription factors are phosphorylated. In mammalian cells, ERK regulates differentiation, migration, proliferation, and survival [24], and activates ER signaling [25]. A previous study found that CYP as an activator of aryl hydrocarbon receptor (AhR) and induces AhR-targeted genes, such as *cytochrome P450 (CYP) 1A1* in ovarian granulosa cells, *HO23*, and potentially affects reproductive function through activating both the AhR and ERK signaling [26]. Additionally, CYP was found to have the potential to affect ER signaling in our previous study in which it promoted ovarian cancer proliferation via the ER-dependent pathway [24]. Therefore, it can be estimated that CYP may act as a cellular physiological disrupter in the human body.

The present study was conducted to investigate the CYP's action as an endocrine disrupter by examining its xenoestrogenic effects on cancer cell proliferation, EMT, and metastasis by using an ER-dependent and estrogen-responsive Ishikawa endometrial cancer cell line, which is a well-differentiated adenocarcinoma cell line derived from the human endometrial epithelium that expresses functional ER [27]. In addition, anti-estrogenic and anti-cancer effects of DIM were investigated using this cancer model.

2. Results

2.1. Effects of CYP Exposure on Cell Viability of Ishikawa Endometrial Cancer Cells

This experiment was conducted to identify the effects of E2, CYP, and DIM on cell viability of Ishikawa cells and determine the optimal concentrations of E2, CYP, and DIM for subsequent experiments. As shown in Figure 1A, E2 (10^{-9} M) and CYP (10^{-11}–10^{-6} M) augmented cell viability when compared with 0.1% DMSO as a control. Moreover, CYP increased cell viability in a concentration-dependent manner in the concentration range of 10^{-10}–10^{-6} M, implying that CYP has an estrogenic effect at these concentrations. Although DIM did not change the cell viability at 10^{-8}, 10^{-7}, or 10^{-6} M, it inhibited E2- or CYP-induced cell viability when combined with E2 or CYP at these concentrations (Figure 1B,C). Based on these results, DIM was considered to have anti-estrogenic activity, contrary to CYP. Among the concentrations of CYP and DIM tested in this experiment, 10^{-8} and 10^{-7} M of CYP and DIM, respectively, were selected to evaluate the in vitro effects of each compound on the processes of EMT and metastasis of Ishikawa cells. Treatment with 10^{-8} M CYP increased the cell viability of Ishikawa cells to the same level as E2, a positive control (Figure 1A). DIM at 10^{-7} M was selected from 10^{-8}, 10^{-7}, and 10^{-6} M of DIM tested because there was no change in E2-induced cell viability at these concentrations (Figure 1C).

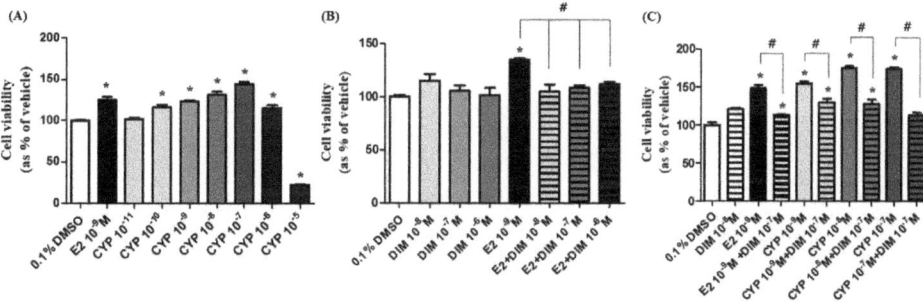

Figure 1. Effects of Cyprodinil (CYP) exposure on cell viability of Ishikawa endometrial cancer cells. Ishikawa cancer cells were treated with 0.1% DMSO as a control, E2 (10^{-9} M), CYP (10^{-11}–10^{-5} M), or 3,3′-Diindolylmethane (DIM) (10^{-8}–10^{-6} M) for six days, after which the cell viability was measured by MTT assay. The experiment was repeated three times, and data were reported as the means ± SD. (A) Effects of E2 and CYP on cell viability. * indicates a significant difference in cell viability by E2 or CYP compared to the control ($p < 0.05$ according to Dunnett's multiple comparison test); (B) Effects of the mixture of E2 and DIM on cell viability. * shows a significant difference in cell viability by E2 or DIM compared to the control ($p < 0.05$ according to Dunnett's multiple comparison test). # shows a significant reduction in cell viability in response to E2 + DIM compared to E2 alone ($p < 0.05$ according to Dunnett's multiple comparison test); (C) Effects of the mixture of CYP and DIM. * shows a significant difference in cell viability in response to E2, DIM, CYP, E2 + DIM, or CYP + DIM compared to the control ($p < 0.05$ according to Dunnett's multiple comparison test). # shows a significant reduction in cell viability in response to E2 + DIM compared to E2 alone or CYP + DIM compared to CYP alone ($p < 0.05$ according to Dunnett's multiple comparison test).

2.2. Morphological Changes in Ishikawa Cells in Response to Treatment with E2 and CYP in the Presence or Absence of ICI or DIM

To investigate the induction of EMT, morphological changes in Ishikawa cells in response to treatment with E2 (10^{-9} M) and CYP (10^{-8} M) in the presence or absence of DIM (10^{-7} M) or ICI 182,780 (10^{-8} M) were observed. After treatment for 24 h, microscopic analysis showed that Ishikawa cells lost cell-to-cell contact and developed a spindle- or a fibroblast-like morphology, which is a phenotype of mesenchymal cells, in response to treatment with E2 and CYP. Conversely, when treatment was applied in conjunction with ICI 182,780, or DIM, most Ishikawa cells maintained a cobblestone-like appearance, which is a typical morphology of epithelial cells (Figure 2). These results indicate that CYP mediated the induction of the EMT process of Ishikawa cells, similar to E2 via ER; however, DIM suppressed E2 or CYP-induced EMT process similar to ICI 182,780, an ER antagonist.

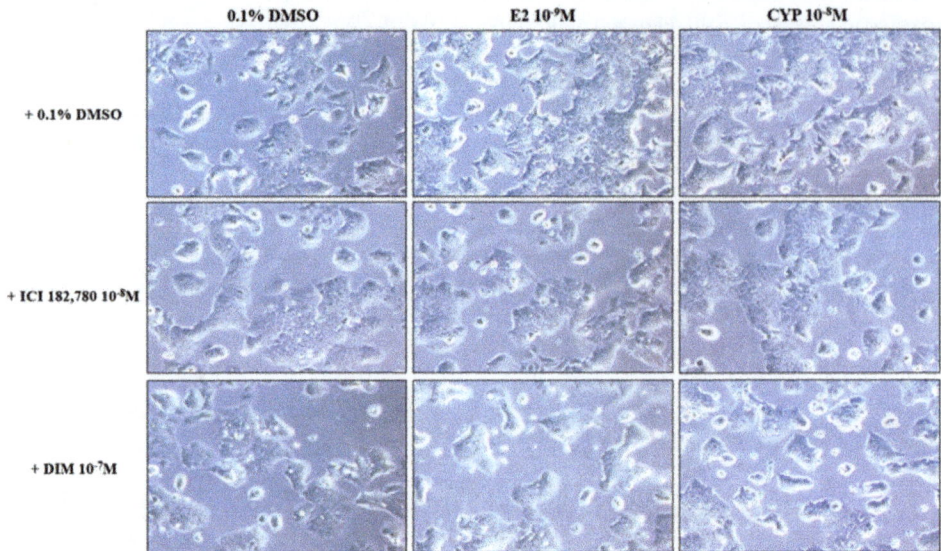

Figure 2. Morphological changes in Ishikawa cells in response to treatment with E2 and CYP in the presence or absence of ICI 182,780 or DIM. Ishikawa cells were cultivated in six-well plates and treated with E2 (10^{-9} M), CYP (10^{-8} M), DIM (10^{-7} M), or ICI 182,780 (10^{-8} M) for 24 h. Ishikawa cells were photographed using a microscope at a magnification of 400×.

2.3. Effects of CYP and DIM on the Expression of EMT Related Genes

The effects of each agent on the protein expressions of EMT-related genes including epithelial and mesenchymal cell markers were identified through Western blot assay. As shown in Figure 3, CYP (10^{-8} M) decreased the protein expression of E-cadherin, a key epithelial marker, by about 50%, which was similar to E2 (10^{-9} M), and by approximately 80% when compared to DMSO as a control (Figure 3A,B). Conversely, when ICI 182,780 (10^{-8} M) or DIM (10^{-7} M) was administered in conjunction with E2 (10^{-9} M) or CYP (10^{-8} M), the expression of E-cadherin was restored to the control level. Moreover, CYP (10^{-8} M) increased the protein expression of N-cadherin and Snail, which are mesenchymal markers, by about 45%, similar to E2 (10^{-9} M), which increased N-cadherin and Snail expression by 53% and 24%, respectively, compared to DMSO (Figure 3A,B). However, when applied in conjunction with ICI 182,780 (10^{-8} M) or DIM (10^{-7} M), the expression of N-cadherin and Snail returned to the control level. These results indicate that E2 and CYP induced the EMT process of Ishikawa cells by regulating the protein expression of EMT-related genes, such as E-cadherin, N-cadherin, and Snail, via the ER-dependent signaling pathway and that DIM inhibited the induction of the EMT process by neutralizing the effects of E2 and CYP on the protein expression of these genes.

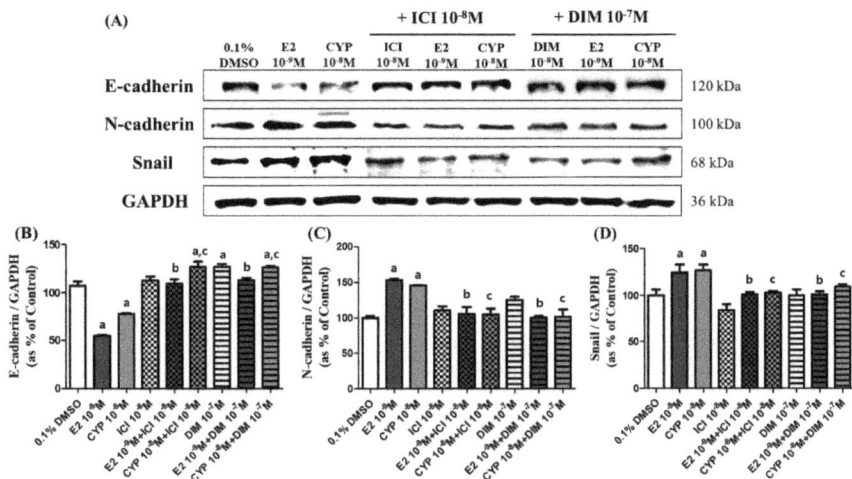

Figure 3. Effects of E2, CYP, ICI 182,780, and DIM on the expression of EMT related genes. Ishikawa cells were treated with 0.1% DMSO, E2 (10^{-9} M), CYP (10^{-8} M), a mixture of E2 (10^{-9} M) or CYP (10^{-8} M) and ICI (10^{-8} M), or a mixture of E2 (10^{-9} M) or CYP (10^{-8} M) and DIM (10^{-7} M), respectively, for 72 h. Total proteins were extracted and analyzed by Western blot. (**A**) Band images correspond to E-cadherin, N-cadherin, and Snail proteins. Quantification of bands corresponding to (**B**) E-cadherin, (**C**) N-cadherin, and (**D**) Snail proteins was conducted using Luminograph II. The experiment was repeated three times, and data are presented as the means ± SD. a: A significant augmentation or reduction in expression of each protein by E2 and CYP compared to the control ($p < 0.05$ according to Dunnett's multiple comparison test); b: a significant reduction in the expression of each protein by the mixture with DIM or ICI and E2 compared to E2 alone ($p < 0.05$ according to Dunnett's multiple comparison test); and c: a significant reduction in expression of each protein by the mixture with DIM or ICI and CYP compared to CYP alone ($p < 0.05$ according to Dunnett's multiple comparison test).

2.4. Suppression of DIM on CYP-Induced Ishikawa Endometrial Cancer Cell Migration

Changes in migration activity of Ishikawa cells treated with E2, CYP, DIM, and ICI 182,780 were identified by cell scratch assay. After the cells were treated with 0.1% DMSO as a control, E2 (10^{-9} M), CYP (10^{-8} M), DIM (10^{-7} M), or ICI 182,780 (10^{-8} M) and scratched using a 1 mL micropipette tip, wounded areas were photographed at 0, 24, and 48 h. Application of E2 or CYP reduced unrecovered wound areas in a time-dependent manner when compared to those of the control (Figure 4A), implying that CYP promoted the migration of Ishikawa cells as did E2.

After Ishikawa cells were treated with a combination of ICI 182,780 (10^{-8} M) or DIM (10^{-7} M) and E2 (10^{-9} M) or CYP (10^{-8} M), unrecovered areas were unchanged at 48 h (Figure 4B,C). According to these results, CYP may induce the migration of Ishikawa cells via the ER-dependent signaling pathway and DIM can inhibit the E2 or CYP-induced cell migration.

2.5. Suppression of DIM on CYP-Induced Ishikawa Endometrial Cancer Cell Invasion

To check the altered invasion capacity of Ishikawa cells in response to treatment with E2, CYP, DIM, and ICI 182,780, a transwell assay was conducted. After cells in the upper chamber of a transwell were treated with E2 (10^{-9} M) or CYP (10^{-8} M) for 24 h, the number of Ishikawa cells that moved from the top chamber to the bottom chamber was significantly augmented (Figure 5). Conversely, when treated with a mixture of ICI 182,780 (10^{-8} M) or DIM (10^{-7} M) and E2 (10^{-9} M) or CYP (10^{-8} M), the number of intruded cells was reduced to the control level (Figure 5A,B). These results indicate that

CYP enhanced the invasion capacity of Ishikawa cells through an ER-dependent signaling pathway, as did E2, and that DIM has the capacity to restrain E2 or CYP-induced invasion of Ishikawa cells.

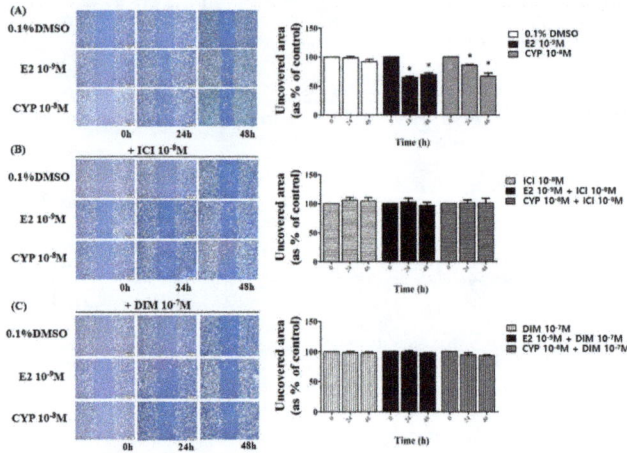

Figure 4. Effects of ICI 182,780 or DIM on E2- or CYP-induced Ishikawa endometrial cancer cell migration. Cells were treated with (**A**) 0.1% DMSO, E2 (10^{-9} M), CYP (10^{-8} M), (**B**) a mixture of E2 (10^{-9} M) or CYP (10^{-8} M) and ICI (10^{-8} M), or (**C**) a mixture of E2 (10^{-9} M) or CYP (10^{-8} M) and DIM (10^{-7} M), respectively, then scratched with a 1 mL micropipette tip. The images presenting the recovery of wounded area were captured at 0, 24, and 48 h using a microscope at a magnification of 40×. The percentage of the wound recovery area at each time point was calculated. The experiment was repeated three times, and data are presented as the means ± SD. *: Mean values were significantly differentiated from 0 h of each treatment, $p < 0.05$ (Dunnett's multiple comparison test).

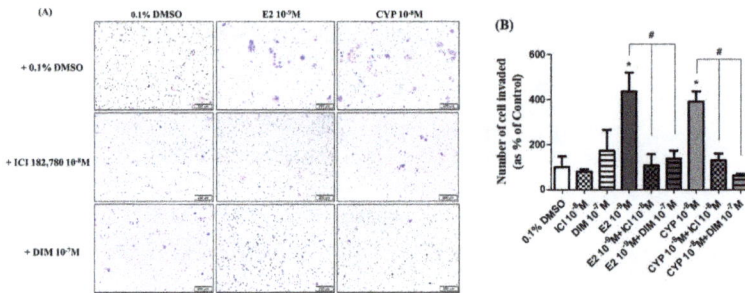

Figure 5. Effects of ICI 182,780 or DIM on E2- or CYP-induced Ishikawa endometrial cancer cell invasion. Ishikawa cells (1×10^5 cells) were cultured in transwells with the bottom surface covered with fibronectin in each well of a 24-well plate for 24 h. Cells were treated with 0.1% DMSO, E2 (10^{-9} M), CYP (10^{-8} M), a mixture of E2 (10^{-9} M) or CYP (10^{-8} M) and ICI (10^{-8} M) or a mixture of E2 (10^{-9} M) or CYP (10^{-8} M) and DIM (10^{-7} M), respectively, for 24 h. The cells attached to the bottom surface of the transwell were fixed with 10% formalin solution and stained with crystal violet. (**A**) The stained cells were detected under a microscope, and (**B**) the number of invading cells was counted. The experiment was repeated three times, and data were presented as the means ± SD. *: Mean values were significantly different from 0.1% DMSO (control), $p < 0.05$ (Dunnett's multiple comparison test). #: Mean values of the mixture of ICI 182,780 or DIM and E2 and the mixture of ICI 182,780 or DIM and CYP were significantly reduced from E2 or CYP alone ($p < 0.05$ according to Dunnett's multiple comparison test).

2.6. Effects of CYP and DIM on the Expression of Metastasis Related Genes

To clarify the effects of E2 and CYP on protein expression of metastasis-related genes, such as Cathepsin D and MMP-9, a Western blot assay was conducted. In cells treated with CYP (10^{-8} M), the protein expression of Cathepsin D and MMP-9 increased by 67% (Cathepsin D) and by 79% (MMP-9), similar to E2 (10^{-9} M; 47% for Cathepsin D and 55% for MMP-9) compared to a control (Figure 6). Conversely, when cells were co-treated with ICI 182,780 (10^{-8} M) or DIM (10^{-7} M), the expression of Cathepsin D and MMP-9 was restored to the control level (Figure 6A–C). These results indicate that the metastasis of Ishikawa cancer cells may be induced by E2 or CYP through increased expression of Cathepsin D and MMP-9 protein in Ishikawa cells via the ER-dependent signaling pathway, and that DIM can suppress the metastatic potential of Ishikawa cells.

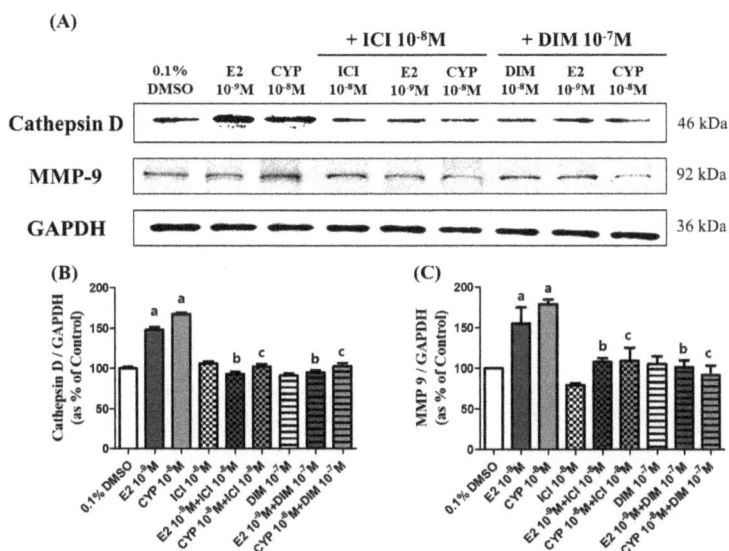

Figure 6. Effects of E2, CYP, ICI 182,780, and DIM on the expression of metastasis related genes. Ishikawa cells were treated with 0.1% DMSO, E2 (10^{-9} M), CYP (10^{-8} M), a mixture of E2 (10^{-9} M) or CYP (10^{-8} M) and ICI (10^{-8} M), or a mixture of E2 (10^{-9} M) or CYP (10^{-8} M) and DIM (10^{-7} M), respectively, for 72 h. Total proteins were extracted and analyzed by Western blot. (**A**) Band images correspond to Cathepsin D and MMP-9 proteins. Quantification of bands corresponding to (**B**) Cathepsin D and (**C**) MMP-9 proteins was conducted using Luminograph II. The experiment was repeated three times, and data are presented as the means ± SD. a: significant augmentation or reduction in expression of each protein by E2 and CYP compared to the control ($p < 0.05$ according to Dunnett's multiple comparison test); b: significant reduction in expression of each protein by the mixture with DIM or ICI and E2 compared to E2 alone ($p < 0.05$ according to Dunnett's multiple comparison test); and c: significant reduction in expression of each protein by the mixture with DIM or ICI and CYP compared to CYP alone ($p < 0.05$ according to Dunnett's multiple comparison test).

3. Discussion

Cancer metastasis, which is the spread of cancer cells by a cancerous tumor within the body, is the primary cause of cancer mortality [28]. In the initiation step of the metastatic process, EMT enables tumor cells to acquire migratory and invasive capabilities through the formation of motile characteristics [28,29]. In estrogen-dependent cancers, E2 was found to increase the metastatic potential by inducing EMT, migration, and invasion of cancer cells via the ER-dependent pathway [21,30,31]. In this regard, EDCs having estrogenic activity are also implicated with cancer progression and metastasis of estrogen-dependent cancers [30,32]. As typical EDCs, bisphenol A, and nonylphenol were reported to enhance the EMT process and migration of ovarian cancer cells via the ER-dependent pathway [12]. Conversely, phytoestrogens exerted anti-metastatic effects by inhibiting EMT, migration and the invasion of estrogen-responsive cancer cells, which is associated with their anti-estrogenic activity. For instance, genistein suppressed E2-induced EMT and the migration of ER-positive BG-1 ovarian cancer cells [33]. Moreover, kaempferol restrained E2-induced EMT and the metastatic behaviors of ER-positive MCF-7 breast cancer cells [10].

In the present study, we investigated the concurrent effects of CYP as an EDC and DIM as a phytoestrogen on the cell viability, migration, and invasion capacities of Ishikawa endometrial cancer cells that are estrogen responsive. A cell viability assay showed that treatment with E2 (10^{-9} M) or CYP (10^{-10}–10^{-6} M) increased the level of cell viability of Ishikawa cells. In addition, E2 (10^{-9} M) and CYP (10^{-8} M) changed the cell morphology of Ishikawa cells from a cobblestone appearance, which is a typical morphology of epithelial cells, to a spindle-shaped morphology or a fibroblast-like morphology, which is typical of mesenchymal cells in the ER-dependent pathway. In the present study, ER dependency of E2 and CYP was identified by co-treatment with ICI 182,780, an ER antagonist, which counteracted the effects of E2, as well as CYP. In addition, E2 and CYP decreased the protein expression of E-cadherin, but increased the expression of N-cadherin and Snail. E-cadherin as a typical epithelial cell marker is a transmembrane protein that is responsible for the adherens junction [34]. During the progression of invasive carcinoma, E-cadherin loss is permitted for a crucial stage causing the EMT event [35]. However, N-cadherin and Snail as mesenchymal cell markers assign an invasive capacity for metastasis to the cancer cells [36–38]. Over-expression of N-cadherin is associated with an invasive capacity of breast tumor by increasing the interactions between tumor cells and stromal cells [39]. Based on the ability to induce the EMT process, E2 and CYP were found to promote the migration and invasion of Ishikawa cancer cells and to increase the protein expression of metastasis-related genes, such as Cathepsin D and MMP-9 [40,41], in the ER-dependent pathway. Therefore, these results indicate that CYP may induce metastatic processes of endometrial cancer cells including EMT, migration, and invasion, similar to E2. In our previous study, CYP was found to enhance cell cycle progression and cell migration in an estrogen-responsive ovarian cancer model in an ER signaling-dependent manner [24].

On the contrary, when DIM was co-treated with E2 or CYP, DIM withdrew E2 and CYP-induced cell viability, EMT, migration, and invasion of Ishikawa endometrial cancer cells, even at the low concentration of 10^{-7} M. This effect of co-treatment of DIM was similar to that of co-treatment of ICI 182,780 with E2 or CYP, indicating that DIM, as a phytoestrogen, has an anti-estrogenic activity that is associated with its anti-metastatic potential to suppress E2 or CYP-induced metastasis of estrogen-dependent endometrial cancer. A previous study reported that dietary I3C, a precursor substance of DIM, prevents the development of estrogen-enhanced cancers as a negative regulator of estrogen [42]. As anti-estrogens, I3C and DIM are known to have anti-tumorigenic properties by targeting ER-alpha (ER-α), and DIM was more effective than I3C at depressing mRNA expression of ER-α in MCF-7 breast cancer cells [43]. Additionally, in a study using thyroid cancer model, DIM was found to inhibit E2-induced proliferation and clone formation of cancer cells in a similar fashion to ICI 182,780 and act as an anti-estrogen by possibly targeting E2-ER signaling pathways [44]. Although the more detailed mechanism for anti-estrogenic properties of DIM in connection with its anti-EMT and anti-metastatic potential in endometrial cancer was not identified in the present study, DIM was found to suppress endometrial cancer metastasis by abrocating the effects of E2 and CYP in a similar way to anti-estrogen.

In summary, as shown in Figure 7, CYP was shown to work as a xenoestrogen by stimulating an increase in cell viability of Ishikawa cells. Moreover, CYP promoted the ability of metastasis of Ishikawa cells by causing the EMT process, cell migration, and invasion through the regulation of E-cadherin, N-cadherin, and Snail as EMT-related markers and Cathepsin D, as well as MMP-9, as metastasis-related markers through the pathway of the ER-dependent signaling. Therefore, the present study indicated that CYP is a risk factor for endometrial cancer progression through activating ER signaling. Conversely, DIM was shown to act as an anti-cancer agent by mimicking the function of ICI 182,780 as an ER-antagonist by reducing the cancer progression effect of endogenous estrogen and exogenous EDCs. However, more studies are needed to elucidate the molecular mechanisms underlying the two conflicting effects of CYP and DIM revealed in endometrial cancer progression.

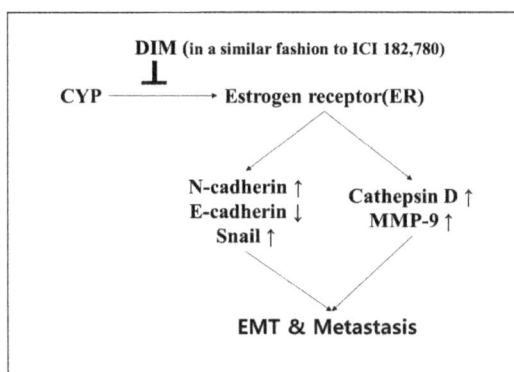

Figure 7. Suppressive behaviors of DIM on E2- or CYP-induced EMT and metastasis of Ishikawa cells. CYP was presented by acting as xenoestrogens via acceleration of the proliferation of estrogen-responsive Ishikawa endometrial cancer cells. CYP also enhanced EMT, migration, and invasion of Ishikawa cells by regulating EMT-related genes, such as *E-cadherin*, *N-cadherin*, and *Snail*, as well as metastasis-related genes, including *Cathepsin D* and *MMP-9* in an ER-dependent manner, as did E2. Conversely, DIM was found to significantly suppress E2 and CYP-induced proliferation, EMT, migration, and invasion of Ishikawa cancer cells, implying that while CYP has the capacity to enhance the metastatic potential of estrogen-responsive endometrial cancer, DIM has an anti-estrogenic chemopreventive effect that withdraws the cancer-enhancing effect of E2 and CYP (⊥; decrease or inhibit, arrows; increase or promote).

4. Materials and Methods

4.1. Reagents and Chemicals

17β-estradiol (E2), CYP, and DIM were purchased from Sigma-Aldrich Corp. (St. Louis, MO, USA), while fulvestrant (ICI 182,780) was purchased from Tocris Bioscience (Avon, Bristol, UK). All chemicals were dissolved in 100% dimethyl sulfoxide (DMSO; Junsei Chemical Co., Tokyo, Japan) and stored at room temperature.

4.2. Cell Culture and Media

The Ishikawa cell line was obtained from E.B. Jeung (College of Veterinary Medicine, Chungbuk National University, Cheongju, Chungbuk, Korea). Ishikawa cells were cultivated in Dulbecco's modified Eagle's medium (DMEM; HyClone Laboratories Inc., Logan, UT, USA) replenished with 10% heat-inactivated fetal bovine serum (FBS; RMBIO, Missoula, MT, USA), 2% penicillin, streptomycin (Capricorn Scientific, Ebsdorfergrund, Germany), and 1% HEPES (Thermofisher Scientific, Waltham, MA, USA) at 37 °C in a humidified atmosphere of 95% air-5% CO_2. To exclude estrogenic components from DMEM and FBS, phenol red-free DMEM with 5% charcoal-dextran processed FBS (CD-FBS) was utilized to cultivate Ishikawa cells and to estimate the estrogenicity of EDCs. The CD-FBS was made in the laboratory as follows. Approximately 40 mL of distilled water (DW) was added to 2.2 g of charcoal in a 50 mL conical tube (SPL Life Science, Seoul, Korea), mixed strongly, and centrifuged at 300 rpm for 5 min. After dropping DW into the tube, 40 mL of the new DW was added. This process was repeated

20 times, after which the DW was discarded and 0.22 g of dextran was added to the tube. Next, 40 mL of DW was added and centrifuged for 5 min at 300 rpm with strong inverting. After discarding all DW in the tube, 40 mL of new DW was added. This process was repeated 20 times. Once clear, all DW was discarded. Next, 42 mL of inactivated FBS was added and the samples were inverted strongly. Samples were then filtered twice with a 0.22 μm bottle filter (Millipore, Billerica, MA, USA), after which they were stored at $-20\,°C$ until use. Ishikawa cells were cultured in phenol red-free DMEM with 5% CD-FBS for conducting the diverse assays tested in the present study. The cells were detached with 0.05% Trypsin-EDTA (Life Technologies, Carlsbad, CA, USA).

4.3. Cell Viability Assay

A cell viability assay was conducted to estimate the influence of E2, CYP, and DIM on Ishikawa cell proliferation. Ishikawa cells were implanted in 96-well plates (SPL Life Science) at a density of 3×10^3 cells per well at 37 °C in a humidified atmosphere supplemented with 5% CO_2. For 48 h, the cells were cultivated in phenol red-free DMEM with 5% CD-FBS. Samples were then treated with diverse concentrations of E2, CYP, or DIM (E2: 10^{-9} M, CYP: 10^{-11}–10^{-5} M, or DIM: 10^{-8}–10^{-6} M) in phenol red-free DMEM with 5% CD-FBS for six days. The media were switched, replaced with identical new media every two days during this period. When adding chemicals to the media, 0.1% DMSO was utilized as a vehicle. Cell viability was detected by the addition of EZ-cytox (DOGEN, Cheongju, Chungbuk, Korea). Briefly, EZ-cytox solution diluted 1:10 was added to each well of a 96-well plate, after which samples were incubated for 90 min at 37 °C in a humidified atmosphere supplemented with 5% CO_2. The optical density (OD) per well was monitored at 450 nm using an Epoch (BioTek, Winooski, VT, USA) to determine the number of viable cells.

4.4. Protein Extraction and Western Blot Assay

Ishikawa cells were cultivated in 100 mm dishes to a density of 1.0×10^6 cells, then treated with 0.1% DMSO (control), E2 (10^{-9} M), CYP (10^{-8} M), DIM (10^{-7} M), or ICI 182,780 (10^{-8} M) or combinations of ICI 182,780 (10^{-8} M) and E2, CYP or DIM. After treatment with chemicals, the proteins from Ishikawa cells were yielded with RIPA lysis buffer (pH 8.0, 50 mM Tris-HCl; 0.1% SDS, 0.5% deoxycholic acid, 1% NP-40, and 150 mM NaCl). Total protein concentrations were measured through utilization of bicinchoninic acid (BCA; Sigma-Aldrich Corp.). Briefly, proteins on 10% SDS-PAGE gel were transferred to a polyvinylidene fluoride (PVDF) membrane (BioRad Laboratories, Hercules, CA, USA). The membrane was then cultivated with primary antibody (Table 1) at 4 °C overnight. Primary antibody binding was identified using horseradish peroxidase (HRP) conjugated with secondary antibody (anti-rabbit lgG (H + L) or goat anti-mouse lgG (H + L); 1:5000 dilution, BioRad Laboratories). Aimed proteins were detected using WSE-7120 EzWestLumi plus (ATTO, Motoasakusa, Taito-ku, Tokyo, Japan). Individual proteins were quantified by scanning the band density on a transfer membrane using Lumino Graph II (ATTO).

Table 1. Antibodies utilized in this study.

Protein	Company	Cat No.	Description	Dilution Ratio
E-cadherin	Abcam	Ab15148	Rabbit pAb	1:500
Occludin	Santa Cruz	Sc-5562	Rabbit pAb	1:1000
N-cadherin	Abcom	Ab98952	Mouse mAb	1:2000
Snail	Cell signaling	3895S	Mouse mAb	1:1000
Cathepsin D	Abcam	Ab75852	Rabbit mAb	1:2000
MMP-9	Abcam	Ab76003	Rabbit mAb	1:1000
GAPDH	Abcam	Ab8245	Mouse mAb	1:2000

4.5. Effects of E2, CYP, or DIM on Ishikawa Cells Morphology

Ishikawa cells were seeded into 6-well plates, then treated with E2 (10^{-9} M), CYP (10^{-8} M), or combinations of ICI 182,780 (10^{-8} M) or DIM (10^{-7} M) and E2 or CYP for 24 h. Before and after treatment, samples were viewed under a microscope (Olympus IX-73 Inverted Microscopy, Olympus, Tokyo, Japan) at $400\times$ magnification.

4.6. Scratch-Wound Healing Assay

Ishikawa cells were cultivated in six-well plates at 37 °C in a humidified atmosphere supplemented with 5% CO_2 until over 70% confluent (approximately 1.0×10^{-6} cells). Monolayers of Ishikawa cells implanted in wells were scratched to the same width and length using a 1 mL micropipette tip, then treated with media including 5% CD-FBS with 0.1% DMSO as a control, E2 (10^{-9} M), CYP (10^{-8} M), DIM (10^{-7} M), or ICI 182,780 (10^{-8} M), or a combination of E2 (10^{-9} M), CYP (10^{-8} M), DIM (10^{-7} M), or ICI 182,780 (10^{-8} M), respectively, then incubated for 48 h. In each treatment group, the images were viewed under $40\times$ magnification using an Olympus IX-73 Inverted Microscope (Olympus).

4.7. Data Analysis

All experiments were repeated at least three times, and the data were analyzed using the Graph-pad Prism software (San Diego, CA, USA). Data were presented as the means $\pm$ SD and statistically analyzed as one-way analysis of variance (ANOVA) followed by Dunnett's multiple comparison test. p-Values < 0.05 were regarded as statistically significant.

Acknowledgments: This work was supported by a National Research Foundation of Korea (NRF) grant funded by the Ministry of Education, Science and Technology (MEST) of the Republic of Korea (2017R1D1A1A09000663). In addition, this study was also supported by the Global Research and Development Center (GRDC) Program through the National Research Foundation of Korea (NRF) funded by the Ministry of Education, Science, and Technology (2017K1A4A3014959).

Author Contributions: Bo-Gyoung Kim, Jin-Wook Kim, Kyung-A Hwang, and Kyung-Chul Choi conceived the research; Bo-Gyoung Kim, Jin-Wook Kim, Soo-Min Kim, and Ryeo-Eun Go designed and performed the experiments; Soo-Min Kim, Ryeo-Eun Go, Kyung-A Hwang, and Kyung-Chul Choi analyzed the data; Bo-Gyoung Kim, Jin-Wook Kim, Kyung-A Hwang, and Kyung-Chul Choi wrote the paper.

Conflicts of Interest: The authors declare no conflict of interest.

References

1. Dutta, S.; Kharkar, P.S.; Sahu, N.U.; Khanna, A. Molecular docking prediction and in vitro studies elucidate anti-cancer activity of phytoestrogens. *Life Sci.* **2017**, *185*, 73–84. [CrossRef] [PubMed]
2. Murkies, A.L.; Wilcox, G.; Davis, S.R. Clinical review 92: Phytoestrogens. *J. Clin. Endocrinol. Metab.* **1998**, *83*, 297–303. [PubMed]
3. Lee, G.A.; Hwang, K.A.; Choi, K.C. Roles of Dietary Phytoestrogens on the Regulation of Epithelial-Mesenchymal Transition in Diverse Cancer Metastasis. *Toxins* **2016**, *8*, 162. [CrossRef] [PubMed]
4. Hwang, K.A.; Choi, K.C. Anticarcinogenic Effects of Dietary Phytoestrogens and Their Chemopreventive Mechanisms. *Nutr. Cancer* **2015**, *67*, 796–803. [CrossRef] [PubMed]
5. Qadir, M.I.; Cheema, B.N. Phytoestrogens and Related Food Components in the Prevention of Cancer. *Crit. Rev. Eukaryot. Gene Expr.* **2017**, *27*, 99–112. [CrossRef] [PubMed]
6. Smith, S.; Sepkovic, D.; Bradlow, H.L.; Auborn, K.J. 3,3′-Diindolylmethane and genistein decrease the adverse effects of estrogen in LNCaP and PC-3 prostate cancer cells. *J. Nutr.* **2008**, *138*, 2379–2385. [CrossRef] [PubMed]
7. Thomson, C.A.; Ho, E.; Strom, M.B. Chemopreventive properties of 3,3′-diindolylmethane in breast cancer: Evidence from experimental and human studies. *Nutr. Rev.* **2016**, *74*, 432–443. [CrossRef] [PubMed]
8. Cao, L.; Gao, H.; Gui, S.; Bai, G.; Lu, R.; Wang, F.; Zhang, Y. Effects of the estrogen receptor antagonist fulvestrant on F344 rat prolactinoma models. *J. Neurooncol.* **2014**, *116*, 523–531. [CrossRef] [PubMed]

9. Lee, G.A.; Hwang, K.A.; Choi, K.C. Inhibitory effects of 3,3′-diindolylmethane on epithelial-mesenchymal transition induced by endocrine disrupting chemicals in cellular and xenograft mouse models of breast cancer. *Food Chem. Toxicol.* **2017**, *109 Pt 1*, 284–295. [CrossRef] [PubMed]

10. Lee, G.A.; Choi, K.C.; Hwang, K.A. Kaempferol, a phytoestrogen, suppressed triclosan-induced epithelial-mesenchymal transition and metastatic-related behaviors of MCF-7 breast cancer cells. *Environ. Toxicol. Pharmacol.* **2017**, *49*, 48–57. [CrossRef] [PubMed]

11. Maxwell, T.; Chun, S.Y.; Lee, K.S.; Kim, S.; Nam, K.S. The anti-metastatic effects of the phytoestrogen arctigenin on human breast cancer cell lines regardless of the status of ER expression. *Int. J. Oncol.* **2017**, *50*, 727–735. [CrossRef] [PubMed]

12. Kim, Y.S.; Hwang, K.A.; Hyun, S.H.; Nam, K.H.; Lee, C.K.; Choi, K.C. Bisphenol A and nonylphenol have the potential to stimulate the migration of ovarian cancer cells by inducing epithelial-mesenchymal transition via an estrogen receptor dependent pathway. *Chem. Res. Toxicol.* **2015**, *28*, 662–671. [CrossRef] [PubMed]

13. Chen, Q.; Yang, D.; Zong, H.; Zhu, L.; Wang, L.; Wang, X.; Zhu, X.; Song, X.; Wang, J. Growth-induced stress enhances epithelial-mesenchymal transition induced by IL-6 in clear cell renal cell carcinoma via the Akt/GSK-3beta/beta-catenin signaling pathway. *Oncogenesis* **2017**, *6*, e375. [CrossRef] [PubMed]

14. Wei, H.; Liang, F.; Cheng, W.; Zhou, R.; Wu, X.; Feng, Y.; Wang, Y. The mechanisms for lung cancer risk of PM2.5: Induction of epithelial-mesenchymal transition and cancer stem cell properties in human non-small cell lung cancer cells. *Environ. Toxicol.* **2017**, *32*, 2341–2351. [CrossRef] [PubMed]

15. Wang, S.S.; Jiang, J.; Liang, X.H.; Tang, Y.L. Links between cancer stem cells and epithelial-mesenchymal transition. *Onco Targets Ther.* **2015**, *8*, 2973–2980. [PubMed]

16. Heerboth, S.; Housman, G.; Leary, M.; Longacre, M.; Byler, S.; Lapinska, K.; Willbanks, A.; Sarkar, S. EMT and tumor metastasis. *Clin. Transl. Med.* **2015**, *4*, 6. [CrossRef] [PubMed]

17. In, S.J.; Kim, S.H.; Go, R.E.; Hwang, K.A.; Choi, K.C. Benzophenone-1 and nonylphenol stimulated MCF-7 breast cancer growth by regulating cell cycle and metastasis-related genes via an estrogen receptor alpha-dependent pathway. *J. Toxicol. Environ. Health A* **2015**, *78*, 492–505. [CrossRef] [PubMed]

18. Garcia, M.; Platet, N.; Liaudet, E.; Laurent, V.; Derocq, D.; Brouillet, J.P.; Rochefort, H. Biological and clinical significance of cathepsin D in breast cancer metastasis. *Stem Cells* **1996**, *14*, 642–650. [CrossRef] [PubMed]

19. Bretschneider, N.; Kangaspeska, S.; Seifert, M.; Reid, G.; Gannon, F.; Denger, S. E2-mediated cathepsin D (CTSD) activation involves looping of distal enhancer elements. *Mol. Oncol.* **2008**, *2*, 182–190. [CrossRef] [PubMed]

20. Shin, S.; Go, R.E.; Kim, C.W.; Hwang, K.A.; Nam, K.H.; Choi, K.C. Effect of benzophenone-1 and octylphenol on the regulation of epithelial-mesenchymal transition via an estrogen receptor-dependent pathway in estrogen receptor expressing ovarian cancer cells. *Food Chem. Toxicol.* **2016**, *93*, 58–65. [CrossRef] [PubMed]

21. Kim, J.Y.; Choi, H.G.; Lee, H.M.; Lee, G.A.; Hwang, K.A.; Choi, K.C. Effects of bisphenol compounds on the growth and epithelial mesenchymal transition of MCF-7 CV human breast cancer cells. *J. Biomed. Res.* **2017**, *31*, 358–369. [PubMed]

22. Karadag, H.; Ozhan, F. Effect of cyprodinil and fludioxonil pesticides on bovine liver catalase activity. *Biotechnol. Biotechnol. Equip.* **2015**, *29*, 40–44. [CrossRef] [PubMed]

23. Kanetis, L.; Forster, H.; Jones, C.A.; Borkovich, K.A.; Adaskaveg, J.E. Characterization of genetic and biochemical mechanisms of fludioxonil and pyrimethanil resistance in field isolates of *Penicillium digitatum*. *Phytopathology* **2008**, *98*, 205–214. [CrossRef] [PubMed]

24. Go, R.E.; Kim, C.W.; Choi, K.C. Effect of fenhexamid and cyprodinil on the expression of cell cycle- and metastasis-related genes via an estrogen receptor-dependent pathway in cellular and xenografted ovarian cancer models. *Toxicol. Appl. Pharmacol.* **2015**, *289*, 48–57. [CrossRef] [PubMed]

25. Huang, X.; Jin, Y.; Zhou, D.; Xu, G.; Huang, J.; Shen, L. IQGAP1 modulates the proliferation and migration of vascular smooth muscle cells in response to estrogen. *Int. J. Mol. Med.* **2015**, *35*, 1460–1466. [CrossRef] [PubMed]

26. Fang, C.C.; Chen, F.Y.; Chen, C.R.; Liu, C.C.; Wong, L.C.; Liu, Y.W.; Su, J.G. Cyprodinil as an activator of aryl hydrocarbon receptor. *Toxicology* **2013**, *304*, 32–40. [CrossRef] [PubMed]

27. Tamm-Rosenstein, K.; Simm, J.; Suhorutshenko, M.; Salumets, A.; Metsis, M. Changes in the transcriptome of the human endometrial Ishikawa cancer cell line induced by estrogen, progesterone, tamoxifen, and mifepristone (RU486) as detected by RNA-sequencing. *PLoS ONE* **2013**, *8*, e68907. [CrossRef] [PubMed]

28. Guan, X. Cancer metastases: challenges and opportunities. *Acta Pharm. Sin. B* **2015**, *5*, 402–418. [CrossRef] [PubMed]
29. Lo, U.G.; Lee, C.F.; Lee, M.S.; Hsieh, J.T. The Role and Mechanism of Epithelial-to-Mesenchymal Transition in Prostate Cancer Progression. *Int. J. Mol. Sci.* **2017**, *18*, 2079. [CrossRef] [PubMed]
30. Lee, H.M.; Hwang, K.A.; Choi, K.C. Diverse pathways of epithelial mesenchymal transition related with cancer progression and metastasis and potential effects of endocrine disrupting chemicals on epithelial mesenchymal transition process. *Mol. Cell. Endocrinol.* **2017**, *457*, 103–113. [CrossRef] [PubMed]
31. Kim, S.H.; Hwang, K.A.; Choi, K.C. Treatment with kaempferol suppresses breast cancer cell growth caused by estrogen and triclosan in cellular and xenograft breast cancer models. *J. Nutr. Biochem.* **2016**, *28*, 70–82. [CrossRef] [PubMed]
32. Scsukova, S.; Rollerova, E.; Bujnakova Mlynarcikova, A. Impact of endocrine disrupting chemicals on onset and development of female reproductive disorders and hormone-related cancer. *Reprod. Biol.* **2016**, *16*, 243–254. [CrossRef] [PubMed]
33. Kim, Y.S.; Choi, K.C.; Hwang, K.A. Genistein suppressed epithelial-mesenchymal transition and migration efficacies of BG-1 ovarian cancer cells activated by estrogenic chemicals via estrogen receptor pathway and downregulation of TGF-beta signaling pathway. *Phytomedicine* **2015**, *22*, 993–999. [CrossRef] [PubMed]
34. Xiao, D.; He, J. Epithelial mesenchymal transition and lung cancer. *J. Thorac. Dis.* **2010**, *2*, 154–159. [PubMed]
35. Zeisberg, M.; Neilson, E.G. Biomarkers for epithelial-mesenchymal transitions. *J. Clin. Investig.* **2009**, *119*, 1429–1437. [CrossRef] [PubMed]
36. Hazan, R.B.; Phillips, G.R.; Qiao, R.F.; Norton, L.; Aaronson, S.A. Exogenous expression of N-cadherin in breast cancer cells induces cell migration, invasion, and metastasis. *J. Cell Biol.* **2000**, *148*, 779–790. [CrossRef] [PubMed]
37. Herrera, A.; Herrera, M.; Pena, C. The emerging role of Snail1 in the tumor stroma. *Clin. Transl. Oncol.* **2016**, *18*, 872–877. [CrossRef] [PubMed]
38. Brzozowa, M.; Michalski, M.; Wyrobiec, G.; Piecuch, A.; Dittfeld, A.; Harabin-Slowinska, M.; Boron, D.; Wojnicz, R. The role of Snail1 transcription factor in colorectal cancer progression and metastasis. *Contemp. Oncol. (Pozn.)* **2015**, *19*, 265–270. [CrossRef] [PubMed]
39. Nakajima, S.; Doi, R.; Toyoda, E.; Tsuji, S.; Wada, M.; Koizumi, M.; Tulachan, S.S.; Ito, D.; Kami, K.; Mori, T.; et al. N-cadherin expression and epithelial-mesenchymal transition in pancreatic carcinoma. *Clin. Cancer Res.* **2004**, *10*, 4125–4133. [CrossRef] [PubMed]
40. Paksoy, M.; Hardal, U.; Caglar, C. Expression of cathepsin D and E-cadherin in primary laryngeal cancers correlation with neck lymph node involvement. *J. Cancer Res. Clin. Oncol.* **2011**, *137*, 1371–1377. [CrossRef] [PubMed]
41. Wang, J.; Xu, J.; Xing, G. Lycorine inhibits the growth and metastasis of breast cancer through the blockage of STAT3 signaling pathway. *Acta Biochim. Biophys. Sin. (Shanghai)* **2017**, *49*, 771–779. [CrossRef] [PubMed]
42. Auborn, K.J.; Fan, S.; Rosen, E.M.; Goodwin, L.; Chandraskaren, A.; Williams, D.E.; Chen, D.; Carter, T.H. Indole-3-carbinol is a negative regulator of estrogen. *J. Nutr.* **2003**, *133* (Suppl. S7), 2470S–2475S. [PubMed]
43. Wang, T.T.; Milner, M.J.; Milner, J.A.; Kim, Y.S. Estrogen receptor alpha as a target for indole-3-carbinol. *J. Nutr. Biochem.* **2006**, *17*, 659–664. [CrossRef] [PubMed]
44. Rajoria, S.; Suriano, R.; George, A.; Shanmugam, A.; Schantz, S.P.; Geliebter, J.; Tiwari, R.K. Estrogen induced metastatic modulators MMP-2 and MMP-9 are targets of 3,3′-diindolylmethane in thyroid cancer. *PLoS ONE* **2011**, *6*, e15879. [CrossRef] [PubMed]

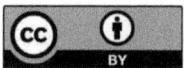

International Journal of
Molecular Sciences

MDPI

Article

In Vivo Imaging of Prostate Cancer Tumors and Metastasis Using Non-Specific Fluorescent Nanoparticles in Mice

Coralie Genevois [1], Arnaud Hocquelet [1], Claire Mazzocco [1], Emilie Rustique [2],
Franck Couillaud [1,*] and Nicolas Grenier [1,*]

[1]   Imagerie Moléculaire et Thérapies Innovantes en Oncologie, IMOTION, EA 7435, Bordeaux University,
      F33076 Bordeaux, France; coralie.genevois@u-bordeaux.fr (C.G.); arnaud.hocquelet@gmail.com (A.H.);
      cmazzocco@immusmol.com (C.M.)
[2]   CEA Grenoble, LETI-DTBS, MINATEC Campus, F38054 Grenoble, France; Emilie.RUSTIQUE@cea.fr
*   Correspondance: franck.couillaud@u-bordeaux.fr (F.C.); nicolas.gernier@chu-bordeaux.fr (N.G.);
      Tel.: +33-(0)5-5757-4750 (F.C.)

Received: 18 October 2017; Accepted: 29 November 2017; Published: 1 December 2017

Abstract: With the growing interest in the use of nanoparticles (NPs) in nanomedicine, there is a crucial need for imaging and targeted therapies to determine NP distribution in the body after systemic administration, and to achieve strong accumulation in tumors with low background in other tissues. Accumulation of NPs in tumors results from different mechanisms, and appears extremely heterogeneous in mice models and rather limited in humans. Developing new tumor models in mice, with their low spontaneous NP accumulation, is thus necessary for screening imaging probes and for testing new targeting strategies. In the present work, accumulation of LipImage[TM] 815, a non-specific nanosized fluorescent imaging agent, was compared in subcutaneous, orthotopic and metastatic tumors of RM1 cells (murine prostate cancer cell line) by in vivo and ex vivo fluorescence imaging techniques. LipImage[TM] 815 mainly accumulated in liver at 24 h but also in orthotopic tumors. Limited accumulation occurred in subcutaneous tumors, and very low fluorescence was detected in metastasis. Altogether, these different tumor models in mice offered a wide range of NP accumulation levels, and a panel of in vivo models that may be useful to further challenge NP targeting properties.

Keywords: prostate cancer; fluorescence imaging; bioluminescence imaging; fluorescence tomography; enhanced permeability and retention (EPR) effect; LipImage[TM]

1. Introduction

New probes for tumor imaging and local therapies are an important clinical need. Currently, clinical developments are mainly based on new radionuclides for positron emission tomography (PET). However, there is growing interest in nanoparticles (NPs), because they offer various specific properties, including high surface-to-volume ratio, high surface energy, and a wide range of additional mechanical, thermal, electrical, magnetic, and optical properties [1–3]. NPs further offer possibilities to combine several contrast agents for multimodal imaging, to be decorated with various biological and chemical moieties and to cargo therapeutic agents.

Determining the distribution of nanocarriers within the body following systemic administration in order to achieve high accumulation of NPs in tumors with low background in other tissues is the major challenge for nanomedicine. NP characteristics have an impact on their pharmacokinetics [4,5], and longer plasmatic half-life favors higher accumulation within the tumor. Such accumulation of NPs in tumors results from different mechanisms, either specific or nonspecific, and involves different cell populations, including cancer and stroma cells [6,7].

The enhanced permeability and retention (EPR) effect [8,9] has been suggested to be the major underlying mechanism of passive NP accumulation in tumors. The EPR effect, although efficient in mice, appears to be extremely heterogeneous—or possibly totally ineffective—in humans [10,11], resulting in low or no accumulation of NPs in human tumors. Since the EPR effect fails in the clinic, new tumor models with low spontaneous NP accumulation are required to screen imaging probes and to test new targeting strategies.

Fluorescent imaging on mice models is a convenient way to initiate the screening process of NP-based imaging probes and to provide key information about NP properties. Although in vivo fluorescence imaging does not discriminate between the different mechanisms involved in NP accumulation in tumors, it allows for rapid evaluation of the overall targeting efficiency [12]. In order to develop new tumor models in mice, the aim of the present work is to study NP accumulation for a single tumor cell line according to different tumor locations. For this purpose, RM1, a murine prostate cancer cell line, was used at different implantation sites to generate subcutaneous, orthotopic and metastatic tumors. LipImage™ 815, a non-specific nanosized (80-nm diameter) fluorescent imaging agent, was injected intravenously to compare NP accumulation in the various tumor locations and types.

2. Results

2.1. In Vivo Imaging of LipImage™ 815 in Mice Bearing RM1-Subcutaneous Tumors

RM1-CMV/Fluc cells were injected subcutaneously (2×10^6 cells/100 µL) into the posterior right leg of the mice ($n = 3$). One week after injection of cells, tumors were monitored by bioluminescence imaging (BLI) (Figure 1A). LipImage™ 815 was then injected into the mice (14×10^{12} particles) via the tail vein and could be monitored by live fluorescence imaging (Figure 1B and Video S1).

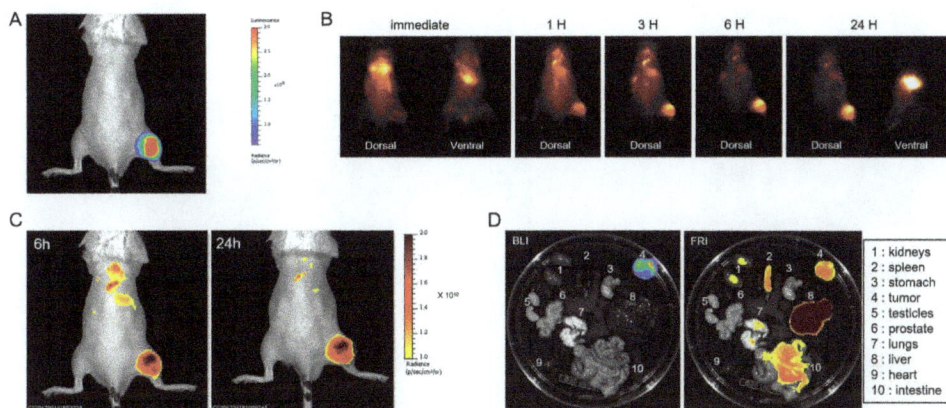

Figure 1. In vivo detection of LipImage™ 815 accumulation in subcutaneous tumors. (**A**) Bioluminescence image (BLI) of a representative mouse; (**B**) Fluorescence reflectance imaging (FRI) of a representative mouse at different time after LipImage™ 815 injection; (**C**) FRI of a representative mouse 6 h and 24 h after LipImage™ 815 injection, respectively; (**D**) Ex vivo BLI and FRI of mouse organs 24 h after LipImage™ 815 injection.

The fluorescent signal was immediately detectable in vasculature, and within a few seconds in the kidney. Hyper-vascularization revealed by instant fluorescence reflectance imaging (FRI) was the first indication of the presence of a tumor on the right leg (Video S1). After 1 h, (Figure 1B), the fluorescent signal had accumulated in the liver and in the tumor. At 6 h and 24 h, both instant FRI (Figure 1B) and dark box FRI (Figure 1C) revealed a high fluorescent signal resulting from LipImage™

815 accumulation in the subcutaneous tumors and in the liver, with limited background fluorescence in other tissues. As shown in Figure S1, LipImage^{TM} 815 accumulation did not interfere with the BLI signal, which increased as the tumor grew. Mice were euthanized 24 h after LipImage^{TM} 815 injection, and organs were imaged by BLI and FRI (Figure 1D). BLI revealed the presence of tumor cells exclusively in the tumor sample. Quantification of FRI signal for ex vivo samples is expressed as photons·s^{-1}·cm^{-2}·sr^{-1}. The highest fluorescent signal from LipImage^{TM} 815 was found in the liver ($1.47 \times 10^{10} \pm 3.14 \times 10^9$ ph·s^{-1}·cm^{-2}·sr^{-1}; $n = 3$). Lower levels were detected in the tumor ($4.55 \times 10^9 \pm 4.22 \times 10^8$ ph·s^{-1}·cm^{-2}·sr^{-1}; $n = 3$), but also in the intestines, kidneys, lungs and spleen.

2.2. In Vivo Imaging of LipImage^{TM} 815 in Mice Bearing RM1-Prostate Tumors

RM1-CMV/Fluc cells ($5 \times 10^5/10$ µL per lobe) were injected into prostate lobes during open surgery ($n = 5$). Tumor growth was monitored by BLI (Figure 2A). Four days after surgery, LipImage^{TM} 815 was injected into the mice (14×10^{12} particles) via the tail vein, and the fluorescence signal was followed by FRI and Fluorescence molecular tomography (FMT) 6 and 24 h after injection. As shown in Figure 2B, FRI revealed a fluorescence signal on the ventral face in regions corresponding to the location of the liver and prostate. FMT provided 3D images of the fluorescent signals in the prostate (Figure 2C) and allowed quantification (Figure 2D). Mice were sacrificed 24 h after LipImage^{TM} 815 injection, and the excised prostates were immediately imaged by BLI (Figure 3A) and FRI (Figure 3B). The fluorescent signal from LipImage^{TM} 815 corresponded to the BLI signal from RM1 cells. The fluorescence signal from LipImage^{TM} 815 in the RM1 tumors was quantified ($1.65 \times 10^{10} \pm 4.22 \times 10^8$ ph·s^{-1}·cm^{-2}·sr^{-1}; $n = 5$). Prostates were further processed for histology. Hematoxylin-eosin-safran (HES) staining (Figure 3C) revealed cancer cells and NIR microscopy (Figure 3D) revealed the presence of the NIR fluorophore.

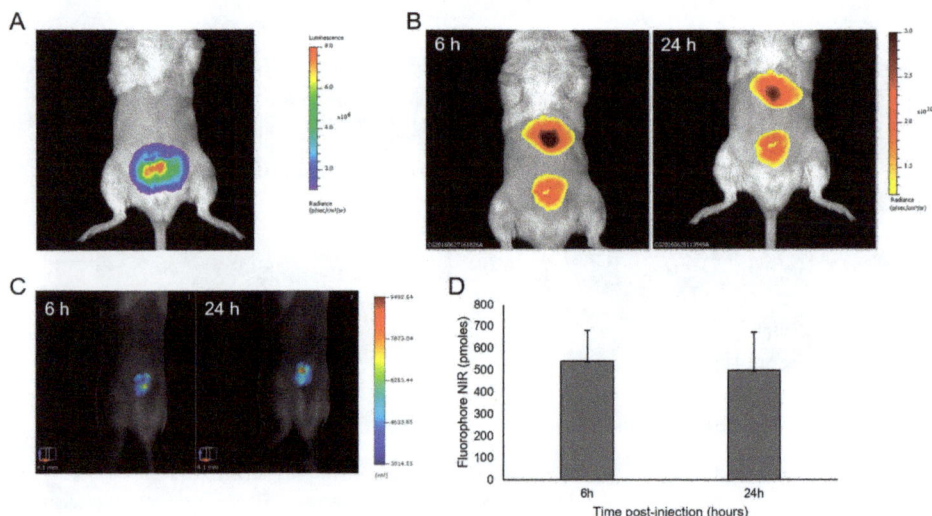

Figure 2. In vivo detection of LipImage^{TM} 815 accumulation in orthotopic prostate tumors. (**A**) Bioluminescence image of a representative mouse; (**B**) FRI and (**C**) FMT of a representative mouse 6 h and 24 h after LipImage^{TM} 815 injection; (**D**) FMT-based quantification of LipImage^{TM} 815 accumulation in the prostate tumor. Mean ± standard deviation.

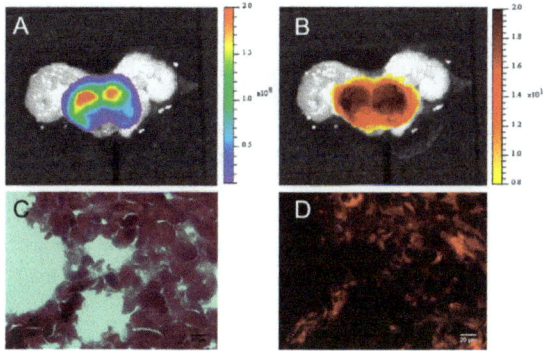

Figure 3. Ex vivo imaging and histology of LipImage™ 815 accumulation in prostate tumors. Prostates were excised and imaged (**A**) by BLI and (**B**) by FRI; (**C**) HES coloration revealed tumor cells and (**D**) epifluorescence revealed fluorescent signals from LipImage™ 815 in prostate cancer cryosection.

2.3. In Vivo Imaging of Metastasis with LipImage™ 815

Intra-cardiac echography-guided injection of RM1-CMV/Fluc cells (10^5/100 μL) in the left ventricle (Video S2) resulted in metastatic dissemination. First metastasis was able to be detected by BLI as soon as 7 days after cells injection (Figure S3; but in the present work, mice were assayed 13 days after injection (Figure 4A,B) (*n* = 11). Six (Figure 4A; *n* = 6) and 24 h (Figure 4B; *n* = 5) after LipImage™ 815 intravenous injection, the main fluorescence location detected was in the liver, but other locations were also detected without a consistent fit with BLI metastasis location (Figure 4A,B, 1st column).

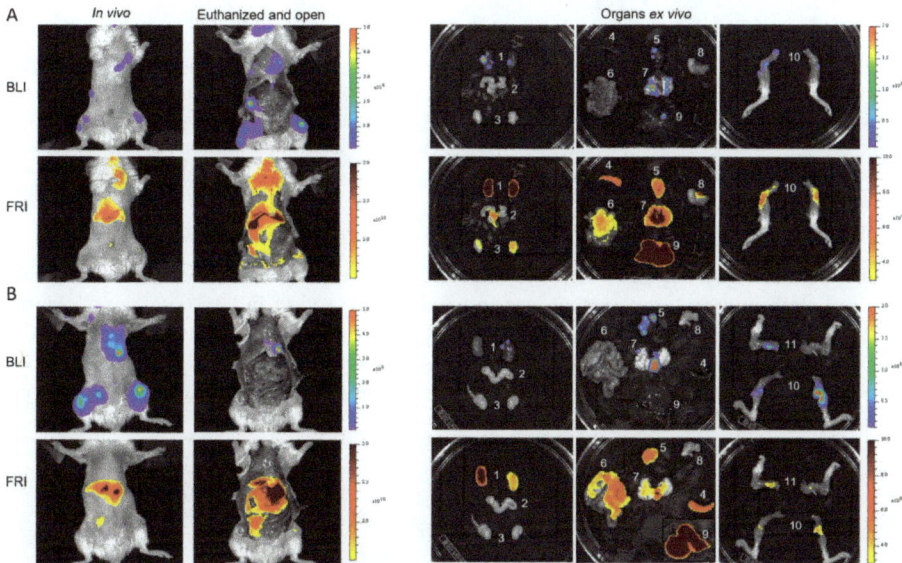

Figure 4. In vivo detection of metastasis. BLI and FRI after LipImage™ 815 injection of 2 representative mice bearing metastatic tumors. Images were taken (**A**) 6 h or (**B**) 24 h after LipImage™ 815 injection first in vivo (column 1), then in euthanized and open mice (column 2). Individual organs were removed and observed by BLI and FRI (columns 3–5). 1: kidneys, 2: prostate, 3: testicles, 4: splenic tumor, 5: heart, 6: intestines, 7: lungs, 8: stomach, 9: liver, 10: posterior legs, 11: anterior legs.

Mice were sacrificed 6 or 24 h after LipImage™ 815 injection. The peritoneal cavity was opened and the skin was removed before BLI and FRI. Again, the liver remained the most fluorescent organ detected (Figure 4A,B, 2nd column). Organs and regions exhibiting a BLI signal were dissected and imaged for BLI and FRI (Figure 4A,B, columns 3–5). Apart from the legs (bone metastasis), the fluorescent signal of NPs did not match the metastatic locations as revealed by BLI. As shown on Figure 5, organs such as the liver and kidneys exhibited high background fluorescence signals throughout the entire organ, and did not exhibit enhancement related to the location of cancer cells. For other organs, such as the stomach or testicles, the fluorescence background was low, and hot spots of fluorescent signal perfectly fitted with metastatic locations revealed by BLI. Nevertheless, the fluorescence level in metastasis remained low, irrespective of location, nearing the background level at $2.31 \times 10^9 \pm 1.44 \times 10^9$ ph·s^{-1}·cm^{-2}·sr^{-1} ($n = 11$).

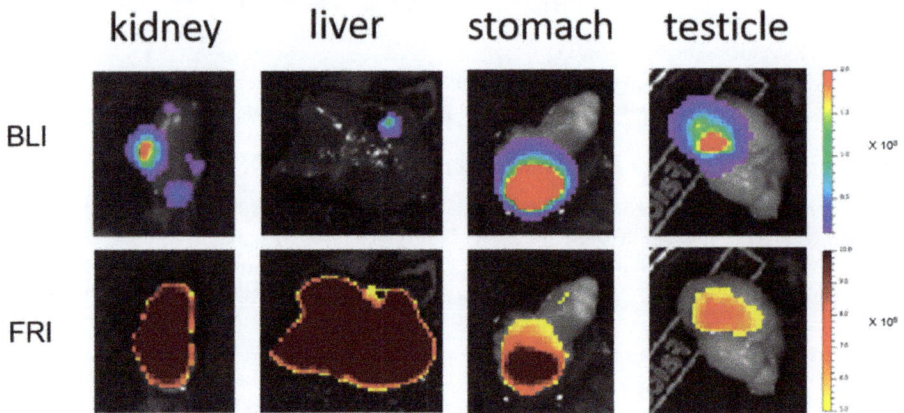

Figure 5. Ex vivo imaging of LipImage™ 815 accumulation in organs containing metastasis. BLI revealed the tumor location and FRI revealed LipImage™ 815 accumulation 6 h or 24 h after intravenous injection. In the kidneys and liver, LipImage™ 815 resulted in a disperse fluorescence signal without detectable accumulation in the metastasis; while in the stomach and testicles, fluorescence coincided with metastasis location. The FRI display scale is identical for all images.

2.4. Ex Vivo Quantification of LipImage™ 815 Accumulation in Tumors and Organs

Quantification of fluorescence signals in tumors and organs from mice bearing subcutaneous tumors, orthotopic tumors, or metastasis was assessed by FRI ex vivo and the data plotted (Figure 6). The highest fluorescence level from LipImage™ 815 at 24 h was found in healthy livers and orthotopic tumors. The fluorescence level in orthotopic tumors was very high compared with subcutaneous tumors, which was, in turn, higher than metastasis. The fluorescence level in metastasis was very low; lower than the fluorescence level in healthy organs.

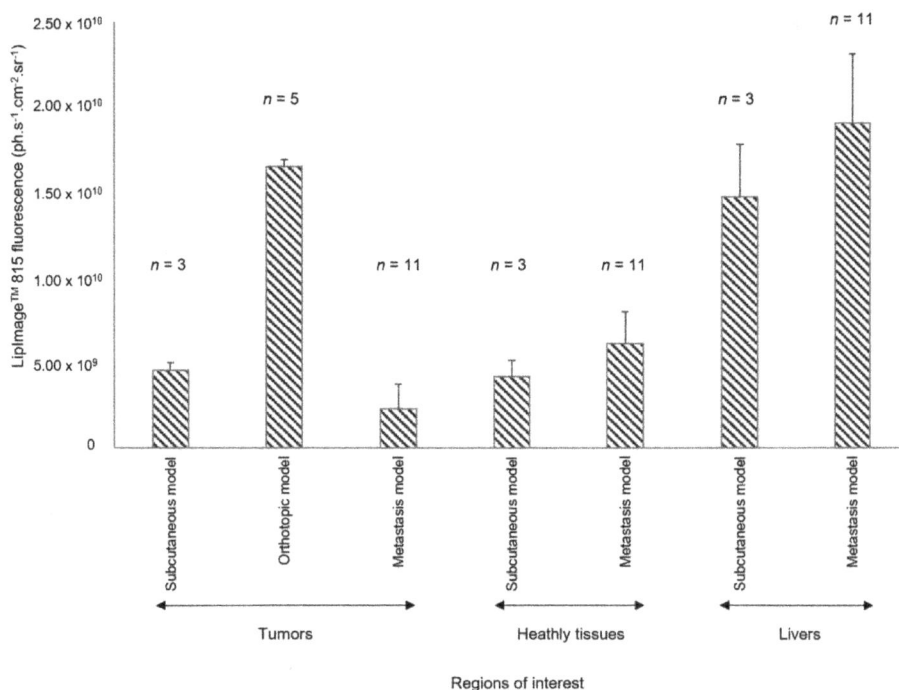

Figure 6. Quantification of fluorescent signal in organs ex vivo, 24 h after intravenous LipImage^{TM} 815 injection. Mean $\pm$ standard deviation, (n) = number of mice.

3. Discussion

Using a single murine prostate cancer cell line (RM1), via different routes, to generate various types of tumors (orthotopic, subcutaneous and metastatic), a constant dose of NPs and a wide panel of in vivo and ex vivo fluorescence imaging techniques, we demonstrated here that the non-specific labeling pattern varied according to tumor type. LipImage^{TM} 815 accumulation was highly predominant in orthotopic tumors when compared with subcutaneous tumors and disseminated metastasis.

RM1 is a mouse prostate cancer cell line syngenic in C57BL/6 mice [13]. It was genetically modified to produce a constitutive Fluc reporter gene and to make in vivo detection by BLI possible, even for small or deep tumors in mice. The BLI signal was not only used to follow tumor growth, but also to compare BLI and fluorescence imaging patterns. As luciferase activity requires oxygen and intraperitoneal injected luciferin (M_W = 280 D) as a substrate, the BLI signal further confirms that the tumors are not hypoxic, and are properly vascularized. RM1 tumors are very fast-growing, providing significant orthotopic prostate tumors in 4 days, subcutaneous tumors in 7 days, and metastasis in 13 days. Thus, the present RM1 models provided a complete panel of different tumor types exhibiting different levels of NP accumulation, making wide screening of NPs possible in a short period of time. On the other hand, the rapid growth of RM1 tumors is not favorable for long term studies, as tumors rapidly reached ethical endpoints. Finally, as RM1 is syngenic in C57BL/6 mice, the tumors grew in a microenvironment more representative of the clinical physio-pathological context. The rapid growth of RM1 tumors is a convenient feature for experimental purposes, but clearly diverges from a human tumor growth rate that may influence tumor properties. In the current work, however, the level of NP accumulation in RM1 tumors is not correlated with growing time.

Present data showed that the level of NP accumulation in a tumor was not a characteristic of the tumor cells, but involved other parameters, including tumor location. As a limitation of the present study, the different tumor locations required different implantation methods, which may influence NP accumulation. For metastasis, however, the fluorescence level is low, irrespective of location.

The fluorescent signal in tumors may result from several mechanisms, including retention in extracellular space, binding to or internalization in tumor cells, and tumor microenvironment components [6,7]. Variations in NP accumulation in tumors are often attributed to variations in EPR effect. The EPR effect results from hyper-permeability of the tumor blood vessels and dysfunction of intra-tumoral lymphatics drainage; the first mechanism enables nanoparticles to enter the tumor interstitial space, while the second one allows particles to stay in the tumor for a longer time [14]. In the present work, solid evidence that accumulation results from a true EPR effect is lacking. Vascularization is a key parameter for NP accumulation in different tumors types; but in the present work, no information—such as pericytes coverage or fenestration sizes—is available. Regardless of the mechanism involved, our results confirmed that the resulting non-specific accumulation of NPs in tumors is highly variable. Conversely, accumulation found in some other normal tissues demonstrates that these mechanisms are no more efficient within metastasis or subcutaneous tumors than in healthy tissues.

LipImage^{TM} 815 NPs (50 nm) have previously been characterized for their optical and pharmacokinetic characteristics [15], and have been shown to display a long shelf life, as well as colloidal and optical stabilities, with high brightness and strong and long accumulation in subcutaneous tumors in mice [15]. Injection of these NPs in immunodeficient Swiss nude mice with implanted human prostate cancer PC3 resulted in strong and long-term fluorescent labeling of the tumor [15], but data are lacking concerning NP stability. LipImage^{TM} 815 NPs (80 nm) also accumulated in RM1 subcutaneous tumors at 24 h, but their long-term residence could not be confirmed, as tumors grew very quickly, requiring rapid euthanasia of the mice. The post-mortem analysis of individual organs excised 24 h post NP injection showed high accumulation in the liver, but the fluorescent signal in the tumor was about 4 times less, and was not clearly different from those in organs such as the kidneys, intestines or spleen. As subcutaneous tumors grew on the surface, fluorescence from NP accumulation was easily detected, and changes in the fluorescence signal could be quantified. That makes this model quite attractive, as small chemical modifications in NPs induced changes in NP accumulation in the tumor that could be easily monitored by FRI [12].

RM1 orthotopic tumors are deep in the body and thus detection of the fluorescence signal was impaired by photon absorption by the tissues. However, a deep tumor location is more favorable for fluorescence tomography, and FMT allowed for fluorescence detection and absolute in-depth quantification. Both in vivo and ex vivo imaging methods confirmed high levels of accumulation of LipImage^{TM} 815 in RM1 orthotopic tumors. Because they grow in an original microenvironment, orthotopic tumors are relevant from a physio-pathological point of view; but, as they exhibit a high level of passive NP accumulation, they behave quite differently from the clinical context.

LipImage^{TM} 815 accumulation in disseminated metastasis is low at 24 h. Combined with in-depth localization, the fluorescence signal is not detectable by in vivo fluorescence imaging. Tumor localization is made possible by BLI, and a fluorescence signal is detectable by ex vivo FRI only in organs with low background. The low level of LipImage^{TM} 815 accumulation in RM1 metastasis may be relevant for screening new strategies dedicated to circumventing EPR failures currently reported in a clinical context [16].

The choice of animal model necessary for rapid and extensive evaluation of NPs requires improvement towards a more clinically-relevant model for imaging probe evaluation. As illustrated by this study using LipImage^{TM} 815, even when using a single NP and a single cell line, non-specific accumulation clearly depends on a lot of factors, including tumor type and location. Other factors, such as tumor size, injection routes, doses and injection scheme, may further influence NP accumulation. Although it is not wholly representative of the clinical context, each tumor type may be useful for challenging NP properties.

4. Materials and Methods

4.1. Animal Handling and Tumor Generation

Animal manipulations, approved by the local ethical committee (CEEA 50) under agreement A50120196, were performed in agreement with French and European directives on the care and use of animals. B6 Albino (B6N-Tyr^{c-Brd}/BrdCrCrl) mice (6- to 8-weeks-old) were maintained in standard conditions under a 12-h light/dark cycle with water and food provided ad libitum at the University of Bordeaux animal facilities. Manipulations were performed on anesthetized animals using 2% isoflurane (Belamont, Nicholas Piramal Limited, London, UK) in air.

Orthotopic tumors were induced by cell injection within the prostate on anesthetized mice. The skin and the abdominal muscles were incised by a short section and the seminal glands were pulled back outside the body. Cells (5×10^5/10 μL per lobe) were injected in the two dorsal prostate lobes and the seminal glands returned to the abdomen. The incision was then closed with sutures. Metastasis was induced by intra-cardiac cell injection (1×10^5/100 μL) in the left ventricle with ultrasound guidance on anesthetized mice. Subcutaneous tumors were generated by cell injection (2×10^6/100 μL) in the posterior right leg. Before the imaging session, regions to be imaged were shaved with clippers and depilatory cream. LipImage^{TM} 815 (31.5 μM of NIR fluorophore) were injected via the tail vein. After in vivo imaging, organs were removed from euthanized mice and placed in cold phosphate-buffered saline (PBS) in a petri dish and imaged ex vivo.

4.2. LipImage^{TM} 815 Synthesis and Characterization

The IR780-lipid dye was first synthetized [15]. An oil premix with, respectively, 85, 255, and 65 mg of oil, Suppocire NB™ (Gattefosse S.A., Saint-Priest, France) and lecithin was prepared. IR780-lipid dye solution (10 mg/mL; 200 μL) in ethanol was poured into a 5-mL vial and mixed with the oil premix melted at 50 °C. The mixture was homogenized and the solvent was then evaporated under argon flux. After homogenization at 50 °C, the continuous aqueous phase, composed of 345 mg of Myrj^{TM} S40 (Croda Uniquema; Chocques, France) and the appropriate amount of aqueous solution (154 mM NaCl qs 2 mL), was introduced. The mixture was placed in a water bath at 50 °C and was then sonicated for 5 min using a VCX750 Ultrasonic processor (power output 190 W, 3-mm probe diameter, Sonics). LipImage^{TM} 815 solution was dialyzed against 1000 times their volume in the appropriate aqueous buffer overnight at room temperature (12 to 14,000 Da M_W cut off membranes, ZelluTrans, Carl Roth, France). The nanoparticle dispersion was finally sterilized by filtration through a 0.22 μm Millipore membrane. Size distribution of LipImage^{TM} 815 was measured with a Zetasizer (Nano ZS, Malvern instrument, Worcestershire, UK) (Figure S2). The number of particles was calculated by dividing the total volume of lipids (total mass of oil, wax, lecithin and PEG assuming an overall density of 1.05 g·cm^{-3}) divided by the individual volume of LipImage^{TM} 815 nanoparticles (size = 74.4 nm; Figure S2).

4.3. Cell Line Generation and Culture

Murine prostate cancer cell line RM1, initially obtained from Dr. T.C. Thompson (Baylor College of Medicine, Houston, TX, USA), was genetically engineered for constitutive expression of firefly luciferase (RM1-CMV/Fluc) as previously described [12], and was maintained in Dulbecco's modified Eagle's medium (Invitrogen, Carlsbad, CA, USA) supplemented with 10% fetal bovine serum (Invitrogen), 1% antimycotic-antibiotic mix (PSA, Invitrogen) and blasticidin (10 μg/mL, Euromedex, Souffelweyersheim, France). Cell line was maintained in a humidified 5% CO_2 incubator at 37 °C.

4.4. Bioluminescence Imaging (BLI)

BLI was performed at Vivoptic (UMS 3767—Univ. Bordeaux) using Lumina LT (Perkin Elmer Inc., Boston, MA, USA). Mice received an intra-peritoneal injection of D-luciferin (2.9 mg in 100 μL PBS, Promega, Madison, WI, USA), and were anesthetized 5 min later. Bioluminescence images (1 min,

4 × 4 binning) and photographs (100 ms) were acquired successively 8 min after D-luciferin injection. Images acquisition and analysis were performed using Living Image software.

4.5. Fluorescence Reflectance Imaging (FRI)

FRI was performed using the Lumina LT apparatus (Perkin Elmer, Boston, MA, USA) with the 745 nm excitation filter and the 810–875 nm emission filter. Fluorescence images (1 s, 4 × 4 binning) and photographs (100 ms) were acquired successively, and analyzed using Living Image software. FRI signal is expressed as photons·s^{-1}·cm^{-2}·sr^{-1}.

FRI was also performed using the per-operatory camera system Fluobeam® (Fluoptics, Grenoble, France) at a spectral window of excitation of 780 nm and with an emission of 820 nm. The image was analyzed using Image J software.

4.6. Fluorescence Molecular Tomography (FMT)

Mice were imaged in a Fluorescence Molecular Tomograph (FMT®) 4000 (Perkin Elmer, Boston, MA, USA). Scanning was performed using the 745 channel, and the fluorescence signal was filtered with the 770–800 nm filter emission. The images were reconstructed and analyzed using the TrueQuant software.

4.7. Histology and Microscopic Imaging

Tumors were frozen and stored at −80 °C. Tumor slices (10 μm) were obtained, fixed with 4% paraformaldehyde (10 min, room temperature), and hematoxylin-eosin-safran staining was performed. LipImage™ 815 fluorescence detection was performed using Leica DM 5500 microscope fitted with pE-100 (Ex 770 nm) Cool LED and a indocyanine (775/845 nm) filter (Leica Microsystems, Wetzlar, Germany).

Supplementary Materials: Supplementary materials can be found at www.mdpi.com/1422-0067/18/12/2584/s1.

Acknowledgments: We thank Pierre Costet and Laetitia Medan (Univ. Bordeaux) for animal breeding and care. This work was supported in part by public grants from the French Agence Nationale de la Recherche: BITUM (ANR-10-IANN-007), Labex TRAIL (ANR-10-LABX-57), France Life Imaging (ANR-11-INBS-006) and Ligue Nationale contre le Cancer (Comité Aquitaine).

Author Contributions: Coralie Genevois performed mouse handling and imaging experiments. Emilie Rustique performed LipImage™ 815 synthesis and characterization, Claire Mazocco generated cell lines and Arnaud Hocquelet performed image-guided cardiac injection. Coralie Genevois, Franck Couillaud and Nicolas Grenier wrote the manuscript with input from all authors. All authors conceived and designed the experiments, and read and approved the final manuscript.

Conflicts of Interest: The authors declare no conflict of interest.

References

1. Burda, C.; Chen, X.; Narayanan, R.; El-Sayed, M.A. Chemistry and properties of nanocrystals of different shapes. *Chem. Rev.* **2005**, *105*, 1025–1102. [CrossRef] [PubMed]
2. Chen, G.; Roy, I.; Yang, C.; Prasad, P.N. Nanochemistry and Nanomedicine for Nanoparticle-based Diagnostics and Therapy. *Chem. Rev.* **2016**, *116*, 2826–2885. [CrossRef] [PubMed]
3. Li, X.; Zhang, X.-N.; Li, X.-D.; Chang, J. Multimodality imaging in nanomedicine and nanotheranostics. *Cancer Biol. Med.* **2016**, *13*, 339–348. [CrossRef] [PubMed]
4. Sanhai, W.R.; Sakamoto, J.H.; Canady, R.; Ferrari, M. Seven challenges for nanomedicine. *Nat. Nanotechnol.* **2008**, *3*, 242–244. [CrossRef] [PubMed]
5. Bertrand, N.; Wu, J.; Xu, X.; Kamaly, N.; Farokhzad, O.C. Cancer nanotechnology: The impact of passive and active targeting in the era of modern cancer biology. *Adv. Drug Deliv. Rev.* **2014**, *66*, 2–25. [CrossRef] [PubMed]

6.   Siegler, E.L.; Kim, Y.J.; Wang, P. Nanomedicine targeting the tumor microenvironment: Therapeutic strategies to inhibit angiogenesis, remodel matrix, and modulate immune responses. *J. Cell. Immunother.* **2016**, *2*, 69–78. [CrossRef]

7.   Kanapathipillai, M.; Brock, A.; Ingber, D.E. Nanoparticle targeting of anti-cancer drugs that alter intracellular signaling or influence the tumor microenvironment. *Adv. Drug Deliv. Rev.* **2014**, *79–80*, 107–118. [CrossRef] [PubMed]

8.   Matsumura, Y.; Maeda, H. A New Concept for Macromolecular Therapeutics in Cancer Chemotherapy: Mechanism of Tumoritropic Accumulation of Proteins and the Antitumor Agent Smancs. *Cancer Res.* **1986**, *46*, 6387–6392. [PubMed]

9.   Maeda, H. Macromolecular therapeutics in cancer treatment: The EPR effect and beyond. *J. Controll. Release* **2012**, *164*, 138–144. [CrossRef] [PubMed]

10.   Nichols, J.W.; Bae, Y.H. EPR: Evidence and fallacy. *J. Controll. Release* **2014**, *190*, 451–464. [CrossRef] [PubMed]

11.   Danhier, F. To exploit the tumor microenvironment: Since the EPR effect fails in the clinic, what is the future of nanomedicine? *J. Controll. Release* **2016**, *244*, 108–121. [CrossRef] [PubMed]

12.   Adumeau, L.; Genevois, C.; Roudier, L.; Schatz, C.; Couillaud, F.; Mornet, S. Impact of surface grafting density of PEG macromolecules on dually fluorescent silica nanoparticles used for the in vivo imaging of subcutaneous tumors. *Biochim. Biophys. Acta* **2017**, *1861*, 1587–1596. [CrossRef] [PubMed]

13.   Baley, P.A.; Yoshida, K.; Qian, W.; Sehgal, I.; Thompson, T.C. Progression to androgen insensitivity in a novelin vitro mouse model for prostate cancer. *J. Steroid Biochem. Mol. Biol.* **1995**, *52*, 403–413. [CrossRef]

14.   Stylianopoulos, T.; Jain, R.K. Design considerations for nanotherapeutics in oncology. *Nanomed. Nanotechnol. Biol. Med.* **2015**, *11*, 1893–1907. [CrossRef] [PubMed]

15.   Jacquart, A.; Kéramidas, M.; Vollaire, J.; Boisgard, R.; Pottier, G.; Rustique, E.; Mittler, F.; Navarro, F.P.; Boutet, J.; Coll, J.-L.; et al. LipImageTM 815: Novel dye-loaded lipid nanoparticles for long-term and sensitive in vivo near-infrared fluorescence imaging. *J. Biomed. Opt.* **2013**, *18*, 101311. [CrossRef] [PubMed]

16.   Khawar, I.A.; Kim, J.H.; Kuh, H.-J. Improving drug delivery to solid tumors: Priming the tumor microenvironment. *J. Controll. Release* **2015**, *201*, 78–89. [CrossRef] [PubMed]

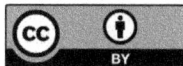

International Journal of
Molecular Sciences

MDPI

Article

SMAD2 Inactivation Inhibits CLDN6 Methylation to Suppress Migration and Invasion of Breast Cancer Cells

Yan Lu [1,†], Liping Wang [1,2,†], Hairi Li [3], Yanru Li [1], Yang Ruan [1], Dongjing Lin [1], Minlan Yang [1], Xiangshu Jin [1], Yantong Guo [1], Xiaoli Zhang [1] and Chengshi Quan [1,*]

[1] The Key Laboratory of Pathobiology, Ministry of Education, College of Basic Medical Sciences, Jilin University, Changchun 130021, China; luyanw87@gmail.com (Y.L.); wlp1008@qmu.edu.cn (L.W.); hairili@ucsd.edu (H.L.); liyr@jlu.edu.cn (Y.L.); dynee@jlu.edu.cn (Y.R.); luyan13@mails.jlu.edu.cn (D.L.); yangml14@mails.jlu.edu.cn (M.Y.); jinxs14@mails.jlu.edu.cn (X.J.); guoyt16@mails.jlu.edu.cn (Y.G.); xiaoli16@mails.jlu.edu.cn (X.Z.)

[2] Clinical Pathology Research Center, Department of Pathobiology, Qiqihar Medical University, Qiqihaer 161006, China

[3] Department of Cellular and Molecular Medicine, University of California, San Diego, La Jolla, CA 92093-0651, USA; lihairi@yahoo.com

* Correspondence: quancs@jlu.edu.cn; Tel.: +86-431-8561-9481; Fax: +86-431-8561-9469

† These authors contributed equally to this work.

Received: 23 May 2017; Accepted: 22 August 2017; Published: 30 August 2017

Abstract: The downregulation of tight junction protein CLDN6 promotes breast cancer cell migration and invasion; however, the exact mechanism underlying CLDN6 downregulation remains unclear. CLDN6 silence is associated with DNA methyltransferase 1 (DNMT1) mediated DNA methylation, and DNMT1 is regulated by the transforming growth factor beta (TGFβ)/SMAD pathway. Therefore, we hypothesized that TGFβ/SMAD pathway, specifically SMAD2, may play a critical role for CLDN6 downregulation through DNA methyltransferase 1 (DNMT1) mediated DNA methylation. To test this hypothesis, we blocked the SMAD2 pathway with SB431542 in two human breast cancer cell lines (MCF-7 and SKBR-3). Our results showed that treatment with SB431542 led to a decrease of DNMT1 expression and the binding activity for CLDN6 promoter. The methylation level of CLDN6 promoter was decreased, and simultaneously CLDN6 protein expression increased. Upregulation of CLDN6 inhibited epithelial to mesenchymal transition (EMT) and reduced the migration and invasion ability of both MCF-7 and SKBR-3 cells. Furthermore, knocked down of CLDN6 abolished SB431542 effects on suppression of EMT associated gene expression and inhibition of migration and invasion. Thus, we demonstrated that the downregulation of CLDN6 is regulated through promoter methylation by DNMT1, which depends on the SMAD2 pathway, and that CLDN6 is a key regulator in the SMAD2/DNMT1/CLDN6 pathway to inhibit EMT, migration and invasion of breast cancer cells.

Keywords: CLDN6; DNMT1; methylation; SMAD2; breast cancer

1. Introduction

Claudins (CLDNs) are small transmembrane proteins, and 27 members have been identified for this protein family [1–3]. Claudin 6 (CLDN6) is a component of tight junctions (TJs), which maintain cell–cell junctions in epithelial cell sheets. In previous studies, we demonstrated that CLDN6 mitigated the malignant phenotype of MCF-7 breast cancer cells, and the expression of CLDN6 was undetectable or at low levels in human breast cancer cells [4]. Similarly, silencing of CLDN6 enhanced migration ability of the human breast epithelium cell line HBL-100 [5]. Epithelial to mesenchymal transition

(EMT) is one of the mechanisms of tumor migration and invasion [6–8]. During the initial stage of EMT, the expression of epithelial genes is suppressed, whereas mesenchymal marker expression is increased [9]. We believe that CLDN6 may inhibit migration and invasion of cancer cells via EMT suppression. However, the exact mechanism underlying CLDN6 downregulation remains unclear.

DNA methyltransferases (DNMTs) lead to ectopic methylation and gene silencing. De novo methylation is established by DNA methyltransferase 3 alpha (DNMT3A) and DNA methyltransferase 3 beta (DNMT3B) in early development. Once established, the methylation patterns are faithfully maintained by DNA methyltransferase 1 (DNMT1) [10,11]. Our previous study showed that CLDN6 silencing in breast cancer cells was associated with DNMT1 mediated DNA methylation [12]. Furthermore, DNMT1 is regulated by transforming growth factor (TGF)β/SMADs pathway. In this pathway, TGFβ regulates the transcription of downstream genes via the translocation of SMAD2/3 into the nucleus and then the formation of transcriptional complexes [13]. Therefore, we hypothesize that SMAD2 plays a critical role in regulating the expression and activity of DNMT1, the upregulation of which leads to CLND6 promoter hypermethylation and downregulation of CLDN6 expression, which promote EMT and enhancesmigration and invasion ability of breast cancer cells. Our results presented in current study provided evidence in support of the above hypothesis.

2. Results

2.1. SMAD2 Signaling Suppresses CLDN6 in MCF-7 and SKBR-3 Cells

To understand the mechanisms by which CLDN6 is regulated, we used SB431542, which efficiently inhibits the activity of activated activin receptor-like kinase 4 (ALK4), ALK5, and ALK7 to phosphorylate SMAD2, to inhibit the activity of SMAD2 [14,15]. As shown in Figure 1, dose dependent and time dependent effects of SB431542 on the reduction of P-SMAD2 were observed. In both MCF-7 and SKBR-3 cells, the optimal concentration of SB431542 was 10 μM (Figure 1A,C), and the optimal time was 24 h (Figure 1B,D). In all of the following experiments, 10 μM SB431542 was used for 24 h. Simultaneously, substantial increases of CLDN6 protein was observed in a dose and time dependent manner, which is very well correlated with the decrease of SMAD2 phosphorylation levels (Figure 1A–D). We also examined the phosphorylated SMAD3 proteins in the two cell lines by Western blot analysis (Figure 1E). Similarly, P-SMAD3 was also considerably downregulated by SB431542. These results suggest that SMAD pathways regulate the expression of CLDN6, and inactivation of SMAD2/3 proteins restore CLDN6 expression in breast cancer cells.

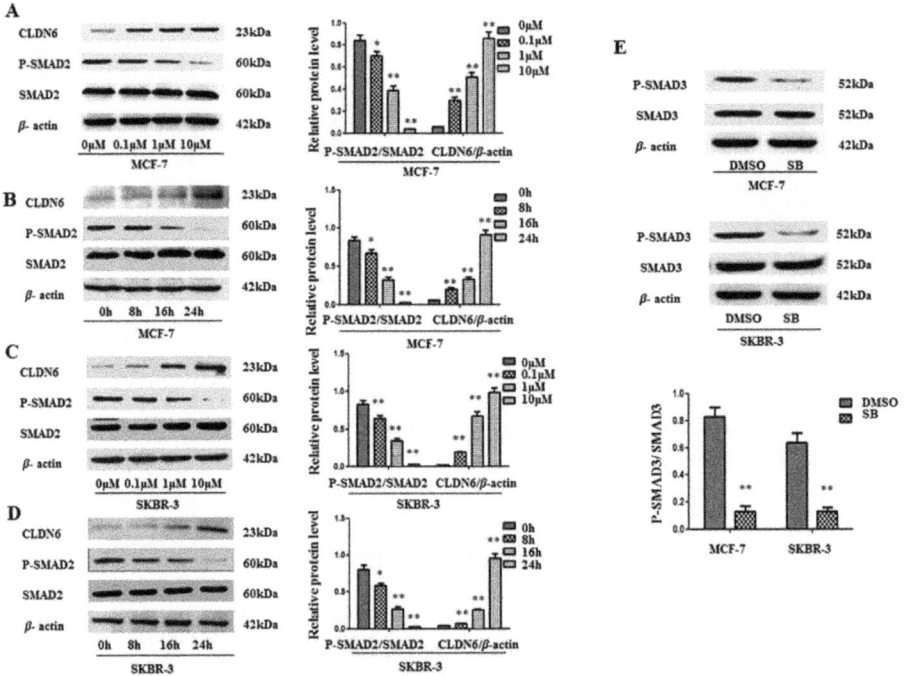

Figure 1. SB431542 inactivated SMAD2 signaling, and suppressed CLDN6 in MCF-7 and SKBR-3 cells. (A–D) SB431542 downregulated P-SMAD2 expression in a time- and dose-dependent manner. SB431542 treatment increased CLDN6 and decreased P-SMAD2. (A,C) MCF-7 and SKBR-3 cells were incubated with SB431542 for 24 h at the indicated concentrations. (B,D) MCF-7 and SKBR-3 cells were incubated with SB431542 at 10 μM for the indicated time (E) P-SMAD3 expression was decreased by SB431542 treatment. Immunoblot analysis was used to determine the expression of P-SMAD2, CLDN6, and P-SMAD3. Results of densitometry analysis of relative expression levels of P-SMAD2 and P-SMAD3 after normalization to SMAD2 and SMAD3 and CLDN6 expression levels after normalization to loading control β-actin are presented (* $p < 0.05$ and ** $p < 0.01$ are considered statistically significant and highly statistically significant, respectively). Bars represent mean ± SE ($n = 3$).

2.2. SMAD2 Downregulated CLDN6 through DNA Methyltransferase 1 (DNMT1) Mediated Methylation

In order to determine whether SMAD2 suppresses CLDN6 expression through DNMT1 mediated methylation, we measured the changes in DNMT1 levels and activity and CLDN6 expression in MCF-7 and SKBR-3 cells after SB431542 treatment. As expected, addition of SB431542 to these cells decreased the expression of DNMT1 and increased the expression of CLDN6 at both mRNA and protein levels (Figure 2A,B), and the activity of DNMT1 was also decreased by 63.76 and 57.14% in MCF-7 and SKBR-3 cells, respectively (Figure 2C). To determine whether SB431542 altered the methylation status of the CLDN6 promoter, we performed methylation-specific PCR (MSP) analysis and demonstrated a decrease in methylation specific regions of CLDN6 promoter in MCF-7 and SKBR-3 cells treated with SB431542 (Figure 2D). We also measured CpG island methylation within the CLDN6 promoter region −300 bp~+200 bp by bisulfite sequencing PCR and found that DNA demethylation occurred at the CLDN6 promoter following SB431542 treatment (Figure 2E). To validate the impact of SB431542 on CLDN6 promoter demethylation by targeting DNMT1, we performed the chromatin immunoprecipitation (ChIP) assay to detect changes in the binding of DNMT1 to the CLDN6 promoter after treatment with SB431542. Consistent with our previous observation [12], DNMT1 bound to the CLDN6 promoter and enhanced its methylation. More importantly, SB431542 treatment substantially reduced the binding ability of DNMT1 to the CLDN6 promoter (Figure 2F). Thus, our results suggest that SMAD2 may regulate CLDN6 through DNMT1 mediated methylation.

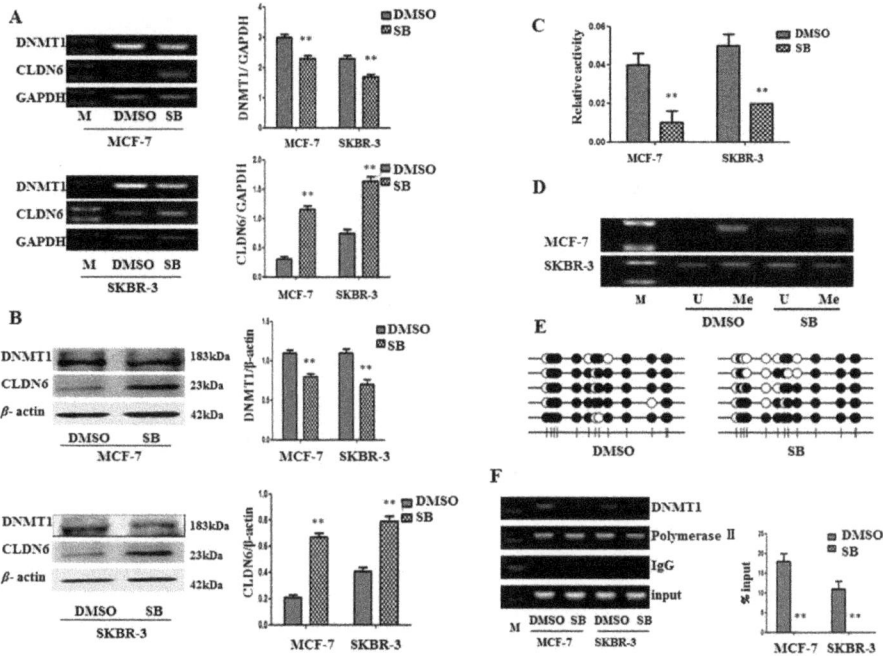

Figure 2. DNA methyltransferase 1 (DNMT1)-mediated upregulation of CLDN6 expression by SB431542. (**A**,**B**) Real-time polymerase chain reaction (RT-PCR) and immunoblot analysis of DNMT1 and CLDN6, and densitometric analysis of relative gene expression levels after normalization to loading controls GAPDH and β-actin are presented. (**C**) DNMT1 activity assays. (**D**) Methylation-specific PCR (MSP) analysis of CpG island of CLDN6 promoter using bisulfite-treated genomic DNA isolated from MCF-7 and SKBR-3 cells. (**E**) CpG island methylation within the CLDN6 promoter region was measured by bisulfite sequencing in SKBR-3 cells. "Me" stands for methylated, and "U" stands for unmethylated. (**F**) Chromatin immunoprecipitation-polymerase chain reaction (ChIP-PCR) assay to detect the binding of DNMT1 to the promoter of CLDN6 (** $p < 0.01$). The lane "M" stands for marker; bars represent mean ± SE ($n = 3$).

2.3. Inactivation of SMAD2 Suppressed Epithelial to Mesenchymal Transition (EMT) and Inhibited Migration and Invasion of Breast Cancer Cells

To explore the outcome of SMAD2 inactivation on CLDN6 regulation, we first detected cellular morphological alterations after treatment with SB431542. It is known that CLDN6 participates in cellular TJ formation and TJ stability [16]. Thus, downregulation of CLDN6 could lead to a more invasive phenotype in cancer cells. Indeed, after SB431542 treatment, cell migration and invasion were examined and significant inhibition of both migration and invasion were found in SB431542 treated breast cancer cells; 38.54 and 35.92% migration reduction and 72.84 and 77.01% cells invasion inhibition were observed for MCF-7 and SKBR-3 cells, respectively (Figure 3A,B). To investigate the mechanism by which migration and invasion were inhibited, we examined the changes in EMT associated genes in MCF-7 and SKBR-3 cells after treatment with SB431542. SNAIL, vimentin, and N-cadherin were found to be downregulated, while E-cadherin was upregulated at both mRNA (Figure 3C) and protein (Figure 3D,E) levels following SB431542 treatment. Therefore, inactivation of SMAD2 upregulated CLDN6 suppressed EMT, and subsequently inhibited the migration and invasion of breast cancer cells.

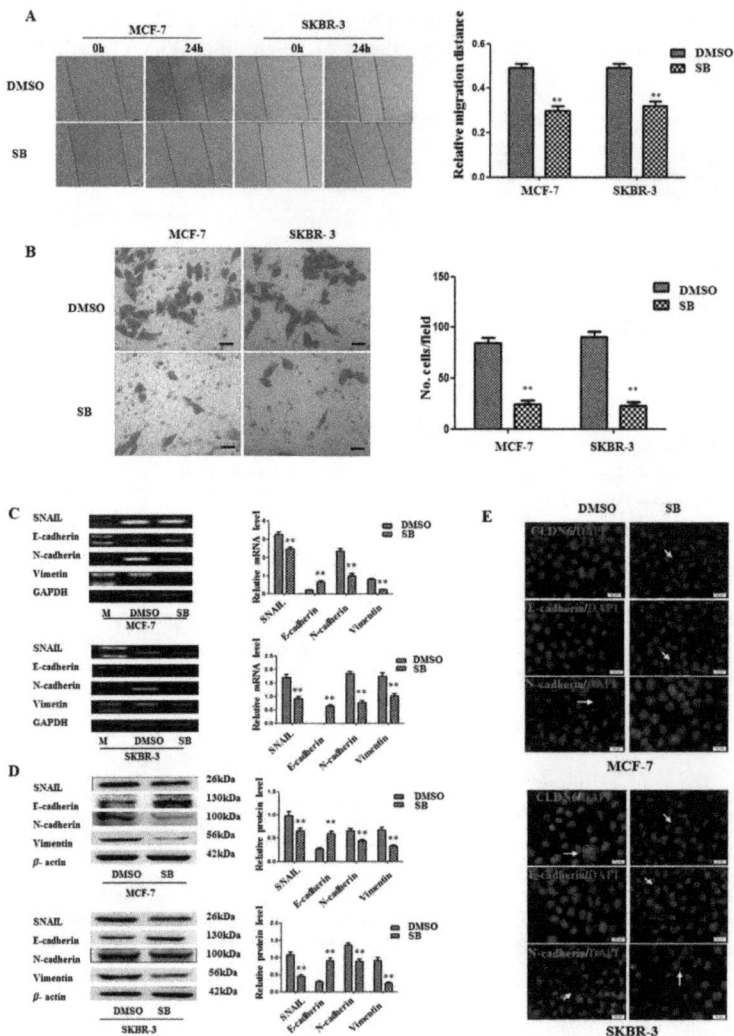

Figure 3. DNMT1-regulated CLDN6 expression inhibited tumor cell migration and invasion by blocking epithelial to mesenchymal transition (EMT). (**A**) Representative light microscope images of wound-healing assays for MCF-7 and SKBR-3 cells after treatment with or without SB431542 to evaluate their migration rate into the cell-free area (bar, 200 μm). (**B**) Matrigel invasion assay. Cells that invaded through the Matrigel were stained with Giemsa and counted. All results are presented as the average of cells counted in 10 fields per condition (bar, 50 μm). (**C**) RT-PCR; and (**D**) Western blotting analysis was used to determine the expression of EMT-related genes (SNAIL, E-cadherin, N-cadherin, and vimentin) in MCF-7 and SKBR-3 cells. Results of densitometric analysis of relative expression levels after normalization to loading control GAPDH or β-actin are presented. (**E**) Immunofluorescence analysis of the expression levels of EMT markers in MCF-7 and SKBR-3 cells. Representative immunofluorescence images (200×) generated using anti-E-cadherin, anti-N-cadherin, and CLDN6 primary and FITC-conjugated secondary antibodies in the breast cancer cells. Blue, cell nuclei were stained with 4,6-diamidino-2-phenylindole. Localization of E-cadherin, N-cadherin, and CLDN6 (red) at the cell–cell junctions is indicated by white arrows (bar, 20 μm). ** $p < 0.01$. Bars represent mean ± SE ($n = 3$).

2.4. Deregulation of CLND6 Is Necessary for SMAD2 Induced EMT and Tumor Cell Migration and Invasion

The observations that SB431542 upregulated CLDN6, inhibited EMT, and suppressed migration and invasion led us to ask whether SB431542 induced cellular phenotype changes were mediated by CLDN6. Knocking down CLDN6 by shRNA (Figure 4A) leads to morphological change of MCF-7 cells into a spindle-shaped cells, but morphological change is not obvious in SKBR-3 cell line (Figure 4B). Furthermore, knocking down CLDN6 abrogated SB431542 mediated inhibition of migration and invasion, as measured by wound healing and transwell migration assays (Figure 4C,D), as well as suppressed the expression of EMT associated genes (Figure 4E–G). Thus, CLDN6 is the key regulator in the SMAD2/DNMT1/CLDN6 pathway to inhibit EMT and migration and invasion of breast cancer cells.

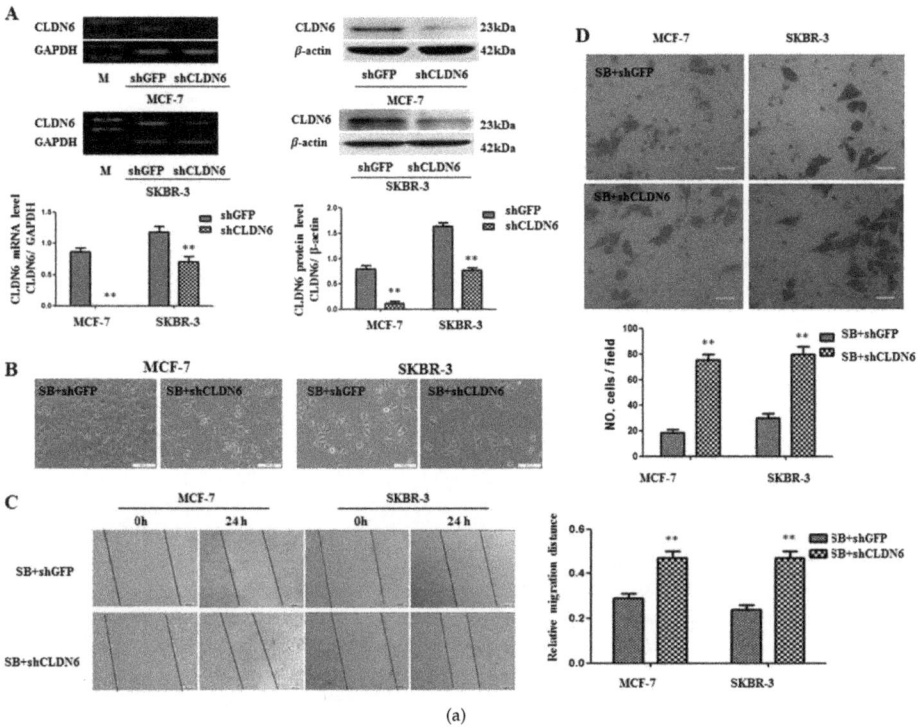

(a)

Figure 4. *Cont.*

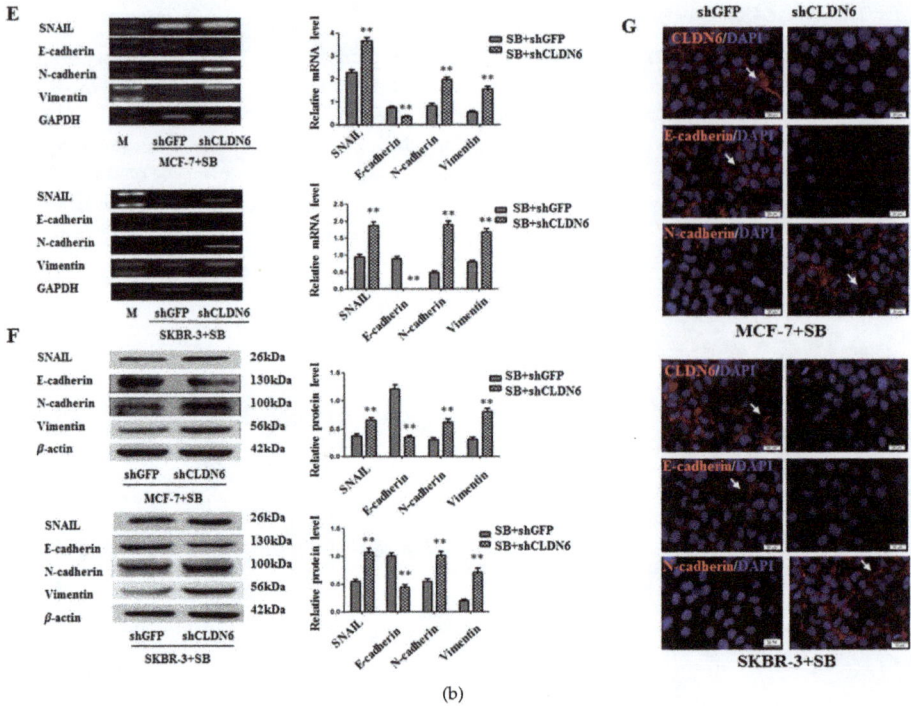

(b)

Figure 4. CLDN6 was required to inhibit EMT and tumor migration and invasion. Cells were stimulated with 10 μM SB431542 for 24 h. (**A**) RT-PCR and immunoblot expression analyses of CLDN6 in MCF-7-shGFP, MCF-7-shCLDN6, SKBR-3-shGFP, and SKBR-3-shCLDN6 cells, and densitometric analysis of relative expression levels after normalization to loading control GAPDH or β-actin are presented. (**B**) The effect of knocking down CLDN6 on cell morphology of SB431542 treated MCF-7 and SKBR-3 cells (bar, 100 μm). (**C**) Representative light microscope images of wound-healing assays for MCF-7 and SKBR-3 cells treated with SB431542 to evaluate the impact of CLDN6 on their migration rate into the cell-free area (bar, 200 μm). (**D**) Matrigel invasion assay. Cells that invaded the Matrigel were stained with Giemsa and counted. All results are presented as the average of cells counted in 10 fields per condition (bar, 50 μm). Results of: (**E**) RT-PCR; and (**F**) Western blotting analyses to determine the impact of CLDN6 on the expression of EMT-related genes (SNAIL, E-cadherin, N-cadherin, and vimentin) in MCF-7 and SKBR-3 cells treated with SB431542, and densitometric analysis of relative gene expression levels after normalization to the loading control GAPDH or β-actin are presented. (**G**) Immunofluorescence analysis to evaluate the impact of CLDN6 on the expression levels of EMT markers in MCF-7 and SKBR-3 cells treated with SB431542. Representative immunofluorescence images (200×) generated using anti-E-cadherin, anti-N-cadherin, and CLDN6 primary and FITC-conjugated secondary antibodies in the breast cancer cells. Blue, cell nuclei were stained with 4,6-diamidino-2-phenylindole. Localization of E-cadherin, N-cadherin, and CLDN6 (red) at the cell–cell junctions is indicated by white arrows (bar, 20 μm). ** $p < 0.01$. Bars represent mean ± SE ($n = 3$).

3. Discussion

In earlier studies, we found that CLDN6 overexpression inhibited the migration and invasion of MCF-7 cells in vitro [4], while the expression of CLDN6 was undetectable or low in several human cancer cells [17,18]. The exact mechanism leading to CLDN6 downregulation, however, remains unclear. We and others also demonstrated that the silencing of CLDN6 was linked to DNMT1 mediated

DNA methylation [12], and that DNMT1was regulated by TGFβ/SMADs pathways [19,20]. DNMT1 possesses a unique capability of identifying the hemimethylated portion of newly replicated DNA. This feature might explain why DNMT1 mediated methylation could be an epigenetic mechanism maintaining the status quo [21,22]. It has been shown that DNMT1 maintains DNA methylation and results in the silencing of tumor suppressor genes [23,24]. Biniszkiewicz and colleagues reported that increased DNMT1 activity led to hypermethylation of CpG islands both in vivo and in vitro [25]. Hypermethylation of CpG islands is also frequently observed in cancer and has been shown to be involved in the silencing of tumor suppressor genes [26]. A recent report showed that DNMT1 plays a key role in the regulation of CLDN4 and CLDN7 by means of the SMAD signaling pathway [19]. Expression of CLDNs epithelial cells is a dynamic equilibrium pattern, high expression of some CLDN member proteins leads to a low expression of other members of the CLDN family [27]. We also found that, compared to immortalized breast epithelial cell line HBL-100, SMAD2 showed a higher expression in breast cancer cells, whereas CLDN6 had a lower expression level in these cells.

In the current study, we aimed to explore the mechanism by which upstream signaling downregulates CLDN6 during mammary cancer progression. The two different breast cancer cell lines used, MCF-7 and SKBR-3, are luminal subtypes of metastatic adenocarcinoma. The MCF-7 cell line is estrogen receptor (ER)$^+$, progesterone receptor (PR)$^+$, and ERBB2/HER2$^-$, while the SKBR-3 cell line is ER$^-$, PR$^-$, and ERBB2/HER2$^+$ [28]. After treating the two breast cancer cell lines with SB431542, a TGFβ type I receptor inhibitor that specifically inhibits SMAD2 and SMAD3 phosphorylation [14,29,30], which leads to down regulation of DNMT1 and upregulation of CLDN6. Furthermore, both DNMT1 enzyme activity and capacity to CLNDN6 promoter were reduced, and simultaneously, the CLDN6 promoter methylation status also decreased significantly. We also measured CpG island methylation within the CLDN6 promoter region by bisulfite sequencing and found that DNA demethylation occurred at the CLDN6 promoter following SB431542 treatment. Our data demonstrated that, in breast cancer cells, the low expression of CLDN6 was regulated by DNMT1 mediated methylation, which was in turn regulated by the SMAD2 pathway.

Similar to our current results, CLDN6 has been found to be silenced by methylation in esophageal squamous cell carcinoma [31]. Besides DNA methylation, CLDN6 also can be regulated by histone modification [32]. Furthermore, in our previous study, we demonstrated that DNA methylation of CLDN6 enhanced breast cancer cell migration and invasion by recruiting methyl CpG binding protein 2 (MeCP2) and deacetylating histone 3 acetylation (H3Ac) and histone 4 acetylation (H4Ac) [12]. Our current study, we showed that DNMT1 could directly regulate CLDN6 through binding to its promoter region. Papageorgis and colleagues showed that DNMT1 played a key role in the regulation of CLDN4 and CLDN7 via the SMAD2 signaling pathway and that the depletion of SMAD2 led to a significant decrease in the amount of DNMT1 bound to the promoter of the target genes, but it did not decrease the expression level of DNMT1 [19], which is different with our current results. Furthermore, SMAD pathways and many major signaling pathways, including those involving Wnt and extracellular signal–regulated kinase (ERK)/Mitogen-activated protein kinase (MAPK), have been reported to be involved in DNA methylation [20,33–36].

CLDNs are the main components of TJs, which have barrier and fence functions and maintain cell polarity, cell adhesion, and cell signal transduction [37,38], and dysfunction of TJs was found to be closely related to tumor development, e.g., CLDN6 overexpression inhibited the migration and invasion of MCF-7 cells in vitro [4]. One of the mechanisms of migration and invasion in epithelium-derived carcinoma was EMT [39] which led to the loss of epithelial cell adhesion and the induction of a mesenchymal phenotype [40,41]. Recent reports have shown that EMT, which is characterized by the loss of epithelial markers such as E-cadherin and the induction of mesenchymal markers, including vimentin, N-cadherin, and fibronectin [42], plays a pivotal role in breast cancer progression [43–45]. In the present study, CLDN6 expression in breast cancer cells was upregulated by SB431542 treatment, and, subsequently, the invasion and migration were suppressed, along with the upregulation of epithelial marker E-cadherin and the downregulation of mesenchymal markers

SNAIL, N-cadherin, and vimentin. Thus, we demonstrated that CLDN6 inhibited invasion and migration by reversing EMT.

Consistent with our data, CLDN3, CLDN4 [46], and CLDN7 [47] have been shown to suppress EMT in ovarian carcinoma cells and lung cancer cells. However, CLDN1 suppressed E-cadherin and subsequently induced EMT in hepatocellular carcinoma cells [48]. The levels of CLDN3 and CLDN4 were frequently elevated in pancreatic adenocarcinoma, ovarian cancer, endometrioid adenocarcinoma, and prostate cancer [49–52], while CLDN7 has been found to be decreased in invasive ductal carcinomas of the breast [53]. This can be attributed to tissue and cell specificity of expression and distribution of CLDNs, which is the main reason for different TJ functions in different types of epithelial tissues [54]. Similarly, the distribution of CLDNs differs greatly in different structures within the same organization [55,56].

TGFβ was first described as an EMT inducer in normal mammary epithelial cells [57] and has been recognized as an EMT master regulator in different cell types [40]. In the current study, we demonstrated that SB431542 inhibited EMT and suppressed migration and invasion of MCF-7 and SKBR-3 cells by upregulating CLDN6 but not the direct effect of inactivation of TGFβ/SMAD pathway. To verify this assumption, we knocked down CLDN6 in SB431542-treated MCF-7 and SKBR-3 cells and found knocking down CLDN6 abrogated the inhibitory effects of SB431542 on EMT, migration and invasion of breast cancer cells, indicating CLDN6 is the key regulator downstream of the SMAD2/DNMT1/CLDN6 pathway. CLDN6 is also an epithelial marker, which was upregulated when EMT was inhibited. It may be confused whether EMT was suppressed before the upregulation of CLDN6. The results in Figure 4 demonstrated that CLDN6 was upregulated and then suppressed EMT in SB431542-treated MCF-7 and SKBR-3 cells.

In conclusion, SMAD2 downregulated CLDN6 via DNMT1 mediated DNA methylation to promote EMT, thereby accelerating the migration and invasion of breast cancer cells.

4. Materials and Methods

4.1. Cell Culture and Reagents

The human breast cancer cell lines MCF-7 and SKBR-3 were obtained from the Cell Bank of the Chinese Academy of Sciences (Shanghai, China) and maintained in DMEM (Gibco, Carlsbad, CA, USA) supplemented with 10% fetal bovine serum (Hyclone, Logan, UT, USA) and 100 units/mL penicillin and streptomycin (Invitrogen, Carlsbad, CA, USA). All the cell lines were grown in a humidified incubator at 37 °C and 5% CO_2. SB431542 was purchased from Sigma (St. Louis, MO, USA).

4.2. Reverse Transcription Polymerase Chain Reaction

Total RNA was extracted from cells using TRIzol (Invitrogen) following the manufacturer's instructions. One microgram of total RNA was subjected to reverse transcription to synthesize cDNA using Moloney murine leukemia virus reverse transcriptase (TaKaRa, Osaka, Japan) at 42 °C for 1 h, and 0.5 μg cDNA was used for PCR. SMAD2, CLDN6, DNMT1, SNAIL, E-cadherin, and N-cadherin were amplified along with glyceraldehyde-3-phosphate dehydrogenase (GAPDH) as an endogenous control following the instructions of the Premix LA Taq Kit (TaKaRa). The PCR conditions and primer sequences are shown in Table 1. After electrophoresis, the gel was imaged and analyzed by an imaging system (Syngene, Cambridge, UK).

Table 1. Details of primers used for real-time polymerase chain reaction (RT-PCR), methylation-specific PCR (MSP), and chromatin immunoprecipitation (ChIP) analyses.

Primer Name	Primer Sequence	Annealing Temp (°C)	Cycles	Length (bp)
CLDN6	TTCATCGGCAACAGCATCGT GGTTATAGAAGTCCCGGATGA	58	35	345
DNMT1	GAGGAAGCTGCTAAGGACTAGTTC ACTCCACAATTTGATCACTAAATC	56	30	141
SMAD2	ATTTGCTGCTCTTCTGGCTCAG ACTTGTTACCGTCTGCCTTCG	56	30	101
SNAIL	GCCTAGCGAGTGGTTCTTCTG TAGGGCTGCTGGAAGGTAAA	56	30	203
E-cadherin	ATTCTGGGGATTCTTGGAGG GGTCAGTATCAGCCGCTTTC	56	30	337
N-cadherin	GTGCCATTAGCCAAGGGAATTCAGC GCGTTCCTGTTCCACTCATAGGAGG	56	30	370
Vimentin	AGCAGG AGTCCACTGAGTACCG GTGACGAGCCATTTCCTCCTTC	56	30	200
GAPDH	TGTTGCCATCAATGACCCCTT CTCCACGACGTACTCAGCG	56	25	178
CLDN6 U (MSP)	TGGATGTTTGTTAGTTTGAGGT ATAACCACAACC CAAATTCACA	58	35	500
CLDN6 M (MSP)	ACGTTTGTTAGTTCGAGGC ATAACCGCAACCCGAATTC	58	35	502
CLDN6 (BSP)	GAGGGGTAGAGATTTTGTTTTTGA AATTAAATAAATTCCCCATATCACC	53	30	210
CLDN6 (ChIP)	GCCACCTGGATGGCCGAGTC GAGGGTTCCCAATTTGCGGG	51	40	191

4.3. Western Blotting Analysis

Western blotting analyses were performed as described previously [12]. Anti-P-SMAD2, SMAD2, P-SMAD3, SMAD3, and vimentin antibodies were purchased from Cell Signaling Technology (Beverly, MA, USA); E-cadherin and SNAIL antibodies were from Bioworld Technology (Dublin, OH, USA); and N-cadherin, DNMT1, and CLDN6 antibodies were from Abcam (Cambridge, UK). The anti-β actin antibody was obtained from Santa Cruz (Santa Cruz, CA, USA). Primary and secondary antibodies were diluted to 1:1000. The blots were stained using an ECL Western blotting system (GE, Fairfield, CT, USA).

4.4. Immunofluorescence

An immunofluorescence assay was performed to evaluate expression as previously described [58]. Cells were incubated with primary antibodies against CLDN6 (1:400), E-cadherin (1:400), and N-cadherin (1:250) at 4 °C overnight. The secondary antibody was Alexa Fluor 647 anti-mouse IgG (1:200 dilution; Cell Signaling Technology, Beverly, MA, USA). Cells were visualized with a fluorescence microscope (Olympus, Tokyo, Japan).

4.5. DNA Methylation Analysis

MSP based on bisulfite conversion was performed. Genomic DNA from cells was isolated using the DNA extraction kit (Qiagen, Valencia, CA, USA), and the methylSEQr™ Bisulfite Conversion Kit (Applied Biosystems, Grand Island, NY, USA) was used for sodium bisulfite treatment of the genomic

DNA according to the manufacturer's protocol. MSP primers were designed with the aid of the Methyl Primer Express v1.0 software (Applied Biosystems, Lincoln, CA, USA) (Table 1). PCR products were purified from 1.5% agarose gels using a Gel Extraction Kit (Qiagen) and cloned into the pGEM-T Easy vector (Promega, Madison, WI, USA). Five randomly selected clones from each sample were chosen for sequencing.

4.6. DNA Methyltransferase 1 (DNMT1) Activity Assays

Nuclear protein was isolated using the Nuclear Protein Extraction Kit (BSP009; GeneChem Co. Ltd., Shanghai, China). The DNMT1 Activity Assay Kit (GMS50080; GenMed, Plymouth, MN, USA) was used for detection of DNMT1 activity according to the manufacturer's protocol. Replicates of each sample (20 µg nucleoprotein, including blank and positive control) were analyzed to validate the signal generated. The DNMT activity data were presented as OD/h/mg.

4.7. Wound Healing Assays

Cells (1×10^6) were grown overnight in 60 mm dishes to reach confluency, and a wound was introduced using a Q tip. Images were obtained using a microscope (Olympus) at 0 and 24 h after wounding to determine the width of the wounded area. The relative migration distance (percent of recovery) was calculated as $(W_0 - W_{24})/W_0 \times 100\%$ (W_0 indicates wound width at 0 h, and W_{24} indicates wound with at 24 h).

4.8. Matrigel Invasion Assays

Matrigel invasion assays were performed using Transwells containing 8.0 µm pore membranes (Corning, Lowell, MA, USA). MCF-7 and SKBR-3 cells were placed in the upper chamber of the Transwell, and 48 h later, the chambers were washed twice with phosphate buffer solution (PBS). The filter side of the upper chamber was cleaned with a cotton swab. Next, the membrane was cut out of the insert. Cells were fixed in methanol and stained with 5% Giemsa for 30 min at room temperature.

4.9. Chromatin Immunoprecipitation Assay

Chromatin immunoprecipitation (ChIP) assay was performed using the EZ Magna ChIP G Chromatin Immunoprecipitation kit (Millipore, Billerica, MA, USA) using chromatin isolated from 1×10^6 cells per condition, according to the manufacturer's protocol. Antibodies included anti-DNMT1 (1:500, Cell Signaling Technology), anti-IgG (Millipore), and anti-DNA polymerase II (Millipore); anti-IgG was the negative control and anti-DNA polymerase II was the positive control.

4.10. Transfection With Short Hairpin RNA

Cells were transfected with short hairpin RNA (shRNA) by using Lipofectamine 2000 (Invitrogen), following the procedure recommended by the manufacturer. shRNA targeting of CLDN6 (5'-GTGCAAGGTGTACGACTCA-3') and a negative control shRNA were purchased from GeneChem Co. Ltd.

4.11. Statistical Analysis

All computations were carried out using the SPSS version 19.0 for Windows (SPSS Inc., Chicago, IL, USA). Unpaired *t*-tests were performed to evaluate data for target mRNA and protein. The data are presented as means ± standard error from at least three independent experiments. $p < 0.05$ was considered statistically significant.

Acknowledgments: This study was supported by the National Natural Science Foundation of China (Grant No. 81172499), Science and Technology Development Plan of the Office of Science and Technology Project in Jilin Province (Grant No. 20140414036GH). We would like to thank the Key Laboratory of Natural Resources of Changbai Mountain & Functional Molecules, Ministry of Education, Yanbian University, China, for the help

Int. J. Mol. Sci. **2017**, *18*, 1863

in the total experiment, and thank William Orr, Department of Pathology, University of Manitoba, Canada, for critical review and editing of the manuscript.

Author Contributions: The study was designed by Chengshi Quan. Yan Lu and Liping Wang carried out most of the experiments, performed the statistical analysis, and drafted the manuscript. Hairi Li helped with manuscript preparation. Dongjing Lin, Yanru Li, Yang Ruan, Minlan Yang, Xiangshu Jin, Yantong Guo and Xiaoli Zhang assisted with the experiments and helped edit the paper. All authors have read and approved the final manuscript.

Conflicts of Interest: The authors declare no conflict of interest.

References

1. Turksen, K.; Troy, T.C. Junctions gone bad: Claudins and loss of the barrier in cancer. *Biochim. Biophys. Acta* **2011**, *1816*, 73–79. [CrossRef] [PubMed]
2. Mineta, K.; Yamamoto, Y.; Yamazaki, Y.; Tanaka, H.; Tada, Y.; Saito, K.; Tamura, A.; Igarashi, M.; Endo, T.; Takeuchi, K.; et al. Predicted expansion of the claudin multigene family. *FEBS Lett.* **2011**, *585*, 606–612. [CrossRef] [PubMed]
3. Turksen, K.; Troy, T.C. Claudin-6: A novel tight junction molecule is developmentally regulated in mouse embryonic epithelium. *Dev. Dyn.* **2001**, *222*, 292–300. [CrossRef] [PubMed]
4. Wu, Q.; Liu, Y.; Ren, Y.; Xu, X.; Yu, L.; Li, Y.; Quan, C. Tight junction protein, claudin-6, downregulates the malignant phenotype of breast carcinoma. *Eur. J. Cancer Prev.* **2010**, *19*, 186–194. [CrossRef] [PubMed]
5. Ren, Y.; Wu, Q.; Liu, Y.; Xu, X.; Quan, C. Gene silencing of claudin6 enhances cell proliferation and migration accompanied with increased MMP2 activity via p38 MAPK signaling pathway in human breast epithelium cell line HBL100. *Mol. Med. Rep.* **2013**, *8*, 1505–1510. [CrossRef] [PubMed]
6. Deckers, M.; van Dinther, M.; Buijs, J.; Que, I.; Lowik, C.; van der Pluijm, G.; ten Dijke, P. The tumor suppressor Smad4 is required for transforming growth factor beta-induced epithelial to mesenchymal transition and bone metastasis of breast cancer cells. *Cancer Res.* **2006**, *66*, 2202–2209. [CrossRef] [PubMed]
7. Viloria-Petit, A.M.; David, L.; Jia, J.Y.; Erdemir, T.; Bane, A.L.; Pinnaduwage, D.; Roncari, L.; Narimatsu, M.; Bose, R.; Moffat, J.; et al. A role for the TGFbeta-Par6 polarity pathway in breast cancer progression. *Proc. Natl. Acad. Sci. USA* **2009**, *106*, 14028–14033. [CrossRef] [PubMed]
8. Xu, J.; Lamouille, S.; Derynck, R. TGF-beta-induced epithelial to mesenchymal transition. *Cell Res.* **2009**, *19*, 156–172. [CrossRef] [PubMed]
9. Yang, J.; Weinberg, R.A. Epithelial-mesenchymal transition: At the crossroads of development and tumor metastasis. *Dev. Cell* **2008**, *14*, 818–829. [CrossRef]
10. Law, J.A.; Jacobsen, S.E. Establishing, maintaining and modifying DNA methylation patterns in plants and animals. *Nat. Rev. Genet.* **2010**, *11*, 204–220. [CrossRef] [PubMed]
11. Bhutani, N.; Burns, D.M.; Blau, H.M. DNA demethylation dynamics. *Cell* **2011**, *146*, 866–872. [CrossRef] [PubMed]
12. Liu, Y.; Jin, X.; Li, Y.; Ruan, Y.; Lu, Y.; Yang, M.; Lin, D.; Song, P.; Guo, Y.; Zhao, S.; et al. DNA methylation of claudin-6 promotes breast cancer cell migration and invasion by recruiting MeCP2 and deacetylating H3Ac and H4Ac. *J. Exp. Clin. Cancer Res. CR* **2016**, *35*, 120. [CrossRef] [PubMed]
13. Massague, J.; Seoane, J.; Wotton, D. Smad transcription factors. *Genes Dev.* **2005**, *19*, 2783–2810. [CrossRef] [PubMed]
14. Inman, G.J.; Nicolas, F.J.; Callahan, J.F.; Harling, J.D.; Gaster, L.M.; Reith, A.D.; Laping, N.J.; Hill, C.S. SB-431542 is a potent and specific inhibitor of transforming growth factor-beta superfamily type I activin receptor-like kinase (ALK) receptors ALK4, ALK5, and ALK7. *Mol. Pharmacol.* **2002**, *62*, 65–74. [CrossRef] [PubMed]
15. Laping, N.J.; Grygielko, E.; Mathur, A.; Butter, S.; Bomberger, J.; Tweed, C.; Martin, W.; Fornwald, J.; Lehr, R.; Harling, J.; et al. Inhibition of transforming growth factor (TGF)-beta1-induced extracellular matrix with a novel inhibitor of the TGF-beta type I receptor kinase activity: SB-431542. *Mol. Pharmacol.* **2002**, *62*, 58–64. [CrossRef] [PubMed]
16. Sugimoto, K.; Ichikawa-Tomikawa, N.; Satohisa, S.; Akashi, Y.; Kanai, R.; Saito, T.; Sawada, N.; Chiba, H. The tight-junction protein claudin-6 induces epithelial differentiation from mouse F9 and embryonic stem cells. *PLoS ONE* **2013**, *8*, e75106. [CrossRef] [PubMed]

17. Quan, C.; Lu, S.J. Identification of genes preferentially expressed in mammary epithelial cells of Copenhagen rat using subtractive hybridization and microarrays. *Carcinogenesis* **2003**, *24*, 1593–1599. [CrossRef] [PubMed]

18. Gonzalez-Mariscal, L.; Betanzos, A.; Nava, P.; Jaramillo, B.E. Tight junction proteins. *Prog. Biophys. Mol. Biol.* **2003**, *81*, 1–44. [CrossRef]

19. Papageorgis, P.; Lambert, A.W.; Ozturk, S.; Gao, F.; Pan, H.; Manne, U.; Alekseyev, Y.O.; Thiagalingam, A.; Abdolmaleky, H.M.; Lenburg, M.; et al. Smad signaling is required to maintain epigenetic silencing during breast cancer progression. *Cancer Res.* **2010**, *70*, 968–978. [CrossRef] [PubMed]

20. You, H.; Ding, W.; Rountree, C.B. Epigenetic regulation of cancer stem cell marker CD133 by transforming growth factor-beta. *Hepatology* **2010**, *51*, 1635–1644. [CrossRef] [PubMed]

21. Chen, T.; Hevi, S.; Gay, F.; Tsujimoto, N.; He, T.; Zhang, B.; Ueda, Y.; Li, E. Complete inactivation of DNMT1 leads to mitotic catastrophe in human cancer cells. *Nat. Genet.* **2007**, *39*, 391–396. [CrossRef] [PubMed]

22. Di Ruscio, A.; Ebralidze, A.K.; Benoukraf, T.; Amabile, G.; Goff, L.A.; Terragni, J.; Figueroa, M.E.; De Figueiredo Pontes, L.L.; Alberich-Jorda, M.; Zhang, P.; et al. DNMT1-interacting RNAs block gene-specific DNA methylation. *Nature* **2013**, *503*, 371–376. [CrossRef] [PubMed]

23. Robert, M.F.; Morin, S.; Beaulieu, N.; Gauthier, F.; Chute, I.C.; Barsalou, A.; MacLeod, A.R. DNMT1 is required to maintain CpG methylation and aberrant gene silencing in human cancer cells. *Nat. Genet.* **2003**, *33*, 61–65. [CrossRef] [PubMed]

24. Xiang, J.; Luo, F.; Chen, Y.; Zhu, F.; Wang, J. si-DNMT1 restore tumor suppressor genes expression through the reversal of DNA hypermethylation in cholangiocarcinoma. *Clin. Res. Hepatol. Gastroenterol.* **2014**, *38*, 181–189. [CrossRef] [PubMed]

25. Biniszkiewicz, D.; Gribnau, J.; Ramsahoye, B.; Gaudet, F.; Eggan, K.; Humpherys, D.; Mastrangelo, M.A.; Jun, Z.; Walter, J.; Jaenisch, R. DNMT1 overexpression causes genomic hypermethylation, loss of imprinting, and embryonic lethality. *Mol. Cell. Biol.* **2002**, *22*, 2124–2135. [CrossRef] [PubMed]

26. Szyf, M.; Knox, D.J.; Milutinovic, S.; Slack, A.D.; Araujo, F.D. How does DNA methyltransferase cause oncogenic transformation? *Ann. N. Y. Acad. Sci.* **2000**, *910*, 156–177. [CrossRef]

27. Gunzel, D.; Yu, A.S. Claudins and the modulation of tight junction permeability. *Physiol. Rev.* **2013**, *93*, 525–569. [CrossRef] [PubMed]

28. Kao, J.; Salari, K.; Bocanegra, M.; Choi, Y.L.; Girard, L.; Gandhi, J.; Kwei, K.A.; Hernandez-Boussard, T.; Wang, P.; Gazdar, A.F.; et al. Molecular profiling of breast cancer cell lines defines relevant tumor models and provides a resource for cancer gene discovery. *PLoS ONE* **2009**, *4*, e6146. [CrossRef] [PubMed]

29. Piek, E.; Heldin, C.H.; Ten Dijke, P. Specificity, diversity, and regulation in TGF-beta superfamily signaling. *FASEB J.* **1999**, *13*, 2105–2124. [PubMed]

30. Jornvall, H.; Blokzijl, A.; ten Dijke, P.; Ibanez, C.F. The orphan receptor serine/threonine kinase ALK7 signals arrest of proliferation and morphological differentiation in a neuronal cell line. *J. Biol. Chem.* **2001**, *276*, 5140–5146. [CrossRef] [PubMed]

31. Tsunoda, S.; Smith, E.; De Young, N.J.; Wang, X.; Tian, Z.Q.; Liu, J.F.; Jamieson, G.G.; Drew, P.A. Methylation of CLDN6, FBN2, RBP1, RBP4, TFPI2, and TMEFF2 in esophageal squamous cell carcinoma. *Oncol. Rep.* **2009**, *21*, 1067–1073. [CrossRef]

32. Li, Q.; Zhu, F.; Chen, P. MiR-7 and miR-218 epigenetically control tumor suppressor genes RASSF1A and claudin-6 by targeting HoxB3 in breast cancer. *Biochem. Biophys. Res. Commun.* **2012**, *424*, 28–33. [CrossRef] [PubMed]

33. Bruna, A.; Darken, R.S.; Rojo, F.; Ocana, A.; Penuelas, S.; Arias, A.; Paris, R.; Tortosa, A.; Mora, J.; Baselga, J.; et al. High TGFbeta-Smad activity confers poor prognosis in glioma patients and promotes cell proliferation depending on the methylation of the PDGF-B gene. *Cancer Cell* **2007**, *11*, 147–160. [CrossRef] [PubMed]

34. Kesari, S.; Jackson-Grusby, L.; Stiles, C.D. "Smad" eningly erratic: Target gene methylation determines whether TGFbeta promotes or suppresses malignant glioma. *Dev. Cell* **2007**, *12*, 324–325. [CrossRef] [PubMed]

35. Lu, R.; Wang, X.; Chen, Z.F.; Sun, D.F.; Tian, X.Q.; Fang, J.Y. Inhibition of the extracellular signal-regulated kinase/mitogen-activated protein kinase pathway decreases DNA methylation in colon cancer cells. *J. Biol. Chem.***2007**, *282*, 12249–12259. [CrossRef]

36. Su, H.Y.; Lai, H.C.; Lin, Y.W.; Liu, C.Y.; Chen, C.K.; Chou, Y.C.; Lin, S.P.; Lin, W.C.; Lee, H.Y.; Yu, M.H. Epigenetic silencing of SFRP5 is related to malignant phenotype and chemoresistance of ovarian cancer through wnt signaling pathway. *Int. J. Cancer* **2010**, *127*, 555–567. [CrossRef]

37. Furuse, M.; Fujita, K.; Hiiragi, T.; Fujimoto, K.; Tsukita, S. Claudin-1 and -2: Novel integral membrane proteins localizing at tight junctions with no sequence similarity to occludin. *J. Cell Biol.* **1998**, *141*, 1539–1550. [CrossRef] [PubMed]
38. Cereijido, M.; Contreras, R.G.; Shoshani, L.; Flores-Benitez, D.; Larre, I. Tight junction and polarity interaction in the transporting epithelial phenotype. *Biochim. Biophys. Acta* **2008**, *1778*, 770–793. [CrossRef] [PubMed]
39. Tsai, J.H.; Yang, J. Epithelial-mesenchymal plasticity in carcinoma metastasis. *Genes Dev.* **2013**, *27*, 2192–2206. [CrossRef] [PubMed]
40. Zavadil, J.; Bottinger, E.P. TGF-beta and epithelial-to-mesenchymal transitions. *Oncogene* **2005**, *24*, 5764–5774. [CrossRef] [PubMed]
41. Thiery, J.P.; Sleeman, J.P. Complex networks orchestrate epithelial-mesenchymal transitions. *Nat. Rev. Mol. Cell Biol.* **2006**, *7*, 131–142. [CrossRef] [PubMed]
42. Huber, M.A.; Kraut, N.; Beug, H. Molecular requirements for epithelial-mesenchymal transition during tumor progression. *Curr. Opin. Cell Biol.* **2005**, *17*, 548–558. [CrossRef] [PubMed]
43. Marques, F.R.; Fonsechi-Carvasan, G.A.; De Angelo Andrade, L.A.; Bottcher-Luiz, F. Immunohistochemical patterns for alpha- and beta-catenin, E- and N-cadherin expression in ovarian epithelial tumors. *Gynecol. Oncol.* **2004**, *94*, 16–24. [CrossRef] [PubMed]
44. Conacci-Sorrell, M.; Simcha, I.; Ben-Yedidia, T.; Blechman, J.; Savagner, P.; Ben-Ze'ev, A. Autoregulation of E-cadherin expression by cadherin-cadherin interactions: The roles of beta-catenin signaling, slug, and MAPK. *J. Cell Biol.* **2003**, *163*, 847–857. [CrossRef] [PubMed]
45. Hartsock, A.; Nelson, W.J. Adherens and tight junctions: Structure, function and connections to the actin cytoskeleton. *Biochim. Biophys. Acta* **2008**, *1778*, 660–669. [CrossRef] [PubMed]
46. Lin, X.; Shang, X.; Manorek, G.; Howell, S.B. Regulation of the epithelial-mesenchymal transition by claudin-3 and claudin-4. *PLoS ONE* **2013**, *8*, e67496. [CrossRef] [PubMed]
47. Lu, Z.; Ding, L.; Hong, H.; Hoggard, J.; Lu, Q.; Chen, Y.H. Claudin-7 inhibits human lung cancer cell migration and invasion through ERK/MAPK signaling pathway. *Exp. Cell Res.* **2011**, *317*, 1935–1946. [CrossRef] [PubMed]
48. Suh, Y.; Yoon, C.H.; Kim, R.K.; Lim, E.J.; Oh, Y.S.; Hwang, S.G.; An, S.; Yoon, G.; Gye, M.C.; Yi, J.M.; et al. Claudin-1 induces epithelial-mesenchymal transition through activation of the c-Abl-ERK signaling pathway in human liver cells. *Oncogene* **2013**, *32*, 4873–4882. [CrossRef]
49. Long, H.; Crean, C.D.; Lee, W.H.; Cummings, O.W.; Gabig, T.G. Expression of clostridium perfringens enterotoxin receptors claudin-3 and claudin-4 in prostate cancer epithelium. *Cancer Res.* **2001**, *61*, 7878–7881. [PubMed]
50. Michl, P.; Barth, C.; Buchholz, M.; Lerch, M.M.; Rolke, M.; Holzmann, K.H.; Menke, A.; Fensterer, H.; Giehl, K.; Lohr, M.; et al. Claudin-4 expression decreases invasiveness and metastatic potential of pancreatic cancer. *Cancer Res.* **2003**, *63*, 6265–6271. [PubMed]
51. Rangel, L.B.; Agarwal, R.; D'Souza, T.; Pizer, E.S.; Alo, P.L.; Lancaster, W.D.; Gregoire, L.; Schwartz, D.R.; Cho, K.R.; Morin, P.J. Tight junction proteins claudin-3 and claudin-4 are frequently overexpressed in ovarian cancer but not in ovarian cystadenomas. *Clin. Cancer Res.* **2003**, *9*, 2567–2575. [PubMed]
52. Pan, X.Y.; Wang, B.; Che, Y.C.; Weng, Z.P.; Dai, H.Y.; Peng, W. Expression of claudin-3 and claudin-4 in normal, hyperplastic, and malignant endometrial tissue. *Int. J. Gynecol. Cancer* **2007**, *17*, 233–241. [CrossRef] [PubMed]
53. Kominsky, S.L.; Argani, P.; Korz, D.; Evron, E.; Raman, V.; Garrett, E.; Rein, A.; Sauter, G.; Kallioniemi, O.P.; Sukumar, S. Loss of the tight junction protein claudin-7 correlates with histological grade in both ductal carcinoma in situ and invasive ductal carcinoma of the breast. *Oncogene* **2003**, *22*, 2021–2033. [CrossRef] [PubMed]
54. Itoh, M.; Bissell, M.J. The organization of tight junctions in epithelia: Implications for mammary gland biology and breast tumorigenesis. *J. Mammary Gland Biol. Neoplasia* **2003**, *8*, 449–462. [CrossRef] [PubMed]
55. Rahner, C.; Mitic, L.L.; Anderson, J.M. Heterogeneity in expression and subcellular localization of claudins 2, 3, 4, and 5 in the rat liver, pancreas, and gut. *Gastroenterology* **2001**, *120*, 411–422. [CrossRef] [PubMed]
56. Kiuchi-Saishin, Y.; Gotoh, S.; Furuse, M.; Takasuga, A.; Tano, Y.; Tsukita, S. Differential expression patterns of claudins, tight junction membrane proteins, in mouse nephron segments. *J. Am. Soc. Nephrol. JASN* **2002**, *13*, 875–886. [PubMed]

57. Miettinen, P.J.; Ebner, R.; Lopez, A.R.; Derynck, R. TGF-beta induced transdifferentiation of mammary epithelial cells to mesenchymal cells: Involvement of type I receptors. *J. Cell Biol.* **1994**, *127*, 2021–2036. [CrossRef]

58. Lu, Y.; Yu, L.; Yang, M.; Jin, X.; Liu, Z.; Zhang, X.; Wang, L.; Lin, D.; Liu, Y.; Wang, M.; et al. The effects of shRNA-mediated gene silencing of transcription factor SNAI1 on the biological phenotypes of breast cancer cell line MCF-7. *Mol. Cell. Biochem.* **2014**, *388*, 113–121. [CrossRef] [PubMed]

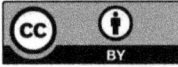

International Journal of
Molecular Sciences

MDPI

Review

Arachidonic Acid Metabolite as a Novel Therapeutic Target in Breast Cancer Metastasis

Thaiz F. Borin *, Kartik Angara, Mohammad H. Rashid, Bhagelu R. Achyut and Ali S. Arbab

Tumor Angiogenesis Laboratory, Georgia Cancer Center, Department of Biochemistry and Molecular Biology, Augusta University, Augusta, GA 30912, USA; kangara@augusta.edu (K.A.); mrashid@augusta.edu (M.H.R.); bachyut@augusta.edu (B.R.A.); aarbab@augusta.edu (A.S.A.)
* Correspondence: tborin@augusta.edu; Tel.: +1-706-721-4375

Received: 1 November 2017; Accepted: 6 December 2017; Published: 8 December 2017

Abstract: Metastatic breast cancer (BC) (also referred to as stage IV) spreads beyond the breast to the bones, lungs, liver, or brain and is a major contributor to the deaths of cancer patients. Interestingly, metastasis is a result of stroma-coordinated hallmarks such as invasion and migration of the tumor cells from the primary niche, regrowth of the invading tumor cells in the distant organs, proliferation, vascularization, and immune suppression. Targeted therapies, when used as monotherapies or combination therapies, have shown limited success in decreasing the established metastatic growth and improving survival. Thus, novel therapeutic targets are warranted to improve the metastasis outcomes. We have been actively investigating the cytochrome P450 4 (CYP4) family of enzymes that can biosynthesize 20-hydroxyeicosatetraenoic acid (20-HETE), an important signaling eicosanoid involved in the regulation of vascular tone and angiogenesis. We have shown that 20-HETE can activate several intracellular protein kinases, pro-inflammatory mediators, and chemokines in cancer. This review article is focused on understanding the role of the arachidonic acid metabolic pathway in BC metastasis with an emphasis on 20-HETE as a novel therapeutic target to decrease BC metastasis. We have discussed all the significant investigational mechanisms and put forward studies showing how 20-HETE can promote angiogenesis and metastasis, and how its inhibition could affect the metastatic niches. Potential adjuvant therapies targeting the tumor microenvironment showing anti-tumor properties against BC and its lung metastasis are discussed at the end. This review will highlight the importance of exploring tumor-inherent and stromal-inherent metabolic pathways in the development of novel therapeutics for treating BC metastasis.

Keywords: breast cancer metastasis; cytochrome P450; 20-HETE

1. Introduction

Breast cancer (BC) is composed of multiple subtypes with distinct morphologies and clinical implications. Histologically, BC can be classified according to tissue morphology into ductal and tubular types, which are further divided into benign or invasive subtypes [1]. Additionally, four major molecular categories are used to classify BC according to their steroid hormone receptor status and the presence or absence of the human epidermal growth factor receptor 2 (HER2). The luminal A subtype is characterized by the presence of an estrogen receptor (ER) and/or progesterone receptor (PR); luminal B is ER+ and/or PR+ and HER2+. The HER2-enriched tumors are positive for HER2+ expression and negative for both steroid hormone receptors. The basal-like or triple-negative breast cancer (TNBC) subtype is negative for all three receptors. Other molecular classifications can be used to complement distinctive gene and protein expression signatures such as claudin (low or high), Ki67 rates, or mesenchymal and epithelial marker status to predict personalized treatment and prognosis for BC patients. The percentage of each subtype presenting clinically, as well as their associated prognosis, is summarized in Table 1.

Table 1. Breast cancer subtypes classified according to immunohistochemical characterization. The details of prevalence, prognosis, and treatment of each subtype are presented. Data were obtained from the *Susan G. Komen Foundation* website [1] and the literature.

Subtypes	Molecular Characterization	Prevalence	Prognosis	Treatment
Luminal A	Estrogen receptor (ER)–positive, Progesterone receptor (PR)–positive or negative, Human epidermal growth factor receptor 2 (HER2)–negative	30–70% [2–7]	Best prognosis, high survival rates, and low recurrence rates [3–5,8]	Treatment for these tumors often includes chemotherapy and anti-hormone therapy
Luminal B	ER-positive, PR-positive or negative, HER2-positive	10–20% [2–7] Luminal B tumors are often diagnosed at a younger age than luminal A tumors [7–9]	Luminal B tumors tend to have factors that lead to a poorer prognosis, compared to luminal A tumors, including poorer tumor grade, larger tumor size and lymph node-positivity [3–5,8–11] Patients with luminal B tumors tend to have fairly high survival rates, although not as high as those with luminal A tumors [4,8]	The treatment for luminal B tumors includes anti-hormone therapy, anti-HER2 therapies and radiation, depending on tumor grade and lymph nodes status
HER2-enriched	ER-negative, PR-negative, HER2-positive	5–15% [3,5,7] HER2-type tumors may be diagnosed at a younger age than luminal A and luminal B tumors [8]	HER2-type tumors tend to have lymph node-positivity and poorer tumor grade [3–5,8,10]	HER2-type breast cancers can be treated with anti-HER2 drugs such as trastuzumab (Herceptin), lapatinib, capecitabine. Before these drugs were available, HER2-type tumors had a fairly poor prognosis [3,12]
Basal-like or Triple-negative breast cancer	ER-negative, PR-negative, HER2-negative	15–20% [2–7] These tumors tend to occur more often in younger women [5,9]	Triple-negative/basal-like tumors are often aggressive and have a poorer prognosis compared to ER-positive subtypes (luminal A and luminal B tumors) [3,5]	Triple-negative tumors can be treated successfully with chemotherapy and radiation, depending on tumor grade, lymph nodes status and disease stage

[1] https://ww5.komen.org/BreastCancer/SubtypesofBreastCancer.html.

Remarkably, these molecular subtypes are strongly associated with survival: luminal A tumors have the most favorable prognosis; luminal B, HER2-positive, and basal-like tumors are associated with the shortest relapse-free and overall survival rates [13]. Molecular subtypes also predict treatment response, with HER2-positive and TNBC tumors being more sensitive to preoperative chemotherapy than the luminal tumors [14]. BC has a propensity for distant metastasis to the bones, lungs, brain, and liver [15–18]. Bone metastasis is the first most common site of distant spread, having the longest median survival duration of about two to five years. However, patients with brain metastasis (BM) have the shortest survival of around four to seven months [16,19,20]. It has been reported that up to 15–30% of metastatic BC patients will eventually develop BM during the course of the disease [21,22]. Luminal A and B subtypes have a low risk of BM, of 2–9% and 4–10%, respectively [20,23,24], while HER2-enriched and TNBCs exhibited high rates of brain, lung, bone, and distant nodal metastases of 15–30%, 20–30%, 10–25%, and 17.2%, respectively [7,10,11]. Not all BC cells in primary tumors possess metastatic potential, and only a small subpopulation of cells can home to distant tissues or organs [25]. Metastasis remains one of the major causes of mortality in BC; however, no standardized therapy is available. Since the outcomes of tumor cell-targeted therapies are poor, tumor-associated stroma could be targeted to inhibit BC metastasis.

Interestingly, BC has been shown to thrive in the tumor microenvironment (TME), which consists of a pro-tumorigenic pathological immunosuppressive niche not only for BC cells themselves, but also for a significant amount of surrounding stroma and tumor-associated cells. Diverse components of the BC microenvironment, such as suppressive immune cells, re-programmed fibroblast cells, pathological neovascular structures, altered extracellular matrix, and certain soluble factors, synergistically impede an effective anti-tumor response and promote BC progression and metastasis [26]. BC cells recruit tumor infiltrated lymphocytes such as T-regulatory cells, myeloid-derived suppressor cells (MDSCs), and M2-macrophages to induce a pro-tumorigenic environment that attenuates anti-tumor immunity [27,28]. Aberrant expansion and accumulation of MDSCs have been extensively reported in BC. MDSCs are a heterogeneous population of immature granulocytes, macrophages, and dendritic cells [29] that are recruited to the primary tumor as well as the metastatic site and play a crucial role in inhibiting innate and adaptive immune responses by suppressing CD4+ T-cells, CD8+ T-cells, and natural killer (NK) cells [30–32]. In clinical scenarios, circulating MDSCs have been shown to have a positive correlation with BC stage and metastatic tumor burden [33]. In addition, increased numbers of MDSCs are correlated with the rate of recurrence and metastasis of BC [28,34–37].

Another important pro-tumorigenic myeloid subset in the TME are the macrophages, which are either residents or derived from the spleen or bone marrow [38,39]. Tumor-associated macrophages (TAMs) can be present as an M1 subtype that produces type 1 pro-inflammatory cytokines promoting the anti-tumorigenic role and an M2 subtype that produces type 2 anti-inflammatory cytokines that facilitate a pro-tumorigenic environment [40]. In the hypoxic tumor core, M1 macrophages polarize and switch phenotypes to M2 macrophages to promote pathological angiogenesis, thereby making the tumor more aggressive and invasive [41]. Furthermore, a metastatic subpopulation of TAMs was observed in a mouse model to promote the extravasation, invasion, and colonization of BC cells in the metastatic site [38,42]. Current therapies, including chemotherapy and targeted therapies, are failing due to the immunosuppression caused largely by MDSCs and TAMs in the primary tumor or the metastatic sites [43]. It is therefore important to understand the mechanisms causing this therapy resistance, tumor relapse, and refractoriness.

Recently, we observed that targeting the arachidonic acid (AA) pathway by inhibiting the synthesis of 20-hydroxy-eicosatetraenoic acid (20-HETE) resulted in the decreased migration and invasion of metastatic BC cells. In addition, in the same study, we found a synergistic reduction of the granulocytic MDSC (g-MDSCs: CD11b+Ly6G+) populations in the metastatic niches [44]. In our previous studies, we have been able to demonstrate a decrease in the levels of pro-angiogenic factors that are responsible for the communication between tumor cells and the microenvironment with a selective 20-HETE inhibitor, N-hydroxy-N'-(4-butyl-2 methyl phenyl) formamidine (HET0016), alone or in combination with anti-angiogenic therapies. Anti-20-HETE therapy was able to decrease breast and glioma tumor sizes [45,46]. Interestingly, the anti-AA pathway therapy was more effective at reducing tumor volume, the level of pro-angiogenic factors, and extent of metastasis than the antiangiogenic therapies used. It is therefore important for researchers to focus on and understand the role of metabolic pathways in tumors and their interplay with the stroma. In the current review, we have focused exclusively on the AA-20-HETE pathway and its implications in modeling the TME.

2. Arachidonic Acid Metabolism

AA is a polyunsaturated w-6 fatty acid present in the phospholipids of cell membranes, which is abundant in the brain, muscles, and liver [47–49]. The main precursors (fatty acids) of AA are obtained through the diet and its synthesis involves the expression of enzymes regulated in situ [50] after the activation of phospholipase A2 (PLA2) by neuroeffectors such as norepinephrine, angiotensin II, and bradykinin [51]. AA produces different biologically active metabolites through three different enzymatic pathways (Figure 1): the cyclooxygenase (COX), lipoxygenase (LOX), and cytochrome P450 (CYP) pathways [52]. These metabolic products can modulate renal, pulmonary, and cardiovascular functions, vascular tone, and inflammatory responses as paracrine factors and second messengers [53–55]. The COX pathway has two main enzymes, COX-1 and COX-2, which are critical in the regulation of inflammation and tissue homeostasis. Both COX-1 and COX-2 enzymes act on the AA synthesized from the cell membrane phospholipid by PLA2, and then metabolize AA into an intermediate prostaglandin (PG) H2 through PGG_2 (Figure 1) [56,57]. PGH_2 is an unstable endoperoxide that is catalyzed by specific synthases and generates five major prostanoids such as PGD_2, PGE_2, $PGF_{2\alpha}$, PGI_2 (prostacyclin), and thromboxane A_2 that have an important role in cancer-associated inflammation, tumor progression, and metastasis [57,58]. COX-1 is constitutively expressed in almost all tissues and inflammatory cells, and generates PGs that control homeostasis [56,57]. COX-2 is transiently and highly expressed in response to growth factors and endotoxins and is often involved in inflammation, cell proliferation, and differentiation [56]. The COX-2 pathway has also been targeted in many cancer studies, including colon cancer, colorectal cancer, breast cancer, gliomas, prostate cancer, esophageal carcinoma, pancreatic cancer, and lung carcinoma, due to its increased expression and correlation with the reduction of survival rates in cancer patients [56–58]. It is already known that most cancerous tissues show signs of inflammation in the pre-cancer stages, and chronic stimulation by innate immune cells, cytokines, and chemokines lead to malignant transformation and tumor progression [58]. COX-2 inhibitors have been extensively studied through their properties to inhibit tumor growth by suppressing inflammation and angiogenesis. However, patients treated with celecoxib, a COX-2 inhibitor, in clinical trials demonstrated gastrointestinal complications, a higher risk of cardiovascular toxicity, and death [58]. Even then, the toxicities of COX-2 inhibitors do not exclude the importance of this treatment as an adjuvant in cancer therapy.

A third isoform of COX enzymes has been identified primarily in canine samples and then confirmed in human tissue. COX-3 contains all of the COX-1 protein information, except for the retained intron sequence that alters its enzymatic properties, significantly generating PGE_2 [59]. The functional COX-3 biosynthesis is an important concept that can help to explain the prostaglandin-independent, anti-inflammatory actions previously attributed to the reactivation of COX-2 activity at a later stage in enhancing inflammatory resolution [60,61]. However, further studies showing whether there is a unique human COX-3 that acts independently of COX-1 and COX-2 and to determine the role of COX-3 in tumor growth and development are still lacking.

The LOX pathway produces different leukotrienes (LTs), lipoxins (LXs), hepoxillins (HOs), and hydroxy-eicosatetraenoic acids (HETEs), causing inflammation, allergic reactions, bronchoconstriction, and vasoconstriction (Figure 1). The principal lipoxygenases expressed in humans are 5-lipoxygenase (5-LOX), 8-lipoxygenase (8-LOX), 12-lipoxygenase (12-LOX), and 15-lipoxygenase (15-LOX) type 1 and 2. In general, the LOX pathway catalyzes the oxygenation of AA into hydroperoxy-eicosatetraenoic acid (HPETE) and converts HPETEs to LTs, LXs, Hos, and HETEs through the reduction of HPETE to HETE [62]. The four distinct enzymes insert oxygen at the specific carbons 5, 8, 12, or 15 of AA, generating 5-, 8-, 12-, or 15-HPETE, which can be further reduced by glutathione peroxidase (GPx) to the hydroxy forms (5-, 8-, 12-, 15-HETE), respectively [63]. The 5-LOX pathway synthesizes the key pro-inflammatory LT mediators such as leukotriene A4 (LTA_4) and leukotriene B4 (LTB_4) [58]. LTA_4 is an unstable LT that can be converted into LTB_4 or cysteinyl LTs (LTC_4, LTD_4, and LTE_4) [57]. High levels of LTB_4, the main product of the 5-LOX pathway, were found in prostate cancer samples [64], and its receptors were found to be overexpressed in gastric cancer compared to normal tissue [65]. Interestingly, an LTB_4 receptor antagonist in combination with chemotherapy was able to decrease tumor growth and metastasis in vitro and in vivo in colon cancer and pancreatic cancer models [66]. However, this combination did not change the survival rates in pancreatic or lung cancer clinical trials [67]. 8-LOX and its products 8-HPETE and 8-HETE are expressed in skin, mainly after irritation, but their importance in tumorigenesis remains unclear and poorly reported [63].

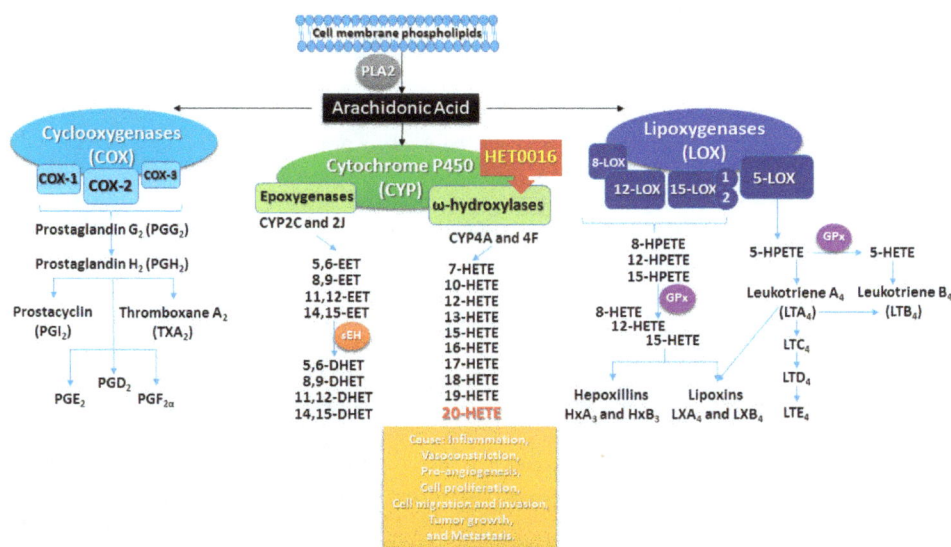

Figure 1. Schematic representation of phospholipid-arachidonic acid metabolites produced via the major enzymes cyclooxygenase (COX), lipoxygenase (LOX), and cytochrome P450 (CYP4A). CYP4A produced 20-hydroxy-eicosatetraenoic acids (20-HETE) metabolite, which is known to promote tumor growth. Legend: phospholipase A2 (PLA2); epoxy-eicosatrienoic acids—(EETs); epoxide hydrolase (sEH); dihydroxy-eicosatrienoic acids (DHETs); hydroperoxy-eicosatetraenoic acid (HPETE); glutathione peroxidase (GPx).

12-LOX also has a critical role in tumor angiogenesis, motility, invasion, and metastasis [68]. 12-LOX is the main human 12-HETE-generating enzyme and can synthesize 12S-HPETE through AA or either 12S- or 15S-HPETE through linoleic acid metabolism [57,63]. Three isoforms of the 12-LOX enzyme have been identified, including the leukocyte and platelet type (named as S) and epidermal type (named as R), expressed in various types of cells such as leukocytes, platelets, smooth muscle cells, endothelial cells, and keratinocytes [57]. Evidence shows that both the leukocyte- and platelet-types of 12-LOXs have been found in cancer tissues such as melanoma, prostate, and epidermal cancers and promote cell proliferation and survival [69]. 12-LOX inhibition can decrease the proliferation and induce apoptosis in human gastric cancer cells, prostate cancer cells, and carcinosarcoma cells [56,70,71]. 12S-LOX also converts AA to HOs by reducing 12S-HETE into 8-hydroxy-11,12-epoxy-eicosatetraenoic acid (HxA$_3$) and 10-hydroxy-11,12-epoxy-eicosatrienoic acid (HxB$_3$) or by its isomerization [72]. HOs exhibit vast biological activities including the stimulation of insulin secretion by glucose induction, an increase of intracellular calcium levels in pancreatic islets cells, and the induction of hyperpolarization of the membrane potential in neurons [72].

15-LOX is subdivided into two isoforms, 15-LOX-1 and 15-LOX-2. They are widely distributed in the tissues and mainly expressed in reticulocytes, eosinophils, pulmonary epithelial cells, and macrophages [57]. 15-LOX has an ambiguous activity, being pro- or anti-tumorigenic depending on its subtype. 15-LOX-1 metabolizes linoleic acid to 3-hydroxy-octadecadienoic acid (13S-HODE) and metabolizes AA to 15S-HETE. However, 15-LOX-2 mainly converts AA to 15S-HETE [57,63].

Lipoxins are trihydroxy-eicosatetraenoic acids derived from three different pathways of AA metabolism. They can be synthesized by the platelet–leukocyte interaction that involves the production of LTA$_4$ by 5-LOX in neutrophils and its conversion to lipoxin A4 (LXA$_4$) and lipoxin B4 (LXB$_4$) by 12-LOX in platelets upon their adherence to leukocytes. Without this interaction the production of LXs does not happen [73]. The generation of LXs can also be achieved through the oxygenation of AA in the presence of 15-LOX, generating 15S-HPETE, which serves as a substrate for 5-LOX, or through COX-2 acetylation, which generates COX-2-derived HETE and is converted by 5-LOX to 15-epi-lipoxin A4, also known as aspirin-triggered lipoxin (ATL) and 15 epi-lipoxin B4 [73,74]. Lipoxins and epi-lipoxins show anti-inflammatory effects through signals engendered by binding to G protein-coupled lipoxin A4 receptor (ALX)/formyl peptide receptor (FPR2) [74]. Lipoxins have been shown to downregulate NFκB expression and could be used as a potential treatment for several cancer types [74]. LXA$_4$ can decrease cell proliferation, inhibits cell invasion, and suppresses tumor growth, exhibiting anti-inflammatory properties in cancer cells [58]. Since LXs can target a variety of inflammatory and angiogenic molecules, inhibitors of LTA$_4$ hydrolase could be potentially used in a combination therapy along with standard chemotherapeutic drugs to treat cancer [58,74]. Further in vivo studies are required to corroborate the idea of whether LXs could be used as an adjuvant in preventing cancer progression.

The COX and LOX pathways represent two major routes of AA metabolism that controls the biosynthesis and activity of LTs, LXs, HOs, and HETEs or intermediary products such as HPETEs. These products can act as effectors in inflammatory responses or activate the production of second messengers such as reactive oxygen species (ROS) through interaction with cognate G protein-coupled cell-surface receptors or nuclear receptors such as peroxisome proliferator activated receptors (PPARs) [75]. CYP enzymes require nicotinamide adenine dinucleotide phosphate (NADPH) reductase and CYPb5 as cofactors and are a major source of superoxide ions, releasing a significant amount of oxygen radicals in the vasculature, which makes the metabolism of AA by CYP enzymes an important contributor to oxidative stress [53]. Oxidative stress activates a host of pro-inflammatory cytokines and chemokines such as TNF-α and IL-8 and adhesion molecules such as ICAM-1, E-selectin, or P-selectin. The metabolic end products generated as a result of the peroxidation of lipids also serve as potent chemoattractants for inflammatory cells [76]. Two key inducible cytochrome P450 enzymes, CYP2E1 and CYP4A, involved in lipid peroxidation function complementarily, and this may lead to interactions in the regulation of these enzymes [77,78]. CYP2E1 and CYP4A have been demonstrated to function as leaky enzymes that are capable of undergoing "futile cycling". During this process, even in the absence of a substrate, these enzymes are capable of producing ROS such as superoxide anions, hydroxyl radicals, and hydrogen peroxides [79–81]. Reduction in the levels of a key antioxidant such as glutathione (GSH) by inhibiting GSH synthesis with buthionine sulfoximine (BSO) dramatically upregulated the AA levels, causing toxicity. Overexpression of the antioxidant enzyme catalase countered the pro-oxidant activity of CY2E1 [82]. In response to cell mediated injury by AA metabolism, especially in CYP2E1-overexpressing cells, antioxidant molecules such as GSH were high due to the upregulation of γ-glutamylcysteine synthetase [83], GSH S-transferases, and catalase [84]. The contributions of these pathways in cancer development and their interaction and deregulation are still open for discussion. More extensive investigation is needed to delineate how COX and LOX inhibitors could be more effective in decreasing tumor growth and metastasis. In this review, our main focus is the CYP pathway and its metabolites in relation to various aspects of inflammation and cancer.

The cytochrome P450 (*CYP*) gene family consists of a complex 18 gene families that encode more than 103 functional genes in mice and 57 genes in humans [85,86]. The *CYP2*, *CYP3*, and *CYP4* families encode more genes than the remaining 15 families in human as well as in rodent genomes [86]. The majority of the genes found in the *CYP1*, *CYP2*, *CYP3*, and *CYP4* families encode enzymes involved in eicosanoid metabolism and are inducible by diet, chemical inducers, drugs, pheromones, and other factors [86]. Their function is predominantly in the detoxification of drugs, toxic compounds, chemotherapies, xenobiotics, and products of endogenous metabolism such as bilirubin in the liver [85,86]. The *CYP2* and *CYP3* families are the most redundant, mutated, or defective in one or more genes compared to the other 16 gene families that might be responsible for the CYP-related diseases that will be directly involved in their critical life functions [86].

The CYP pathway is an enzymatic pathway divided into ω-hydroxylase and epoxygenase pathways that use AA as a substrate to produce eicosanoids. Derivatives of the ω-hydroxylase pathway (HETEs) cause inflammation, vasoconstriction, vascular remodeling, and cellular proliferation. Metabolites of the epoxygenase pathways (epoxy-eicosatrienoic acids—EETs) resolve inflammation and cause vasodilation, the protection of cardiac function, and cell proliferation [85,87,88]. In mammalian cells, the most studied and effective subfamily to produce 20-HETE is CYP4A [53]. In rats, there are four isoforms identified: CYP4A1, CYP4A2, CYP4A3, and CYP4A8 [89]. These isoforms share 66–98% homology and common catalytic activity and are expressed in the liver, kidney, and brain [90]. CYP4A1 has the highest catalytic efficiency to convert AA into 20-HETE, followed by CYP4A2 and CYP4A3; however, CYP4A8 did not catalyze AA or linoleic acid [91]. In mice, CYP4A10, CYP4A12a, CYP4A12b, and CYP4A14 are the principal isoforms that catalyze AA ω-hydroxylation to 20-HETE [92]. CYP4A10 has a lower catalytic activity for 20-HETE production than the CYP4A12 isoforms. CYP4A12a and CYP4A12b have similar hydroxylase activity, constituting the major source of 20-HETE synthesis [92]. Particularly, in addition to the CYP4A enzymes, the CYP4F isoforms are also significant for 20-HETE production [90]. In humans, the isoforms CYP4A11, CYP4A22, CYP4F2, and CYP4F3 are the most important in the production of 20-HETE, predominantly CYP4F2, followed by CYP4A11 [93]. The isoforms and their species-specific expression are summarized in Table 2.

Table 2. CYP ω-hydroxylases that produce 20-HETE in mice, rats, rabbits, and humans. Data have been obtained from Roman [48].

Species	20-HETE Production
Mouse	CYP4A10; CYP4A12a; CYP4A12b; CYP4A14
Rat	CYP4A1; CYP4A2; CYP4A3
Rabbit	CYP4A4; CYP4A6; CYP4A7
Human	CYP4A11; CYP4A22; CYP4F2; CYP4F3

The ω-hydroxylases from the CYP family 4, subfamily A (*CYP4A*), and F (*CYP4F*) genes convert AA into 7-, 10-, 12-, 13-, 15-, 16-, 17-, 18-, 19-, and 20-HETEs, and the epoxygenases mainly encoded by the *CYP* family 2 subfamilies C and J genes generate 5,6-EET, 8,9-EET, 11,12-EET, and 14,15-EET, which will be further metabolized into the less active dihydroxy-eicosatrienoic acids (DHETs) through epoxide hydrolase (sEH) [58,85]. All four EETs and their metabolite DHET can act as a long-chain of fatty acids and stimulate the peroxisome proliferator response element to bind to PPAR [85]. 20-HETE is the principal pro-inflammatory metabolite produced by the ω-hydroxylase enzymes and regulates vascular remodeling and neovascularization under ischemic or hypoxic conditions [94–96]. 20-HETE synthesis can be controlled through the activation of calcium/calmodulin-dependent kinase II and mitogen-activated protein kinase (MAPK) in smooth muscle cells [97]. 20-HETE can be incorporated into endothelial lipids through a coenzyme A-dependent process and is further metabolized by ω-oxidation or β-oxidation to 20-carboxy-arachidonic acid (20-COOH-AA) [98]. The metabolism of

20-HETE can also be regulated through COX-mediated pathways into 20-hydroxy-prostaglandin G2 and H2 [99]. 20-HETE stimulates the activation of the nuclear factor κB (NFκB) and MAPK/ERK pathways, mediating pro-inflammatory effects, and also has an important role in epidermal growth factor (EGF), hypoxia-inducible factor (HIF), and vascular endothelial growth factor (VEGF) activation, showing pro-angiogenic effects and the stimulation of endothelial cell proliferation, migration, and cell survival [94,100]. Recently, molecular studies highlighting the relationship between aberrant AA metabolism through 20-HETE downstream signaling pathway activation and carcinogenesis have provided novel molecular targets for cancer chemoprevention and treatments.

3. Cytochrome P450 Mechanisms in Obesity and Breast Cancer

Dysregulated energy metabolism is already known to be a hallmark of cancer [101]. One of the main examples of dysregulated energy metabolism is obesity, which has been associated with high levels of aromatase in breast tumors and undifferentiated adipose tissue [102]. Aromatase is a CYP19 enzyme responsible for the critical steps in the synthesis of estrogens [103] that are most related to breast cancer risks. Several drugs, in particular anti-diabetic drugs, have shown effects in decreasing tumor growth, breast cancer recurrence, and metastasis [102,104]. Metformin, for example, can inhibit aromatase expression via 5′ AMP-activated protein kinase (AMPK) in breast adipose stromal cells [105]. In breast cancer, adipose tissue provides structural and paracrine support for tumor development and growth. In addition to adipose tissue in the breast, other stromal cells can provide crucial metabolites through the CYP-mediated lipid peroxidation pathway to favor tumor growth and the production of pro-tumorigenic eicosanoids.

AA and its metabolites have been strongly implicated in the pathogenesis of obesity and related complications in peripheral tissues and organs owing to their ability to provide fatty acids for the production of pro-inflammatory cytokines [106]. The constituent expression of all the molecular players crucial for the 5-LOX pathway to generate leukotrienes and the receptors (two LTB$_4$ [BLT1 and BLT2] receptors and two cysteinyl LT [CysLT-R1 and CysLT-R2]) receptors in the adipocyte and the stromal vascular fraction highlight the importance of this pathway in obesity. LTB$_4$ signaling plays a crucial role in mediating the differentiation of preadipocytes to mature adipocytes, and 5-LOX-derived leukotrienes are elevated in the obese adipose tissue [107–112]. 5-LOX has also been indicated in the modulation of lipid metabolism to provide free fatty acids as substrates for the production of pro-inflammatory eicosanoids [110]. In our studies, we have demonstrated that HET0016 is a selective CYP4A and CYP4F ω-hydroxylase inhibitor that does not have any possible effects on the 5-LOX signaling pathway to control obesity. However, a recent study by Park et al. [113] showed the effects of the inhibition of CYP4A enzyme activity in type 2 diabetes mellitus (T2DM) in obese mice. The authors reported that obesity is one of the important causes of elevated endoplasmic reticulum stress in obese mice and identified 54 novel CYP4A enzyme isoforms that were upregulated in obesity-induced T2DM in the *db/db* mice model, of which CYP4A10 and CYP4A14 levels were significantly upregulated [113]. Since HET0016 has specificity for the inhibition of CYP4A enzymes, it can be strongly hypothesized that the effects of HET0016 can be observed in animals. Animals fed with a high-fat diet and treated with HET0016 for 12 weeks presented a significantly decreased body weight and total fat-pad mass, and improved glucose tolerance and insulin sensitivity compared with animals that were not fed the high-fat diet [113]. The fasting blood glucose concentration in obese animals was comparable to the levels observed in normal-diet-fed animals [113]. We did not find any evidence of studies in humans. The specificity of CYP4A for ω-oxidation facilitates the degradation of long-chain fatty acids, therefore providing a secondary metabolic pathway for the metabolism of fatty acids when levels of these substrates increase during the physiological processes of lipolysis and hepatic fatty acid uptake. It would be fascinating to investigate the other mechanisms involved in the inhibition of the CYP4A-mediated control of obesity in these animals. However, the current review is focused on presenting evidence as to how the inhibition of 20-HETE, an AA metabolite, might be a novel therapeutic target in BC metastasis.

4. Arachidonic Acid Pathway and 20-HETE in Primary Tumors and Metastasis

In tumors, the CYP4A/20-HETE axis promotes inflammation, endothelial cell migration, and neovascularization [114–119]. When *N*-hydroxy-*N'*-(4-butyl-2 methyl phenyl) formamidine (HET0016), a highly selective inhibitor of 20-HETE synthesis, was used alone in tumor-bearing animals, a decrease in tumor growth was observed via impaired tumor neovascularization [44–46,120]. HET0016 is also shown to decrease MAPK signaling, pSTAT1, EGFR, and HIF-1α in glioblastoma (GBM) tumor lysates [121]. When the expression of different pro- and anti-angiogenic factors and inflammatory cytokines in the tumor lysates were analyzed, there were significant changes following HET0016 treatments compared to that of vehicle-treated tumors [46,121]. When the extravascular extracellular space (EES), different vascular parameters, and neovascularization were examined, HET0016 treatment significantly decreased EES, tumor blood volume, permeability, and neovascularization [46,121]. We also reported that HET0016 decreased vascular mimicry, a phenomenon where tumor cells make blood vessel-like structures [120,122]. We found that the CYP4A/20-HETE axis plays a critical role in metastasis in a syngeneic model of BC-mediated pulmonary metastasis. Targeting 20-HETE production also decreased pulmonary metastasis in an aggressive BC model [44]. When applied at the pre-metastatic stage, HET0016 significantly decreased pulmonary metastatic growth through decreasing a survival pathway (p-AKT), inflammation pathway (canonical NFκB signaling), migration pathway (matrix metalloproteinase-2 and -9, MMP2 and 9), and mesenchymal cancer stem cell markers (CD44 and *N*-cadherin) in the metastatic lung niche [44]. In cancer studies, 20-HETE mediated effects have been studied in the context of tumor cells and endothelial progenitor cells (EPCs). Investigations regarding the contribution of tumor-associated stromal cells such as myeloid cells are rare. The following sections will discuss the role of stromal and myeloid cell-mediated 20-HETE production and its effects on tumor growth and metastasis.

5. Role of 20-HETE in Stromal Cells and Tumor Cells

Initially, the entirety of cancer research was focused on the idea that tumor growth and metastasis were tumor-cell inherent/autonomously driven by mutations arising in these tumor cells to meet with their metabolic and nutritional needs. This dogma has been refuted to incorporate the idea of a "tumor microenvironment" comprised of stromal cells such as endothelial cells, fibroblasts, and pericytes and also infiltrating myeloid cells such as monocytes, macrophages, and MDSCs to favor tumor growth and metastasis [123–127]. The non-tumor cell-dependent contribution to tumor growth and progression has gained immense popularity, thanks to the landmark hypothesis of tumor angiogenesis proposed by Folkman in 1971 [128]. Tumor neovascularization has now been extended to include vasculogenesis, intussusception, tumor cell transdifferentiation to endothelial phenotypes, and vascular mimicry [129,130].

The ω-hydroxylation of therapeutic drugs, as well as endogenous compounds, e.g., fatty acids, by the CYP4 family members functions to metabolically activate and further eliminate these compounds. Eicosanoids, derived from AA, are key substrates of this cytochrome P450-dependent oxidation reaction. Human CYP4 enzymes such as CYP4A11, CYP4F2, and CYP4F3B, hydroxylate AA at the omega position to form 20-HETE. 20-HETE has already been shown to have hallmark effects in tumor progression, angiogenesis, and inflammatory processes associated with tumor growth and metastasis. The processes of tumor-associated angiogenesis and inflammation driving the immunosuppression go hand-in-hand and thus exert significant influence on tumor growth and metastasis. The pro-inflammatory cytokines and pro-growth factors work to promote tumor growth; the tumor thereby releases various chemokines/cytokines that promote the recruitment of MDSCs, neutrophils, macrophages, and other myeloid cells to facilitate the development of an immunosuppressive niche conducive to tumor growth [131–133].

The first evidence pointing towards the role of the CYP4A/20-HETE axis in angiogenesis was pointed out by Sa et al. in their study, where they reported that FGF-2-mediated activation of cytosolic phospholipase A2 is responsible for AA production and CYP4A stimulation in endothelial cells [134]. Recent studies have shown that the CYP4A/F-20-HETE and VEGF pathways have a positive feedback regulation in circulating EPCs. Both hypoxia and VEGF induced expression of the CY4A11 gene and protein in EPCs, and 20-HETE and VEGF had a synergistic effect on EPC proliferation. Moreover, 20-HETE induced the expression of Very Late Antigen-4 (VLA-4) and CXCR4 in EPCs, thereby promoting their role in neovascularization, and targeting the 20-HETE pathway attenuated EPC-induced angiogenesis in a Matrigel plug angiogenesis assay [114]. 20-HETE offers a survival advantage to bovine pulmonary artery endothelial cells by activating the pro-survival PI3-kinase and Akt pathways, NADPH oxidase activation, and NADPH oxidase-derived superoxide, and thereby protects these cells from undergoing apoptosis [135]. There is a dynamic interplay between the tumor cells and the tumor stroma in regulating tumor growth, invasion, and metastasis, as shown in Figure 2. A bi-directional synergism comes into play to meet the metabolic and nutrient demands of the tumors and also to counter therapeutic resistance in the face of insult by chemotherapy and antiangiogenic therapy (AAT).

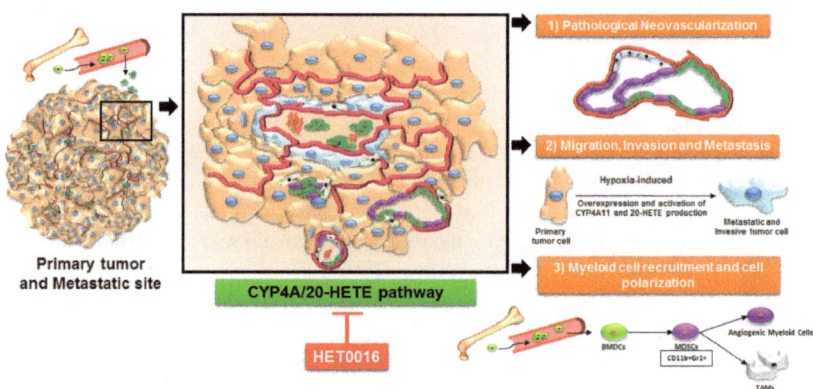

Figure 2. Schematic representation of the involvement of the CYP4A/20-HETE pathway in the primary tumor microenvironment and its potential metastatic site. (**1**) The CYP4A/20-HETE pathway is overexpressed in myeloid-derived suppressor cells (MDSCs) recruited to the primary tumor and in the tumor-associated stroma cells, promoting polarization to a g-MDSC phenotype; (**2**) The CYP4A/20-HETE pathway increases pathological neovascularization in the tumor microenvironment (TME); (**3**) The CYP4A/20-HETE pathway induces the expression of HIF1a, VEGF, MMP2, MMP9, and other factors to increase migration, invasion, and metastasis. HET0016, a selective inhibitor of 20-HETE in the CYP4A pathway, decreases the metastatic potential of tumor cells, normalizes the blood flow, and controls abnormal neovascularization. The red boundary defines the tumor-associated vascular structure.

Our laboratory has shown that using HET0016, a 20-HETE inhibitor, decreased the level of several pro-angiogenic factors in a mouse model of TNBC, thereby affecting tumor growth [45]. T47D and BT-474 human BC cells overexpressing CYP4Z1 enhanced proliferation, migration, and tube formation of human umbilical vein endothelial cells (HUVECs), and promoted angiogenesis in the zebrafish embryo and chorioallantoic membrane of the chick embryo [136]. CYP4A1 expression in U251 glioma cells induced hyperproliferation both in vitro and in vivo, possibly due to the production of 20-HETE [117]. The CYP4A/20-HETE axis significantly increased tumor weight, microvessel density (MVD), and lung metastasis by upregulating VEGF and MMP in non-small cell lung cancer [137]. Many studies designed to understand tumor growth, the development of resistance to therapies, and metastasis have focused on tumor neovascularization as a primary target. A novel neovascularization mechanism that has gained widespread popularity amidst controversy is vascular mimicry [130,138,139]. Studies from our laboratory have demonstrated the efficacy of targeting the

CYP4A/20-HETE axis in controlling vascular mimicry-dependent AAT resistance [120,122]. In light of the aforementioned evidence, studies of the CYP4A/20-HETE axis in mediating tumor growth, invasion, and metastasis serve to be an exciting domain of investigation.

Reports on the emerging role of the CYP4A/20-HETE axis in immune regulatory myeloid cells are building up. For the very first time, our laboratory has recently shown that pharmacological targeting of the CYP4A/20-HETE axis through HET0016 decreased g-MDSCs in the metastatic niche [44]. The growth factors and cytokines released by g-MDSCs can inhibit an effective T-cell response and promote the growth of disseminated tumor cells [37,140,141]. Chen et al. in a similar context, have shown that TAMs overexpressing a CYP4A10 variant can increase pre-metastatic niche formation and pulmonary metastasis [142]. Similarly, a novel flavonoid FLA-16, through inhibiting CYP4A pathways, normalized the tumor vasculature and improved survival. This was accompanied by the decreased secretion of 20-HETE, VEGF, and transforming growth factor beta (TGF-β) in TAMs and EPCs [143]. Altogether, CYP4A in TAMs is crucial for the tumor-dependent macrophage phenotype shift, and its inhibition by HET0016 or FLA-16 decreased tumor-associated phenotypes [142,143]. Moreover, these reports strongly suggest a critical role of the myeloid cell-produced 20-HETE metabolite in tumor growth and metastasis. In the future, more experimental investigations are needed to explore its role in other stromal cell types such as heterogeneous myeloid subsets, e.g., MDSCs and T cell subsets, which display a profound role in tumor and metastatic microenvironments (shown schematically in Figure 2). Since the TME is modeled around the availability of neovascular structures to meet the nutrient and metabolic demands of the tumor, the following section will highlight the role of the 20-HETE pathway in tumor and tumor-associated stromal cells with a special emphasis on endothelial cells.

6. HET0016 as a Novel Therapeutic Agent in Treatment of Metastasis

Currently, there is a dearth of studies investigating the CYP4A/20-HETE axis and its involvement in tumor growth and metastasis in patients. Increased levels of 12-HETE and 20-HETE were found in patients with prostate cancer and with myeloid leukemia [52,144]. In fact, various human cancer cells show the upregulation of 20-HETE-producing enzymes of CYP4A/F families including BC, colon and ovary cancer, and melanoma [142,145]. Our laboratory has extensively employed HET0016, a selective 20-HETE synthesis inhibitor, as a treatment to reduce the hyperproliferation of glioma [121,146,147] and BC cells [44,45].

Recently, we have shown that the growth of human glioblastoma was dwindled by an intravenous (IV) formulation of HET0016. We optimized the route of administration of the drug by making a novel IV formulation of HET0016 with 2-hydroxypropyl β cyclodextrin (HPβCD) to enhance bioavailability (resulting in a seven-fold higher level in plasma and 3.6-fold higher level in the tumor in the first hour compared to treatment via an intraperitoneal route) and to deliver an effective dose of the drug to the tumor site with reduced off-target effects and rapid clearance. We saw significantly reduced tumor growth with the IV HET0016 treatment in athymic nude rats that were orthotopically implanted with U251 cells. Similar growth inhibition was observed in the syngeneic GL261 GBM immunocompetent mouse model. Using magnetic resonance imaging (MRI), we evaluated the vascular kinetics in the TME, which showed that the delayed IV HET0016-treated animals have significantly lower v_p (blood plasma pool), v_e (extracellular space or interstitial volume), and K^{trans} (forward permeability transfer constant), and increased and normalized blood flow compared to that of the corresponding vehicle-treated groups. We observed a reduced expression of markers of cell proliferation (Ki67) and neovascularization (laminin, MVD, and αSMA), downregulation of pro-angiogenic proteins such as VE-cadherin (vascular endothelial cadherin-vasculogenesis), bFGF (basic fibroblast growth factor), IL-8 (chemokine CXCL8), SDF-1α (stromal cell-derived factor-1), and MCP-1 (a CCL2 ligand), and increased expression of anti-angiogenic proteins such as Tie-2, angiostatin, and angiopoietin-2/Tie-1 in the IV HET0016 treatment group. We determined the expression of different proteins by western blot and confirmed that HET0016 treatment decreases the level of markers of cellular proliferation (pERK), survival, migration, invasion (pAKT), inflammation (COX-1/2, p-NFκB), and angiogenesis (HIF-1α, EGFR, VEGF, and MMP2). Furthermore, we observed significantly improved survival in patient-derived xenograft (PDX) tumor models of GBM811 and HF2303 with HET0016 treatment alone or in combination with temozolomide (TMZ) in irradiated animals. Overall survival was prolonged to 26 weeks after combined treatment with HET0016 plus TMZ and radiation, while control animals survived for only 10 weeks in the GBM811 model while survival was prolonged to 26 weeks vs. 17 weeks for the irradiated control in the PDX model of HF2303 [121].

In one of our studies to understand the role of HET0016 in controlling metastasis, we have shown that HET0016 decreases migration and invasion in the metastatic TNBC cell line from both human (MDA-MB-231) and mouse (4T1) models in vitro. We also showed that IV HET0016 treatment reduces primary tumor growth and lung metastasis in 4T1 bearing immunocompetent Balb/c mice. Other studies have similarly observed a diminished expression of pro-inflammatory cytokines such as EGF, Fas, SDF-1α, IL-1β, IL-4, IL-17A, MMP-2, and MMP-9, which led us to investigate the downstream signaling mechanisms that could be affected by HET0016 [137,142,148–150]. The PI3K/Akt and MAPK signaling pathways are thought to be climacteric to regulate proliferation, invasion, angiogenesis, and metastasis ability [151–153]. Previously, it was found that 20-HETE is involved in activation of ERK1/2 and PI3K/Akt in endothelial cells [116] and also alters cell growth in U251 human gliomas by a mechanism that initially involves activation of the ERK1/2 pathway [117]. A schematic of the signaling pathway presented by Shankar et al. [46] from our research group summarizes the possible therapeutic actions of HET0016 in Figure 3. Yu et al. also showed that CYP ω-hydroxylase overexpression enhanced the lung metastasis of A549 cells in the nude mouse by upregulating VEGF and MMP-9 expression via the PI3K and ERK1/2 signaling pathway [137]. Our results showed reduced protein levels of pAKT, total AKT, pERK1/2, and pNFκB in lungs of animals treated with HET0016 compared to 4T1-bearing control mice. In recent years, many studies have shown the pivotal role of MDSCs in downregulating anti-tumor immunity and promoting tumor growth and metastasis [154–156]. We reported a novel role of HET0016 in impeding metastasis by decreasing the g-MDSCs polarization in the metastatic site [44].

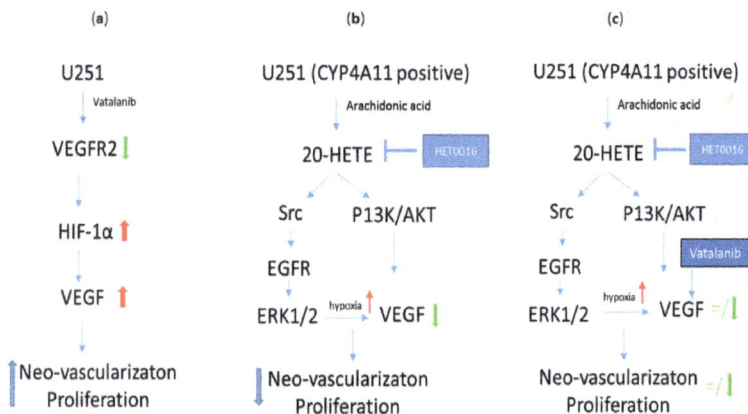

Figure 3. A possible mode of action of HET0016 in relation to growth factor pathways. (a) Treatment with vatalanib causes a decrease in expression of vascular endothelial growth factor receptor 2 (VEGFR2), but increases the expression of hypoxia-inducible factor 1 α (HIF-1α) and VEGF, which will cause increased neovascularization and tumor growth; (b) When HET0016 alone is used, VEGF expression is decreased through different signaling pathways, which will cause decreased neovascularization and tumor growth; (c) When HET0016 and vatalanib are used together some of the effects of vatalanib (increased VEGF, increased neovascularization and tumor growth) can be attenuated. Data obtained from Shankar et al. [46].

Int. J. Mol. Sci. **2017**, *18*, 2661

7. Conclusions

Considering the evidence provided by studies from our and other research groups, the CYP4A/20-HETE axis has a multi-faceted role in promoting tumor growth and metastasis. This axis has also been highly activated in myeloid cells mediating immunosuppression in the TME. The tumor stroma consisting of tumor-associated endothelial cells proliferate and lay down neovascular structures induced by 20-HETE production. However, the CYP4A/20-HETE axis has been a neglected pathway in the development of novel therapeutics. We have successfully employed HET0016 in controlling glioma and breast tumor growth and metastasis. Therefore, novel therapeutics targeting the CYP4A/20-HETE axis should gain considerable importance in translational medicine, either as monotherapy or in combination with established chemotherapeutic and radiotherapeutic approaches.

Acknowledgments: This work was supported by grants from the National Institutes of Health (NIH) R01CA160216 and R01CA172048 and from startups from the Georgia Cancer Center. The authors thank Georgia Cancer Center core facilities at Augusta University and at Henry Ford Hospital System for their assistance during the years wherein the data for this review were produced.

Author Contributions: All the authors wrote and revised the entire manuscript.

Conflicts of Interest: The authors declare no conflict of interest.

Abbreviations

20-HETE	20-Hydroxy-eicosatetraenoic acid
4T1	Triple negative metastatic murine breast cancer cell line
ALX/FPR2	Lipoxin A4 receptor/formyl peptide receptor
AA	Arachidonic acid
AAT	Antiangiogenic therapy
AKT	Protein kinase B
AMPK	5′ AMP-activated protein kinase
BC	Breast cancer
BM	Brain metastasis
BSO	Buthionine sulfoximine
BT-474	Breast cancer luminal B subtype cell line
COX	Cyclooxygenase enzyme
CXCR4	C-X-C chemokine receptor type 4 also known as fusion or CD184;
CYP	Cytochrome P450
CYP4A	Cytochrome P450, family 4, subfamily A
CYP4F	Cytochrome P450, family 4, subfamily F
DHETs	Dihydroxy-eicosatrienoic acids
EES	Extravascular extracellular space
EETs	Epoxy-eicosatrienoic acids
EGF	Epidermal growth factor
EGFR	Epidermal growth factor receptor
sEH	Epoxide hydrolase
EPCs	Endothelial progenitor cells
ER	Estrogen receptor
ERK	Extracellular signal-regulated kinases
Fas	Fas ligand or CD95 ligand
FGF-2	Basic fibroblast growth factor 2
FLA-16	Novel flavonoid
GBM	Glioblastoma
GBM811	Glioblastoma-derived from patient
GL261	Murine glioblastoma cell line

GM-CSF	Granulocyte-macrophage colony-stimulating factor
GSH	Glutathione
GPx	Glutathione peroxidase
HER2	Human epidermal growth factor receptor2
HET0016	N-hydroxy-N'-(4-butyl-2 methyl phenyl) formamidine
HF2303	Glioblastoma-derived from patient
HIF-1α	Hypoxia-inducible factor 1 α
HO	Hepoxillin
HPβCD	2-Hydroxypropyl β-cyclodextrin
HPETE	Hydroperoxy-eicosatetraenoic acid
HUVEC	Human umbilical vein endothelial cells
IL	Interleukin
IV	Intravenous
Ki67	Proliferation marker
Ktrans	Forward permeability transfer constant
LOX	Lipoxygenase
LT	Leukotriene
LX	Lipoxin
MAPK	Mitogen-Activated Protein Kinase
MCP-1	Monocyte Chemoattractant Protein-1
MDA-MB-231	Triple negative metastatic human breast cancer cell line
MDSCs	Myeloid-derived suppressor cells
MMPs	Matrix metalloproteinases
MRI	Magnetic resonance imaging
MVD	Microvessel density
NADPH	Nicotinamide adenine dinucleotide phosphate
NFκB	Nuclear factor kappa-light-chain-enhancer of activated B cells
eNOS	Endothelial nitric oxide synthase
PDX	Patient-derived xenograft
PET	Polyethylene terephthalate
PG	Prostaglandin
PI3K	Phosphatidylinositol-3-kinases
PLA2	Phospholipase A2
PPARs	Peroxisome proliferator-activated receptors
PR	Progesterone receptor
ROS	Reactive oxygen species
SCF	Stem cell factor
SDF-1α	Stromal cell-derived factor 1 α
STAT1	Signal transducer and activator of transcription 1
T2DM	Type 2 diabetes mellitus
T47D	Breast cancer luminal A subtype cell line
TAMs	Tumor-associated macrophages
TGF-β	Transforming growth factor β 1
Tie-2	Transmembrane tyrosine-protein kinase receptor
TME	Tumor microenvironment
TMZ	Temozolomide
TNBC	Triple-negative breast cancer
TNFα	Tumor necrosis factor α
U251	Human glioblastoma cell line
ve	extracellular space or interstitial volume
VE-cadherin	Vascular endothelial cadherin
VEGF	Vascular endothelial growth factor
VLA-4	Very late antigen-4
vp	Blood plasma pool
α-SMA	α-smooth muscle actin

References

1. Flemban, A.; Qualtrough, D. The potential role of hedgehog signaling in the luminal/basal phenotype of breast epithelia and in breast cancer invasion and metastasis. *Cancers* **2015**, *7*, 1863–1884. [CrossRef] [PubMed]
2. Caan, B.J.; Sweeney, C.; Habel, L.A.; Kwan, M.L.; Kroenke, C.H.; Weltzien, E.K.; Quesenberry, C.P., Jr.; Castillo, A.; Factor, R.E.; Kushi, L.H.; et al. Intrinsic subtypes from the pam50 gene expression assay in a population-based breast cancer survivor cohort: Prognostication of short- and long-term outcomes. *Cancer Epidemiol. Biomark. Prev. Publ. Am. Assoc. Cancer Res. Cospons. Am. Soc. Prev. Oncol.* **2014**, *23*, 725–734. [CrossRef] [PubMed]
3. Sestak, I.; Cuzick, J.; Dowsett, M.; Lopez-Knowles, E.; Filipits, M.; Dubsky, P.; Cowens, J.W.; Ferree, S.; Schaper, C.; Fesl, C.; et al. Prediction of late distant recurrence after 5 years of endocrine treatment: A combined analysis of patients from the austrian breast and colorectal cancer study group 8 and arimidex, tamoxifen alone or in combination randomized trials using the pam50 risk of recurrence score. *J. Clin. Oncol. Off. J. Am. Soc. Clin. Oncol.* **2015**, *33*, 916–922.
4. Tamimi, R.M.; Baer, H.J.; Marotti, J.; Galan, M.; Galaburda, L.; Fu, Y.; Deitz, A.C.; Connolly, J.L.; Schnitt, S.J.; Colditz, G.A.; et al. Comparison of molecular phenotypes of ductal carcinoma in situ and invasive breast cancer. *Breast Cancer Res.* **2008**, *10*, R67. [CrossRef] [PubMed]
5. Clark, S.E.; Warwick, J.; Carpenter, R.; Bowen, R.L.; Duffy, S.W.; Jones, J.L. Molecular subtyping of dcis: Heterogeneity of breast cancer reflected in pre-invasive disease. *Br. J. Cancer* **2011**, *104*, 120–127. [CrossRef] [PubMed]
6. Fan, C.; Oh, D.S.; Wessels, L.; Weigelt, B.; Nuyten, D.S.; Nobel, A.B.; van't Veer, L.J.; Perou, C.M. Concordance among gene-expression-based predictors for breast cancer. *N. Engl. J. Med.* **2006**, *355*, 560–569. [CrossRef] [PubMed]
7. Society, A.C. *Breast Cancer Facts & Figures 2015–2016*; American Cancer Society, Inc.: Atlanta, GA, USA, 2015.
8. Howlader, N.; Altekruse, S.F.; Li, C.I.; Chen, V.W.; Clarke, C.A.; Ries, L.A.; Cronin, K.A. US incidence of breast cancer subtypes defined by joint hormone receptor and her2 status. *J. Natl. Cancer Inst.* **2014**, *106*. [CrossRef] [PubMed]
9. Arvold, N.D.; Taghian, A.G.; Niemierko, A.; Abi Raad, R.F.; Sreedhara, M.; Nguyen, P.L.; Bellon, J.R.; Wong, J.S.; Smith, B.L.; Harris, J.R. Age, breast cancer subtype approximation, and local recurrence after breast-conserving therapy. *J. Clin. Oncol. Off. J. Am. Soc. Clin. Oncol.* **2011**, *29*, 3885–3891. [CrossRef] [PubMed]
10. Voduc, K.D.; Cheang, M.C.; Tyldesley, S.; Gelmon, K.; Nielsen, T.O.; Kennecke, H. Breast cancer subtypes and the risk of local and regional relapse. *J. Clin. Oncol. Off. J. Am. Soc. Clin. Oncol.* **2010**, *28*, 1684–1691. [CrossRef] [PubMed]
11. Metzger-Filho, O.; Sun, Z.; Viale, G.; Price, K.N.; Crivellari, D.; Snyder, R.D.; Gelber, R.D.; Castiglione-Gertsch, M.; Coates, A.S.; Goldhirsch, A.; et al. Patterns of recurrence and outcome according to breast cancer subtypes in lymph node-negative disease: Results from international breast cancer study group trials viii and ix. *J. Clin. Oncol. Off. J. Am. Soc. Clin. Oncol.* **2013**, *31*, 3083–3090. [CrossRef] [PubMed]
12. Couch, F.J.; Hart, S.N.; Sharma, P.; Toland, A.E.; Wang, X.; Miron, P.; Olson, J.E.; Godwin, A.K.; Pankratz, V.S.; Olswold, C.; et al. Inherited mutations in 17 breast cancer susceptibility genes among a large triple-negative breast cancer cohort unselected for family history of breast cancer. *J. Clin. Oncol. Off. J. Am. Soc. Clin. Oncol.* **2015**, *33*, 304–311. [CrossRef] [PubMed]
13. Toft, D.J.; Cryns, V.L. Minireview: Basal-like breast cancer: From molecular profiles to targeted therapies. *Mol. Endocrinol.* **2011**, *25*, 199–211. [CrossRef] [PubMed]
14. Rouzier, R.; Perou, C.M.; Symmans, W.F.; Ibrahim, N.; Cristofanilli, M.; Anderson, K.; Hess, K.R.; Stec, J.; Ayers, M.; Wagner, P.; et al. Breast cancer molecular subtypes respond differently to preoperative chemotherapy. *Clin. Cancer Res.* **2005**, *11*, 5678–5685. [CrossRef] [PubMed]
15. Sihto, H.; Lundin, J.; Lundin, M.; Lehtimaki, T.; Ristimaki, A.; Holli, K.; Sailas, L.; Kataja, V.; Turpeenniemi-Hujanen, T.; Isola, J.; et al. Breast cancer biological subtypes and protein expression predict for the preferential distant metastasis sites: A nationwide cohort study. *Breast Cancer Res.* **2011**, *13*, R87. [CrossRef] [PubMed]

16. Yücel, B.; Bahar, S.; Kaçan, T.; Şeker, M.; Celasun, M. Importance of metastasis site in survival of patients with breast cancer. *Austin J. Med. Oncol.* **2014**, *1*, 1–7.

17. Kimbung, S.; Loman, N.; Hedenfalk, I. Clinical and molecular complexity of breast cancer metastases. *Semin. Cancer Biol.* **2015**, *35*, 85–95. [CrossRef] [PubMed]

18. Weidle, U.H.; Birzele, F.; Kollmorgen, G.; Ruger, R. Molecular basis of lung tropism of metastasis. *Cancer Genom. Proteom.* **2016**, *13*, 129–139.

19. Largillier, R.; Ferrero, J.M.; Doyen, J.; Barriere, J.; Namer, M.; Mari, V.; Courdi, A.; Hannoun-Levi, J.M.; Ettore, F.; Birtwisle-Peyrottes, I.; et al. Prognostic factors in 1,038 women with metastatic breast cancer. *Ann. Oncol. Off. J. Eur. Soc. Med. Oncol. ESMO* **2008**, *19*, 2012–2019. [CrossRef] [PubMed]

20. Soni, A.; Ren, Z.; Hameed, O.; Chanda, D.; Morgan, C.J.; Siegal, G.P.; Wei, S. Breast cancer subtypes predispose the site of distant metastases. *Am. J. Clin. Pathol.* **2015**, *143*, 471–478. [CrossRef] [PubMed]

21. Rostami, R.; Mittal, S.; Rostami, P.; Tavassoli, F.; Jabbari, B. Brain metastasis in breast cancer: A comprehensive literature review. *J. Neuro-Oncol.* **2016**, *127*, 407–414. [CrossRef] [PubMed]

22. Witzel, I.; Oliveira-Ferrer, L.; Pantel, K.; Muller, V.; Wikman, H. Breast cancer brain metastases: Biology and new clinical perspectives. *Breast Cancer Res.* **2016**, *18*, 8. [CrossRef] [PubMed]

23. Kennecke, H.; Yerushalmi, R.; Woods, R.; Cheang, M.C.; Voduc, D.; Speers, C.H.; Nielsen, T.O.; Gelmon, K. Metastatic behavior of breast cancer subtypes. *J. Clin. Oncol. Off. J. Am. Soc. Clin. Oncol.* **2010**, *28*, 3271–3277. [CrossRef] [PubMed]

24. Smid, M.; Wang, Y.; Zhang, Y.; Sieuwerts, A.M.; Yu, J.; Klijn, J.G.; Foekens, J.A.; Martens, J.W. Subtypes of breast cancer show preferential site of relapse. *Cancer Res.* **2008**, *68*, 3108–3114. [CrossRef] [PubMed]

25. Luo, M.; Brooks, M.; Wicha, M.S. Epithelial-mesenchymal plasticity of breast cancer stem cells: Implications for metastasis and therapeutic resistance. *Curr. Pharm. Des.* **2015**, *21*, 1301–1310. [CrossRef] [PubMed]

26. Yu, T.; Di, G. Role of tumor microenvironment in triple-negative breast cancer and its prognostic significance. *Chin. J. Cancer Res.* **2017**, *29*, 237–252. [CrossRef] [PubMed]

27. Duechler, M.; Peczek, L.; Zuk, K.; Zalesna, I.; Jeziorski, A.; Czyz, M. The heterogeneous immune microenvironment in breast cancer is affected by hypoxia-related genes. *Immunobiology* **2014**, *219*, 158–165. [CrossRef] [PubMed]

28. Shou, D.; Wen, L.; Song, Z.; Yin, J.; Sun, Q.; Gong, W. Suppressive role of myeloid-derived suppressor cells (mdscs) in the microenvironment of breast cancer and targeted immunotherapies. *Oncotarget* **2016**, *7*, 64505–64511. [CrossRef] [PubMed]

29. Filipazzi, P.; Valenti, R.; Huber, V.; Pilla, L.; Canese, P.; Iero, M.; Castelli, C.; Mariani, L.; Parmiani, G.; Rivoltini, L. Identification of a new subset of myeloid suppressor cells in peripheral blood of melanoma patients with modulation by a granulocyte-macrophage colony-stimulation factor-based antitumor vaccine. *J. Clin. Oncol. Off. J. Am. Soc. Clin. Oncol.* **2007**, *25*, 2546–2553. [CrossRef] [PubMed]

30. Sinha, P.; Clements, V.K.; Ostrand-Rosenberg, S. Reduction of myeloid-derived suppressor cells and induction of m1 macrophages facilitate the rejection of established metastatic disease. *J. Immunol.* **2005**, *174*, 636–645. [CrossRef] [PubMed]

31. Kusmartsev, S.A.; Li, Y.; Chen, S.H. Gr-1+ myeloid cells derived from tumor-bearing mice inhibit primary t cell activation induced through cd3/cd28 costimulation. *J. Immunol.* **2000**, *165*, 779–785. [CrossRef] [PubMed]

32. Suzuki, E.; Kapoor, V.; Jassar, A.S.; Kaiser, L.R.; Albelda, S.M. Gemcitabine selectively eliminates splenic gr-1+/cd11b+ myeloid suppressor cells in tumor-bearing animals and enhances antitumor immune activity. *Clin. Cancer Res.* **2005**, *11*, 6713–6721. [CrossRef] [PubMed]

33. Diaz-Montero, C.M.; Salem, M.L.; Nishimura, M.I.; Garrett-Mayer, E.; Cole, D.J.; Montero, A.J. Increased circulating myeloid-derived suppressor cells correlate with clinical cancer stage, metastatic tumor burden, and doxorubicin-cyclophosphamide chemotherapy. *Cancer Immunol. Immunother.* **2009**, *58*, 49–59. [CrossRef] [PubMed]

34. Solito, S.; Falisi, E.; Diaz-Montero, C.M.; Doni, A.; Pinton, L.; Rosato, A.; Francescato, S.; Basso, G.; Zanovello, P.; Onicescu, G.; et al. A human promyelocytic-like population is responsible for the immune suppression mediated by myeloid-derived suppressor cells. *Blood* **2011**, *118*, 2254–2265. [CrossRef] [PubMed]

35. Waight, J.D.; Netherby, C.; Hensen, M.L.; Miller, A.; Hu, Q.; Liu, S.; Bogner, P.N.; Farren, M.R.; Lee, K.P.; Liu, K.; et al. Myeloid-derived suppressor cell development is regulated by a stat/irf-8 axis. *J. Clin. Investig.* **2013**, *123*, 4464–4478. [CrossRef] [PubMed]

36. Bergenfelz, C.; Larsson, A.M.; von Stedingk, K.; Gruvberger-Saal, S.; Aaltonen, K.; Jansson, S.; Jernstrom, H.; Janols, H.; Wullt, M.; Bredberg, A.; et al. Systemic monocytic-mdscs are generated from monocytes and correlate with disease progression in breast cancer patients. *PLoS ONE* **2015**, *10*, e0127028. [CrossRef] [PubMed]

37. Ouzounova, M.; Lee, E.; Piranlioglu, R.; El Andaloussi, A.; Kolhe, R.; Demirci, M.F.; Marasco, D.; Asm, I.; Chadli, A.; Hassan, K.A.; et al. Monocytic and granulocytic myeloid derived suppressor cells differentially regulate spatiotemporal tumour plasticity during metastatic cascade. *Nat. Commun.* **2017**, *8*, 14979. [CrossRef] [PubMed]

38. Arvelo, F.; Sojo, F.; Cotte, C. Tumour progression and metastasis. *Ecancermedicalscience* **2016**, *10*, 617. [CrossRef] [PubMed]

39. Qian, B.Z.; Pollard, J.W. Macrophage diversity enhances tumor progression and metastasis. *Cell* **2010**, *141*, 39–51. [CrossRef] [PubMed]

40. Biswas, S.K.; Mantovani, A. Macrophage plasticity and interaction with lymphocyte subsets: Cancer as a paradigm. *Nat. Immunol.* **2010**, *11*, 889–896. [CrossRef] [PubMed]

41. Escribese, M.M.; Casas, M.; Corbi, A.L. Influence of low oxygen tensions on macrophage polarization. *Immunobiology* **2012**, *217*, 1233–1240. [CrossRef] [PubMed]

42. Qian, B.Z.; Li, J.; Zhang, H.; Kitamura, T.; Zhang, J.; Campion, L.R.; Kaiser, E.A.; Snyder, L.A.; Pollard, J.W. Ccl2 recruits inflammatory monocytes to facilitate breast-tumour metastasis. *Nature* **2011**, *475*, 222–225. [CrossRef] [PubMed]

43. Achyut, B.R.; Arbab, A.S. Myeloid cell signatures in tumor microenvironment predicts therapeutic response in cancer. *OncoTargets Ther.* **2016**, *9*, 1047–1055.

44. Borin, T.F.; Shankar, A.; Angara, K.; Rashid, M.H.; Jain, M.; Iskander, A.; Ara, R.; Lebedyeva, I.; Korkaya, H.; Achyut, B.R.; et al. HET0016 decreases lung metastasis from breast cancer in immune-competent mouse model. *PLoS ONE* **2017**, *12*, e0178830. [CrossRef] [PubMed]

45. Borin, T.F.; Zuccari, D.A.; Jardim-Perassi, B.V.; Ferreira, L.C.; Iskander, A.S.; Varma, N.R.; Shankar, A.; Guo, A.M.; Scicli, G.; Arbab, A.S. HET0016, a selective inhibitor of 20-hete synthesis, decreases pro-angiogenic factors and inhibits growth of triple negative breast cancer in mice. *PLoS ONE* **2014**, *9*, e116247. [CrossRef] [PubMed]

46. Shankar, A.; Borin, T.F.; Iskander, A.; Varma, N.R.; Achyut, B.R.; Jain, M.; Mikkelsen, T.; Guo, A.M.; Chwang, W.B.; Ewing, J.R.; et al. Combination of vatalanib and a 20-hete synthesis inhibitor results in decreased tumor growth in an animal model of human glioma. *OncoTargets Ther.* **2016**, *9*, 1205–1219.

47. Bosisio, E.; Galli, C.; Galli, G.; Nicosia, S.; Spagnuolo, C.; Tosi, L. Correlation between release of free arachidonic acid and prostaglandin formation in brain cortex and cerebellum. *Prostaglandins* **1976**, *11*, 773–781. [CrossRef]

48. Bergstroem, S.; Danielsson, H.; Samuelsson, B. The enzymatic formation of prostaglandin e2 from arachidonic acid prostaglandins and related factors 32. *Biochim. Biophys. Acta* **1964**, *90*, 207–210. [CrossRef]

49. Rahman, M.; Wright, J.T., Jr.; Douglas, J.G. The role of the cytochrome p450-dependent metabolites of arachidonic acid in blood pressure regulation and renal function: A review. *Am. J. Hypertens.* **1997**, *10*, 356–365. [CrossRef]

50. Bazinet, R.P.; Laye, S. Polyunsaturated fatty acids and their metabolites in brain function and disease. *Nat. Rev. Neurosci.* **2014**, *15*, 771–785. [CrossRef] [PubMed]

51. Kroetz, D.L.; Xu, F. Regulation and inhibition of arachidonic acid omega-hydroxylases and 20-hete formation. *Ann. Rev. Pharmacol. Toxicol.* **2005**, *45*, 413–438. [CrossRef] [PubMed]

52. Zhu, Q.F.; Hao, Y.H.; Liu, M.Z.; Yue, J.; Ni, J.; Yuan, B.F.; Feng, Y.Q. Analysis of cytochrome p450 metabolites of arachidonic acid by stable isotope probe labeling coupled with ultra high-performance liquid chromatography/mass spectrometry. *J. Chromatogr. A* **2015**, *1410*, 154–163. [CrossRef] [PubMed]

53. Roman, R.J. P-450 metabolites of arachidonic acid in the control of cardiovascular function. *Physiol. Rev.* **2002**, *82*, 131–185. [CrossRef] [PubMed]

54. Fleming, I. The factor in edhf: Cytochrome p450 derived lipid mediators and vascular signaling. *Vasc. Pharmacol.* **2016**, *86*, 31–40. [CrossRef] [PubMed]

55. Zhao, H.; Qi, G.; Han, Y.; Shen, X.; Yao, F.; Xuan, C.; Gu, Y.; Qian, S.Y.; Zeng, Q.; O'Rourke, S.T.; et al. 20-hydroxyeicosatetraenoic acid is a key mediator of angiotensin ii-induced apoptosis in cardiac myocytes. *J. Cardiovasc. Pharmacol.* **2015**, *66*, 86–95. [CrossRef] [PubMed]

56. Matsuyama, M.; Yoshimura, R. Arachidonic acid pathway: A molecular target in human testicular cancer (review). *Mol. Med. Rep.* **2009**, *2*, 527–531. [PubMed]

57. Koontongkaew, S.; Leelahavanichkul, K. Arachidonic acid metabolism and its implication on head and neck cancer. In *Head and Neck Cancer*; Agulnik, D.M., Ed.; InTech: London, UK, 2012.

58. Greene, E.R.; Huang, S.; Serhan, C.N.; Panigrahy, D. Regulation of inflammation in cancer by eicosanoids. *Prostaglandins Other Lipid Mediat.* **2011**, *96*, 27–36. [CrossRef] [PubMed]

59. Chandrasekharan, N.V.; Dai, H.; Roos, K.L.; Evanson, N.K.; Tomsik, J.; Elton, T.S.; Simmons, D.L. Cox-3, a cyclooxygenase-1 variant inhibited by acetaminophen and other analgesic/antipyretic drugs: Cloning, structure, and expression. *Proc. Natl. Acad. Sci. USA* **2002**, *99*, 13926–13931. [CrossRef] [PubMed]

60. Schwab, J.M.; Schluesener, H.J.; Meyermann, R.; Serhan, C.N. Cox-3 the enzyme and the concept: Steps towards highly specialized pathways and precision therapeutics? *Prostaglandins Leukot. Essent. Fat. Acids* **2003**, *69*, 339–343. [CrossRef]

61. Willoughby, D.A.; Moore, A.R.; Colville-Nash, P.R. Cox-1, cox-2, and cox-3 and the future treatment of chronic inflammatory disease. *Lancet* **2000**, *355*, 646–648. [CrossRef]

62. Moore, G.Y.; Pidgeon, G.P. Cross-talk between cancer cells and the tumour microenvironment: The role of the 5-lipoxygenase pathway. *Int. J. Mol. Sci.* **2017**, *18*. [CrossRef] [PubMed]

63. Ding, X.Z.; Hennig, R.; Adrian, T.E. Lipoxygenase and cyclooxygenase metabolism: New insights in treatment and chemoprevention of pancreatic cancer. *Mol. Cancer* **2003**, *2*, 10. [CrossRef] [PubMed]

64. Larre, S.; Tran, N.; Fan, C.; Hamadeh, H.; Champigneulles, J.; Azzouzi, R.; Cussenot, O.; Mangin, P.; Olivier, J.L. Pge2 and ltb4 tissue levels in benign and cancerous prostates. *Prostaglandins Other Lipid Mediat.* **2008**, *87*, 14–19. [CrossRef] [PubMed]

65. Venerito, M.; Kuester, D.; Harms, C.; Schubert, D.; Wex, T.; Malfertheiner, P. Upregulation of leukotriene receptors in gastric cancer. *Cancers* **2011**, *3*, 3156–3168. [CrossRef] [PubMed]

66. Hennig, R.; Ventura, J.; Segersvard, R.; Ward, E.; Ding, X.Z.; Rao, S.M.; Jovanovic, B.D.; Iwamura, T.; Talamonti, M.S.; Bell, R.H., Jr.; et al. Ly293111 improves efficacy of gemcitabine therapy on pancreatic cancer in a fluorescent orthotopic model in athymic mice. *Neoplasia* **2005**, *7*, 417–425. [CrossRef] [PubMed]

67. Adrian, T.E.; Hennig, R.; Friess, H.; Ding, X. The role of ppargamma receptors and leukotriene b(4) receptors in mediating the effects of ly293111 in pancreatic cancer. *PPAR Res.* **2008**, *2008*, 827096. [CrossRef] [PubMed]

68. Tang, K.; Honn, K.V. 12(s)-hete in cancer metastasis. *Adv. Exp. Med. Biol.* **1999**, *447*, 181–191. [PubMed]

69. Steele, V.E.; Holmes, C.A.; Hawk, E.T.; Kopelovich, L.; Lubet, R.A.; Crowell, J.A.; Sigman, C.C.; Kelloff, G.J. Lipoxygenase inhibitors as potential cancer chemopreventives. *Cancer Epidemiol. Biomark. Prev. Publ. Am. Assoc. Cancer Res. Cospons. Am. Soc. Prev. Oncol.* **1999**, *8*, 467–483.

70. Wong, B.C.; Wang, W.P.; Cho, C.H.; Fan, X.M.; Lin, M.C.; Kung, H.F.; Lam, S.K. 12-lipoxygenase inhibition induced apoptosis in human gastric cancer cells. *Carcinogenesis* **2001**, *22*, 1349–1354. [CrossRef] [PubMed]

71. Tang, D.G.; Honn, K.V. Apoptosis of w256 carcinosarcoma cells of the monocytoid origin induced by ndga involves lipid peroxidation and depletion of gsh: Role of 12-lipoxygenase in regulating tumor cell survival. *J. Cell. Physiol.* **1997**, *172*, 155–170. [CrossRef]

72. Nigam, S.; Patabhiraman, S.; Ciccoli, R.; Ishdorj, G.; Schwarz, K.; Petrucev, B.; Kuhn, H.; Haeggstrom, J.Z. The rat leukocyte-type 12-lipoxygenase exhibits an intrinsic hepoxilin a3 synthase activity. *J. Biol. Chem.* **2004**, *279*, 29023–29030. [CrossRef] [PubMed]

73. Janakiram, N.B.; Mohammed, A.; Rao, C.V. Role of lipoxins, resolvins, and other bioactive lipids in colon and pancreatic cancer. *Cancer Metastasis Rev.* **2011**, *30*, 507–523. [CrossRef] [PubMed]

74. Chandrasekharan, J.A.; Sharma-Walia, N. Lipoxins: Nature's way to resolve inflammation. *J. Inflamm. Res.* **2015**, *8*, 181–192. [PubMed]

75. Pidgeon, G.P.; Lysaght, J.; Krishnamoorthy, S.; Reynolds, J.V.; O'Byrne, K.; Nie, D.; Honn, K.V. Lipoxygenase metabolism: Roles in tumor progression and survival. *Cancer Metastasis Rev.* **2007**, *26*, 503–524. [CrossRef] [PubMed]

76. Curzio, M.; Esterbauer, H.; Poli, G.; Biasi, F.; Cecchini, G.; Di Mauro, C.; Cappello, N.; Dianzani, M.U. Possible role of aldehydic lipid peroxidation products as chemoattractants. *Int. J. Tissue React.* **1987**, *9*, 295–306. [PubMed]

77. Wan, Y.Y.; Cai, Y.; Li, J.; Yuan, Q.; French, B.; Gonzalez, F.J.; French, S. Regulation of peroxisome proliferator activated receptor alpha-mediated pathways in alcohol fed cytochrome p450 2e1 deficient mice. *Hepatol. Res. Off. J. Jpn. Soc. Hepatol.* **2001**, *19*, 117–130. [CrossRef]

78. Robertson, G.; Leclercq, I.; Farrell, G.C. Nonalcoholic steatosis and steatohepatitis. Ii. Cytochrome p-450 enzymes and oxidative stress. *Am. J. Physiol. Gastrointest. Liver Physiol.* **2001**, *281*, G1135–G1139. [PubMed]

79. Bell, L.C.; Guengerich, F.P. Oxidation kinetics of ethanol by human cytochrome p450 2e1. Rate-limiting product release accounts for effects of isotopic hydrogen substitution and cytochrome b5 on steady-state kinetics. *J. Biol. Chem.* **1997**, *272*, 29643–29651. [CrossRef] [PubMed]

80. Gorsky, L.D.; Koop, D.R.; Coon, M.J. On the stoichiometry of the oxidase and monooxygenase reactions catalyzed by liver microsomal cytochrome p-450. Products of oxygen reduction. *J. Biol. Chem.* **1984**, *259*, 6812–6817. [PubMed]

81. Ekstrom, G.; Ingelman-Sundberg, M. Rat liver microsomal nadph-supported oxidase activity and lipid peroxidation dependent on ethanol-inducible cytochrome p-450 (p-450iie1). *Biochem. Pharmacol.* **1989**, *38*, 1313–1319. [CrossRef]

82. Wu, D.; Cederbaum, A.I. Removal of glutathione produces apoptosis and necrosis in hepg2 cells overexpressing cyp2e1. *Alcohol. Clin. Exp. Res.* **2001**, *25*, 619–628. [CrossRef] [PubMed]

83. Mari, M.; Cederbaum, A.I. Cyp2e1 overexpression in hepg2 cells induces glutathione synthesis by transcriptional activation of gamma-glutamylcysteine synthetase. *J. Biol. Chem.* **2000**, *275*, 15563–15571. [CrossRef] [PubMed]

84. Mari, M.; Cederbaum, A.I. Induction of catalase, alpha, and microsomal glutathione s-transferase in cyp2e1 overexpressing hepg2 cells and protection against short-term oxidative stress. *Hepatology* **2001**, *33*, 652–661. [CrossRef] [PubMed]

85. Panigrahy, D.; Kaipainen, A.; Greene, E.R.; Huang, S. Cytochrome p450-derived eicosanoids: The neglected pathway in cancer. *Cancer Metastasis Rev.* **2010**, *29*, 723–735. [CrossRef] [PubMed]

86. Nebert, D.W.; Wikvall, K.; Miller, W.L. Human cytochromes p450 in health and disease. *Philos. Trans. R. Soc. Lond. Ser. B Biol. Sci.* **2013**, *368*, 20120431. [CrossRef] [PubMed]

87. Nie, D.; Che, M.; Zacharek, A.; Qiao, Y.; Li, L.; Li, X.; Lamberti, M.; Tang, K.; Cai, Y.; Guo, Y.; et al. Differential expression of thromboxane synthase in prostate carcinoma: Role in tumor cell motility. *Am. J. Pathol.* **2004**, *164*, 429–439. [CrossRef]

88. Medhora, M.; Dhanasekaran, A.; Gruenloh, S.K.; Dunn, L.K.; Gabrilovich, M.; Falck, J.R.; Harder, D.R.; Jacobs, E.R.; Pratt, P.F. Emerging mechanisms for growth and protection of the vasculature by cytochrome p450-derived products of arachidonic acid and other eicosanoids. *Prostaglandins Other Lipid Mediat.* **2007**, *82*, 19–29. [CrossRef] [PubMed]

89. Wang, J.S.; Zhang, F.; Jiang, M.; Wang, M.H.; Zand, B.A.; Abraham, N.G.; Nasjletti, A.; Laniado-Schwartzman, M. Transfection and functional expression of cyp4a1 and cyp4a2 using bicistronic vectors in vascular cells and tissues. *J. Pharmacol. Exp. Ther.* **2004**, *311*, 913–920. [CrossRef] [PubMed]

90. Huang, H.; Al-Shabrawey, M.; Wang, M.H. Cyclooxygenase- and cytochrome p450-derived eicosanoids in stroke. *Prostaglandins Other Lipid Mediat.* **2016**, *122*, 45–53. [CrossRef] [PubMed]

91. Nguyen, X.; Wang, M.H.; Reddy, K.M.; Falck, J.R.; Schwartzman, M.L. Kinetic profile of the rat cyp4a isoforms: Arachidonic acid metabolism and isoform-specific inhibitors. *Am. J. Physiol.* **1999**, *276*, R1691–R1700. [PubMed]

92. Muller, D.N.; Schmidt, C.; Barbosa-Sicard, E.; Wellner, M.; Gross, V.; Hercule, H.; Markovic, M.; Honeck, H.; Luft, F.C.; Schunck, W.H. Mouse cyp4a isoforms: Enzymatic properties, gender- and strain-specific expression, and role in renal 20-hydroxyeicosatetraenoic acid formation. *Biochem. J.* **2007**, *403*, 109–118. [CrossRef] [PubMed]

93. Hoopes, S.L.; Garcia, V.; Edin, M.L.; Schwartzman, M.L.; Zeldin, D.C. Vascular actions of 20-hete. *Prostaglandins Other Lipid Mediat.* **2015**, *120*, 9–16. [CrossRef] [PubMed]

94. Chen, L.; Joseph, G.; Zhang, F.F.; Nguyen, H.; Jiang, H.; Gotlinger, K.H.; Falck, J.R.; Yang, J.; Schwartzman, M.L.; Guo, A.M. 20-hete contributes to ischemia-induced angiogenesis. *Vasc. Pharmacol.* **2016**, *83*, 57–65. [CrossRef] [PubMed]

95. Garcia, V.; Joseph, G.; Shkolnik, B.; Ding, Y.; Zhang, F.F.; Gotlinger, K.; Falck, J.R.; Dakarapu, R.; Capdevila, J.H.; Bernstein, K.E.; et al. Angiotensin ii receptor blockade or deletion of vascular endothelial ace does not prevent vascular dysfunction and remodeling in 20-hete-dependent hypertension. *Am. J. Physiol. Regul. Integr. Comp. Physiol.* **2015**, *309*, R71–R78. [CrossRef] [PubMed]

96. Seki, T.; Wang, M.H.; Miyata, N.; Laniado-Schwartzman, M. Cytochrome p450 4a isoform inhibitory profile of N-hydroxy-N'-(4-butyl-2-methylphenyl)-formamidine (het0016), a selective inhibitor of 20-hete synthesis. *Biol. Pharm. Bull.* **2005**, *28*, 1651–1654. [CrossRef] [PubMed]

97. Muthalif, M.M.; Benter, I.F.; Karzoun, N.; Fatima, S.; Harper, J.; Uddin, M.R.; Malik, K.U. 20-hydroxyeicosatetraenoic acid mediates calcium/calmodulin-dependent protein kinase ii-induced mitogen-activated protein kinase activation in vascular smooth muscle cells. *Proc. Natl. Acad. Sci. USA* **1998**, *95*, 12701–12706. [CrossRef] [PubMed]

98. Kaduce, T.L.; Fang, X.; Harmon, S.D.; Oltman, C.L.; Dellsperger, K.C.; Teesch, L.M.; Gopal, V.R.; Falck, J.R.; Campbell, W.B.; Weintraub, N.L.; et al. 20-hydroxyeicosatetraenoic acid (20-hete) metabolism in coronary endothelial cells. *J. Biol. Chem.* **2004**, *279*, 2648–2656. [CrossRef] [PubMed]

99. Schwartzman, M.L.; Falck, J.R.; Yadagiri, P.; Escalante, B. Metabolism of 20-hydroxyeicosatetraenoic acid by cyclooxygenase. Formation and identification of novel endothelium-dependent vasoconstrictor metabolites. *J. Biol. Chem.* **1989**, *264*, 11658–11662. [PubMed]

100. Garcia, V.; Shkolnik, B.; Milhau, L.; Falck, J.R.; Schwartzman, M.L. 20-hete activates the transcription of angiotensin-converting enzyme via nuclear factor-kappab translocation and promoter binding. *J. Pharmacol. Exp. Ther.* **2016**, *356*, 525–533. [CrossRef] [PubMed]

101. Hanahan, D.; Weinberg, R.A. Hallmarks of cancer: The next generation. *Cell* **2011**, *144*, 646–674. [CrossRef] [PubMed]

102. Zahid, H.; Simpson, E.R.; Brown, K.A. Inflammation, dysregulated metabolism and aromatase in obesity and breast cancer. *Curr. Opin. Pharmacol.* **2016**, *31*, 90–96. [CrossRef] [PubMed]

103. Bulun, S.E.; Chen, D.; Moy, I.; Brooks, D.C.; Zhao, H. Aromatase, breast cancer and obesity: A complex interaction. *Trends Endocrinol. Metab.* **2012**, *23*, 83–89. [CrossRef] [PubMed]

104. Leonel, C.; Ferreira, L.C.; Borin, T.F.; Moschetta, M.G.; Freitas, G.S.; Haddad, M.R.; de Camargos Pinto Robles, J.A.; Aparecida Pires de Campos Zuccari, D. Inhibition of epithelial-mesenchymal transition in response to treatment with metformin and y27632 in breast cancer cell lines. *Anticancer Agents Med. Chem.* **2017**, *17*, 1113–1125. [CrossRef] [PubMed]

105. Brown, K.A.; Hunger, N.I.; Docanto, M.; Simpson, E.R. Metformin inhibits aromatase expression in human breast adipose stromal cells via stimulation of amp-activated protein kinase. *Breast Cancer Res. Treat.* **2010**, *123*, 591–596. [CrossRef] [PubMed]

106. Patterson, E.; Wall, R.; Fitzgerald, G.F.; Ross, R.P.; Stanton, C. Health implications of high dietary omega-6 polyunsaturated fatty acids. *J. Nutr. Metab.* **2012**, *2012*, 539426. [CrossRef] [PubMed]

107. Horrillo, R.; Gonzalez-Periz, A.; Martinez-Clemente, M.; Lopez-Parra, M.; Ferre, N.; Titos, E.; Moran-Salvador, E.; Deulofeu, R.; Arroyo, V.; Claria, J. 5-lipoxygenase activating protein signals adipose tissue inflammation and lipid dysfunction in experimental obesity. *J. Immunol.* **2010**, *184*, 3978–3987. [CrossRef] [PubMed]

108. Hirata, K.; Wada, K.; Murata, Y.; Nakajima, A.; Yamashiro, T.; Kamisaki, Y. Critical role of leukotriene b4 receptor signaling in mouse 3t3-l1 preadipocyte differentiation. *Lipids Health Dis.* **2013**, *12*, 122. [CrossRef] [PubMed]

109. Li, P.; Oh, D.Y.; Bandyopadhyay, G.; Lagakos, W.S.; Talukdar, S.; Osborn, O.; Johnson, A.; Chung, H.; Maris, M.; Ofrecio, J.M.; et al. Ltb4 promotes insulin resistance in obese mice by acting on macrophages, hepatocytes and myocytes. *Nat. Med.* **2015**, *21*, 239–247. [CrossRef] [PubMed]

110. Curat, C.A.; Miranville, A.; Sengenes, C.; Diehl, M.; Tonus, C.; Busse, R.; Bouloumie, A. From blood monocytes to adipose tissue-resident macrophages: Induction of diapedesis by human mature adipocytes. *Diabetes* **2004**, *53*, 1285–1292. [CrossRef] [PubMed]

111. Sartipy, P.; Loskutoff, D.J. Monocyte chemoattractant protein 1 in obesity and insulin resistance. *Proc. Natl. Acad. Sci. USA* **2003**, *100*, 7265–7270. [CrossRef] [PubMed]

112. Kaaman, M.; Ryden, M.; Axelsson, T.; Nordstrom, E.; Sicard, A.; Bouloumie, A.; Langin, D.; Arner, P.; Dahlman, I. Alox5ap expression, but not gene haplotypes, is associated with obesity and insulin resistance. *Int. J. Obes.* **2006**, *30*, 447–452. [CrossRef] [PubMed]

113. Park, E.C.; Kim, S.I.; Hong, Y.; Hwang, J.W.; Cho, G.S.; Cha, H.N.; Han, J.K.; Yun, C.H.; Park, S.Y.; Jang, I.S.; et al. Inhibition of cyp4a reduces hepatic endoplasmic reticulum stress and features of diabetes in mice. *Gastroenterology* **2014**, *147*, 860–869. [CrossRef] [PubMed]

114. Chen, L.; Ackerman, R.; Saleh, M.; Gotlinger, K.H.; Kessler, M.; Mendelowitz, L.G.; Falck, J.R.; Arbab, A.S.; Scicli, A.G.; Schwartzman, M.L.; et al. 20-hete regulates the angiogenic functions of human endothelial progenitor cells and contributes to angiogenesis in vivo. *J. Pharmacol. Exp. Ther.* **2014**, *348*, 442–451. [CrossRef] [PubMed]

115. Guo, A.M.; Janic, B.; Sheng, J.; Falck, J.R.; Roman, R.J.; Edwards, P.A.; Arbab, A.S.; Scicli, A.G. The cytochrome p450 4a/f-20-hydroxyeicosatetraenoic acid system: A regulator of endothelial precursor cells derived from human umbilical cord blood. *J. Pharmacol. Exp. Ther.* **2011**, *338*, 421–429. [CrossRef] [PubMed]

116. Guo, A.M.; Arbab, A.S.; Falck, J.R.; Chen, P.; Edwards, P.A.; Roman, R.J.; Scicli, A.G. Activation of vascular endothelial growth factor through reactive oxygen species mediates 20-hydroxyeicosatetraenoic acid-induced endothelial cell proliferation. *J. Pharmacol. Exp. Ther.* **2007**, *321*, 18–27. [CrossRef] [PubMed]

117. Guo, A.M.; Sheng, J.; Scicli, G.M.; Arbab, A.S.; Lehman, N.L.; Edwards, P.A.; Falck, J.R.; Roman, R.J.; Scicli, A.G. Expression of cyp4a1 in u251 human glioma cell induces hyperproliferative phenotype in vitro and rapidly growing tumors in vivo. *J. Pharmacol. Exp. Ther.* **2008**, *327*, 10–19. [CrossRef] [PubMed]

118. Chen, L.; Ackerman, R.; Guo, A.M. 20-hete in neovascularization. *Prostaglandins Other Lipid Mediat.* **2012**, *98*, 63–68. [CrossRef] [PubMed]

119. Guo, A.M.; Scicli, G.; Sheng, J.; Falck, J.C.; Edwards, P.A.; Scicli, A.G. 20-hete can act as a nonhypoxic regulator of hif-1{alpha} in human microvascular endothelial cells. *Am. J. Physiol. Heart Circ. Physiol.* **2009**, *297*, H602–H613. [CrossRef] [PubMed]

120. Angara, K.; Rashid, M.H.; Shankar, A.; Ara, R.; Iskander, A.; Borin, T.F.; Jain, M.; Achyut, B.R.; Arbab, A.S. Vascular mimicry in glioblastoma following anti-angiogenic and anti-20-hete therapies. *Histol. Histopathol.* **2017**, *32*, 917–928. [PubMed]

121. Jain, M.; Gamage, N.H.; Alsulami, M.; Shankar, A.; Achyut, B.R.; Angara, K.; Rashid, M.H.; Iskander, A.; Borin, T.F.; Wenbo, Z.; et al. Intravenous formulation of het0016 decreased human glioblastoma growth and implicated survival benefit in rat xenograft models. *Sci. Rep.* **2017**, *7*, 41809. [CrossRef] [PubMed]

122. Angara, K.; Borin, T.F.; Arbab, A.S. Vascular mimicry: A novel neovascularization mechanism driving anti-angiogenic therapy (aat) resistance in glioblastoma. *Transl. Oncol.* **2017**, *10*, 650–660. [CrossRef] [PubMed]

123. Folkman, J. What is the evidence that tumors are angiogenesis dependent? *J. Natl. Cancer Inst.* **1990**, *82*, 4–6. [CrossRef] [PubMed]

124. McAllister, S.S.; Weinberg, R.A. Tumor-host interactions: A far-reaching relationship. *J. Clin. Oncol. Off. J. Am. Soc. Clin. Oncol.* **2010**, *28*, 4022–4028. [CrossRef] [PubMed]

125. Panigrahy, D.; Huang, S.; Kieran, M.W.; Kaipainen, A. Ppargamma as a therapeutic target for tumor angiogenesis and metastasis. *Cancer Biol. Ther.* **2005**, *4*, 687–693. [CrossRef] [PubMed]

126. Bhowmick, N.A.; Neilson, E.G.; Moses, H.L. Stromal fibroblasts in cancer initiation and progression. *Nature* **2004**, *432*, 332–337. [CrossRef] [PubMed]

127. Orimo, A.; Gupta, P.B.; Sgroi, D.C.; Arenzana-Seisdedos, F.; Delaunay, T.; Naeem, R.; Carey, V.J.; Richardson, A.L.; Weinberg, R.A. Stromal fibroblasts present in invasive human breast carcinomas promote tumor growth and angiogenesis through elevated sdf-1/cxcl12 secretion. *Cell* **2005**, *121*, 335–348. [CrossRef] [PubMed]

128. Folkman, J. Tumor angiogenesis: Therapeutic implications. *N. Engl. J. Med.* **1971**, *285*, 1182–1186. [PubMed]

129. Carmeliet, P.; Jain, R.K. Molecular mechanisms and clinical applications of angiogenesis. *Nature* **2011**, *473*, 298–307. [CrossRef] [PubMed]

130. Maniotis, A.J.; Folberg, R.; Hess, A.; Seftor, E.A.; Gardner, L.M.; Pe'er, J.; Trent, J.M.; Meltzer, P.S.; Hendrix, M.J. Vascular channel formation by human melanoma cells in vivo and in vitro: Vasculogenic mimicry. *Am. J. Pathol.* **1999**, *155*, 739–752. [CrossRef]

131. Lin, E.Y.; Pollard, J.W. Role of infiltrated leucocytes in tumour growth and spread. *Br. J. Cancer* **2004**, *90*, 2053–2058. [CrossRef] [PubMed]

132. De Visser, K.E.; Eichten, A.; Coussens, L.M. Paradoxical roles of the immune system during cancer development. *Nat. Rev. Cancer* **2006**, *6*, 24–37. [CrossRef] [PubMed]

133. Marvel, D.; Gabrilovich, D.I. Myeloid-derived suppressor cells in the tumor microenvironment: Expect the unexpected. *J. Clin. Investig.* **2015**, *125*, 3356–3364. [CrossRef] [PubMed]

134. Sa, G.; Murugesan, G.; Jaye, M.; Ivashchenko, Y.; Fox, P.L. Activation of cytosolic phospholipase a2 by basic fibroblast growth factor via a p42 mitogen-activated protein kinase-dependent phosphorylation pathway in endothelial cells. *J. Biol. Chem.* **1995**, *270*, 2360–2366. [CrossRef] [PubMed]

135. Dhanasekaran, A.; Bodiga, S.; Gruenloh, S.; Gao, Y.; Dunn, L.; Falck, J.R.; Buonaccorsi, J.N.; Medhora, M.; Jacobs, E.R. 20-hete increases survival and decreases apoptosis in pulmonary arteries and pulmonary artery endothelial cells. *Am. J. Physiol. Heart Circ. Physiol.* **2009**, *296*, H777–H786. [CrossRef] [PubMed]

136. Yu, W.; Chai, H.; Li, Y.; Zhao, H.; Xie, X.; Zheng, H.; Wang, C.; Wang, X.; Yang, G.; Cai, X.; et al. Increased expression of cyp4z1 promotes tumor angiogenesis and growth in human breast cancer. *Toxicol. Appl. Pharmacol.* **2012**, *264*, 73–83. [CrossRef] [PubMed]

137. Yu, W.; Chen, L.; Yang, Y.Q.; Falck, J.R.; Guo, A.M.; Li, Y.; Yang, J. Cytochrome p450 ω-hydroxylase promotes angiogenesis and metastasis by upregulation of vegf and mmp-9 in non-small cell lung cancer. *Cancer Chemother. Pharmacol.* **2011**, *68*, 619–629. [CrossRef] [PubMed]

138. Folberg, R.; Hendrix, M.J.; Maniotis, A.J. Vasculogenic mimicry and tumor angiogenesis. *Am. J. Pathol.* **2000**, *156*, 361–381. [CrossRef]

139. Folberg, R.; Maniotis, A.J. Vasculogenic mimicry. *Acta Pathol. Microbiol. Immunol. Scand.* **2004**, *112*, 508–525. [CrossRef] [PubMed]

140. Youn, J.I.; Collazo, M.; Shalova, I.N.; Biswas, S.K.; Gabrilovich, D.I. Characterization of the nature of granulocytic myeloid-derived suppressor cells in tumor-bearing mice. *J. Leukoc. Biol.* **2012**, *91*, 167–181. [CrossRef] [PubMed]

141. Yang, W.C.; Ma, G.; Chen, S.H.; Pan, P.Y. Polarization and reprogramming of myeloid-derived suppressor cells. *J. Mol. Cell Biol.* **2013**, *5*, 207–209. [CrossRef] [PubMed]

142. Chen, X.W.; Yu, T.J.; Zhang, J.; Li, Y.; Chen, H.L.; Yang, G.F.; Yu, W.; Liu, Y.Z.; Liu, X.X.; Duan, C.F.; et al. Cyp4a in tumor-associated macrophages promotes pre-metastatic niche formation and metastasis. *Oncogene* **2017**, *36*, 5045–5057. [CrossRef] [PubMed]

143. Wang, C.; Li, Y.; Chen, H.; Zhang, J.; Zhang, J.; Qin, T.; Duan, C.; Chen, X.; Liu, Y.; Zhou, X.; et al. Inhibition of cyp4a by a novel flavonoid fla-16 prolongs survival and normalizes tumor vasculature in glioma. *Cancer Lett.* **2017**, *402*, 131–141. [CrossRef] [PubMed]

144. Nithipatikom, K.; Isbell, M.A.; See, W.A.; Campbell, W.B. Elevated 12- and 20-hydroxyeicosatetraenoic acid in urine of patients with prostatic diseases. *Cancer Lett.* **2006**, *233*, 219–225. [CrossRef] [PubMed]

145. Alexanian, A.; Miller, B.; Roman, R.J.; Sorokin, A. 20-hete-producing enzymes are up-regulated in human cancers. *Cancer Genom. Proteom.* **2012**, *9*, 163–169.

146. Guo, M.; Roman, R.J.; Fenstermacher, J.D.; Brown, S.L.; Falck, J.R.; Arbab, A.S.; Edwards, P.A.; Scicli, A.G. 9l gliosarcoma cell proliferation and tumor growth in rats are suppressed by N-hydroxy-N′-(4-butyl-2-methylphenol) formamidine (het0016), a selective inhibitor of cyp4a. *J. Pharmacol. Exp. Ther.* **2006**, *317*, 97–108. [CrossRef] [PubMed]

147. Guo, M.; Roman, R.J.; Falck, J.R.; Edwards, P.A.; Scicli, A.G. Human u251 glioma cell proliferation is suppressed by HET0016 [N-hydroxy-N′-(4-butyl-2-methylphenyl)formamidine], a selective inhibitor of cyp4a. *J. Pharmacol. Exp. Ther.* **2005**, *315*, 526–533. [CrossRef] [PubMed]

148. Zheng, H.; Li, Y.; Wang, Y.; Zhao, H.; Zhang, J.; Chai, H.; Tang, T.; Yue, J.; Guo, A.M.; Yang, J. Downregulation of cox-2 and cyp 4a signaling by isoliquiritigenin inhibits human breast cancer metastasis through preventing anoikis resistance, migration and invasion. *Toxicol. Appl. Pharmacol.* **2014**, *280*, 10–20. [CrossRef] [PubMed]

149. Jiang, J.G.; Ning, Y.G.; Chen, C.; Ma, D.; Liu, Z.J.; Yang, S.; Zhou, J.; Xiao, X.; Zhang, X.A.; Edin, M.L.; et al. Cytochrome p450 epoxygenase promotes human cancer metastasis. *Cancer Res.* **2007**, *67*, 6665–6674. [CrossRef] [PubMed]

150. Panigrahy, D.; Edin, M.L.; Lee, C.R.; Huang, S.; Bielenberg, D.R.; Butterfield, C.E.; Barnes, C.M.; Mammoto, A.; Mammoto, T.; Luria, A.; et al. Epoxyeicosanoids stimulate multiorgan metastasis and tumor dormancy escape in mice. *J. Clin. Investig.* **2012**, *122*, 178–191. [CrossRef] [PubMed]

151. Jiang, B.H.; Liu, L.Z. Akt signaling in regulating angiogenesis. *Curr. Cancer Drug Targets* **2008**, *8*, 19–26. [CrossRef] [PubMed]

152. Qiao, M.; Sheng, S.; Pardee, A.B. Metastasis and akt activation. *Cell Cycle* **2008**, *7*, 2991–2996. [CrossRef] [PubMed]

153. Reddy, K.B.; Nabha, S.M.; Atanaskova, N. Role of map kinase in tumor progression and invasion. *Cancer Metastasis Rev.* **2003**, *22*, 395–403. [CrossRef] [PubMed]

Int. J. Mol. Sci. **2017**, *18*, 2661

154. Parker, K.H.; Beury, D.W.; Ostrand-Rosenberg, S. Myeloid-derived suppressor cells: Critical cells driving immune suppression in the tumor microenvironment. *Adv. Cancer Res.* **2015**, *128*, 95–139. [PubMed]
155. Kumar, V.; Patel, S.; Tcyganov, E.; Gabrilovich, D.I. The nature of myeloid-derived suppressor cells in the tumor microenvironment. *Trends Immunol.* **2016**, *37*, 208–220. [CrossRef] [PubMed]
156. Umansky, V.; Blattner, C.; Gebhardt, C.; Utikal, J. The role of myeloid-derived suppressor cells (mdsc) in cancer progression. *Vaccines* **2016**, *4*. [CrossRef] [PubMed]

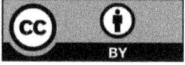

International Journal of
Molecular Sciences

MDPI

Communication

The Differential Distribution of RAPTA-T in Non-Invasive and Invasive Breast Cancer Cells Correlates with Its Anti-Invasive and Anti-Metastatic Effects

Ronald F. S. Lee [1], Stéphane Escrig [2], Catherine Maclachlan [3], Graham W. Knott [3], Anders Meibom [2,4], Gianni Sava [5,*] and Paul J. Dyson [1]

[1] Institute of Chemical Sciences and Engineering, Swiss Federal Institute of Technology (EPFL), CH-1015 Lausanne, Switzerland; ronald.lee@epfl.ch (R.F.S.L.); paul.dyson@epfl.ch (P.J.D.)
[2] Laboratory for Biological Geochemistry, Ecole Polytechnique Fédérale de Lausanne (EPFL), CH-1015 Lausanne, Switzerland; stephane.escrig@epfl.ch (S.E.); anders.meibom@epfl.ch (A.M.)
[3] Interdisciplinary Centre for Electron Microscopy, Ecole Polytechnique Fédérale de Lausanne (EPFL), CH-1015 Lausanne, Switzerland; catherine.maclaclan@epfl.ch (C.M.); graham.knott@epfl.ch (G.W.K.)
[4] Center for Advanced Surface Analysis, Institute of Earth Sciences, University of Lausanne, CH-1015 Lausanne, Switzerland
[5] Callerio Foundation Onlus, via A. Fleming 22, 34127 Trieste, Italy
* Correspondence: gsava@units.it

Received: 27 July 2017; Accepted: 24 August 2017; Published: 29 August 2017

Abstract: Nanoscale secondary ion mass spectrometry (NanoSIMS) combined with transmission electron microscopy (TEM) can be a powerful approach to visualize the exact distribution of drugs at the sub-cellular level. In this work, we exploit this approach to identify the distribution and localisation of the organometallic ruthenium(II)-arene drug $Ru(\eta^6\text{-}C_6H_5Me)(pta)Cl_2$, termed RAPTA-T, in MDA-MB-231 and MCF-7 human breast cancer cells. These cell lines have been chosen because the former cell lines are highly invasive and resistant to most chemotherapeutic agents and the latter ones are very sensitive to hormonal-based therapies. In the MDA-MB-231 cells, RAPTA-T was found to predominantly localise on the cell membrane and to a lesser extent in the nucleolus. These findings are consistent with the previously reported anti-metastatic properties of RAPTA-T and the observation that once internalized RAPTA-T is associated with chromatin. RAPTA-T shows a lack of membrane accumulation on the non-invasive MCF-7 cells, which correlates well with its selective anti-metastatic properties on invasive cell lines.

Keywords: breast cancer; invasion; metastasis; ruthenium

1. Introduction

Platinum-based drugs are widely used in the clinic [1,2]. However, in recent years, an increasing number of ruthenium complexes, with profoundly different properties compared with the currently used platinum drugs, e.g., higher cancer cell selectivity leading to reduced side-effects in vivo [3], have been (pre-)clinically evaluated [4–7]. All these drugs possess the classical coordination complexes structure, but there is now considerable interest in the anticancer properties of organometallic complexes, i.e., those containing direct metal-to-carbon bonds [8,9]. Of these organometallic compounds, the ruthenium(II)-arene drugs (Scheme 1), $Ru(\eta^6\text{-arene})(pta)Cl_2$ where pta = 1,3,5-triaza-7-phosphaadamantane, termed RAPTA compounds, are the most advanced in pre-clinical studies, and many derivatives have been prepared and tested [10]. Specifically, $Ru(\eta^6\text{-}C_6H_5Me)(pta)Cl_2$ (RAPTA-T) possesses anti-metastatic properties in an in vitro model mimicking the detachment, invasion, migration, and re-attachment steps of metastasis formation [11]. This effect is much more evident on the invasive MDA-MB-231 breast cancer cells than on non-invasive MCF-7 breast cancer cells [11]. The in vitro studies were validated in an in vivo syngeneic, spontaneously metastasizing mammary carcinoma murine model, which showed RAPTA-T treatment to be effective, resulting in a reduction of lung metastasis formation of these tumours [12].

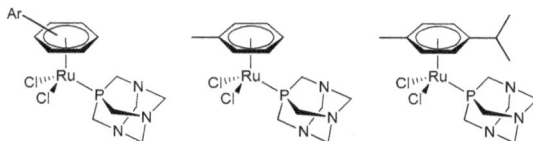

Scheme 1. Generic RAPTA (Ru(η^6-arene)(pta)Cl$_2$) structure (left) and the structures of RAPTA-T (centre) and RAPTA-C (where the arene = *p*-cymene) (right).

RAPTA-T is not the only compound of this family that has the capacity to reduce metastasis formation in experimental models [12]. However, RAPTA-T has other favourable physico-chemical and biological characteristics, i.e., particularly good water solubility and an intrinsic cancer cell selectivity demonstrated by a cytotoxicity difference between tumorigenic (74 μM) and non-tumorigenic (>1000 μM) cells [12], making it suitable for pharmacological development.   Nevertheless, the development of RAPTA-T is also dependent on knowledge about its biological and pharmacological mode of action. Although RAPTA-T was not derived from a targeted approach, but essentially from the upgrading of clinically used platinum drugs [13], its mode of action is profoundly different, binding preferentially to proteins rather than DNA [14]. It is therefore necessary to acquire as much data as possible on the behaviour of RAPTA-T in cells as a function of cellular characteristics and of their response to treatment.

An approach that produces visual distribution maps of metal-based drugs in cells, nanoscale secondary ion mass spectrometry (NanoSIMS) [15] is attracting increasing attention [16] and has been used to image RAPTA-T in cisplatin-resistant human ovarian cancer (A2780CR) cells [17]. Consequently, the aim of the present study is to determine the distribution of RAPTA-T in MDA-MB-231 and MCF-7 cells and to probe whether any difference in distribution exists between these cells possessing different metastatic phenotypes.   Both MCF-7 and MDA-MB-231 are breast cancer adenocarcinomas isolated from pleural effusions [18].   MDA-MB-231 are a triple-negative cell line lacking oestrogen and progesterone receptors in which the human epidermal growth factor receptor 2 (HER2/Neu) is not amplified, making it resistant to most chemotherapeutic agents. These characteristics differ to MCF-7 cells, which are positive for both oestrogen and progesterone receptors, and are therefore sensitive to hormonal-based therapies [19].

2. Results

Secondary ion maps of $^{13}C^{12}C^-/^{12}C_2^-$, $^{14}N^{12}C^-/^{12}C_2^-$, $^{15}N^{12}C^-/^{14}N^{12}C^-$, $^{31}P^-/^{12}C_2^-$, $^{34}S^-/^{12}C_2^-$, and $^{102}Ru^-/^{12}C_2^-$, as well as transmission electron microscopy (TEM) images of MDA-MB-231 cells treated with $^{15}N/^{13}C$-labelled RAPTA-T (500 μM, 24 h), are shown in Figure 1. As observed previously in A2780CR cells treated with $^{15}N+^{13}C$-labelled RAPTA-T [17], ^{13}C enrichment was not observed in RAPTA-T treated MDA-MB-231 and MCF-7 cells indicating that the sample preparation dilutes the ^{13}C-isotopic enrichment from the ^{13}C-enriched toluene ligand to below the detection limit [20]. In the MDA-MB-231 cells, all Ru hotspots found were co-enriched with ^{15}N (Figure 1, green boxes), suggesting that the phosphine (PTA) ligand remains coordinated to the Ru centre. However, there were several ^{15}N-enriched hotspots that did exhibit Ru enrichment, most likely due to detachment of PTA from Ru.

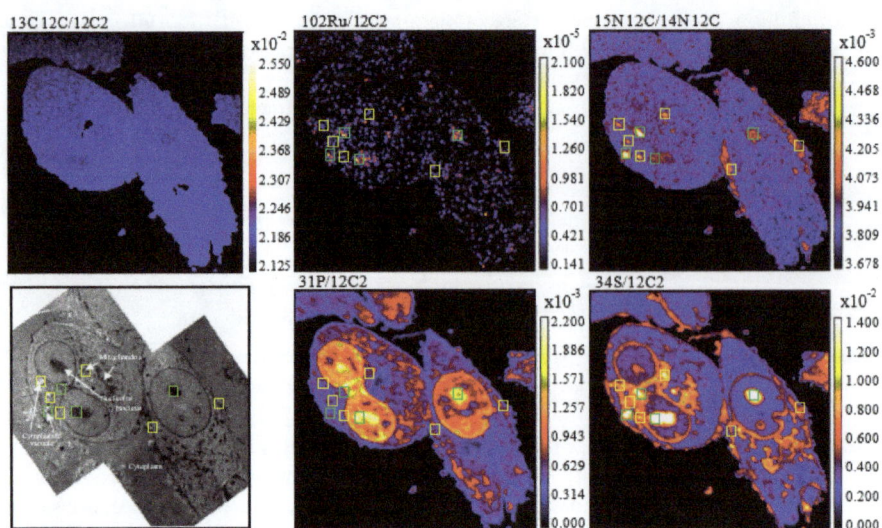

Figure 1. NanoSIMS secondary ion maps of $^{31}P^-/^{12}C_2^-$, $^{34}S^-/^{12}C_2^-$, $^{14}N^{12}C^-/^{12}C_2^-$, $^{15}N^{12}C^-/^{14}N^{12}C^-$, $^{102}Ru^-/^{12}C_2^-$, and $^{13}C^{12}C^-/^{12}C_2^-$ and TEM images of MDA-MB-231 cells treated with $^{15}N/^{13}C$-labelled RAPTA-T (500 µM, 24 h). Blue boxes indicate Ru-enriched hotspots, yellow boxes indicate ^{15}N-enriched hotspots, and green boxes indicate hotspots co-enriched with ^{15}N and Ru. Cellular organelles are labeled in the TEM image.

RAPTA-T was found to accumulate in the nucleolus of MDA-MB-231 cells (Figure 1). This observation is consistent with other studies in which RAPTA-T has been shown to interact with the histone proteins that package and order DNA into nucleosomes [21]. Accumulation of RAPTA-T was also observed on the cell membrane of MDA-MB-231 cells where it could interact with extracellular cell adhesion proteins implicated in its anti-metastatic activity [11]. Overlaying the $^{102}Ru^-$ and $^{12}C^{15}N^-$ maps with TEM images reveals that RAPTA-T also accumulate partially in cytoplasmic vacuoles, which are potential drug targets [22,23], and in mitochondria. The distribution and action of RAPTA-T in mitochondria has been reported previously, where treatment with the drug resulted in an appreciable accumulation in mitochondrial fractions from A2780CR cells [24] and results in perturbation of the expression of several mitochondrial proteins [25]. RAPTA-T accumulation tends to correlate with the sulphur-rich regions of the MDA-MB-231 cells, which is not surprising considering that most organelles in which RAPTA-T is distributed contain sulphur-rich biomolecules.

In MCF-7 cells, the accumulation profile of RAPTA-T is in part similar to that in MDA-MB-231 cells, i.e., with accumulation in the nucleolus and a general co-accumulation of the drug at sulphur-rich hotspots (Figure 2). However, in contrast to MDA-MB-231 cells, accumulation of RAPTA-T was not observed in the nucleus or on the cell membrane of MCF-7 cells. From the overlaid TEM images, RAPTA-T was also found to accumulate partially in mitochondria and cytoplasmic vacuoles. The lack of distribution in the nucleus and membrane of MCF-7 cells could partially explain the weaker activity of RAPTA-T in preventing migration, detachment, and reattachment of these cells compared to MDA-MB-231 cells.

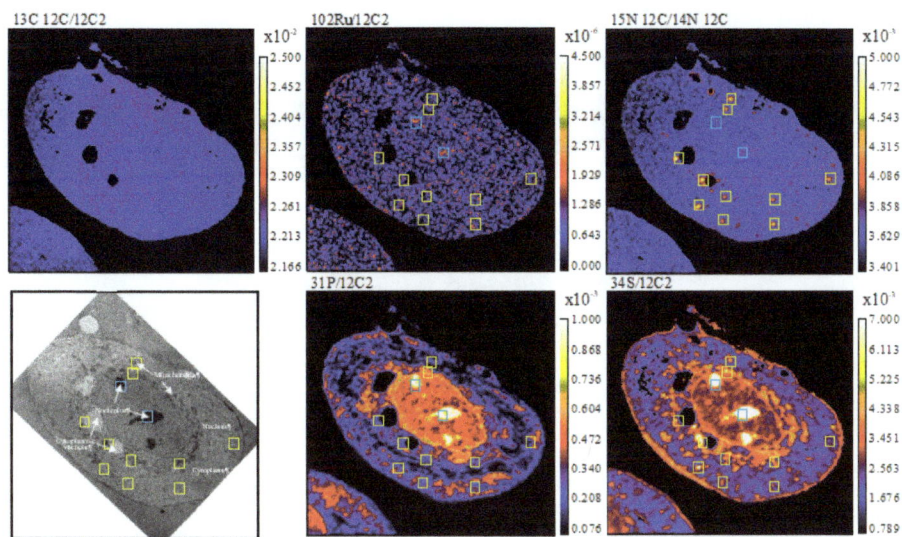

Figure 2. NanoSIMS secondary ion maps of $^{31}P^-/^{12}C_2^-$, $^{34}S^-/^{12}C_2^-$, $^{14}N^{12}C^-/^{12}C_2^-$, $^{15}N^{12}C^-/^{14}N^{12}C^-$, $^{102}Ru^-/^{12}C_2^-$, and $^{13}C^{12}C^-/^{12}C_2^-$ and TEM of MCF-7 cells treated with ^{15}N and ^{13}C-labelled RAPTA-T (500 µM, 24 h). Blue boxes indicate Ru enriched hotspots, yellow boxes indicate ^{15}N enriched hotspots and green boxes indicate hotspots co-enriched with ^{15}N and Ru. Cellular organelles are labeled in the TEM image.

3. Discussion

Accumulation of RAPTA-T in the membrane of human breast cancer cell lines is significantly higher in the invasive MDA-MB-231 cell line compared to MCF-7 cells. Such differences in RAPTA-T accumulation must be due to differences in the cell type and phenotype. It has been shown previously that A2780CR cells, unlike their cisplatin-sensitive (A2780) counterparts, undergo metastasis and shorten survival rates of mice xenografted with these cells [26]. Hence, both A2780CR and MDA-MB-231 cells are highly invasive, and the selective membrane association of RAPTA-T with these cell lines might be correlated with the anti-metastatic properties of the compound. This selectivity is exemplified by the lack of membrane accumulation of RAPTA-T on the less invasive MCF-7 cells. Notably, in the A2780CR and MDA-MB-231 cell lines, the amount of RAPTA-T associated with the membrane exceeds that inside the cells.

The distribution of RAPTA-T inside both cell lines is largely associated with accumulation in the nucleolus. Interestingly, RAPTA-C, a closely related compound to RAPTA-T, has been shown to reduce proliferation, migration, and tube formation in endothelial cells and also stimulate apoptosis [27]. These effects may be attributed to interactions of RAPTA-C with the endothelial cell membrane and to epigenetic factors.

Overall, the differences observed in the NanoSIMS studies provide new insights into how RAPTA-T distribution correlates with the phenotypic changes induced by its activity on cancer cells. These data emphasise the role of targeting molecules to the cell membrane for the control of metastasis of solid tumours. This aspect has already been stressed for the ruthenium(III) drug, NAMI-A, another potent anti-metastatic drug, which has been shown to bind to integrins [28]. If it is found that RAPTA-T is also able to target integrins, integrin modulation could become a highly attractive approach for tumour control with metal-based drugs. Such a mechanism, which is profoundly different to the development of DNA-damaging metal-based drugs [29], would stimulate the search for novel, selective drugs to control tumour malignancy.

4. Materials and Methods

4.1. Synthesis and Characterisation of $^{13}C/^{15}N$ Labelled RAPTA-T

^{15}N enriched 1,3,5,7-tetraazatricyclo[3.3.1.1 (3,7)]decane (PTA) was synthesized according to a literature method [30], with minor modifications consisting in the replacement of ^{14}NH$_4$OH with ^{15}NH$_4$OH in the described procedure [31]. ^{13}C labelled metyl-cyclohexadiene was prepared from a birch reduction of toluene-(phenyl-^{13}C6) and used to prepare ^{15}N/^{13}C-RAPTA-T (Scheme 2) as described previously [17].

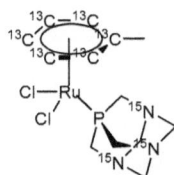

Scheme 2. Structure of ^{15}N/^{13}C labelled RAPTA-T. Characterisation: ^{1}H NMR (400 MHz, Methanol-d_4) = δ 5.95–5.22 (m, 5H), 4.60 (s, 6H), 4.35 (s, 6H), 2.17 (s, 3H). ^{13}C NMR (101 MHz, Methanol-d_4) only enriched ^{13}C = δ 108.33, 88.64–85.31 (m), 77.87–75.73 (m). ^{31}P NMR (162 MHz, Methanol-d_4) = δ 33.43. HRMS (ESI+) m/z calculated for C$_7$^{13}C$_6$H$_{20}$Cl^{15}N$_3$PRu [M-Cl+H]$^+$: 395.0239; found: 395.0242.

4.2. Cell Culture

MDA-MB-231 and MCF-7 (human breast adenocarcinoma) cells were cultured in DMEM medium supplemented with 10% foetal calf serum, penicillin 100 units/mL, and streptomycin 100 μg/mL (Invitrogen, Carlsbad, CA, USA). Cells were incubated at 37 °C in a humid environment containing 5% CO_2.

4.3. Cell Preparation

Cells were seeded 50,000 cells/well in 24-well or 500,000 cells/well in 6-well clear bottom plates fitted with sapphire disks. After 24 h, cell media was aspirated and fresh media containing ^{15}N and ^{13}C-RAPTA-T (500 μM) was added (a high concentration of compound was used due to the reduced incubation time). Upon incubation, the sapphire disks were removed from the media and then high pressure frozen (Leica HPM100, Leica Microsystems, Wetzlar, Germany) with excess 20% BSA solution in 0.01 M PBS (phosphate buffer solution) to avoid any air bubbles becoming trapped and the formation of ice crystals. The frozen cells were then embedded in resin at low temperature [32]. The sapphire discs were placed on a frozen solution of 1% osmium, 0.5% uranyl acetate, 5% water in acetone. The samples where then warmed to room temperature in an ice bucket containing solid carbon dioxide blocks that were allowed to sublime over a period of 2 h until they reached room temperature. At this point the solution was removed and replaced with dry acetone. After washing twice with acetone, the samples were embedded in increasing concentrations of epon resin in acetone. At 100% concentration of resin, the samples were then left overnight to fully infiltrate and then polymerised in a 60 °C oven for at least 12 h. Samples where then glued to empty resin blocks, trimmed, and sections of alternating thickness of 500 nm and 50 nm cut sequentially from the face. The thicker sections were collected onto a glass coverslip stained with 1% toulidine blue and imaged with light microscopy and NanoSIMS. The 50 nm thick sections were collected on to an electron microscopy slot grid ready for imaging with transmission electron microscopy at a final magnification of around 1400 times (Tecnai Spirit, FEI Company, Eindhoven, The Netherlands).

4.4. NanoSIMS Analysis

NanoSIMS measurements were performed at the Laboratory of Biological Geochemistry, EPFL and the University of Lausanne. Prior to NanoSIMS imaging the samples were gold-coated in order to avoid charging effects. Before acquiring an image, Cs^+ ions were implanted into the surface of the sample in order to enhance the ionization of the element of interest. The electron multiplier detectors were set up to measure $^{12}C_2^-$, $^{13}C^{12}C^-$, $^{12}C^{14}N^-$, $^{12}C^{15}N^-$, $^{31}P^-$, $^{34}S^-$, and $^{102}Ru^-$ secondary ions, generated by bombarding the sample with a ~4 pA Cs^+ primary beam focused to a spot size of approximately 160 nm. In order to resolve possible isobaric interferences, the instrument was operated at a mass-resolving power (MRP) of about 10,000. Due to the low signal of $^{102}Ru^-$ obtained from cells, peak-shape and mass resolving power was checked using a Ru standard. Data acquisition was performed by scanning the Cs^+ primary beam over areas of 34 × 34 µm with a 256 × 256 pixel image resolution. The per pixel dwell time of the primary ion beam was 10 ms. The final images are the accumulation of 120 layers obtained by sequential scanning and correspond to a cumulated acquisition time per pixel of 1.2 s. Between every layer, the transmission of the secondary ion beam was optimized and automatic peak centring was performed for $^{12}C_2^-$, $^{13}C^{12}C^-$, $^{12}C^{14}N^-$, $^{12}C^{15}N^-$. The Ru peak could not be centred due to the low count rates. However, post-analysis checks revealed that there was no significant change in the peaks position during the entire acquisition time. The total acquisition time including the centring procedure was 22 h per image.

4.5. Data Extraction and Image Processing

NanoSIMS image processing was performed with L'image (L. Nittler, Carnegie Institution of Washington, Washington, DC, USA). Over the ~20 h of image acquisition, the image drift of a 34 × 34 µm image was less than 7 pixels (i.e., less than 1 µm). The data reduction software can easily correct for such a drift by aligning the positions of identified structures. Regions of interest (ROI) were defined manually based on identifiable cell features on the $^{31}P^-$ elemental map. Images were accumulated from planes where accumulated counts per ROI were stable with $^{12}C^{14}N^-$ used as the alignment mass. All other elements were normalized against $^{12}C_2$, the images of which are essentially flat, to normalize out small ionization variations across the sample surface.

Acknowledgments: We thank the EPFL and Swiss National Science Foundation for financial support.

Author Contributions: Ronald F. S. Lee prepared/characterized the compound, performed incubation with cells and analyzed NanoSIMS data. Stéphane Escrig collected and analyzed NanoSIMS data. Catherine Maclachlan and Graham W. Knott performed cell fixation/embedding and TEM. Anders Meibom, Gianni Sava and Paul J Dyson supervised the research. Ronald F.S. Lee, Anders Meibom, Gianni Sava and Paul J Dyson wrote the manuscript.

Conflicts of Interest: The authors declare no conflict of interest.

References

1. Galanski, M.; Jakupec, M.A.; Keppler, B.K. Update of the preclinical situation of anticancer platinum complexes: Novel design strategies and innovative analytical approaches. *Curr. Med. Chem.* **2005**, *12*, 2075–2094. [CrossRef] [PubMed]
2. Kelland, L. The resurgence of platinum-based cancer chemotherapy. *Nat. Rev. Cancer* **2007**, *7*, 573–584. [CrossRef] [PubMed]
3. Alessio, E. Thirty Years of the Drug Candidate NAMI-A and the myths in the field of ruthenium anticancer compounds: A personal perspective. *Eur. J. Inorg. Chem.* **2017**, *2017*, 1549–1560. [CrossRef]
4. Rademaker-Lakhai, J.M.; van den Bongard, D.; Pluim, D.; Beijnen, J.H.; Schellens, J.H.M. A phase I and pharmacological study with imidazolium-trans-DMSO-imidazole-tetrachlororuthenate, a novel ruthenium anticancer agent. *Clin. Cancer Res.* **2004**, *10*, 3717–3727. [CrossRef] [PubMed]
5. Hartinger, C.G.; Jakupec, M.A.; Zorbas-Seifried, S.; Groessl, M.; Egger, A.; Berger, W.; Zorbas, H.; Dyson, P.J.; Keppler, B.K. KP1019, a new redox-active anticancer agent—preclinical development and results of a clinical Phase I study in tumor patients. *Chem. Biodivers.* **2008**, *5*, 2140–2155. [CrossRef] [PubMed]

6. Trondl, R.; Heffeter, P.; Kowol, C.R.; Jakupec, M.A.; Berger, W.; Keppler, B.K. NKP-1339, the first ruthenium-based anticancer drug on the edge to clinical application. *Chem. Sci.* **2014**, *5*, 2925–2932. [CrossRef]

7. Leijen, S.; Burgers, S.A.; Baas, P.; Pluim, D.; Tibben, M.; van Werkhoven, E.; Alessio, E.; Sava, G.; Beijnen, J.H.; Schellens, J.H. Phase I/II study with ruthenium compound NAMI-A and gemcitabine in patients with non-small cell lung cancer after first line therapy. *Investig. New Drugs* **2015**, *33*, 201–214. [CrossRef] [PubMed]

8. Hillard, E.A.; Jaouen, G. Bioorganometallics: Future trends in drug discovery, analytical chemistry, and catalysis. *Organometallics* **2011**, *30*, 20–27. [CrossRef]

9. Hanif, M.; Babak, M.V.; Hartinger, C.G. Development of anticancer agents: Wizardry with osmium. *Drug Discov. Today* **2014**, *19*, 1640–1648. [CrossRef] [PubMed]

10. Murray, B.S.; Babak, M.V.; Hartinger, C.G.; Dyson, P.J. The development of RAPTA compounds for the treatment of tumors. *Coord. Chem. Rev.* **2016**, *306*, 86–114. [CrossRef]

11. Bergamo, A.; Masi, A.; Dyson, P.J.; Sava, G. Modulation of the metastatic progression of breast cancer with an organometallic ruthenium compound. *Int. J. Oncol.* **2008**, *33*, 1281–1289. [CrossRef] [PubMed]

12. Scolaro, C.; Bergamo, A.; Brescacin, L.; Delfino, R.; Cocchietto, M.; Laurenczy, G.; Geldbach, T.J.; Sava, G.; Dyson, P.J. In vitro and in vivo evaluation of ruthenium (II)-arene PTA complexes. *J. Med. Chem.* **2005**, *48*, 4161–4171. [CrossRef] [PubMed]

13. Johnstone, T.C.; Suntharalingam, K.; Lippard, S.J. The next generation of platinum drugs: Targeted Pt(II) agents, nanoparticle delivery, and Pt(IV) prodrugs. *Chem. Rev.* **2016**, *116*, 3436–3486. [CrossRef] [PubMed]

14. Adhireksan, Z.; Palermo, G.; Riedel, T.; Ma, Z.; Muhammad, R.; Rothlisberger, U.; Dyson, P.J.; Davey, C.A. Allosteric cross-talk in chromatin can mediate drug-drug synergy. *Nat. Commun.* **2017**, *8*, 14860. [CrossRef] [PubMed]

15. Hoppe, P.; Cohen, S.; Meibom, A. NanoSIMS: Technical aspects and applications in cosmochemistry and biological geochemistry. *Geostand. Geoanal. Res.* **2013**, *37*, 111–154. [CrossRef]

16. Lee, R.F.S.; Theiner, S.; Meibom, A.; Koellensperger, G.; Keppler, B.K.; Dyson, P.J. Application of imaging mass spectrometry approaches to facilitate metal-based anticancer drug research. *Metallomics* **2017**, *9*, 365–381. [CrossRef] [PubMed]

17. Lee, R.F.; Escrig, S.; Croisier, M.; Clerc-Rosset, S.; Knott, G.W.; Meibom, A.; Davey, C.A.; Johnsson, K.; Dyson, P.J. NanoSIMS analysis of an isotopically labelled organometallic ruthenium(II) drug to probe its distribution and state in vitro. *Chem. Commun.* **2015**, *51*, 16486–16489. [CrossRef] [PubMed]

18. Lacroix, M.; Leclercq, G. Relevance of breast cancer cell lines as models for breast tumours: An update. *Breast Cancer Res. Treat.* **2004**, *83*, 249–289. [CrossRef] [PubMed]

19. Neve, R.M.; Chin, K.; Fridlyand, J.; Yeh, J.; Baehner, F.L.; Fevr, T.; Clark, L.; Bayani, N.; Coppe, J.P.; Tong, F.; et al. A collection of breast cancer cell lines for the study of functionally distinct cancer subtypes. *Cancer Cell* **2006**, *10*, 515–527. [CrossRef] [PubMed]

20. Kopf, S.H.; McGlynn, S.E.; Green-Saxena, A.; Guan, Y.; Newman, D.K.; Orphan, V.J. Heavy water and ^{15}N labelling with NanoSIMS analysis reveals growth rate-dependent metabolic heterogeneity in chemostats. *Environ. Microbiol.* **2015**, *17*, 2542–2556. [CrossRef] [PubMed]

21. Adhireksan, Z.; Davey, G.E.; Campomanes, P.; Groessl, M.; Clavel, C.M.; Yu, H.; Nazarov, A.A.; Yeo, C.H.F.; Ang, W.H.; Dröge, P.; et al. Ligand substitutions between ruthenium–cymene compounds can control protein versus DNA targeting and anticancer activity. *Nat. Commun.* **2014**, *5*, 3462. [CrossRef] [PubMed]

22. Shubin, A.V.; Demidyuk, I.V.; Komissarov, A.A.; Rafieva, L.M.; Kostrov, S.V. Transformation of cells by rous sarcoma virus: Cytoplasmic vacuolization. *Oncotarget* **2016**, *7*, 55863–55889. [CrossRef] [PubMed]

23. Aki, T.; Nara, A.; Uemura, K. Cytoplasmic vacuolization in cell death and survival. *Cell Biol. Toxicol.* **2012**, *28*, 125–131. [CrossRef] [PubMed]

24. Groessl, M.; Zava, O.; Dyson, P.J. Cellular uptake and subcellular distribution of ruthenium-based metallodrugs under clinical investigation versus cisplatin. *Met. Integr. Biometal Sci.* **2011**, *3*, 591–599. [CrossRef] [PubMed]

25. Wolters, D.A.; Stefanopoulou, M.; Dyson, P.J.; Groessl, M. Combination of metallomics and proteomics to study the effects of the metallodrug RAPTA-T on human cancer cells. *Metallomics* **2012**, *4*, 1185. [CrossRef] [PubMed]

26. Shaw, T.J.; Senterman, M.K.; Dawson, K.; Crane, C.A.; Vanderhyden, B.C. Characterization of intraperitoneal, orthotopic, and metastatic xenograft models of human ovarian cancer. *Mol. Ther.* **2004**, *10*, 1032–1042. [CrossRef] [PubMed]
27. Berndsen, R.H.; Weiss, A.; Abdul, U.K.; Wong, T.J.; Meraldi, P.; Griffioen, A.W.; Dyson, P.J.; Nowak-Sliwinska, P. Combination of ruthenium(II)-arene complex [Ru(η(6)-p-cymene)Cl2(pta)] (RAPTA-C) and the epidermal growth factor receptor inhibitor erlotinib results in efficient angiostatic and antitumor activity. *Sci. Rep.* **2017**, *7*, 43005. [CrossRef] [PubMed]
28. Pelillo, C.; Mollica, H.; Eble, J.A.; Grosche, J.; Herzog, L.; Codan, B.; Sava, G.; Bergamo, A. Inhibition of adhesion, migration and of $\alpha5 \beta1$ integrin in the HCT-116 colorectal cancer cells treated with the ruthenium drug NAMI-A. *J. Inorg. Biochem.* **2016**, *160*, 225–235. [CrossRef] [PubMed]
29. Bergamo, A.; Sava, G. Linking the future of anticancer metal-complexes to the therapy of tumour metastases. *Chem. Soc. Rev.* **2015**, *44*, 8818–8835. [CrossRef] [PubMed]
30. Eller, K.; Henkes, E.; Rossbacher, R.; Höke, H. *Ullmann's Encyclopedia of Industrial Chemistry*; Wiley-VCH Verlag GmbH & Co. KGaA: Weinheim, Germany, 2000.
31. Daigle, D.J.; Pepperman, A.B.; Vail, S.L. Synthesis of a monophosphorus analog of hexamethylenetetramine. *J. Heterocycl. Chem.* **1974**, *11*, 407–408. [CrossRef]
32. McDonald, K.L.; Webb, R.I. Freeze substitution in 3 h or less. *J. Microsc.* **2011**, *243*, 227–233. [CrossRef] [PubMed]

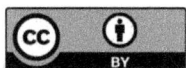

International Journal of
Molecular Sciences

MDPI

Article

Does Locoregional Chemotherapy Still Matter in the Treatment of Advanced Pelvic Melanoma?

Stefano Guadagni [1,*], Giammaria Fiorentini [2], Marco Clementi [3], Giancarlo Palumbo [3],
Paola Palumbo [3], Alessandro Chiominto [3], Stefano Baldoni [3], Francesco Masedu [1],
Marco Valenti [1], Ambra Di Tommaso [3], Bianca Fabi [3], Camillo Aliberti [4], Donatella Sarti [2],
Veronica Guadagni [5] and Cristina Pellegrini [1]

[1]   Department of Applied Clinical Sciences and Biotechnology, University of L'Aquila, 67100 L'Aquila, Italy;
      francesco.masedu@cc.univaq.it (F.M.); marco.valenti@cc.univaq.it (M.V.);
      cristina.pellegrini@cc.univaq.it (C.P.)
[2]   Department of Oncology and Hematology, Ospedali Riuniti Marche Nord, 61121 Pesaro, Italy;
      g.fiorentini@alice.it (G.F.); d.sarti@fastwebnet.it (D.S.)
[3]   Department of Life, Health and Environmental Sciences, University of L'Aquila, 67100 L'Aquila, Italy;
      marco.clementi@univaq.it (M.C.); giancarlo.palumbo@cc.univaq.it (G.P.); paola.palumbo@univaq.it (P.P.);
      alessandro.chiominto@univaq.it (A.C.); stefano.baldoni@univaq.it (S.B.);
      ambra.ditommaso@graduate.univaq.it (A.D.T.); biancafabi@gmail.com (B.F.)
[4]   Department of Radiology, Institute for the Research and Treatment of Cancer, 35128 Padova, Italy;
      camillo.aliberti@ioveneto.it
[5]   Department of Physiology and Pharmacology, Cumming School of Medicine, University of Calgary,
      Calgary, AB T2N 4N1, Canada; vguadagn@ucalgary.ca
*   Correspondence: stefano.guadagni@univaq.it; Tel.: +39-3339-4361-71

Received: 1 September 2017; Accepted: 7 November 2017; Published: 9 November 2017

Abstract: Pelvic Melanoma relapse occurs in 15% of patients with loco regional metastases, and 25% of cases do not respond to new target-therapy and/or immunotherapy. Melphalan hypoxic pelvic perfusion may, therefore, be an option for these non-responsive patients. Overall median survival time (MST), stratified for variables, including BRAF V600E mutation and eligibility for treatments with new immunotherapy drugs, was retrospectively assessed in 41 patients with pelvic melanoma loco regional metastases. They had received a total of 175 treatments with Melphalan hypoxic perfusion and cytoreductive excision. Among the 41 patients, 22 (53.7%) patients exhibited a wild-type *BRAF* genotype, 11 of which were not eligible for immunotherapy. The first treatment resulted in a 97.5% response-rate in the full cohort and a 100% response-rate in the 22 wild-type *BRAF* patients. MST was 18 months in the full sample, 20 months for the 22 wild-type *BRAF* patients and 21 months for the 11 wild-type *BRAF* patients not eligible for immunotherapy. Melphalan hypoxic perfusion is a potentially effective treatment for patients with pelvic melanoma loco regional metastases that requires confirmation in a larger multicenter study.

Keywords: melanoma; *BRAF*; Melphalan; pelvic perfusion; hypoxia; stopflow

1. Introduction

Cutaneous melanoma is one of the most aggressive treatment-resistant cancers [1]. Proto-oncogenes and tumor suppressor genes involved in the Mitogen-Activated Protein Kinase (MAPK) pathway have been implicated in the molecular pathogenesis of cutaneous melanoma, with activating mutations in *BRAF* (v-Raf murine sarcoma viral oncogene homolog B) and *NRAS* (neuroblastoma RAS viral oncogene homolog) encountered in approximately 70% of all melanomas [1]. Somatic *BRAF* mutation in codon 600 of exon 15 occurs in 40–50% of cutaneous melanomas, with V600E the most common mutation. BRAF^{V600E} is now recognized as a validated therapeutic target, although acquired resistance is almost universal [2].

Recently, novel immunotherapies that target negative immune checkpoint molecules have gained a major interest in the treatment of melanoma [2]. Therefore, in the last six years, options for treatment of advanced melanoma patients have significantly changed, thanks to new target therapy and immunotherapy. The new era of effective systemic therapy, also involves patients with pelvic locoregional metastases without lesions in the legs, which are approximately less than 2% of all malignant melanoma patients [3,4].

Unfortunately, target therapy provides a significant overall median survival improvement in only 50% of patients who carry the BRAF^{V600E} mutation, with salvage immunotherapy, following discontinuation of targeted therapy, frequently unsatisfactory [5,6]. Furthermore, these new immunotherapies are effective in only 45% of wild-type *BRAF* melanoma patients, associated with overall median survival times ranging from 11 to 20 months, with adverse events observed in 4–25% of patients [7–9].

An effective treatment for melanoma patients with loco-regional pelvic metastases, who do not respond to target therapy and/or new immunotherapy, remains an important area for clinical research. A recent review has examined the role of surgery and loco-regional chemotherapy in the management of in-transit disease, in the era of effective systemic therapy [10]. A decade ago, standard treatment for patients with loco-regional melanoma metastases resulted in a median survival time of approximately eight months [11,12] and high complex regional chemotherapy procedures containing Melphalan were considered to have potential to improve clinical outcome [4,13–16]. However, techniques were not standardised and results varied according to the experience of each institution. Since then, more feasible procedures associated with lower morbidity and fewer adverse effects have been developed, with particular emphasis on the use of interventional radiology [14]. An important question however, remains to be answered, and that is whether loco-regional chemotherapy, performed by the surgical or percutaneous approach, still has a place in the treatment of advanced stage melanoma?

In this report, we present a retrospective study of the efficacy of Melphalan hypoxic perfusion in patients with pelvic metastatic melanoma stratified for prognostic factors, including *BRAF*.

2. Results

2.1. Patients Characteristics

A total of 41 melanoma patients with metastatic lesions were included in this study (13 males and 28 females). Mean patient age (±SD, standard deviation) was 63.9 years (±13.6), mean male age was 58.2 years (±14.7) and mean female age was 66.3 years (±12.5). Seven lymph node negative patients with loco-regional metastases were classified as stage IIIB and 24 lymph node positive patients were classified as stage IIIC. The ten stage IV patients were classified by the presence of concurrent metastases to the lungs (four patients), bones (four patients) or abdomen (two patients).

2.2. Treatments

A total of 175 perfusions were performed, including 52 surgical procedures and 123 percutaneous procedures. The mean (±SD) number of treatments received by each patient was 4.3 (±3.1) and the median number of treatments received was four (range 2–5). Contemporary palliative cytoreduction was performed in 35 patients (85.4%). With respect to hospitalization, the median length of post-surgical perfusion recovery was 8.8 days, which was significantly longer ($p < 0.01$) than following percutaneous perfusion (4.7 days).

Patients did not experience any technical (i.e., balloon rupture), hemodynamic, or vascular complications, and no deaths occurred during the 175 procedures or during the post-operative period. Hematological toxicity, resulting in the termination of treatment, occurred in three patients following the 4th procedure (9.7%) and in a single patient following the 14th procedure. Procedure-related complications and toxicities are listed in Table 1.

Table 1. Procedure related complications and toxicity after 175 treatments in 41 metastatic melanoma patients.

Complications	Grade	n (%)
Seroma	1	4 (2.3)
Persistent leakage of fluid from the incision	2	14 (8.0)
Wound infection	1	3 (1.7)
Inguinal hematoma	1	7 (4.0)
Wound dehiscence	2	7 (4.0)
Lymphangitis	2	3 (1.7)
Scrotum edema	1	6 (3.4)
Pelvic pain	1	6 (3.4)
Toxicity	**Grade**	**n (%)**
	1	25 (14.3)
Bone marrow hypocellularity	2	18 (10.3)
	3	8 (4.6)
Alopecia	1	7 (4.0)
Nausea and vomiting	1	26 (14.9)

n = numbers of cases.

2.3. BRAF Mutational Status

BRAF gene mutational analysis in the 41 metastatic melanoma tissues, identified the V600E BRAF mutation in 19 metastases (19/41, 46.3%), with 22 samples (22/41, 53.7%) characterized as wild-type *BRAF*. Eleven (11/41, 26.8%) wild-type *BRAF* patients were not suitable for immune check-point therapy, three of which (3/41, 7.3%) were in disease progression after Ipilimumab immunotherapy and 8 of which (19.5%) were ineligible due to hepatitis C (4 patients; 9.7%), human immunodeficiency virus-HIV (one patient; 2.4%) and active inflammatory bowel disease (three patients; 7.3%).

2.4. Tumor Responses

Tumor response was related primarily to perfusion, with minimal contribution made by additional surgical excision. In the full sample cohort, the overall response rate after the first treatment was 97.5%, with a complete response observed in four patients (9.7%), a partial response observed in 36 patients (87.8%) and stable disease observed in one patient (2.4%). No evidence of disease progression was detected within 30 days, following initial treatment. In patients who underwent more than three treatments the overall response rate was 27.3%.

In the 22 wild-type *BRAF* patients, the overall response rate following the initial treatment was 100%, with two complete responses (9.1%) and 20 partial responses (90.9%), recorded. In wild-type *BRAF* patients who underwent more than three treatments, the overall response rate was 33.3%.

With respect to the 11 wild-type *BRAF* patients that were not eligible or non-responsive to immunotherapy, two patients exhibited a complete response (18.2%) and nine patients exhibited a partial response (81.8%), following the initial treatment. Partial responses were recorded for 10% of patients following the second treatment, 11.1% of patients following the 3rd treatment and 16.7% of patients following the fourth treatment.

2.5. Survival

The overall MST for this patient cohort was 18 months (range 9–22) (Figure 1A), with a mean survival time of 27.6 (±35.7) months. The one-year, three-year and five-year survival rates were 63.4%,

17.1% and 9.7%, respectively and the overall median progression free survival (PFS) was 15.5 months (range 6–21), with a mean of 25.7 (±36.3) months.

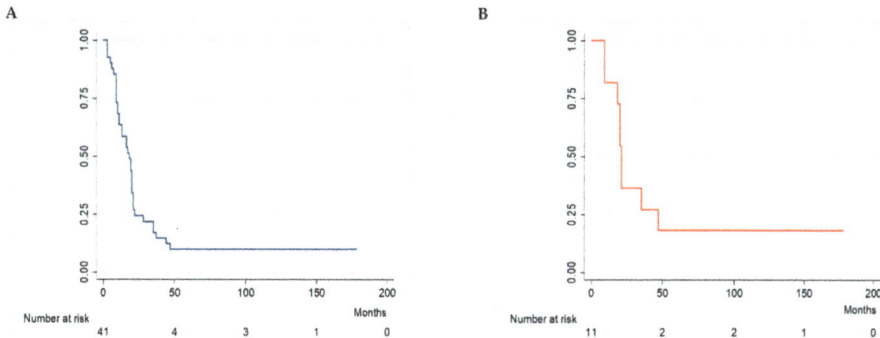

Figure 1. Kaplan-Meyer survival. (**A**) overall; (**B**) 11 wild-type *BRAF* patients not eligible for check-point therapy or non-responsive for progression or adverse events.

Table 2 shows factors associated with survival, including gender, age, stage of disease, number and dimension of nodules, melanin cellular pigmentation, mitosis, associated excision, number of treatments and *BRAF* status.

Table 2. Survival according to age, gender, stage, *BRAF* V600E status, burden, mitosis, associated excision, cellular melanin pigmentation, number of treatments.

Variables (Number of Patients)	MST (Months)	Log-Rank χ²	*p* Value	Cox HR
Age				
<65 (*n* = 18)	17			
≥65 (*n* = 23)	20	0.80	0.371	
Gender				
Female (*n* = 28)	19.5			
Male (*n* = 13)	10	2.31	0.132	
Stage				
IIIB (*n* = 7)	37			
IIIC (*n* = 24)	19			
IV (*n* = 10)	8	21.44	0.001	4.03 [1.91–6.59]
BRAF status				
Wild-type (*n* = 22)	20			
V600E Mutated (*n* = 19)	13	0.36	0.551	
Burden				
Low (*n* = 23)	21			
High (*n* = 18)	16.5	7.61	0.005	2.58 [1.26–5.58]
Mitosis				
<1 (*n* = 17)	20			
≥1 (*n* = 24)	14.5	3.66	0.064	
Associate Excision				
Yes (*n* = 35)	18			
Not (*n* = 6)	17.5	2.41	0.128	
Melanin cellular pigmentation				
Yes (*n* = 15)	20			
Not (*n* = 26)	14.5	0.15	0.691	
Number of treatments				
≤2 (*n* = 7)	5			
>2 (*n* = 34)	19	1.58	0.203	

MST = median survival time; HR = hazard ratio.

Disease stage (*p* = 0.001) (Figure 2A), and "burden" (*p* = 0.005) (Figure 2B) significantly affected survival, whereas gender, age, mitosis, melanin pigmentation, associate excision, number of treatments, and *BRAF* V600E status did not.

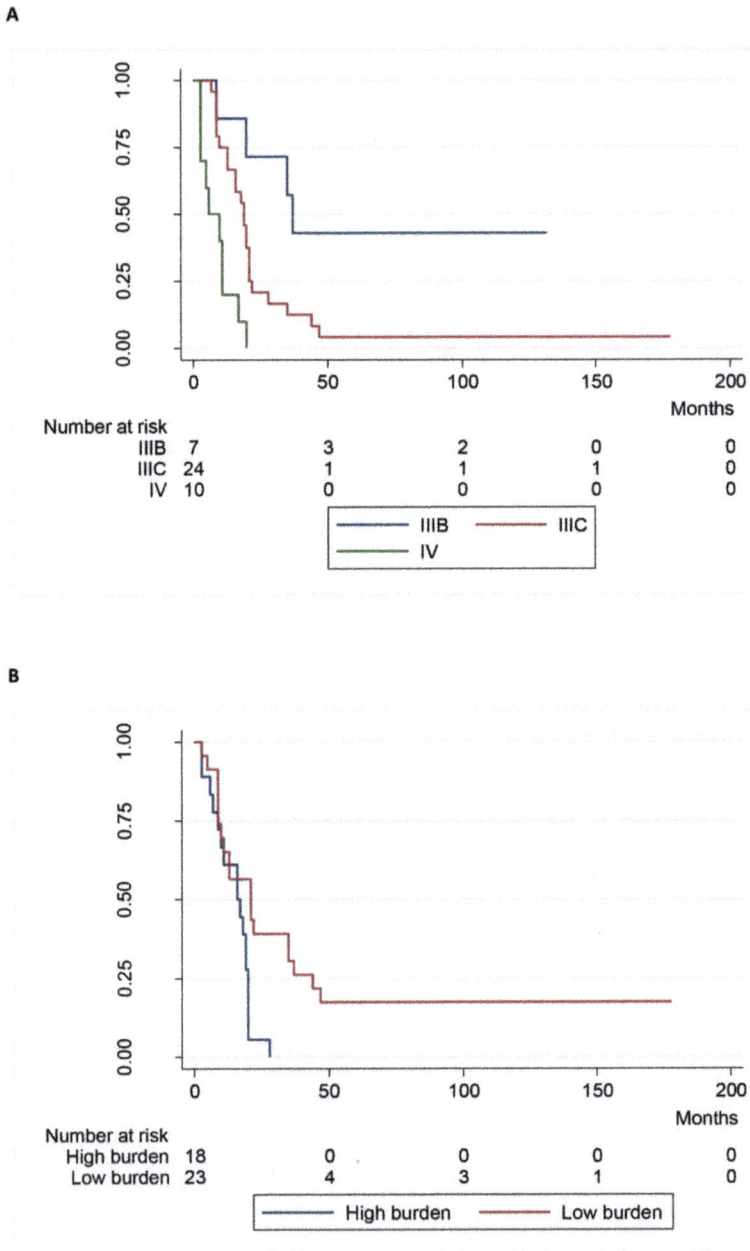

Figure 2. Kaplan-Meyer survival. (**A**) Stratified by Stage; (**B**) stratified by Burden.

In 22 wild-type *BRAF* patients, the MST was 20 months (range 11–21), with a mean survival time of 31.3 (±41.9) months. Gender, the number of treatments and nodule number and dimension (burden) all had an impact on survival that could not be evaluated statistically due to the small number of patients in these sub-groups. The median PFS was 17.7 months (range 9.5–20), with a mean of 29.4 (±42.5) months.

In the 11 wild-type *BRAF* patients that were not eligible or non-responsive to checkpoint therapy, the MST (Figure 1B) was 21 months (range 18–47), with a mean of 46.4 (±55.7) months. The median PFS for this group was 20 months (range 16.5–45), with a mean of 44.4 (±56.8) months.

2.6. Follow-Up

Median follow-up was 18 months (range 9–22), with a mean of 27.6 (±35.7) months. Among the 41 patients studied, four (9.8%) are still alive without evidence of disease after 76, 109, 132 and 178 months, whereas the remaining 37 (90.2%) have deceased as a consequence of melanoma. Therapy was interrupted in one patient due to Melphalan allergy, following the 10th treatment and another patient developed a brain metastasis six-years after the last perfusion. This patient was referred for surgical excision and remains disease-free after nine years.

With respect to the 20 patients who interrupted treatment due to disease progression, the median MST was 10 months, with a mean of 12.1 (±8.6) months, which was significantly shorter ($p < 0.01$) than the MST of the 10 patients who interrupted treatment due to worsening condition (median 20; mean 27.5 ± 11.6 months) or the seven patients who retired the consent (median 20; mean 17.0 ± 5.6 months; $p < 0.04$).

Disease progression in the pelvis was detected in 17 stage IIIC patients (one of which also developed distant site relapse) and in two stage IIIB patients. Distant site relapse was observed in two stage IIIB patients, seven stage IIIC patients and in 10 stage IV patients (one also with pelvic recurrence).

3. Discussion

In this retrospective study, we present evidence that demonstrates the potential efficacy of Melphalan hypoxic pelvic perfusion in patients with pelvic and/or inguinal loco regional melanoma metastases.

Prior to 2013, pelvic perfusion was an option for patients with loco regional melanoma metastases who were non-responsive to standard treatments. Within the last four years, immunotherapy with checkpoint inhibition and MAPK pathway targeted inhibitory therapy have led to important improvements in patient outcomes and has become the first line of therapy. Reports suggest, however, that up to 25% of melanoma patients may not respond to new target and immunotherapeutic drugs [17]. In our retrospective study, melanoma patients received repeated Melphalan hypoxic pelvic perfusions associated with cytoreductive excision between 2002 and 2013. This cohort had several interesting characteristics: (1) patients with loco regional pelvic melanoma metastases with or without leg lesions below mid-thigh level, represent a very rare category (enrollment of three/four patients per year) and the small sample size was a deliberate choice from a single institute in order to minimize procedural and technical bias, consistent with similar sample sizes in previous reports [13–16]; (2) in all 41 patients, lymphocyte invasion into metastatic melanoma tissues was not detected. This condition has been reported recently to associate with melanoma resistance to anti-PD1 antibody therapy [17]. Furthermore, melanomas did not exhibit desmoplasia with malignant spindle cells (DM). The prognosis for melanoma with DM is controversial with a recent report indicating a similar survival rate for case-matched patients with or without DM [18].

Molecular analysis of metastatic melanomas identified a BRAF^{V600E} mutation-rate of 46.3%. This frequency is similar to that commonly found for primary tumours in large series of cases [19] and in other Italian cohorts [20]. It remains unclear, however, whether the primary tumour *BRAF* mutation status is retained in metastases and we are unable to add anything more to this debate, in this study.

Among the 22 wild-type *BRAF* patients, 11 were not eligible for new immunotherapeutic drugs or had therapy interrupted due to disease progression or adverse events. A recent review discusses the reasons for which many patients seen in routine clinical practice do not qualify for immune checkpoint inhibitor clinical trials and have been seriously underrepresented in new immunotherapy trials [21].

In this study, Melphalan mono-therapy was chosen for this patient cohort based upon the rationale that Melphalan cytotoxicity is enhanced 3-fold in conditions of hypoxia-induced acidosis [22] and a previous study reporting grade 3 post-perfusion neutropenia in 18% of patients treated with Melphalan-based poly-chemotherapy [4]. In our study, pelvic perfusion was immediately followed by hemofiltration to protect against toxicity, rather than the use of a pneumatic anti-shock garment [16], which modifies hemodynamic and respiratory parameters but does not prevent leakage.

Long-term MST for Melphalan mono-therapy was 37 months for IIIB patients and 19 months for IIIC patients, who previously progressed following standard therapy and surgery. MST was decreased to eight months in stage IV patients and significantly lower survival characterized the remaining 48.8% of patients who had interrupted perfusion due to disease progression, compared to patients who interrupted treatments by refusing consent or due to general worsening of conditions. One patient developed a skin reaction and mild dyspnea during the 10th Melphalan perfusion, which were resolved by corticosteroid and antihistamine treatment. Allergy to Melphalan is not common but has been reported in approximately 2% of patients [23].

MST in the wild-type *BRAF* cohort was 20 months with a median PFS of 17.7 months, and the MST of the 11 patients not eligible for target therapy or new immunotherapy was 21 months. No other therapy has demonstrated significant clinical efficacy in this wild-type *BRAF* subgroup and the only alternative therapy suggested is systemic chemotherapy. A survival benefit of >10% is required for a new therapeutic regimen or modality to be recommended. Very recently, overall survival of patients with metastatic melanoma treated with new target and immunotherapies in a real-life setting has been compared to an overall survival of 7.4 months in a 95-patients-cohort treated with systemic chemotherapy [24]. In this retrospective study, a survival benefit of >10% was recorded for our procedure in wild type *BRAF* melanoma patients, suggesting a potentially important survival benefit. However, greater numbers will be required to confirm this.

It would be interesting to determine whether Melphalan pelvic perfusion under conditions of hypoxia may generate an immune response that could be augmented by systemic immunotherapy with anti-programmed cell death-ligand protein 1 (PD-L1) antibodies [25]. In this regard, two trials are currently underway to explore the efficacy of Melphalan combined with Ipilimumab, as either adjuvant (NCT01323517) or neo-adjuvant (NCT02115243) systemic immunotherapy.

A major limitation of our study is, however, the small sample size that cannot definitively establish the true benefit of this approach in patients with wild-type *BRAF* metastatic melanoma who are not eligible or non-responsive to new immunotherapeutic drugs. However, we defend our approach as necessary in order to minimize surgical procedure variability. Finally, although hypoxic pelvic perfusion is an expensive procedure, costs are similar to those incurred by isolated limb perfusion or infusion procedures for metastatic melanoma [26].

4. Patients and Methods

4.1. Patients

This project has been performed in accordance with the Declaration of Helsinki and has been approved by the ethics committee of University of L'Aquila, L'Aquila, Italy. Written informed consent was obtained from each patient.

In this retrospective study, in order to respect performance homogeneity, a subset of patients was selected from a larger database, which included melanoma patients from different sites who underwent hypoxic perfusion. Forty-one melanoma patients with pelvic and/or inguinal loco-regional metastases, treated with a total of 175 hypoxic perfusions between September 2002 and January 2013, were included in this study. Table 3 reports patient and tumor characteristics. Patients with associated lesions below mid-thigh level, requiring a larger compartment for perfusion, were excluded from this study. Prior to treatment initiation, all patients were characterised by disease progression after previous therapies, including palliative surgery (39 patients; 95.1%), Dacarbazine-based systemic chemotherapy (19 patients; 46.3%), immunotherapy with Interferon α and/or Interleukin-2 (15 patients; 36.6%), isolated limb perfusion with tumour necrosis factor (4 patients; 9.7%), electro-chemotherapy (two patients; 4.8%), Ipilimumab (3 patients; 7.3%). Patients who had received any kind of chemotherapy, immunotherapy and/or target therapy after the last perfusion treatment were also excluded from this study. Patients with stage IV melanoma were included in this study, as loco-regional therapy was performed in these patients to avoid severe local complications. Informed consent was obtained from all patients who received complete information concerning their disease and the implications of the proposed palliative treatment, as required by the ethical standards committee on human experimentation of our institution.

Table 3. Characteristics of patients and tumors.

Characteristics of Patients		*n* (%)
Gender	Males	13 (31.7)
	Females	28 (68.3)
Stage [27]	IIIB	7 (17.1)
	IIIC	24 (58.5)
	IV	10 (24.4)
Burden [28]	Low Burden *	23 (56.1)
	High Burden **	18 (43.9)
Patients with exclusion criteria for immune check-point therapy	Yes	8 (19.5)
	No	33 (80.5)
Characteristics of tumors		***n* (%)**
Anatomical site	Labia/vagina	2 (4.9)
	Anus	2 (4.9)
	Anterior trunk	2 (4.9)
	Back	3 (9.7)
	Lower extremity	31 (75.6)
Melanin presence	Yes	15 (36.6)
	No	26 (63.4)
Mitotic rate	<1 mitosis per mm^2	17 (41.5)
	>1 mitosis per mm^2	24 (58.5)
BRAF status	wild-type	22 (53.7)
	V600E mutated	19 (46.3)

n = numbers of patients; * <10 nodules; or no lesion >3 cm; ** ≥10 nodules; or one lesion >3 cm.

4.2. Histopathological and Molecular Evaluation

Pathological examination revealed that all surgical specimens had an epithelioid cell pattern. Lesions were classified as "pigmented" or "non-pigmented", based on the presence or absence of melanin-producing cells and lesions were also classified according to mitotic rate (<1 or ≥1 mitosis per mm^2). Tumor-infiltrating lymphocytes were not detected in any of the 41 tumor specimens.

DNA was isolated from five, 10 µm formalin fixed paraffin embedded (FFPE) tissue sections from each excised lesion, using the DNA Mini Kit, as directed by the manufacturer (Qiagen, Hilden, Germany), and DNA concentration and quality determined in a Qubit fluorometer (Thermo-Fisher, Foster City, CA, USA). *BRAF* V600E mutation status was assessed using Competitive Allele Specific hydrolysis probes (TaqMan) and PCR technology (CAST) (Thermo-Fischer Scientific, Waltham, MA, USA) [29].

4.3. Treatment Protocol

The eligibility criteria for hypoxic pelvic perfusion have been previously reported [4]. In particular, all patients were free from renal and/or liver failure, deep venous thrombosis, severe atherosclerosis, or coagulopathy. The clinical protocol provision was for repetitive cycles of perfusion and palliative cytoreductive surgery at 6 to 7-week intervals, with purpose and timing of repetition based on previous pilot studies [4,30]. Criteria for surgical excision and other treatment details have been recently reported [25]. In the case of complete response to treatment, a prolonged treatment repetition interval of 12 weeks was performed in order to gain the clinical result of one-year progression-free survival.

4.4. Hypoxic Pelvic Perfusion Technique and Melphalan Regimen

All 175 perfusions were performed under general anesthesia, as previously reported [4,31]. In 123 procedures (70.3%), a percutaneous technique was adopted; in 52 treatments (29.7%) the method was surgical with 39 femoral-access, 13 iliac-access, and 49 lymphadenectomies. Details of the surgical and percutaneous techniques plus hemofiltration characteristics have been recently reported [25]. Briefly, hypoxic perfusion with hemofiltration included three phases: isolation, perfusion and hemofiltration. In the isolation phase, the blood flow to the aorta and inferior cava vein was blocked by endovascular balloon catheters and at thigh-level by pneumatic cuffs. During the perfusion phase, pelvic perfusion was performed via extracorporeal blood circulation at approximately 100 mL/min. According to previous pilot studies [4,30], 30 mg/m^2 of Melphalan in 250 mL of isotonic sodium chloride solution was administered via the circuit over a 3-min period. The extracorporeal circuit connected to the circulation device contained a heating element and a hemofiltration module controlled by the device during perfusion and subsequent hemofiltration phases [32]. Following perfusion, balloon catheters and pneumatic cuffs were deflated to restore normal circulation and hemofiltration was then administered for 60 min (hemofiltration phase).

4.5. Criteria for Responses and Adverse Events

Tumor response was assessed using Response Evaluation Criteria in Solid Tumors, version 1.1 [33] at 30 days after each loco-regional chemotherapy treatment. Patient responses prior to 2009 were retrospectively re-classified. Computerized tomography (CT), Magnetic Resonance Imaging (MRI), and Position-emission Tomography (PET) were used to evaluate responses for deep masses and inspection with photo comparison employed for the monitoring of superficial lesions. Adverse events were assessed using Common Terminology Criteria for Adverse Events of the National Cancer Institute (CTCAE v4.03).

4.6. Statistical Analysis

Descriptive statistics estimated with 95% confidence are presented as mean ± SD Survival estimates were calculated using the Kaplan-Meier product limit estimator. No patients were lost to follow-up and no patients died of causes other than melanoma. Survival times were stratified according to clinical variables that potentially influence survival. Log-rank tests were used to assess the significant differences between the groups and hazard ratios were estimated using a proportional hazard Cox regression model. Progression free survival time (PFS) was calculated from the first day of loco-regional treatment. Statistical analyses were performed using STATA software, version 14 (Stata Corp., College Station, TX, USA).

5. Conclusions

In conclusion, we propose that Melphalan hypoxic perfusion is a potentially effective treatment for pelvic metastatic melanoma, but this should be confirmed in a larger multicenter prospective controlled trial.

Int. J. Mol. Sci. **2017**, *18*, 2382

Acknowledgments: We would like to thank Aigner Karl Reinhard for his surgical teaching and Mackay Andrew Reay for editing this article.

Author Contributions: In our study, Stefano Guadagni, Marco Clementi, Camillo Aliberti operated the patients, Stefano Guadagni, Giancarlo Palumbo, Giammaria Fiorentini, Marco Valenti, Veronica Guadagni participated in the design of the study, Giancarlo Palumbo, Paola Palumbo, Stefano Baldoni, Alessandro Chiominto, Bianca Fabi, Ambra Di Tommaso, Cristina Pellegrini, Veronica Guadagni performed the clinical analyses, Francesco Masedu, Marco Valenti performed the statistical analyses, Stefano Guadagni, Cristina Pellegrini, Veronica Guadagni, Donatella Sarti drafted of the manuscript. All authors read and approved the final manuscript.

Conflicts of Interest: The authors declare no conflict of interest.

Abbreviations

MST	median survival time
DOAJ	v-Raf murine sarcoma viral oncogene homolog B
FFPE	formalin fixed paraffin embedded
CAST	competitive allele specific technology
CT	Computerized tomography
MRI	Magnetic Resonance Imaging
PET	Position-emission Tomography
CTCAE	common Terminology Criteria for Adverse Events
SD	standard deviation
PFS	progression free survival
MAP	mitogen-activated protein
PD-1	programmed cell death protein 1
PD-L1	programmed cell death-ligand protein 1

References

1. Shain, A.H.; Bastian, B.C. From melanocytes to melanomas. *Nat. Rev. Cancer* **2016**, *16*, 345–358. [CrossRef] [PubMed]
2. Kunz, M.; Hölzel, M. The impact of melanoma genetics on treatment response and resistance in clinical and experimental studies. *Cancer Metastasis Rev.* **2017**, *36*, 53–75. [CrossRef] [PubMed]
3. Trout, A.T.; Rabinowitz, R.S.; Platt, J.F.; Elsayes, K.M. Melanoma metastases in the abdomen and pelvis: Frequency and patterns of spread. *World J. Radiol.* **2013**, *5*, 25–32. [CrossRef] [PubMed]
4. Guadagni, S.; Russo, F.; Rossi, C.R.; Pilati, P.L.; Miotto, D.; Fiorentini, G.; Deraco, M.; Santinami, M.; Palumbo, G.; Valenti, M.; et al. Deliberate hypoxic pelvic and limb chemoperfusion in the treatment of recurrent melanoma. *Am. J. Surg.* **2002**, *83*, 28–36. [CrossRef]
5. Khushalani, N.I.; Sondak, V.K. Are we there yet? Prolonged MAPK inhibition in BRAF V600-mutant melanoma. *Lancet Oncol.* **2016**, *17*, 1178–1179. [CrossRef]
6. Chan, M.M.; Haydu, L.E.; Menzies, A.M.; Azer, M.W.; Klein, O.; Lyle, M.; Clements, A.; Guminski, A.; Kefford, R.F.; Long, G.V. The nature and management of metastatic melanoma after progression on BRAF inhibitors: Effects of extended BRAF inhibition. *Cancer* **2014**, *120*, 3142–3153. [CrossRef] [PubMed]
7. Topollian, S.L.; Sznol, M.; McDermott, D.F.; Kluger, H.M.; Carvajal, R.D.; Sharfman, W.H.; Brahmer, J.R.; Lawrence, D.P.; Atkins, M.B.; Powderly, J.D.; et al. Survival, durable tumor remission, and long-term safety in patients with advanced melanoma receiving nivolumab. *J. Clin. Oncol.* **2014**, *32*, 1020–1030. [CrossRef] [PubMed]
8. Ribas, A.; Hamid, O.; Daud, A.; Hodi, F.S.; Wolchok, J.D.; Kefford, R.; Joshua, A.M.; Patnaik, A.; Hwu, W.J.; Weber, J.S.; et al. Association of pembrolizumab with tumor response and survival among patients with advanced melanoma. *JAMA* **2016**, *315*, 1600–1609. [CrossRef] [PubMed]
9. Daud, A.; Nandoskar, P. Pembrolizumab for melanoma-safety profile and future trends. *Expert Opin. Drug Saf.* **2016**, *15*, 727–729. [CrossRef] [PubMed]
10. Raigani, S.; Cohen, S.; Boland, G.M. The role of surgery for melanoma in an era of effective systemic therapy. *Curr. Oncol. Rep.* **2017**, *19*, 17. [CrossRef] [PubMed]
11. Chapman, P.B.; Einhorn, L.H.; Meyers, M.L.; Saxman, S.; Destro, A.N.; Panageas, K.S.; Begg, C.B.; Agarwala, S.S.; Schuchter, L.M.; Ernstoff, M.S.; et al. Phase III multicenter randomized trial of the Dartmouth

regimen versus dacarbazine in patients with metastatic melanoma. *J. Clin. Oncol.* **1999**, *17*, 2745–2751. [CrossRef] [PubMed]

12. Bhatia, S.; Tykodi, S.S.; Thompson, J.A. Treatment of metastatic melanoma: An overview. *Oncology* **2009**, *23*, 488–496. [PubMed]

13. Stehlin, J.S.; Clark, R.L.; White, E.C.; Smith, J.L.; Griffin, A.C.; Jesse, R.H.; Healey, J.E. Regional chemotherapy for cancer: Experiences with 116 perfusions. *Ann. Surg.* **1960**, *151*, 605–619. [CrossRef] [PubMed]

14. Guadagni, S.; Palumbo, G.; Fiorentini, G.; Clementi, M.; Marsili, L. Surgical versus percutaneous isolated pelvic perfusion (IPP) for advanced melanoma: Comparison in terms of melphalan pharmacokinetic pelvic bio-availability. *BMC Res Notes* **2017**, *10*. [CrossRef] [PubMed]

15. Wanebo, H.J.; Chung, M.A.; Levy, A.I.; Turk, P.S.; Vezeridis, M.P.; Belliveau, J.F. Preoperative therapy for advanced pelvic malignancy by isolated pelvic perfusion with the balloon-occlusion technique. *Ann. Surg. Oncol.* **1996**, *3*, 295–303. [CrossRef] [PubMed]

16. Bonvalot, S.; de Baere, T.; Mendiboure, J.; Paci, A.; Farace, F.; Drouard-Troalen, L.; Bonnet, L.; Hakime, A.; Bonniaud, G.; Raynard, B.; et al. Hyperthermic pelvic perfusion with tumor necrosis factor-α for locally advanced cancers. Encouraging results of a phase II study. *Ann. Surg.* **2012**, *255*, 281–286. [CrossRef] [PubMed]

17. Merlino, G.; Herlyn, M.; Fisher, D.E.; Bastian, B.C.; Flaherty, K.T.; Davies, M.A.; Wargo, J.A.; Curiel-Lewandrowski, C.; Weber, M.J.; Leachman, S.A.; et al. The state of melanoma: challenges and opportunities. *Pigment Cell Melanoma Res.* **2016**, *29*, 404–416. [CrossRef] [PubMed]

18. Murali, R.; Shaw, H.M.; Lai, K.; McCarthy, S.W.; Quinn, M.J.; Stretch, J.R.; Thompson, J.F.; Scolyer, R.A. Prognostic factors in cutaneous Desmoplastic Melanoma: A study of 252 patients. *Cancer* **2010**, *116*, 4130–4138. [CrossRef] [PubMed]

19. Kim, S.Y.; Kim, S.N.; Hahn, H.J.; Lee, Y.W.; Choe, Y.B.; Ahn, K.J. Metaanalysis of BRAF mutations and clinicopathologic characteristics in primary melanoma. *J. Am. Acad. Dermatol.* **2015**, *72*, 1036. [CrossRef] [PubMed]

20. Pellegrini, C.; Di Nardo, L.; Cipolloni, G.; Martorelli, C.; de Padova, M.; Antonini, A.; Maturo, M.G.; del Regno, L.; Strafella, S.; Micantonio, T.; et al. Heterogeneity of Braf, Nras, and Tert-Promoter Mutational Status in Multiple Melanomas and association with Mc1r Genotype: Findings from Molecular and immunohistochemical analysis. *J. Mol. Diagn.* **2017**. [CrossRef] [PubMed]

21. Johnson, D.B.; Sullivan, R.J.; Menzies, A.M. Immune checkpoint inhibitors in challenging populations. *Cancer* **2017**, *123*, 1904–1911. [CrossRef] [PubMed]

22. Pruijn, F.B.; van Daalen, M.; Holford, N.H. Mechanisms of enhancement of the antitumour activity of Melphalan by the tumour-blood-flow inhibitor 5,6-dimethylxanthenone-4-acetic acid. *Cancer Chemother. Pharmacol.* **1997**, *39*, 541–546. [CrossRef] [PubMed]

23. Kroon, H.M.; Lin, D.Y.; Kam, P.C.A.; Thompson, J.F. Efficacy of repeat isolated limb infusion with melphalan and actinomycin D for recurrent melanoma. *Cancer* **2009**, *115*, 1932–1940. [CrossRef] [PubMed]

24. Mangana, J.; Cheng, P.F.; Kaufmann, C. Multicenter, real-life experience with checkpoint inhibitors and targeted therapy agents in advanced melanoma patients in Switzerland. *Melanoma Res.* **2017**, *27*, 358–368. [CrossRef] [PubMed]

25. Guadagni, S.; Fiorentini, G.; Clementi, M.; Palumbo, G.; Chiominto, A.; Cappelli, S.; Masedu, F.; Valenti, M. Melphalan hypoxic perfusion with hemofiltration for melanoma locoregional metastases in the pelvis. *J. Surg. Res.* **2017**, *215*, 114–124. [CrossRef] [PubMed]

26. Ma, Q.; Zhao, Z.; Barber, B.L.; Shilkrut, M. Use patterns and costs of isolated limb perfusion and infusion in the treatment of regional metastatic melanoma: A retrospective database analysis. *Adv. Ther.* **2016**, *33*, 282–289. [CrossRef] [PubMed]

27. Balch, C.M.; Gershenwald, J.E.; Song, S.J.; Thompson, J.F.; Atkins, M.B.; Byrd, D.R.; Buzaid, A.C.; Cochran, A.J.; Coit, D.G.; Ding, S.; et al. Final version of 2009 AJCC melanoma staging and classification. *J. Clin. Oncol.* **2009**, *27*, 6199–6206. [CrossRef] [PubMed]

28. Steinman, J.; Ariyan, C.; Rafferty, B.; Brady, M.S. Factors associated with response, survival, and limb salvage in patients undergoing isolated limb infusion. *J. Surg. Oncol.* **2014**, *109*, 405–409. [CrossRef] [PubMed]

29. Didelot, A.; le Corre, D.; Luscan, A.; Cazes, A.; Pallier, K.; Emile, J.F.; Laurent-Puig, P.; Blons, H. Competitive allele specific TaqMan PCR for KRAS, BRAF and EGFR mutation detection in clinical formalin fixed paraffin embedded samples. *Exp. Mol. Pathol.* **2012**, *92*, 275–280. [CrossRef] [PubMed]

30. Guadagni, S.; Santinami, M.; Patuzzo, R.; Pilati, P.L.; Miotto, D.; Deraco, M.; Rossi, C.R.; Fiorentini, G.; di Filippo, F.; Valenti, M.; et al. Hypoxic pelvic and limb perfusion with Melphalan and mitomycin C for recurrent limb melanoma: A pilot study. *Melanoma Res.* **2003**, *13*, 51–58. [CrossRef] [PubMed]

31. Varrassi, G.; Guadagni, S.; Ciccozzi, A.; Marinangeli, F.; Pozone, T.; Piroli, A.; Marsili, I.; Paladini, A. Hemodynamic variations during thoracic and abdominal stop-flow regional chemotherapy. *Eur. J. Surg. Oncol.* **2004**, *30*, 377–383. [CrossRef] [PubMed]

32. Guadagni, S.; Fiorentini, G.; Clementi, M.; Palumbo, G.; Masedu, F.; Deraco, M.; de Manzoni, G.; Chiominto, A.; Valenti, M.; Pellegrini, C. MGMT methylation correlates with melphalan pelvic perfusion survival in stage III melanoma patients: A pilot study. *Melanoma Res.* **2017**, *27*, 439–447. [CrossRef] [PubMed]

33. Eisenhauer, E.A.; Therasse, P.; Bogaerts, J. New response valuation criteria in solid tumors: Revised RECIST guideline (version 1.1). *Eur. J. Cancer* **2009**, *45*, 228–247. [CrossRef] [PubMed]

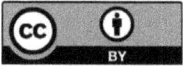

MDPI

St. Alban-Anlage 66

4052 Basel, Switzerland

Tel. +41 61 683 77 34

Fax +41 61 302 89 18

http://www.mdpi.com

International Journal of Molecular Sciences Editorial Office

E-mail: ijms@mdpi.com

http://www.mdpi.com/journal/ijms

www.ingramcontent.com/pod-product-compliance
Lightning Source LLC
Chambersburg PA
CBHW051724210326
41597CB00032B/5594